Therapeutic Modalities

Third Edition

Therapeutic Modalities

Third Edition

Chad Starkey, PhD, ATC
Associate Professor
Bouvé College of Health Sciences
Northeastern University
Boston, Massachusetts

F.A. DAVIS COMPANY • Philadelphia

F. A. Davis Company
1915 Arch Street
Philadelphia, PA 19103
www.fadavis.com

Printed in the United States of America
Last digit indicates print number: 10 9 8 7 6 5 4 3 2

Acquisitions Editor: Christa Fratantoro
Manager, Creative Development: Susan R. Rhyner
Developmental Editor: Kim Wyatt
Developmental Associate: Melissa Reed
Cover Designer: Louis J. Forgione, Design Manager

As new scientific information becomes available through basic and clinical research, recommended treatments and drug therapies undergo changes. The author(s) and publisher have done everything possible to make this book accurate, up to date, and in accord with accepted standards at the time of publication. The author(s), editors, and publisher are not responsible for errors or omissions or for consequences from application of the book, and make no warranty, expressed or implied, in regard to the contents of the book. Any practice described in this book should be applied by the reader in accordance with professional standards of care used in regard to the unique circumstances that may apply in each situation. The reader is advised always to check product information (package inserts) for changes and new information regarding dose and contraindications before administering any drug. Caution is especially urged when using new or infrequently ordered drugs.

Library of Congress Cataloging-in-Publication Data

Starkey, Chad, 1959-
  Therapeutic modalities / Chad Starkey.-- 3rd ed.
      p. ; cm.
  Includes bibliographical references and index.
    ISBN 0-8036-1139-0 (hardcover : alk. paper)
    1. Sports medicine. 2. Athletic trainers. 3. Athletes--Rehabilitation. 4. Sports injuries--Treatment.
    [DNLM: 1. Athletic Injuries--therapy. QT 261 S795t 2004] I. Title.
    RC1210.S785 2004
    617.1'027--dc22

                                                                                    2003019506

Preface to the Third Edition

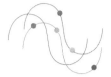

This edition of *Therapeutic Modalities* has been restructured to provide information in student-friendly and instructor-friendly blocks. The text is organized in five sections, with group-related content. Section One describes the body's response to injury as well as treatment planning and administrative considerations when providing patient care. Section Two describes cold modalities and superficial heating agents; the deep-heating modalities therapeutic ultrasound and shortwave diathermy are covered in Section Three. The modalities in Sections Two and Three are covered in two chapters each: one that describes the physics, biophysical effects, and the effects on the injury response process and another that describes the clinical application of the device or devices. In Section Four, electrical stimulation is presented in three chapters: the physics of electricity, electrical stimulation objectives, and clinical application of electrical stimulation. The mechanical agents in Section Five are described in a single chapter per modality.

Several design features have been incorporated into this edition. One of the most visible features is the "At a Glance" box that accompanies each modality and that serves as a quick overview of the effects, treatment parameters, indications, contraindications, and precautions. "Treatment Strategies" boxes have been added to relate the theoretical and physiological material presented in the chapter to direct clinical practice. The Treatment Strategies are not "cookbooks" but rather a conceptual approach about how to affect the problem at hand. "Clinical Techniques" boxes provide general guidelines for outcome-specific modality application. There is also a liberal allocation of informational boxes, tables, and figures, all of which, I hope, will contribute to the comprehension of this material.

I debated for a long time about the inclusion (and exclusion) of some of the modalities and techniques presented in this text. Some, such as contrast baths, have demonstrated relatively little efficacy but are still used clinically. Likewise, some devices such as infrared light are seldom (if ever) used, but some reviewers encouraged me to continue to include them. These devices may soon need to be retired.

I have also included information on "new" devices, although some are not really new. Therapeutic magnets have been included, not because of their efficacy (indeed, there is a striking lack of evidence that these devices work) but because patients frequently ask clinicians about their use and function and self-prescribe their use. The use of the therapeutic laser is still tightly regulated by the U.S. Food and Drug Administration, but exemptions have recently been made for specific uses. Although very few facilities have hyperbaric oxygen equipment designed for orthopedic use, I have included this device because of the potential that it appears to hold for treating musculoskeletal injuries.

A strong emphasis has recently been placed on the importance of evidence-based practice. Although each of the previous editions of this text has attempted to balance clinical practice and research findings, another layer has been added to this concept. Each modality now has a section titled "Controversies in Treatment" that describes contradictions in clinical practice and provides an overview of research findings (which is sorely lacking for most of these modalities). I have attempted to word these sections in a manner that does not confuse or frustrate the reader. I also encourage students and instructors to continue to read current peer-reviewed research regarding therapeutic modalities.

For instructors who adopt this text, a web-based image bank is available through www.fadavis.com. This website is password-protected, so contact your sales representative to obtain access information.

As always, I encourage reader feedback, and I am always willing to respond to questions or help clarify any of this information for instructors or students (but I won't do your homework for you!). Please feel free to contact me at chadstarkey@aol.com

Chad Starkey

Preface to the First Edition

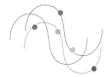

This is an introductory text designed to fill the void between the baseline knowledge of undergraduate student athletic trainers and the information presented in existing therapeutic modality texts. Its scope and content are written in a style that will accommodate a wide range of students with varying educational backgrounds. The presentation of these modalities has a strong slant toward their application but not at the expense of theory and research. Traditional application techniques are supported or refuted based on current literature.

The aim was to write this text to the students in a manner that facilitates their comprehension of the material. The information in this text is presented in a sequential manner. Each chapter begins with the "basics" and progresses to higher levels of information. Terms that may be new to the student are defined on the same page for quick reference, and the text also includes a complete glossary. Chapters conclude with a short quiz to measure the student's learning.

The focal point of this text is Chapter 1, which presents the body's physiological and psychological response to trauma. Each subsequent chapter relates how individual modalities affect the injury response process. Chapter 2 discusses the basic physics involved in the transfer of energy.

Specific modalities are categorized by the manner in which they deliver their energy to the body. Chapter 3 presents thermal agents and the diathermies. Chapter 4 covers the principles, effects, and application of electricity. Chapter 5 deals with mechanical agents. Each modality is prefaced by an introductory section that is followed by the specific effects that the energy has on the injury response process. The unit then progresses to the modalities' instrumentation, set-up, and application and concludes with the indications, contraindications, and precautions of its use.

Chapter 6 introduces clinical decision making through the use of the problem solving approach and is supplemented through the use of case studies. The text concludes with a chapter addressing organizational and administrative concerns in the use of therapeutic modalities.

Chad Starkey

Acknowledgements

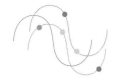

The writing of a text such as this requires the input and careful and critical review of several individuals. I wish to thank the following people for their thoughtful reviews:

Kim Attig-Terrell, MS, ATC
Associate Director of Athletic Medicine
University of Oregon
Eugene, OR

Paul Borsa, PhD, ATC
Department of Kinesiology
University of Michigan
Ann Arbor, MI

Sara D. Brown, MS, ATC
Director
Physical Therapy
Boston University
Boston, MA

Scott T. Doberstein, MS, ATC, CSCS
Head, Athletic Training
Exercise and Sports Science
University of Wisconsin—La Crosse
La Crosse, WI

Linda Gazillo, EdD, ATC, LMT
Associate Professor
Exercise and Movement Science
William Paterson University
Wayne, NJ

Pam Guidry, ATC
Instructor
Athletic Training
McNeese State University
Lake Charles, LA

Christopher D. Ingersoll, PhD, ATC, FACSM
Director
Graduate Program in Sports and Athletics
University of Virginia
Charlottesville, VA

Bentley A. Krause, PhD, ATC
Associate Professor
Athletic Training
Northeastern University
Boston, MA

Steven G. Lesh, PhD, MPA, PT, SCS, ATC
Associate Professor
Physical Therapy
Southwest Baptist University
Bolivar, MO

Mark A. Merrick, PhD, ATC
Program Director
Athletic Training
The Ohio State University
Columbus, OH

Jeff Ryan, PT, ATC
Clinical Director of Sports Medicine
Sports Medicine
Hahnemann University Hospital
Philadelphia, PA

Susan Saliba, PhD, ATC, MPT
Instructor
Orthopedic Surgery
University of Virginia
Charlottesville, VA

Daniel R. Sedory, MS, ATC, NHLAT
Associate Professor
Department of Kinesiology
University of New Hampshire
Durham, NH

Sue Stanley-Green, MS, ATC/L
Assistant Professor
Athletic Training
Florida Southern College
Lakeland, FL

Benito Velasquez, DA, ATC
Associate Professor
Athletic Training
University of Southern Mississippi
Hattiesburg, MS

Stacy E. Walker, PhD, ATC
Associate Professor
Athletic Training/EMS
William Paterson University
Wayne, NJ

I would like to thank the staff at F.A. Davis, especially the Manager of Creative Development, Susan Rhyner; Developmental Associate, Melissa Reed; Acquisitions Editor, Christa Fratantoro; and Developmental Editor, Kim Wyatt. Their efforts in developing the manuscript and page design have truly been remarkable.

Another era at F.A. Davis has passed with the retirement of Ona Kosmos. Ona was with me on this project since its inception and with me and Jeff Ryan during the writing of our evaluation texts. Ona, enjoy your retirement, and thanks for everything!

Having used the theorem "surround yourself with people who are much smarter than you," much credit goes to those individuals who contributed information to this third edition: Jodie Humphrey, PT, ATC, for providing the case studies in the text and the ancillaries and for providing a critical review of Chapter 1; Jeff Ryan, PT, ATC, for once again contributing the problem-solving approach chapter; and Bob Sikes, PhD, who has completely rewritten The Physiology and Psychology of Pain chapter. Mark Merrick, PhD, ATC, must be recognized for his expert reviews and contributions to The Injury Response Process, Therapeutic Ultrasound, and Shortwave Diathermy chapters (and his comments were a blast to read!).

Special thanks go to Christina Roache, an athletic training student at Northeastern University, who read the entire manuscript and provided me with a student's perspective on the information provided. Ms. Roache provided valuable input on how to best present this material. Indeed, the Treatment Strategies boxes were developed based on her input. Incorporating a student as a reviewer was a great decision.

For those of you keeping score, the "curse of Therapeutic Modalities" continues. I don't know what it is with this beast, but there is certainly a cloud that hovers over it. Once again, a huge thanks to all of you who have stood by me and gave me the boosts and laughs that I needed, whether in person or otherwise. Several years ago Gary Numan penned a song called "Are Friends Electric?" All through my college years, I wondered what that meant. Now I know. What I don't know is if there will be a fourth edition.

Contributors

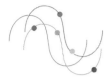

Jodie B. Humphrey, PT, ATC
Performance Physical Therapy
Pawtucket, RI

Jeff Ryan, PT, ATC
Clinical Director of Sports Medicine
Sports Medicine
Hahnemann University Hospital
Philadelphia, PA

Robert W. Sikes, PhD
Associate Professor
Northeastern University
Boston, MA

Contents

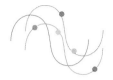

Chapter 4

Administrative Considerations

Section TWO

Therapeutic Cold and Superficial Heating Agents

Chapter 5

Thermal Modalities

Chapter 6

Clinical Application of Thermal Modalities

Section **THREE**

Deep-Heating Agents

Chapter 7

Therapeutic Ultrasound

Chapter 8

Clinical Application of Therapeutic Ultrasound

Chapter 9

Shortwave Diathermy

Chapter 10

Clinical Application of Shortwave Diathermy   192

Section FOUR

Electrical Stimulation

Chapter 11

Principles of Electrical Stimulation   204

Chapter 12

Electrical Stimulation Techniques   220

Chapter 13

Clinical Application of Electrical Agents   240

Section **FIVE**

Mechanical and Light Modalities

Chapter 14
Intermittent Compression   280

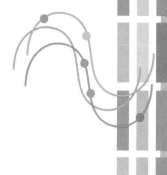

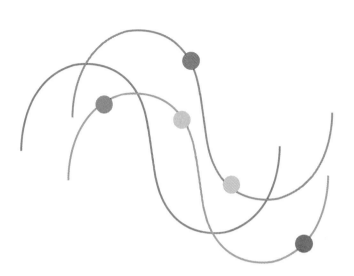

Injury Response and Treatment Planning

This section describes the body's physiological and psychological responses to injury and their subsequent influence on treatment planning. Administrative factors in the planning and delivery of therapy are also discussed.

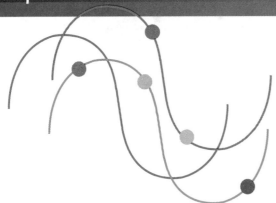

Chapter 1

The Injury Response Process

This chapter provides an overview of the body's physical and psychological reactions to stress and injury. It also introduces many of the terms and concepts used throughout the text. The physiological response to trauma and the subsequent healing process are affected by the therapeutic modalities described later in this book. The response to trauma, pain, is presented in Chapter 2.

Why does a text dealing with therapeutic modalities focus its initial attention on the cell? To understand the purpose and effects of therapeutic modalities, we must first gain a basic knowledge of the body's response to injury. We will see that when therapeutic modalities are applied to living tissue, we are not just treating an ankle or a knee. We are applying **stress ∎** to the cells that will influence their metabolic function.

No modality can actually speed the healing of an injury. The body heals the injury at its own rate. However, by treating an injury with thermal, electrical, or mechanical energy, we attempt to provide the optimal environment for healing to occur. But what is considered a modality? Simply stated, it is the application of some form of stress to the body for the purpose of eliciting an adaptive response.

To illustrate this concept, consider a lacerated finger. If dirt and grime are allowed to enter the cut, an infection occurs and delays the healing process by hindering the normal physiological healing response. If we clean the area, apply an antibiotic ointment, and cover the wound with a dressing, healing progresses relatively unhindered. Therapeutic modalities function similarly; by applying cold, heat, electrical stimulation, or another form of energy, we influence the body's physiological functions to provide the traumatized tissue with the best healing environment.

Defining the term "therapeutic" is needed to understand the principles behind the application of thermal, mechanical, electrical, or chemical energy to the body. To be deemed therapeutic, the stress applied to the body must be conducive to the healing process of the injury in its current healing state. The optimum conditions for healing require a balance between protecting the area from further distresses and restoring tissue function at the earliest

---

Stress: A force that disrupts the normal homeostasis of a system.

possible time.[1] The application of a modality at an improper point in its recovery may hinder, if not set back, the healing process.

■ Stresses Placed on the Cell

Any type of mechanical, chemical, or emotional force placed on the body and its cells may be regarded as stress. Although we often think of stress as being negative, many of the "stresses" in life are positive. Indeed, to be without stress is to be without life.

For example, consider the various types of stressors encountered by an athlete: the cardiovascular benefits associated with conditioning, the physical contact associated with sports such as football, the repeated pounding of the feet when running, and the emotional elation or anguish related to the outcome of a game. If stress, regardless of its nature, is applied at a sufficient magnitude, the body undergoes several physiological changes at both the cellular and **systemic ■** levels.

When a stress is placed on a cell, it reacts in one of three way

- It adapts to the stress.
- It is altered but recovers.
- It dies.

The General Adaptation Syndrome

Hans Selye, a researcher in the early 1900s, observed that hospitalized patients shared a common set of symptoms regardless of their **pathology ■** . These symptoms included diffuse aches and pains in the joints, loss of strength, loss of appetite, and an elevated body temperature. These striking similarities led him to conclude that the body's systems had a common mechanism for coping with stress. Selye termed this phenomenon the general adaptation syndrome and outlined three stages of stress response[2]:

1. Alarm stage
2. Resistance stage
3. Exhaustion stage

The **alarm stage**, best exemplified by the "flight-or-fight response," is the body's initial reaction to a change in **homeostasis ■**. The body's systems spring to life, mobiliz-ing its resources to thwart the effects of the stressor by readying its defensive systems. Increased blood supplies are routed to areas needing the resources by elevating the heart rate, cardiac stroke volume, and the force of **myocardial ■** contractions. The blood supply to nonessential areas is decreased by **vasoconstriction ■** of the superficial and abdominal arteries. **Cortisol ■** is released into the bloodstream to regulate inflammation, stimulate cellular level energy production, and otherwise help to prepare the body to deal with trauma. Proteins are broken down into **amino acids ■** in preparation for long fasting periods to provide a potential energy source in the event that injury does occur.

After the alarm stage, there is a plateau in the body's adaptation to the stress: the **resistance stage**. The body continues to adapt to the stressor by using homeostatic resources to maintain its integrity. This is the longest phase of the general adaptation syndrome, lasting many days, months, or years. During this stage of stress response, the individual achieves physiological resistance or, as it is commonly referred to in exercise, "physical fitness."

When the body can no longer withstand the applied stresses, it reaches the **exhaustion stage**. At this point, one or more of the body's systems cannot tolerate the stress and therefore fails. This stage may also be referred to as the point of distress, stage the stressors placed on the body produce a negative effect. Clinically, the exhaustion stage may show itself in the form of traumatic or overuse injuries.

General Adaptation Syndrome and Its Relationship to Trauma

It should now be apparent that all people experience beneficial or harmful stresses as a part of everyday life. Harmful stresses may take the form of an **acute ■** injury such as a **sprain ■**, **strain ■**, or fracture. In these types of injuries, the body is overwhelmed by too much force in too short a time (macrotrauma). Distresses may also result from repeated, relatively low-intensity forces, as exemplified by stress fractures, **chronic ■** inflammatory conditions, and muscle soreness (microtrauma).

The amount of stress applied to the body must be of a proper intensity and duration for the body to develop phys-

---

Acute: Of recent onset. The period after an injury when the local inflammatory response is still active.
Amino acids: Building blocks of protein.
Chronic: Continuing for a long period; with injury, extending past the primary hemorrhage and inflammation cycle.
Cortisol: A cortisone-like substance produced in the body.
Homeostasis: State of equilibrium in the body and its systems that provides a stable internal environment.
Myocardial: Pertaining to the middle layer of the heart walls.
Pathology: Changes in structure and/or function caused by disease or trauma.
Sprain: A stretching or tearing of ligaments.
Strain: A stretching or tearing of tendons or muscles.
Systemic: Affecting the body as a whole.
Vasoconstriction: Reduction in a blood vessel's diameter. This results in a decrease in blood flow.

iological resistance. If the stimulus is too intense or of too long a duration, the body reacts negatively to the stress, and injury occurs. In the context of exercise, little (if any) physiological benefit occurs if a person trains at an insufficient intensity. Conversely, if the intensity of the workout is too great, the body is placed in the stage of exhaustion, and injury occurs.

The body has certain mechanisms to balance the effects of positive and negative stressors. According to Wolff's law, bone adapts to the forces placed on it (Box 1–1). This remodeling may be exemplified by the deposition of **collagen** ■ fibers and inorganic salts in response to prolonged presence of stressors. This adaptation is based on the balance between the activities of **osteoblasts** ■ and **osteoclasts** ■. For example, the repeated physical stresses associated with running increase the rate of osteoblastic activity along the lines of stress. This increased osteoblastic remodeling results in new areas of structural strength and increased bone density. If this stress is applied too rapidly, osteoclastic activity outweighs osteoblastic activity, resulting in a stress fracture. In contrast, a femur immobilized for 20 days can lose up to 30 percent of its mineral deposits, causing it to become porous and fragile.[3]

The principles presented in the general adaptation syndrome and Wolff's law also apply to the use of therapeutic modalities. If the intensity of the modality application is too low or the treatment duration is too short, little or no benefit is gained. A 60-degree "cold" pack applied for 5 minutes would not penetrate deeply enough into the tissues to effect change. If the magnitude of the modality is too great, such as a moist heat pack with no covering or if it is applied at the wrong point in the healing process (e.g., during the acute state) further injury occurs (see Chapter 5).

■ Types of Soft Tissue Found in the Body

This text focuses on five types of soft tissues: (1) epithelial, (2) adipose, (3) muscular, (4) nervous, and (5) connective. This is also the order through which different forms of therapeutic energy must pass to affect the tissues. Based on

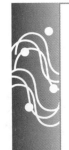

Box 1–1. **Wolff's Law**

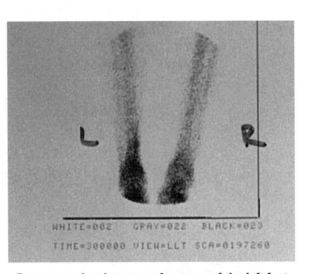

WHITE=002   GRAY=022   BLACK=023
TIME=300000   VIEW=LLT   SCA=0197260

Bone scan showing stress fractures of the left foot.

Bones remodel and adapt to the forces placed on them by increasing their strength along the lines of mechanical stress. Based on fluctuations in the intrinsic piezoelectrical current of bones, the osteoblastic and osteoclastic activity changes in response to the presence or absence of functional stress. Bone is removed from sites of little or no stress and is formed along the sites of new stress.

Most commonly, these stresses are caused by compressive, distractive, or shear forces associated with running, throwing, and so on. However, the removal of these stresses can also result in the bone's remodeling itself. If a limb is immobilized, the daily stresses placed on its bones are removed. As a result, the body adapts to the lack of stress by decreasing bone density.

Collagen: A protein-based connective tissue.
Osteoblast: A cell concerned with the formation of new bone.
Osteoclast: A cell that absorbs and removes unwanted bone.

its cellular structure, each tissue type has unique properties that allow it to reproduce after trauma (Table 1–1). When an injury occurs, the scope and severity of the trauma are generally in direct proportion to the number and type of cells that have been damaged. The regenerative potential and the ability of each of these types of tissues to transmit or absorb various forms of energy must be considered when selecting therapeutic modalities.

Epithelial Tissues

Epithelial tissues line the skin (stratified squamous epithelium), heart and blood vessels (simple squamous epithelium), hollow organs (transitional epithelium), glands, and external openings (Fig. 1–1). This type of tissue is able to secrete and absorb various substances and has the distinction of being devoid of blood vessels. Epithelial tissue has excellent potential to regenerate, a fortunate trait because it is the tissue most commonly injured. Imagine how our bodies would appear if our skin failed to regenerate each time we suffered a minor cut.

The skin's outer layer is formed by the stratum corneum, a layer of flat, densely packed dead cells. Unlike living cells, which are filled with cytoplasm, the stratum corneum cells are filled with keratin, a dry, fibrous protein. This structure forms a barrier that prevents many external substances, such as germs, from entering the body and helps keep the body's fluids inside.

Most forms of energy produced by the therapeutic modalities discussed in this text must pass through the stratum corneum and the remainder of the epidermis, dermis, and adipose tissues to affect the target tissues. Thermal agents initially heat or cool this layer, and the underlying tissues lose or gain heat to each other through **conduction** ■. Ultrasonic energy passes relatively easily through this layer. Because the cells of the stratum corneum are dead and dry, this tissue layer resists electrical stimulating currents and inhibits them from affecting the underlying tissues. **Transdermally** ■ applied medications must pass through the stratum corneum by finding portals surrounding hair follicles and sweat glands.

Adipose Tissue

Immediately underlying the dermis is a layer of adipose tissue that stores fat cells and, in areas such as the heel and palm, protects the underlying structures from hard blows (see Fig. 1–1). The high water content of adipose tissue makes it an ideal medium for ultrasound to pass through and is selectively heated during some forms of **diathermy** ■. Because the body's fat layering also serves as insulation against cold, the effectiveness of thermal agents such as cold packs or moist heat packs is reduced when they are applied over thick layers of adipose tissue.

Muscular Tissues

Muscular tissues have the ability to actively shorten and to be passively lengthened and are classified by the function they serve: smooth muscle, cardiac muscle, and skeletal muscle. Smooth muscle, which is not under voluntary control, is associated with the hollow organs of the body and the vascular system other than the capillaries. Cardiac muscle is responsible for the pumping of blood. Skeletal muscle is responsible for the movement of the body's joints. Muscular tissue possesses little or no ability to reproduce duplicates of lost cells.

Skeletal muscle fiber is classified by the intensity and duration of the contraction it can produce or its proportion of contractile properties (Table 1–2). Type I muscle fibers are slow to fatigue and are prevalent in postural muscles (e.g., the spinal erector muscles, quadriceps femoris group, gastrocnemius and soleus muscles). Type II (fast-twitch) muscle fibers are capable of generating a high amount of force in a short amount of time. Type II fibers are predominant in explosive muscle contractions.

Voluntary muscle contractions are based on the size principle in which small-diameter type I **motor nerves** ■ are recruited into the contraction first. As more tension within the muscle is needed, larger diameter type II motor nerves are brought into the contraction. Increased muscular tension is produced by recruiting more **motor units** ■ or increasing the frequency with which each unit is depolarized.

TABLE 1–1	Types of Cells Found in the Body	
Type	*Tissues Where Found*	*Ability to Regenerate*
Labile cells	Skin, intestinal tract, blood	Good
Stabile cells	Bone	Some
Permanent cells	Muscle	Some
	Peripheral nervous system	Some
	Central nervous system	None

Conduction: The transfer of heat from a high temperature to a low temperature between two objects that are touching each other.

Diathermy: A classification of therapeutic modality that uses high-frequency electrical energy to heat subcutaneous tissues.

Motor nerve: A nerve that provides impulses to muscles.

Motor unit: A group of skeletal muscle fibers that are innervated by a single motor nerve.

Transdermal (Transdermally): Introduction of medication to the subcutaneous tissues through unbroken skin.

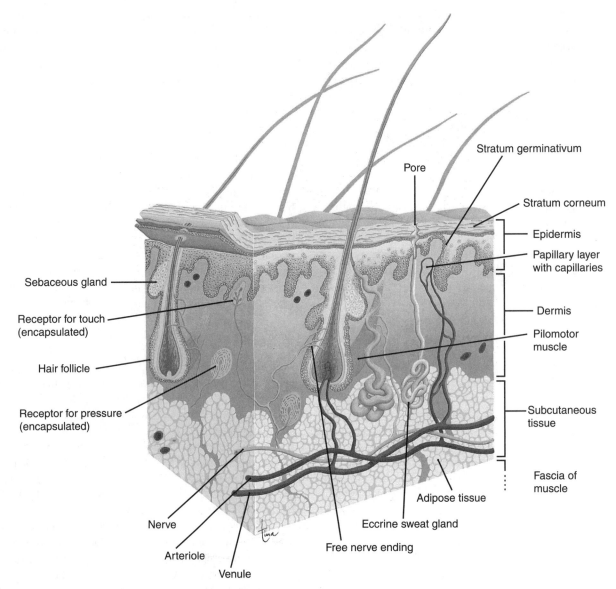

Figure 1–1. **Cross-Section of the Skin.**Therapeutic modalities must first penetrate the epidermis, dermis, and subcutaneous adipose tissue before affecting the deeper tissues, including muscle. (From Scanlon, VC: Essentials of Anatomy and Physiology, ed 4. Philadelphia, FA Davis, 2003, with permission.)

Skeletal muscle is frequently injured during athletics, work, or even by the activities of daily living. Despite this relatively high frequency of injury, muscle tissue only has limited ability to regenerate. Muscular tissues are heated or cooled through conduction with the overlying tissues. The flow of warm blood and increased cell **metabolism** ■, such as that experienced during exercise, also increases the temperature of muscles. Therapeutic ultrasound heats muscle without heating the skin or adipose tissues. In some circumstances, a DC electrical current can cause muscle fibers to shorten, but electrically induced muscle contractions are usually obtained by depolarizing motor nerves.

Nervous Tissue

Nerves are classified as being in the central or peripheral nervous system. The central nervous system (CNS) includes the brain and spinal cord. The peripheral nervous system (PNS) is formed by all nerves leading to or from the CNS. The nerves in the PNS are either traumatized during injury or send a signal—pain—that tissue damage has occurred. The pain system and CNS are described in Chapter 2.

Nervous tissue has the ability to conduct **afferent** ■ and **efferent** ■ impulses. Individual nerve cells, or

---

Afferent: Carrying impulses toward a central structure, for example, the brain.
Efferent: Carrying impulses away from a central structure. Nerves leaving the central nervous system are efferent nerves.
Metabolism: The sum of physical and chemical reactions taking place within the body.

TABLE 1–2 **Types of Skeletal Muscular Tissues**

Type	Fiber Type	Energy Source	Contraction Type
Type I	Slow-twitch	**aerobic** ■	Long-duration, low intensity
Type II	Fast twitch	**anaerobic** ■	Short-duration, high-intensity
Type II-A	Mixture	both	Characteristics of both type I and type II
Type II-X	Fast twitch	anaerobic	Short-duration, high-intensity

neurons, form the basic functional unit of the nervous system, with two distinct segments forming each neuron: (1) dendrites, which transmit impulses toward a cell body, and (2) the axon, which transmits impulses away from the cell body. Nerve impulses are transferred from one nerve to another through a synapse (Fig. 1–2). Although their anatomical and physiological structure and processes are similar, nerves are specialized in terms of their function (Table 1–3). As we see throughout this text, these differences can be exploited by different types of therapeutic modalities for purposes ranging from pain relief to developing stronger muscle contractions.

Synaptic junctions are classified as either electrical or chemical. Electrical synapses are characterized by a gap junction that allows the nerve impulse to be transferred directly to the next nerve in sequence. Nerves that transmit information toward a synapse are termed presynaptic neurons; those that transmit the impulse away from the synapse are postsynaptic neurons. As shown in Figure 1–2, a nerve may be both presynaptic and postsynaptic.

Most of the body's synapses are chemical synapses. Here, a small gap, the synaptic cleft, separates the presynaptic and postsynaptic nerves. A chemical neurotransmitter is released from the presynaptic nerve, spills across the synaptic cleft, and binds into a receptor site on the postsynaptic neuron (Table 1–4). At an excitatory synapse, the neurotransmitter release tends to activate the postsynaptic nerve through an excitatory postsynaptic potential. Activation of an inhibitory synapse increases the postsynaptic nerve's resting polarity, making it more hyperpolar (negative), potentially stopping **propagation** ■ of the impulse.

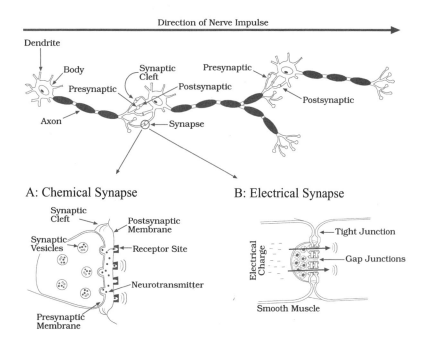

Figure 1–2. **Nerve Transmission.** Nerve impulses originate at the dendrite, pass through the nerve's body, and are transmitted along the axon (see Box 1–2 for a discussion of the propagation of nerve impulses). The junction between two nerves is called a synapse. Inset A depicts a chemical synapse in which the impulse is propagated by the release of a neurotransmitter from the presynaptic nerve that crosses the synaptic cleft and binds to a postsynaptic receptor site. Inset B portrays an electrical synapse in which the depolarization of the presynaptic nerve continues directly to the postsynaptic nerve.

Aerobic: Requiring the presence of oxygen.

Anaerobic: Able to survive in the absence of oxygen. Anaerobic systems derive their energy through the breakdown of adenosine triphosphate (ATP) into adenosine diphosphate (ADP).

Propagation: Transmission through a medium.

TABLE 1–3	Types and Function of Various Peripheral Nerves			
Axon	*Function*		*Diameter*	*Conduction Velocity m/sec*
Afferents				
Ia (A-alpha)	Muscle spindle afferent		12–20 μm ■	70–120
Ib (A-alpha)	Golgi tendon afferent		12–20 μm	70–120
II (A-beta)	Touch/pressure afferent Secondary muscle afferent		6–12 μm	30–70
III (A-delta)	Temperature afferent Sharp pain		1–6 μm	6–30
IV (C)	Temperature afferent Dull pain		<1.5 μm	0.5–2
Efferents				
A-alpha	Skeletal muscle efferent		12–20 μm	70–120
A-gamma	**Muscle spindle** ■ efferent		2–10 μm	10–50
A-beta	Muscle and muscle spindle efferent		8–12 μm	30–50

The nerve cell's semipermeable membrane separates opposite electrical charges. The resting potential is approximately –70 **millivolt (mV)** ■ between the inside and outside of the membrane. A high concentration of potassium (K+) ions creates a net negative charge within the cell. A positive charge is formed outside of the membrane by the presence of sodium (Na$^+$) and chlorine (Cl$^-$). The cell membrane is more permeable to potassium than it is to

TABLE 1–4	Common Neurotransmitters and Their Functions	
Neurotransmitter	*Location*	*Functions*
Acetylcholine	Motor nerves Central nervous system	Transmits motor impulses
Dopamine	Brain stem	Absence results in motor dysfunction Increases blood pressure Increases cardiac output Causes vasoconstriction
Epinephrine	Brain stem	Behavior Bronchial dilation Emotions Mood Vasoconstriction
Norepinephrine	Autonomic nervous system	Arousal (flight-or-fight response) Dreams Mood regulation Vasoconstriction
Serotonin	Platelets Mast cells	Sensory perception Sleep Temperature regulation Vasoconstriction
Substance P	Pain-transmitting nerve fibers	Transmits **noxious** ■ impulses Produces inflammation-like responses in local tissues

---

μm: Micrometer, 1/1,000,000 of a meter.

Millivolt (mV): One millivolt equals 1/1,000 of a volt.

Muscle spindle: An organ located within the muscular tissue that detects the rate and magnitude of a muscle contraction.

Noxious: Harmful, injurious, or painful. Capable of producing pain.

sodium. **Depolarization** of the nerve represents a change in the cell membrane permeability to sodium and potassium that evokes an action potential. During depolarization, there is a loss of the negative internal charge within the cell as potassium moves to the outside of the membrane and sodium moves into the cell (Box 1–2).

Repolarization returns the electrical balance to the cell's resting potential. Using adenosine triphosphatase (ATP) for its energy source, the sodium-potassium pump actively transports two potassium ions from outside of the cell back to the inside for every three sodium ions moved from the inside to the outside, the **refractory period (Fig. 1–3)**.

Cells damaged in the CNS are not replaced, and their functions are lost. Nerve cells damaged in the PNS possess some ability to regenerate. Their functions may also be restored by a collateral system where intact nerves sprout toward the damaged tissues.

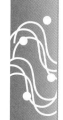

Box 1–2. Propagation of Nerve Impulses

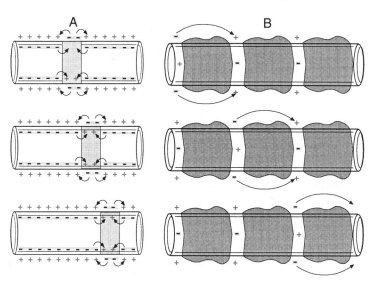

Nerve impulses are created by the depolarization of the nerve's cell membrane. At rest, the outside of the nerve membrane has a positive charge, and the inside has a negative charge. When a stimulus that exceeds the nerve's threshold is received, the nerve depolarizes and the sodium ions (Na^+) rush inside, causing a sequential reversal of the membrane's polarity. In a healthy nerve, this sequence repeats throughout the length of the nerve until the impulse reaches the synapse.

All excitable cell memmbranes have a different electrical charge between the inside and the outside of the membrane, the resting potential. Action potentials that are initiated at the nerve's body or receptor cause a depolarization in the naturally occurring direction (afferently for sensory nerves, efferently for motor nerves). Action potentials that are initiated along the axon will result in the impulse occurring in both directions.

Transmission of impulses in unmyelinated nerves involves depolarization along the length of the axon, a slower and less efficient mechanism than the saltatory conduction mechanism associated with myelinated nerves (*A*). The axons of myelinated nerves are covered by a fatty myelin sheath (Schwann cells) that is interrupted by the nodes of Ranvier, gaps where the cell membrane is exposed. The myelin sheath, which is 80% lipid (fat) and 20% protein, serves as in insulator. Depolarization occurs only at the nodes of Ranvier, jumping from one node to the next (*saltare* is Latin for "leap"). Because only selected areas of the axon are depolarized, transmission along myelinated nerves is faster, more efficient, and requires less metabolic activity than unmyelinated fibers (*B*).

In addition to the nerve's myelin sheath, the nerve's diameter also affects the speed at which the impulse is transmitted. Wider-diameter nerves transmit impulses faster than nerves having a smaller diameter, although small-diameter myelinated nerves have a faster conduction velocity than larger unmyelinated nerves. Small-diameter nerves also have longer refractory periods and lower discharge frequency than wider diameter nerves.

Each impulse is followed by a refractory period, during which the sodium pathways close and the nerve is allowed to repolarize (see Fig. 1–3). Corresponding to the change in sodium permeability, there is an increased charge within the cell, hyperpolarization. The absolute refractory period represents the period of time (approximately 25% of the total refractory period) during which no additional stimulus, regardless of its magnitude, will trigger another action potential. The absolute refractory period ensures that the nerve can completely recharge before the next action potential is initiated, and the length of this period determines the frequency at which the nerve can depolarize in a given length of time. Following the absolute refractory period, there is a relative refractory period during which a stimulus that is stronger than normal can initiate another action potential.

A common local anesthetic, Novocain, works by decreasing the nerves' membrane permeability to sodium, preventing it from depolarizing. The differences in nerve conduction velocities form the basis for the gate-control theory, a fundamental method of pain control. The location of nerves and whether or not they are myelinated also affects their response to thermal modalities. The currents used by electrical stimulators are designed to allow an appropriate amount of time between pulses to allow the nerves to repolarize.

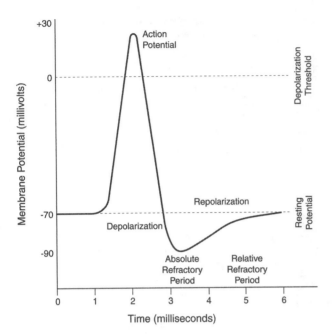

Figure 1–3. **Nerve Depolarization and Repolarization.** Once a stimulus reaches the depolarization threshold, the nerve will evoke an action potential. Following the depolarization there is a repolarization period. No further stimuli will cause depolarization during the absolute refractory period. During the relative refractory period, the membrane is capable of depolarizing, but it requires a more intense stimulus than the initial depolarization until the resting membrane potential is again reached.

Most therapeutic modalities have some affect on nerve function. Thermal agents and ultrasound influence nerve function by altering their conduction velocities. Slowing the rate of painful nerve transmission or activating touch and pressure but not pain impulses can decrease the perception of pain and can reduce muscle spasm. Most forms of electrical stimulation specifically target sensory, motor, or pain nerve fibers. The electrical stimulus causes a depolarization of these nerves in an orderly, predictable manner.

Connective Tissue

Connective tissue (also known as "support cells") is the most abundant type of tissue in the body. Produced by fibroblasts, connective tissue is formed by **ground substance** ■ and collagen fibers that serve as a cement to support and connect the other tissue types.[4] This tissue provides strength, structure, nutrition, and defense for the other tissues. The fundamental types of connective tissue and their function are presented in Table 1–5.

Collagen, the predominant type of connective tissue, is found in high density in fascia, tendons, ligaments, carti-

TABLE 1–5	Types of Connective Tissue and Their Function
Tissue Type	*Function*
Fibroblasts	Secretes **extracellular** ■ matrix components
Chondrocytes	Produces extracellular matrix components in cartilage
Myofibroblasts	Produces extracellular matrix components with contractile properties
Adipocytes	Stores lipids

lage, muscle, and bone. Eleven types of collagen are found in the body and, with the exception of meniscal cartilage, are highly vascular to aid in their repair (Table 1–6).

The connective tissue's elasticity is determined by the ratio of inelastic collagen fibers to elastic yellow elastin fibers. To illustrate the effect of collagen density and elasticity, consider the difference between muscle and tendon. Muscles are highly elastic and contain a much higher percentage of elastin fibers than collagen fibers. Tendons, in contrast to muscles, have very little elasticity because 86 percent of their dry weight is collagen.[5] Collagen is also found in other inelastic tissues such as ligaments, fascia, cartilage, and bone.

The fascial network interconnects the body. The fascial system of the lower leg is connected to that of the femur,

TABLE 1–6	Collagen Fiber Types
Type	*Location*
I	Skin, fascia, tendons, ligaments, bone, fibrous cartilage
II	Hyaline cartilage, elastic cartilage, vertebral disks, vitreous humor (eye)
III	Smooth muscles, nerves, bone marrow, blood vessels (commonly found with type I)
IV	**Basement membranes** ■
V	Smooth muscle, skeletal muscle
VI	Found in most, if not all, of the body's structures
VII	Basement membranes of skin
VIII	Endothelium
IX	Cartilage (primarily found during fetal development)
X	Mineralizing cartilage (growth plates)
XI	Cartilage, heart, skeletal muscle, skin, brain

Basement membrane: Extracellular material that separates the base of epithelial cells from connective tissue.

Extracellular: Outside the cell membrane.

Ground substance: Material occupying the intercellular spaces in fibrous connective tissue, cartilage, or bone (also known as matrix).

which is connected to the hip, which is connected to the torso and so on. Superficial fascia, found between the skin and underlying tissue, normally has a relatively random, loose fibrous arrangement and is not as collagen dense and more elastic than deeper fascia. Superficial fascia contains adipose tissue, nerves, and blood vessels. Deep fascia has a high collagen content and the fibers are arranged along the lines of force. More inelastic than superficial fascia, deep fascia is responsible for transferring physical loads of force.

Collagen can be elongated through stretching, especially when it is heated, and it can be selectively heated by ultrasonic energy. Collagen located in the superficial tissues can also be heated through moist heat.

■ The Injury Process

The body's reaction to injury may be divided into two distinct stages. The primary response to injury is the tissue destruction directly associated with the traumatic force. Secondary damage is cell death caused by a blockage of the oxygen supply to the injured area or caused by enzymatic damage and mitochondrial failure. Just like humans, cells need oxygen to survive. If their oxygen supply is cut off, they will die and continue to perpetuate the injury response process. The damage done during the primary stage is irreversible, and the treatment efforts used after trauma attempt to contain the effects and limit the amount of secondary injury.

Dead and damaged cells release their contents into the area adjacent to the injured site. The presence of these substances causes an inflammatory reaction from the body's tissues. As a result of both the primary trauma and the inflammatory **mediators ■**, **hemorrhage ■**, and **edema ■** occur. The buildup of fluids results in both mechanical pressure on and chemical irritation of the nerve receptors in the area. Because of the clogging of the vasculature, further cell death results from a lack of oxygen in the surviving tissues. A subcycle occurs as a result of pain and **ischemia ■**, causing muscle spasm and increasing the possibility of atrophy over time (Fig. 1–4).

This sequence of events, the injury response cycle, is a self-perpetuating process. For the injury to resolve in the least amount of time, this cycle must be controlled so that healing may occur.

The course of healing is described in three phases: (1) the acute inflammatory response, (2) the proliferation

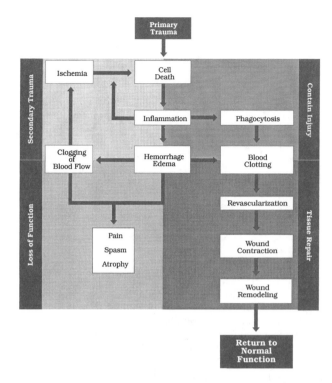

Figure 1–4. **The Injury Response Process.** In traumatic injuries, the primary trauma stems from an outside force and the physical damage inflicted is irreversible. Secondary injury occurs from deprivation of oxygen to the tissues. This, combined with pain, spasm, or atrophy, leads to the tissues or body parts losing the ability to function normally. The body begins its road to repair by first containing the injury and then rebuilding the damaged tissue.

phase, and (3) the maturation phase. Although the central events of each of these phases are marked by distinct responses within a theoretical time frame, an overlap of these stages can, and does, occur (Fig. 1–5).

The acute inflammatory response involves the delivery of **phagocytes ■** and fibroblasts to the area and the formation of **granulation tissue ■** to isolate and localize the trauma. During this time, **histamine ■** released from the traumatized cells increases capillary permeability, resulting in swelling as the proteins follow water out into the tissues. During the proliferation phase, the number and size of fibroblasts increase, causing ground substance and collagen to collect in the traumatized area in preparation to rebuild the damaged tissues. The injury process is completed during the maturation phase, when collagen and

---

Edema: An excessive accumulation of serous fluids.

Granulation tissue: Delicate tissue composed of fibroblasts, collagen, and capillaries formed during the revascularization phase of wound healing.

Hemorrhage: Bleeding from veins, arteries, or capillaries.

Histamine: A blood-thinning chemical released from damaged tissue during the inflammatory process. Its primary function is vasodilation of arterioles and increased vascular permeability in venules.

Ischemia: Local and temporary deficiency of blood supply caused by obstruction of circulation to a part.

Mediators: Chemicals that act through indirect means.

Phagocyte: A classification of scavenger cells that ingest and destroy unwanted substances in the body.

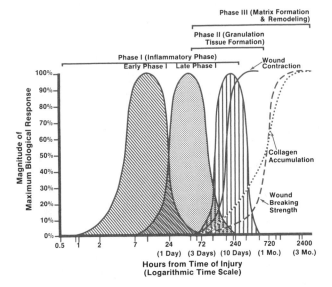

Figure 1–5. **Overlapping Stages of Wound Repair.** There is no clear delineation between the end of one stage of healing and the beginning of the next stage; it is possible for portions of all three stages to overlap. Phase I is the acute inflammatory response stage, phase II is the revascularization stage, and phase III is maturation. (From McCulloch, JM, et al [eds]: Wound Healing: Alternatives in Management, ed 2. FA Davis, Philadelphia, 1995, p 33, with permission.)

fibroblasts align themselves and attempt to adapt to the original tissue orientation and function, although this does not always occur (Table 1–7).[6]

Phagocytosis occurs in several distinct stages. Neutrophils dominate the first 6 to 24 hours of phagocytosis, releasing chemical "cluster bombs" that are intended to destroy bacteria but end up traumatizing all tissues in the area. Macrophages are responsible for restoring the tissues to their original state ("cleaning up the mess") and to stim-

ulate the proliferation stage by releasing growth factors that activate fibroblasts and stimulate the increase in the number of satellite cells and differentiate into myofibers.

Acute Inflammatory Response

Inflammation is the body's natural physiological reaction to injury. Triggered by mechanical trauma such as spraining a ligament, bacterial invasion, chemical irritation, or burns, the acute inflammatory response mobilizes the body's defensive systems and begins to set the stage for healing to occur.[7] The acute inflammatory response is characterized by the release of inflammatory mediators and the migration of fluids and **leukocytes** ■ from the blood into the extravascular tissues of the affected tissues. The inflammatory response can be divided into three phases, but the exact sequence of cellular events associated with these events depends on the number and type of cells involved, the tissue, and individual factors such as age, nutritional status, general health, and so on (Table 1–8).[8]

Inflammation has a bad reputation as an unwanted and unneeded part of the body's response to injury. Nothing could be further from the truth. Inflammation is a necessary part of the healing process. However, if the duration or intensity of the inflammation is excessive, the process becomes detrimental and chronic inflammation becomes a debilitating event. Through the application of therapeutic modalities, we can influence the inflammatory response and deter its unwanted effects.

Inflammation attempts to control the effects of the trauma and prepare the body for healing. In the initial stages, the inflammatory response contains, destroys, and dilutes the injurious agents and attempts to localize the tissue damage. Pain caused by inflammation alerts the individual that tissue damage has occurred and, combined with **muscle guarding** ■ and splinting postures, protects the area from further insult. The movement of plasma and leukocytes to the involved area produces the cardinal signs of inflammation (Box 1–3).

The body is armed with more inflammatory firepower than it normally needs. Whenever trauma occurs, the immune system assumes that a bacterial invasion will also occur and triggers the release of neutrophils to counter this

TABLE 1–7	Phases of Wound Healing
Phase	*Events*
Inflammatory phase	Platelet accumulation, coagulation, leukocyte migration
Proliferation phase	Growth of new tissue (reepithelization), development of new blood vessels (angiogenesis), development of fibrous tissue (fibroplasia), wound contraction, formation of collagen matrix
Maturation phase	Resolution of matrix, deposition of permanent tissues, return to function

TABLE 1–8	Stages of Inflammation After Injury	
Stage	*Process*	*Elapsed Time Since Injury (Days)*
Acute	Reaction to the injury	0–14
Subacute	Symptoms diminish	14–31
Chronic	Unwarranted inflammation	>31 days past the expected resolution

Leukocytes: White blood cells that serve as scavengers.
Muscle guarding: A voluntary or subconscious contraction of a muscle to protect an injured area.

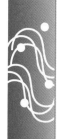

Box 1–3. Cardinal Signs of Inflammation

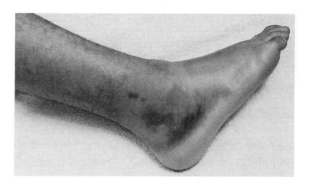

Sign: Associated Inflammatory Events
Heat: Increased blood flow, increased metabolic rate.
Redness: Increased blood flow, increased metabolic rate, histamine release.
Swelling: Leakage of inflammatory mediators into the surrounding tissues, hemorrhage, high concentration of proteins, **gamma globulins ▪**, and **fibrinogen ▪** that block the venous return mechanism; in chronic conditions swelling may represent the proliferation of connective tissue.
Pain: Mechanical pressure on or chemical irritation of nerves, or both; triggered by the release of chemical irritants—bradykinin, histamine, prostaglandin, and other substances—in the inflamed area and increased tissue pressure caused by swelling or muscle spasm, or both.
Loss of function: Primary tissue damage, the sum of preceding signs, muscle guarding.

Five cardinal signs mark the acute inflammatory response. The result of inflammation is the loss of normal function. The magnitude of the patient's inflammation can be clinically quantified based on the amount of swelling, point tenderness, and loss of joint motion.[9] The amount of swelling and loss of range of motion can be measured relative to the uninvolved extremity. Tenderness can be loosely quantified by slight or severe discomfort during palpation, the inability to palpate because of pain, and pain caused by mild stimulation (e.g., blowing on the skin, clothing touching the area). Various blood tests can also accurately determine the biophysical stage of inflammation.

threat. Most musculoskeletal injuries do not have a bacterial component, so that portion of the inflammatory response that attempts to contain bacteria damages otherwise viable tissue instead.

The inflammatory response begins almost immediately following the trauma and persists until the stimulus is removed and the mediators are dissipated or their release into the tissues is inhibited. Acute inflammation may last only a few seconds or may extend for months. Chronic inflammation, discussed later, may persist from months to years. Inflammation and its role in promoting tissue healing and repair, involves a fine balancing act between too much and too little of a response.

Following a traumatic injury, the cells undergo a primary reaction. This primary phase, also known as the reactive or inflammatory phase, is characteristic of the first 2 or 4 days after the injury, although the length of this phase varies. The inflammatory response occurs at two levels: (1) changes in local blood flow (hemodynamic changes) and (2) changes in cellular functioning that balance the presence of proinflammatory mediators and anti-inflammatory mediators of inflammation.

The primary effect of the inflammatory process is increased cell metabolism. Associated with this are changes in cellular function and the appearance of neutrophils and other granulocytes in the tissues. The outcome following injury is influenced by the balance between proinflammatory mediators and anti-inflammatory mediators of inflammation (Box 1–4).[10] We cannot control inflammation caused by the primary trauma, but we can influence the delivery of leukocytes and proinflammatory mediators by the use of thermal modalities or medications. The sequence of the cellular events differs from tissue to tissue.[11]

Neutrophils are the primary source of proinflammatory mediators. Neutrophils, which normally flow in the axial zone, marginate to the plasmatic zone. In a process called pavementing, the neutrophils adhere to the endothelial lining on the **venule ▪** side of the capillary junction.

Fibrinogen: A protein present in the blood plasma and essential for the clotting of blood.
Gamma globulin: An infection-fighting blood protein.
Venule: A small vein exiting from a capillary.

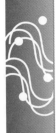

Box 1–4. Mediators of Inflammation

Chemicals released into the area control the inflammatory process. Collectively known as mediators, these chemicals are responsible for a wide range of cellular and vascular events. Mediators either perpetuate the inflammatory response (proinflammatory mediators) or inhibit the inflammatory response (anti-inflammatory mediators). These two types of mediators must be balanced to control the rate and duration of the inflammatory response.

Some mediators are released by the damaged cells. Other mediators are attracted to the area by **chemotaxis** ■. Some mediators cause **vasodilation** ■ of the vessels, increasing both the amount of blood, plasma proteins, and phagocytic leukocytes and the speed with which these products are delivered to the area. Other mediators increase the permeability of the vessels, allowing the movement of blood proteins and blood cells out of the vessels into the surrounding tissues.

- **Heparin:** Inhibits coagulation by preventing the conversion of prothrombin to thrombin.
- **Histamine:** Located in mast cells, basophils, and platelets. The primary function of histamine is vasodilation of arterioles and increased vascular permeability in venules.
- **Kinins:** A group of polypeptides that dilate arterioles, serve as strong chemotactics, and produce pain. They are primarily involved in the inflammatory process in the early stages of inflammatory hemodynamic changes.
- **Neutrophils:** Formed in the bone marrow, neutrophils are released into the bloodstream and serve the first line of cellular defense. Neutrophils are aggressive phagocytes that damage both insulting cells and viable, needed cells.
- **Prostaglandins:** Composed of many different types and are responsible for vasodilation and increased vascular permeability. These are synthesized locally in the injured tissues from fatty acids released from damaged cell membranes. Prostaglandins influence the duration and intensity of the inflammatory process.
    PGE_1: Increases vascular permeability
    PGE_2: Attracts leukocytes.
- **Serotonin:** Causes local vasoconstriction.
- **Leukotrienes:** Fatty acids that cause smooth muscle contraction, increase vascular permeability, and attract neutrophils. Includes slow-reacting substance of anaphylaxis (SRSA).

The presence of proteins changes the osmotic relationship between the blood and the adjacent tissues. During the inflammatory response, the protein content of the plasma decreases while the protein content of the **interstitial** ■ fluid increases.[14] Water tends to follow the blood proteins out of the vessel through osmosis, resulting in edema. Edema, in turn, increases the tissue pressure, irritating the nerve receptors and blocking capillary flow.

These neutrophils then escape to the extravascular space. With more severe trauma, red blood cells may also exit into the extravascular space (diapedesis).

One of the body's first responses to trauma is the localized release of norepinephrine in the traumatized tissues, causing vasoconstriction of the **arterioles** ■ and venules to prevent blood loss in the affected area.[1] Capillaries are not formed by smooth muscle, so they do not constrict or dilate. Although the vessels are in the state of vasoconstriction, the **coagulation** ■ process begins to repair the primary damage. This initial vasoconstriction is transitory, and in as little as 10 minutes after the injury, the

vessels begin to dilate, increasing the volume of blood being delivered to the area.

During normal arteriole flow, blood cells travel in the center of the vessel (axial stream) and plasma flows along the vessel's walls (plasmatic stream), keeping the blood cells away from the walls. After the initial changes in vessel diameter, blood cells flow closer to the walls. As described in the coagulation section of this chapter, this movement of the blood cells toward the vascular walls leads to margination and pavementing of leukocytes.

Gaps form between the **endothelial cells** ■ in the capillary beds. The increased space between the cells

---

Arteriole: A small artery leading to a capillary at its distal end.
Chemotaxis: Movement of living protoplasm toward or away from a chemical stimulus.
Coagulation: The process of blood clotting.
Endothelial cells: Flat cells lining the blood and lymphatic vessels and the heart.
Interstitial: Between the tissues.
Vasodilation: Increase in a blood vessel's diameter. This results in an increase in blood flow.

increases the blood vessel's permeability and allows fluids, proteins, and other substances to escape into the surrounding tissue.

As the volume of blood being delivered to the area increases, a protein-rich **exudate** ■ is formed in the tissues. The prostaglandin PGE₁ increases vascular permeability, and prostaglandin PGE₂ attracts leukocytes to the area.[12] The fluids and proteins leak into the tissue through the newly formed gaps in the capillaries, depositing leukocytes along the site of the injury to localize and remove any harmful substances.

Swelling occurs as a result of the presence of fluids, proteins, and cell debris in the area. As the amount of swelling increases and the extravascular pressure increases, the vascular flow to and from the area is decreased. The venous and lymphatic networks are blocked, causing further clogging of blood flow to the area and perpetuating the process.

Prolonged inflammation damages the connective tissue by depriving it of nutrients, resulting in thickening of the synovial membrane. When unchecked, this condition can lead to the formation of joint adhesions that affect its **range of motion** ■. The release of cortisol, as described in the general adaptation syndrome, is effective in reducing the effects of chronic inflammation because of its cortisone-like anti-inflammatory effects.[13]

Hemorrhage

The initial trauma may tear the local blood vessels or inflammatory mediators may increase their permeability, causing hemorrhage. For hemorrhage to take place, one of two prerequisites must be met: the vessel must (1) lose its continuity (be ruptured) or (2) have a marked increase in permeability so that cells and fluids can escape, or said differently, a gradient must be present in which the pressure inside the vessel is greater than the external pressure.[15] For hemorrhage to stop, the reverse of the two conditions must be met: the vessel must be repaired or the pressure gradient must be equalized.

Subcutaneous ■ hemorrhage is easily recognized by **ecchymosis** ■ of the skin associated with bruising. When hemorrhage occurs deeper in the tissues, a **hematoma** ■ may form. Because of the depth of the bleeding, it may take hours or days for the discoloration to appear in the skin. In the short term, hematomas assist the healing process by equalizing the pressure gradient between the inside and the outside of the injured vessels, limiting the amount of blood

loss. However, the long-term presence of a hematoma in a muscle can restrict motion and hinder the repair process by perpetuating the inflammatory response.

Even in the best possible scenario, the treatment provided immediately after an injury does not affect primary hemorrhaging. By the time the initial injury occurs and the initial evaluation has occurred and ice is applied, several minutes have passed. In most instances, this time is sufficient for the coagulation process to seal the injured vasculature.[1] Application of cold treatments in this time frame helps limit the amount of secondary injury and decrease pain, and the application of an external wrap and elevation helps equalize the pressures inside and outside the vessel.

Coagulation

The inflammatory process encourages the removal of debris and toxic substances from the injured area, and protects the tissues from further damage. Phagocytosis, the body's cellular defense system, involves ingestion of toxic organisms and other foreign particles, and their removal via the lymphatic system. In skin wounds, these wastes may be visible in the form of pus. During this process, scavenger cells, **monocytes** ■, **macrophages** ■, and leukocytes débride the area, devouring toxic and dead tissues by trapping them with armlike appendages and engulfing them (Fig. 1–6). This entrapment occurs by random

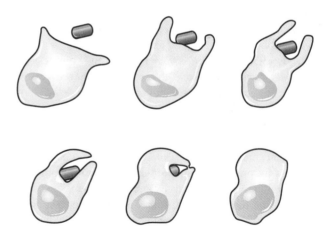

Figure 1–6. **The Process of Phagocytosis.** Scavenger cells randomly collide with vascular debris. Using armlike appendages, the phagocytes surround, devour, and subsequently remove the waste.

Ecchymosis: A blue-black discoloration of the skin caused by movement of blood into the tissues. In the latter stages, the color may appear greenish brown or yellow.

Exudate: Fluid that collects in a cavity and has a high concentration of cells, protein, and other solid matter.

Hematoma: A mass of blood confined to a limited area, resulting from the subcutaneous leakage of blood.

Macrophage: A blood cell having the ability to devour particles; a phagocyte.

Monocyte: A white blood cell that matures to become a macrophage.

Range of motion: The distance, measured in degrees, that a limb moves in one plane (e.g., flexion-extension, adduction-abduction).

Subcutaneous: Beneath the skin.

chance, and the use of pain-free range-of-motion exercises may increases the level of phagocytic activity.

The repair of the blood vessels, coagulation (blood clotting), involves a cascade of enzymes and consists of the formation of a **platelet** ■ plug and the transformation of fibrinogen into **fibrin** ■. This is a complex process and is presented in this text only in its basic form.

When disruption occurs in a vessel, an initial seal is formed by platelets. Margination occurs where the platelets and neutrophilic leukocytes flowing in the bloodstream begin to tumble along the walls of the vessel. Eventually, these substances adhere to collagen exposed by the trauma through the process of pavementing. Because platelets cannot adhere to each other, they must release adenosine diphosphate (ADP), which "glues" one layer of platelets to the other.[8] This series of platelet depositions forms an unstable and leaky patch over the injured site. Further events must occur to form a permanent repair.

The ruptured vessel releases an enzyme that acts as a distress signal to the body, alerting it that an injury has occurred. A subsequent set of reactions, combined with the platelet deposition, results in formation of a permanent seal. **Prothrombin** ■, a free-floating element found in the bloodstream, reacts with the enzyme factor X, converting prothrombin into **thrombin** ■. The presence of thrombin in the area then stimulates fibrinogen to unwind into its individual fibrin elements (Fig. 1–7).

Single, activated fibrin filaments, fibrin monomers, are split from fibrinogen and group together with fibronectin and collagen to form a "fibrin lattice" around the injured area. During this process, the fibrin threads trap red and white blood cells, along with platelets. As these threads contract, they remove the plasma and compress the platelets, forming a "patch" to repair the damaged vessel.

Inflammation serves as both an aid and a deterrent to the coagulation process. In general, the inflammatory process encourages the delivery of prothrombin to the injured area by increasing blood flow. However, one of the chemical mediators, heparin, hinders the coagulation process by preventing prothrombin from being converted to thrombin. A proper balance must be maintained between heparin and the other mediators. Too much heparin could completely inhibit blood coagulation; too little heparin could result in unwanted blood clots.

Proliferation Phase

The proliferation phase is marked by removal of the debris and temporary repair tissue formed during the inflammation stage and by the development of new, permanent replacement tissues. A new vascular framework is

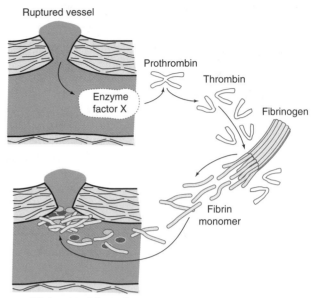

Figure 1–7. **The Process of Coagulation.** Activated by the presence of factor X, prothrombin is broken down into thrombin. In turn, the presence of thrombin causes fibrinogen to unwind into individual fibrin elements. The fibrin monomer deposits itself over the site in the damaged vessel, trapping platelets, red blood cells, and white blood cells. After contraction of the fibrin filaments, a permanent scar is formed.

deposited to supply the repairing tissues with oxygen, nutrients, and the cells needed to restore the area. This framework remains in place until the wound contraction phase. The exact length of transition from the acute inflammatory response to proliferation is unclear, but it is thought to begin approximately 72 hours after the onset of trauma and may last 3 weeks.[16] The final outcome of the injury response process can include resolution, regeneration, or repair (Table 1–9).

Healing occurs by primary intention or secondary intention. When the amount of tissue damage is minimal, healing occurs by primary intention, in which a minimal amount of granulation tissue and scar tissue is deposited across the gap. More significant tissue loss, or the involvement of more complex tissues, requires healing by secondary intention that results in an increased amount of granulation tissue and substantial scar tissue formation.

Repair of an injured structure involves the interaction between two types of cells: (1) the cells belonging to the injured structure and (2) connective tissue's cells. In acute trauma, inflammation is an active process where the rate is controlled by the body's metabolism. In chronic situations,

---

Fibrin: A filamentous protein formed by the action of thrombin on fibrinogen.

Platelet: A free-flowing cell fragment in the bloodstream.

Prothrombin: A chemical found in the blood that reacts with an enzyme to produce thrombin.

Thrombin: An enzyme formed in the blood of a damaged area.

TABLE 1–9	Possible Outcomes of the Injury Response Process

Outcome	Description
Resolution	Dead cells and cellular debris are removed by phagocytosis.
	The tissue is left with its original structure and function intact.
Regeneration	The damaged tissue is replaced by cells of the same type.
	The structure retains some or all of its original structure and function.
Repair	The original tissue is replaced with scar tissue.
	The original structure and function is lost.

inflammation is a passive process in which the body forms new, and possibly unwanted, connective tissues.

Regeneration of tissues occurs when the new cells are of the same type and can perform the same function as the original structure. Replacement of tissues results when a different type of cell substitutes for the damaged cells, such as scar tissue. Excess scar tissue can result in pain and/or loss of function. There is no clear delineation between "repair" and "regeneration." Most tissue trauma is eventually resolved through processes of both regeneration and repair.

The quality of the repair process is related to the number and type of cells that have been damaged. Labile cells (see Table 1–1), such as those found in the skin, have the greatest ability to produce a "clone" of the original tissues. In the case of skeletal muscles, the process involves the deposition of fibrous scar tissue that does not replicate the original structure. Evidence suggests that microregeneration can occur following minor skeletal muscle strains and microscopic meniscal tears.[16]

ATP is a critical factor that regulates the rate and quality of healing. Serving as the cell's primary source of energy, ATP is required to provide the metabolism needed to restore the cell's membrane properties by moving sodium and potassium into and out of the cell, to build new proteins, and to synthesize proteins.

Soft tissue repair occurs through the proliferation of granulation tissue, requiring four separate but related processes[5]: (1) fibroblast formation, (2) synthesis of collagen, (3) tissue remodeling, and (4) tissue alignment. The growth of granulation tissue requires the presence of fibroblasts, **myofibroblasts** ■, and endothelial cells, and is regulated by **growth factors** ■ produced by platelets and macrophages.

Revascularization

The process of repair begins at the periphery, where macrophages and **polymorphs** ■, both of which can withstand the low-oxygen environment, produce new capillary beds and form granulation tissue. Granulation tissue contains newly formed capillary beds that grow around the wound and gradually work their way toward the center of the injured area, forming a scaffold around which new tissue will be formed. Dermal wound repair involves the presence of mast cells. These cells release agents that stimulate fibroblasts and are involved in the remodeling of the extracellular matrix.[17]

Fibroblasts are indirectly attracted to the area by the presence of macrophages. Once in the area, fibroblasts begin laying down collagen to form a seal over the injured structure and creating the wound's extracellular matrix.[18] This deposition of collagen is random, with little order in the fibrous arrangement (Fig. 1–8). Stresses, in the form of gentle joint movements, may cause these fibers to rapidly arrange themselves in a more orderly fashion.[19]

Wound Contraction

Wound contraction occurs following the revascularization of the injured area and is marked by a decrease in size of

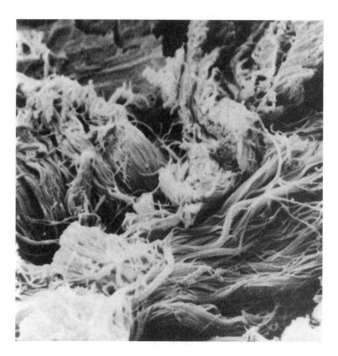

Figure 1–8. **Collagen Replacement.** Shown by means of an electron microscope, new, unorganized collagen can be seen interlacing with older, more densely packed collagen. (From Hunt, TK and Dunphy, JE [eds]: Fundamentals of Wound Management. Appleton-Century-Crofts, New York, 1979, p 38, with permission.)

Growth factors: Substances that stimulate the production of specific types of cells.
Myofibroblasts: Fibroblasts that have contractile properties.
Polymorph: A type of white blood cell; a granulocyte.

the original fibrin clot. Myofibroblasts accumulate at the margins of the wound and begin to move toward the center. Possessing a high **actin ■** filament content, each new myofibroblast shortens to pull the ends of the damaged tissues closer together (Fig. 1–9).[17] Fibroblasts produce weak type III collagen, making the area vulnerable to tensile forces. Water is drawn to the area of repair, and blood vessels, proprioceptive nerves, and sensory nerves begin to develop. In superficial wounds, these events form the characteristic "scar."

As the scar tissue matures, its continuity begins to resemble that of the tissue it is replacing. With time, the strength of the scar is increased by the replacement of the old collagen with a newer, stronger type. Wound contraction should not be confused with a contracture, in which the tissues loss of ability to lengthen results in the limitation of a joint's range of motion. With proper remodeling of the collagen, contractures may be avoided.

Wound Remodeling

The body is constantly remodeling itself. Following trauma, the purpose of the remodeling stage is to develop order in the previously deposited scar tissue. The presence of external stress causes the alignment of the fibers to remodel the wound. Approximately 5 to 11 days following the injury, type III collagen begins to be replaced by stronger type I collagen, resulting in improved **tensile strength ■**.[20, 21]

The use of early range-of-motion exercises can increase the tensile strength of healing ligaments.[22] Initially, the collagen is laid down in a random matrix, causing the scar to be fragile. During remodeling, the fibers form a more organized matrix, thus increasing their strength. However, scar tissue is never as functional as the tissue it replaces.[4] Consider a tear in one of the hamstring muscles. After a small tear, there is usually no residual deficit in strength or range of motion. After a massive tear in which a large amount of scar tissue is needed for repair, the muscle tends to produce less strength and have a decreased range of motion.

Because scar tissue is inelastic, it is more similar in structure and function to ligaments and tendons than it is to muscle. Repair of muscular tissue may be enhanced through a mechanism similar to that which occurs when muscle hypertrophies in response to strength training. Muscle fiber contains **satellite cells ■** that remain dormant in certain muscular tissues. These cells lack the cytoplasm and proteins found in other muscle cells. After an injury, repair of muscular tissue can occur by recruiting satellite cells as the source of nuclei for new muscle cells.[23]

Maturation Phase

The maturation phase marks the conclusion of the proliferation phase of injury response and is characterized by "cleaning up" the area and increased strength of the

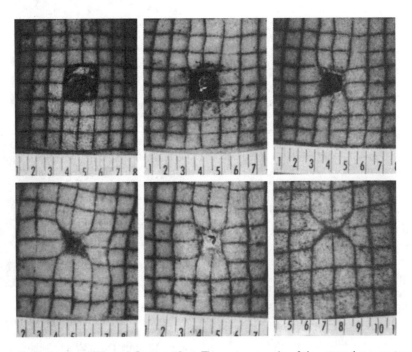

Figure 1–9. **Schematic of Wound Contraction.** The outer margin of the wound moves toward the center, drawing the ends together. (From Fitzpatrick, TB: Dermatology in General Medicine. McGraw-Hill, New York, 1987, p 330, with permission.)

Actin: A contractile muscle protein.

Satellite cell: Spindle-shaped cell that assists in the repair of skeletal muscle.

Tensile strength: The ability of a structure to withstand a pulling force along its length; resistance to tear.

repaired or replaced tissues. This is the final phase of the injury response process and may last a year or more.

At the conclusion of the wound contraction, the number of fibroblasts, myofibroblasts, and macrophages is reduced to the preinjury state. Because these repair agents no longer need to be delivered to the area, the number of capillaries, the overall vascularity of the area, and the water content are reduced. In the case of superficial wounds, these events are indicated by the fading redness of the scar and the eventual return to near-normal skin color and texture.

The proportion of type I collagen continues to increase, replacing the existing type III collagen and other parts of the collagen lattice. As the amount of type I collagen continues to grow, the tissue's tensile strength increases. Because most musculoskeletal injuries are repaired by the replacement of tissues, ever increasing stresses must be applied to the collagen to encourage its proper organization and to allow maximum tensile strength.

Other Possible Consequences of Injury

Depending on the magnitude of the inflammatory response, the tissues involved, and the initial management of the injury, several other consequences of the injury are possible.

Edema
Edema is the buildup of excessive fluid and protein in the interstitial space resulting from the imbalance between the pressures inside and outside the cell membrane, or an obstruction of the **lymphatic return** ■ and venous return mechanisms. This collection of fluids causes the tissues to expand. The amount of edema that accumulates in the injured area is proportional to:

- The severity of the injury (the number and type of cells damaged)
- Changes in vascular permeability
- The amount of primary and secondary hemorrhaging
- High pressure gradients
- The presence of chemical inflammatory mediators

Although they are interrelated, these factors function independently to cause the release of proteins that attract fluids to the injured area.[14]

The movement of fluids across the capillary membrane is contingent on three basic forces described by Starling's law[24]:

1. The vascular hydrostatic pressure and the interstitial fluid colloid osmotic pressure that forces the contents from the capillary outward to the tissues

2. The plasma colloid osmotic pressure that moves fluids from the tissues into the capillaries

3. The limb's hydrostatic pressure that is independently altered by changes in the position of the limb

The formation and removal of edema are based on the relationship among these pressures. Normally, the vascular hydrostatic pressure and the plasma colloid pressure are approximately even, keeping the inflow and outflow equal (a small percentage of normal venous return occurs through the lymphatic system). Capillary permeability increases after injury, making it easier for fluids and solid matter to leave the vessels (Fig. 1–10). If the vascular

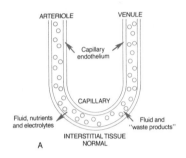

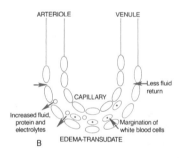

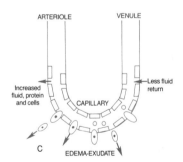

Figure 1–10. **The Formation of Edema.** (A) The normal pressure inside and outside the vessel causes an outward flow of fluids and nutrients at the arteriole end and absorption of wastes at the venule end. (B) The Transudate Stage. Following an injury, inflammatory mediators cause the arterioles to dilate. The increased capillary filtration pressure moves proteins and fluids into the tissues. (C) The Exudate Stage. Increased inflammation forces neutrophils and other blood cells out to the tissues, resulting in a thick, edematous fluid formation. (From Michlovitz, SL [ed]: Thermal Agents in Rehabilitation, ed 2. FA Davis, Philadelphia, 1990, p 7, with permission.)

Lymphatic return: A return process similar to that of the venous network but specializing in the removal of interstitial fluids.

hydrostatic pressure exceeds the plasma colloid osmotic pressure, excessive fluids are forced out of the capillaries into the tissues, and edema results. Likewise, if the plasma colloid osmotic pressure exceeds the vascular hydrostatic pressure, fluids are forced back into the vessels and may then be removed from the area. Most fluids are removed by the venous system, and solids are removed by the lymphatic system.

A limb's hydrostatic pressure depends on the position of the body part. When your arm is hanging at your side, the limb's hydrostatic pressure is increased because gravity is pulling the blood in your vessels distally. The pressure exerted tends to force fluids back out into the interstitial space. When your arm is lifted above your head, the limb hydrostatic pressure decreases. The limb hydrostatic pressure is used to help control and reduce swelling in the extremities. This mechanism is discussed in the following sections.

Lymphatic flow is disrupted by edema when the tissues become so expanded that the flap valves between the endothelial cells in the capillaries become separated. This parting of the valves renders them ineffective, thus allowing the fluids to "slosh" back into the injured area. The expansion of tissues causes further hypoxic injury by clogging the vascular pathways. When the limb is placed in a gravity-dependent position, interstitial pressure increases to the point where the lymphatic vessels collapse, further obstructing outflow from the area (Fig. 1–11).[25]

These events not only prevent the delivery of fresh blood and oxygen to the injured structures but also inhibit venous and lymphatic return from the site, causing perpetuation of the cycle. In addition, the pressure caused by the fluid buildup produces mechanical pain by stimulating mechanical nerve receptors in the area and causes chemically induced pain by depriving the tissues of oxygen. The four basic types of exudates are presented in Table 1–10.

Edema is not only a sign that an injury has occurred, but also contributes to the injury cycle. The edema clogs the vascular and cellular spaces, increasing tissue pressure and preventing oxygen from reaching the tissues and causing further cell death, pain, and restricted joint motion.[26] The healing process itself is slowed by delayed cellular regeneration and improper collagen formation.[27] Collagen deposition is increased in the edematous area and, when uncontrolled, leads to **fibrosis** ■ and joint contractures. These factors lead to a decrease in joint range of motion, decreased muscular strength, loss of normal function, and eventually, atrophy and fibrosis in the afflicted body part.[26]

A primary goal during the early treatment and rehabilitation phase is to reduce the amount of edema that is formed and remove it from the injury site. Ice application reduces the formation of edema. Removal of edema can occur through increased venous return, increased lymphatic flow, or increased blood circulation. The only

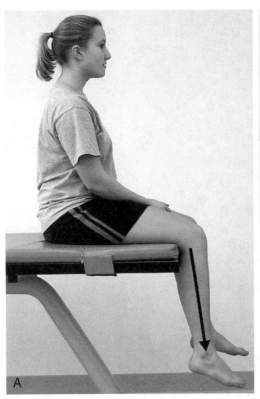
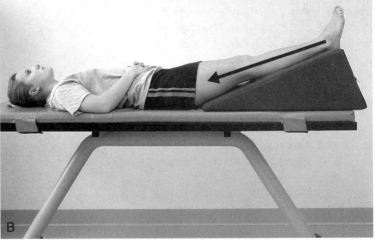

Figure 1–11. **Gravity-Dependent and -Independent Positions.** (A) Gravity-dependent position. Gravity works against venous return. (B) Gravity-independent position. Gravity assists venous return.

Fibrosis: An abnormally large formation of inelastic fibrous tissue..

TABLE 1–10   Types of Exudates

Type	Composition/Characteristic
Serous	Watery consistency common following burns. Also referred to as transudate
Fibrinous	Plasma-rich fluid, especially high in plasma proteins; contains fibrinogen
Suppurative (purulent)	Formation of pus containing dead neutrophils and target organism; abscess
Ulcer	Shredding of inflamed tissue, shedding of epithelia, leaves a crater (ulcer)

mechanism for removing protein from the interstitial space is through the lymphatic system.[28]

Venous or Lymphatic Return

Swelling and edema are reduced only by transporting the fluid and solid wastes away from the area through the venous and lymphatic system (the contents of the lymphatic system eventually return to the venous network through the **thoracic duct ■**).[29] Because the mechanisms of these systems are similar, the function of the venous return system is used to describe the process of returning the contents of the lymphatic system from the extremities to the thorax.

The lymphatic and venous return process is passive relative to the circulatory system. Changes in blood flow, blood pressure, and heart rate do not affect flow within these systems.[30] In contrast to its influence on arterial blood flow in which pressures commonly exceed 80 mm Hg, blood pressure has little effect on returning venous blood to the heart, exerting a pressure of approximately 15 mm Hg on the venous system.[15] Pressures working against the venous system increase 1 mm Hg for every millimeter in distance between the right atrium and the extremity.[31, 32]

Once the blood passes through the capillaries, the body must rely on other mechanisms to return blood to the heart. The respiratory process serves to enhance venous return during both inspiration and expiration. When we take a breath of air, the diaphragm descends and places pressure on the abdominal organs. This pressure is then placed on the veins, partially compressing them and forcing the blood toward the heart. During expiration, a negative pressure gradient is created between the thorax and the abdomen, causing a siphon-like effect that pulls the blood up the venous system, much like sucking on a straw.

During skeletal muscle contraction, the veins are compressed, reducing their diameter. Because of the function of one-way valves, the blood is forced to move out of the extremity toward the heart. As the force of the contrac-

tion is reduced, the one-way valves close, preventing the blood from moving back to its original position (Fig. 1–12). During walking, for instance, contraction of the calf muscles increases the local venous pressure to as high as 200 mm Hg.[31, 33] Certain therapeutic modalities and rehabilitation exercises also can increase venous blood flow (Table 1–11).

Last, gravity serves to return the blood to the heart. The fluids within the venous return system are affected by gravity. Placing the extremity in a dependent position increases the limb's hydrostatic pressure within the peripheral blood vessels and forces fluids into the tissues. When an extremity is placed in a nondependent position (elevated), the venous return system becomes a passive process in which there is a natural downward flow of the fluids in the vessels. The effectiveness of gravity in returning blood to the heart is based on the angle of the extremity relative to the ground, the diameter of the veins, and the **viscosity ■** of the blood.

The maximal effect of gravity on venous return occurs when the limb is perpendicular (90 degrees) to the heart and least effective when the limb is horizontal. The effect that the limb's position has on gravity influencing venous return can be calculated using trigonometric sine function (Fig. 1–13). Gravity is an impediment to venous return when the long axis of the limb drops below horizontal.

The resistance to blood flow is inversely proportional to the fourth power of the vessel's radius ($1/radius^4$) (Fig. 1–14).[15] Consequently, small changes in the vessel's diameter result in great changes in its resistance to flow. Increasing the diameter decreases the resistance; decreasing the diameter increases the resistance to flow. Venules have a smaller diameter than veins; therefore, greater resistance to flow occurs closer to the capillary-venule interface, but the rate of blood flow to the tissues cannot exceed the rate of exchange at this interface.

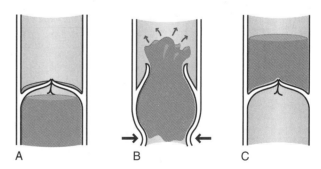

Figure 1–12. **Function of One-Way Valves in Veins.** (A) The position of fluids within the vein when the muscle is relaxed. (B) As the muscle contracts, pressure causes the distal portion of the vein to collapse, opening the one-way valves and forcing blood toward the heart. (C) As the muscle relaxes, the valves close, preventing blood from moving back into the area.

Thoracic duct: A central collection point for the lymphatic system. The contents of the thoracic duct are routed into the left subclavian vein, where they return to the blood system.

Viscosity: The resistance of a fluid to flow.

TABLE 1-11	Rate of Femoral Vein Flow Affected by the Application of Various Modalities

Technique	Femoral Vein Blood Flow (mL/min)
Passive straight-leg raises	1524
Anatomic CPM	1199
Nonanatomic CPM	836
Active ankle dorsiflexion	640
Pneumatic sleeve	586
Manual calf compression	532
Passive dorsiflexion	385

Adapted from Von Schroeder, HP, et al: The changes in intramuscular pressure and femoral vein flow with continuous passive motion, pneumatic compression stockings, and leg manipulations. Clin Orthop 218, May, 1991.

Viscosity is a fluid's resistance to flow. Normally, the viscosity of blood remains constant. However, after injury, the viscosity of blood increases because of the loss of plasma into the surrounding tissues, and the ratio of liquids to solids decreases. Although this change in viscosity is not large enough to affect the systemic flow of blood, it may be sufficient to clog the area adjacent to the injury.

Lymphatic reabsorption is enhanced when the edema is spread over a larger area than when it is concentrated locally. Elevation, edema massage, and compression wraps and pads act to distribute edema and increase the rate of reabsorption.

Secondary Injury

In the primary stage of injury, cell death is the result of physical trauma and affects multiple types of tissues simultaneously. Cell death following the primary injury is the result of secondary hypoxic injury or secondary enzymatic injury caused by ischemia, a decreased oxygen supply to the area, which essentially suffocates the cells.[35]

The primary injury results in ultrastructural changes within the tissues, damaging the cell membrane that leads to a loss of homeostasis and **necrosis** ■. Hemorrhaging from damaged vessels, reduced blood flow caused by increased blood viscosity, **hydropic** ■ swelling of damaged cells, and pressure from the hematoma and muscle spasm can block the supply of fresh blood and result in ischemia. Capillaries in the adjacent areas rupture as a result of swelling in the interstitial space, perpetuating the cycle by obstructing the oxygen supply and killing additional cells. Subsequent cell death continues to block more vascular structures, preventing even more blood and oxygen from being delivered to the site.

This phenomenon, secondary hypoxic injury, results in the cell's inability to use oxygen and places a depend-

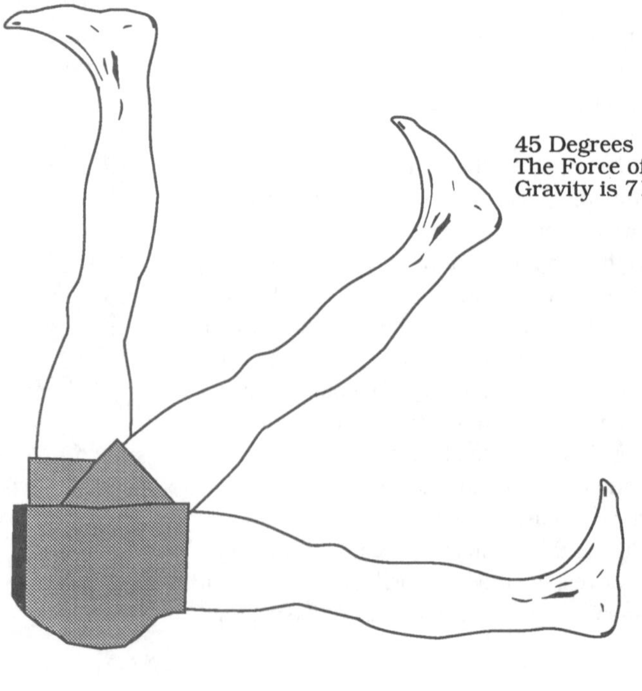

90 Degrees
The Force of
Gravity is 100%

45 Degrees
The Force of
Gravity is 71%

0 Degrees
The Force of
Gravity is 0%

Figure 1–13. **Effect of Gravity on Venous Drainage at Various Limb Positions.** Gravity is most effective when the limb is at 90 degrees and is essentially nonexistent when the limb is parallel to the ground. A compromise between comfort and function is found when the limb is elevated at a 45-degree angle.

Hydropic: Relating to edema; an excessive amount of fluid.
Necrosis: Cell death.

Treatment Strategies
Edema Reduction

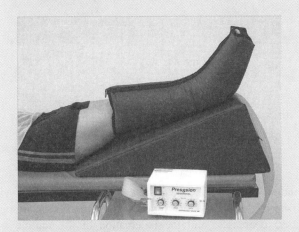

The key to managing edema is preventing it from occurring. Ice, compression, and elevation immediately following trauma discourages the formation of edema (see Chapter 5). The injured structure must be treated with a compression wrap (see Treatment Strategies: Compression Wraps, p 117) between treatment sessions. The patient must be educated regarding the importance of continually wearing the wrap, keeping the extremity elevated whenever possible throughout the day, and sleeping with the limb elevated.

Unfortunately, even the best immediate care does not totally prevent the formation of edema. Once swelling forms, an early treatment goal must be to reduce edema and prevent its other detriments such as pain and decreased range of motion.

The following strategies can be used individually or in tandem to help reduce edema[34]:

- Voluntary muscle contractions
- Compression devices
- Elevation
- Electrically-induced muscle contractions (muscle milking)
- Passive range of motion
- Massage
- Passive motion
- Compression wraps

ence on the **glycolytic pathway** ■ for ATP production. The inefficiency of this system and the ischemia-caused unavailability of needed fuels creates an ATP fuel shortage that results in the failure of the sodium-potassium pump.[35] Secondary hypoxic injury is first seen in the mitochondria within minutes following the primary trauma.[35]

Enzymes released from the dying cells and the inflammatory mediators can cause secondary enzymatic injury.[35] The resulting changes in the cell membrane structure lead to the loss of the resting membrane potential and hydropic swelling, leading to the death of the cell.

Muscle Spasm

Muscle spasm, the involuntary contraction of muscle fibers, is the body's intrinsic mechanism for splinting and protecting the injured area and can result from direct trauma, decreased oxygen supply, or neurological dysfunction.[36] Muscle spasm causes pain by stimulating mechanical and chemical pain receptors. Trigger points are localized areas of muscle spasm (Box 1–5).

The tension produced by the shortened fibers stimulates mechanical pain fibers. The effects of a decreased oxygen supply irritate chemical pain fibers. As muscle spasm persists, irritation of the associated ligaments and tendons occurs.[40] As a result, the amount of muscle spasm increases in an attempt to protect the structures. This becomes a self-perpetuating cycle that is continued by pain, decreased oxygen supply, and a decreased amount of positive stress (in the form of movement).

Atrophy and Muscle Weakness

When a muscle is not used, its fibers become progressively smaller as their actin and **myosin** ■ contents are decreased. Disuse atrophy results when a body part is immobilized by an external splint, is partial weight-bearing, or when the individual consciously or unconsciously refuses to use the extremity because of pain. Denervation atrophy occurs when there is no intact nerve supply to the muscle group. In either case, the resulting changes are similar.

Muscle fibers begin to show physiological changes in as little as 24 hours after immobilization. The size and function of the cells decrease in response to a lack of physical stress and afferent information sent from the injured area.[41] Accordingly, synthesis of protein, energy production, and contractility of the tissues begin to dwindle to the point of degeneration, at which time the muscle's ability to generate force decreases. The postural muscles, composed of slow-twitch (type I) fibers, are the first to show clinical and laboratory signs of atrophy.[42] Bed rest for an illness or unrelated injury also begins the activation of the atrophy process.

The injury response process accelerates the rate of atrophy. Edema and inflammation stimulate Golgi's

---

Glycolytic pathway: A complex chemical reaction that yields adenosine triphosphatase from glucose.
Myosin: Noncontractile muscle protein.

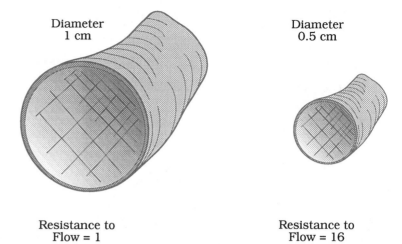

Diameter
1 cm

Diameter
0.5 cm

Resistance to
Flow = 1

Resistance to
Flow = 16

Figure 1–14. **Vessel's Diameter Relative to Resistance to Blood Flow.** Decreasing the diameter of a vessel by one-half increases the resistance to blood flow 16 times.

Treatment Strategies
Preventing Secondary Injury

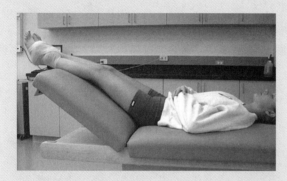

Decreasing the need for oxygen in the injured area and decreasing the amount of blockage of arteriole and venous vessels will limit the amount of secondary injury. The need for oxygen is reduced by decreasing the rate of cellular metabolism through the use of cold application (see Chap. 5). The blockage of the vasculature may be reduced by limiting the amount of fluids that collect in the area via the use of compression and elevation (see Treatment Strategies: Edema Reduction, p 23).

• Cold application: Reduces cell metabolism which reduces the cell's need for oxygen.
• Compression: Decreases hemorrhage and encourages venous return.
• Elevation: Encourages venous and lymphatic uptake and drainage from the extremity.

tendon organs, increasing the rate of atrophy (Box 1–6). As a muscle atrophies, the blood supply to the remaining fibers decreases, and the innervation of the muscle is hindered.[43] The continuing process of atrophy leads to reflex inhibition, in which the effusion and painful impulses create an inhibitory loop that essentially causes the person to "forget" how to contract the muscle, **arthrogenic muscle inhibition**.

Arthrogenic muscle inhibition (AMI) is a presynaptic, reflex inhibition of a muscle caused by joint effusion.[11, 44] Impulses from inhibitory **interneurons** ■ interferes with the recruitment of the motoneurons of muscles crossing the involved joint.[11] In addition to causing atrophy, AMI hinders the rehabilitation process by delaying strength gains and interrupting joint proprioception.[44]

■ Chronic Inflammation

Chronic inflammation, inflammation of prolonged duration, is often provoked by the long-term presence of low-intensity irritants. It is possible for the body to develop chronic inflammation without first going through an acute inflammatory stage significant enough for the patient to seek treatment. The inflammation is there originally but may be at a level insufficient to call attention to it. Often, only when the tissue is near the point of failure does the patient seek assistance.

During chronic inflammation, the body is simultaneously attempting to heal and repair itself. The magnitude of chronic inflammation is based on the balance between the underlying causes and the body's attempt to resolve it. Low concentrations of inflammatory mediators are drawn to the area and, over time, weaken the connective tissue. When it is allowed to persist, chronic inflammation can result in permanent tissue damage.

Interneuron: A neuron connecting two nerves.

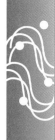

Box 1–5. Trigger Points

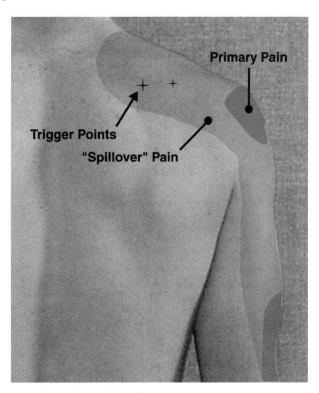

Trigger points of the supraspinatus muscle. The primary pain areas (the diagnostic criteria) are the darkened areas shown in the lateral deltoid and over the lateral epicondyle. Pain may spill over to the surrounding areas (light shaded area).

Localized areas of muscle spasm, trigger points, can be caused by acute trauma, ischemia, **myositis ■**, **dyskinesia ■**, or psychological stress.[37] Clinically, trigger points present themselves as discrete, localized, **hypersensitive ■** areas located in taut bands of skeletal muscle.[38] Local tenderness and referred pain are produced during palpation and can result in limited motion and weakness in the affected muscle. A cross-friction type massage can produce a local twitch muscle contraction. Trigger points typically form along the long axis of postural muscles. Most patients have multiple trigger points.[39] Trigger points are often confused with **fibromyalgia ■**, and are part of the diagnostic criteria for fibromyalgia. However, trigger points can occur in the absence of fibromyalgia.[38, 39] Trigger points are either active or latent.[38] Active trigger points are painful when the body part is at rest. Palpation reproduces the patient's symptoms of referred pain. When palpated or otherwise irritated, active trigger points can activate satellite trigger points.[39] Latent trigger points do not produce pain while at rest, but are painful during palpation and may limit range of motion and muscle strength. Common locations of trigger points and the resulting pain distribution are presented in Appendix A.

The inflammatory response is primarily marked by the loss of function of the body part. During chronic inflammation, the body is still reacting to a stimulus from a delayed hypersensitivity that results in a prolongation of healing and repair, but is doing so in a slower, more protracted manner. The cardinal signs of acute inflammation have given way to the hallmarks of chronic inflammation: production of fibrous connective and granulation

---

Dyskinesia: A defect in the ability to perform voluntary joint movement.

Fibromyalgia: Chronic inflammation of a muscle or connective tissue.

Hypersensitive: Abnormally increased sensitivity, a condition in which there is an exaggerated response by the body to a stimulus.

Myositis: Inflammation of muscular tissue.

tissue and the infiltration of mononuclear cells. The vascular changes associated with acute inflammation, vasodilation and exudation of fluids, are less prominent or absent during chronic inflammation.

Mononuclear cells, leukocytes, lymphocytes, macrophages, and fibroblasts replace the infiltration of neutrophils seen during acute inflammation. Prolonged chronic inflammation also leads to the increased role of plasma cells. Tissue destruction associated with chronic inflammation is caused by cytokines produced by the

mononuclear cells. Tissue healing is promoted by fibroblasts.

Tissue necrosis caused either by the original pathology or the inflammatory process itself occurs and further perpetuates the inflammatory response. The continual deposition of fibrous connective tissue can lead to a hardening of the tissue, **induration.** Fibroblastic activity continues to the point at which large quantities of collagen envelop the affected area, forming a **granuloma** ■. This granuloma affects the function of the involved part, lead-

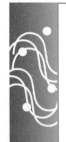

Box 1–6. Misguided Intentions

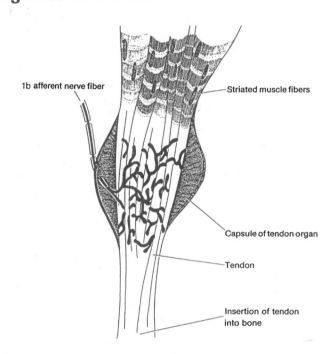

1b afferent nerve fiber — Striated muscle fibers — Capsule of tendon organ — Tendon — Insertion of tendon into bone

Golgi's tendon organs (GTOs) function closely with muscle spindles in monitoring the amount of tension placed on a muscle and its tendon. Located within the muscle belly, projections from the spindle twine around individual muscle fibers. When the muscle contracts, the spindles monitor the rate and magnitude of tension produced.

GTOs divide into several branches, with the highest density being located at the muscle-tendon junction. When the muscle contracts, it places varying amounts of force on the tendon. The GTOs monitor the amount of strain placed on the tendon to prevent damage resulting from too much tension. If the rate of stimulation of GTOs or muscle spindles becomes too great, a nerve impulse is generated that inhibits the muscle contraction. The opposite antagonistic muscle may be facilitated to contract.

During the process of injury response, these nerves can be mechanically stimulated by pressure resulting from muscle spasm or edema, or they can be chemically stimulated by inflammatory mediators. Regardless of the nature of the stimulation, an inhibitory influence is placed on the muscle. If this process is allowed to perpetuate, atrophy of the muscle group occurs.

(Illustration from Ham, AW and Cormack, DH: Histology, ed 8. JB Lippincott, Philadelphia, 1979, p 584, with permission. JB Lippincott)

Granuloma: A hard mass of fibrous tissue.

Treatment Strategies
Muscle Spasm and Trigger Points

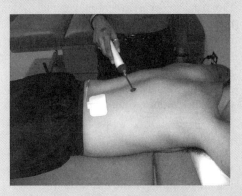

Treatment strategies approach both the symptoms associated with the trigger point and correcting the behavioral, biomechanical, pathological, or ergonomic cause or causes that produce the trigger point or muscle spasm. Relieving pain will decrease the spasm, which will then stop the pain trigger. Massage, cryostretch, electrical stimulation, ultrasound, active exercise, injection of the site, and **iontophoresis** ■ have been successfully used to decrease spasm.

Cold application through ice packs or ice massage is an effective way of desensitizing the local nerve endings. Moist heat packs are effective with superficial spasm. Elongating the tissues along the lines of the muscle fibers also helps decrease the amount of spasm.

Muscle spasm may also be caused by impingement of spinal nerve roots or peripheral nerves. In this case, the treatment approach must be to relieve the pressure at the point on the nerve. For nerve roots, this may take the form of cervical or lumbar traction. For peripheral nerves, it could require the reduction of edema (p 23) that is placing pressure on the nerve or the surgical removal of a bony outgrowth or fibrous sheath that forms around the nerve.

Treatment Strategies
Retarding Atrophy

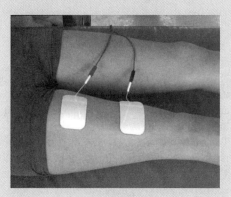

Atrophy occurs when the muscle no longer receives the functional loads to which it is accustomed. The inability to contract the muscle, bear weight, or move the associated joints all decrease the amount of tension which the muscle experiences. When this is prolonged, the absence of this stress sends a signal to start taking away some of the muscle mass because the body (incorrectly) deduces that it is no longer needed.

Rest is a double-edged sword in the treatment and rehabilitation of musculoskeletal injuries. Immobilization is necessary to protect the injured structures, but the lack of physical stress can inhibit proper remodeling of the tissues.[45] If you have ever seen an arm or leg that has been immobilized for a long time, you know that the adverse effects of immobilization are readily apparent.

The atrophy process may be deterred by several methods. Muscles immobilized in a lengthened position are more resistant to atrophy than those immobilized in a shortened position.[46] However, depending on the body part, the structures involved, and the type of injury, it is not always practical to immobilize the muscle in a lengthened position. Isometric contractions or electrical muscle stimulation, or both, can delay the atrophy process (see Chapter 12, p 232).

---

ing to a loss of full function and to development of secondary reactions in associated structures.

Chronic inflammation can also self-perpetuate by altering the body's biomechanics. Pain, restricted motion, or loss of muscular strength can cause the body to substitute compensatory motion for normal motion. The newly acquired mechanics place new loads on the structures and activate an inflammatory response. A baseball pitcher with chronic rotator cuff inflammation may demonstrate this. The presence of a granuloma in the supraspinatus may decrease the range of motion and strength of the muscles. By continuing to pitch, the athlete

---

Iontophoresis: Introduction of ions into the body through the use of an electrical current.

is further irritating the tendon. By changing the pitching motion, forces are distributed to tissues that are not accustomed to this stress, reactivating the inflammatory process.

● Chapter Highlights

- Therapeutic modalities are a form of energy that is applied to evoke an involuntary response and create the best environment for healing to occur.
- "Stress" may have a negative connotation, but it can also be positive. Therapeutic modalities apply a positive stress to the body that promotes healing.
- The body has an amazing ability to adapt to both positive and negative stresses that are placed on it.
- The primary tissue types discussed in this text are epithelial, adipose, muscular, nervous, and connective. Each of these tissues transmits or responds to, or both, different forms of therapeutic energy differently.
- The force causing the body's initial injury is called the primary trauma. The damage that occurs during this stage is irreversible.
- Secondary injury is cell death that occurs as a result of the body's response to the primary trauma. This damage can be limited or prevented.
- The injury response is marked by those cells that are damaged by the primary injury. The dead and dying cells release chemicals that trigger hemorrhage, edema, and pain. This damages more cells, which perpetuates the cycle, leading to the death of more cells.
- The acute inflammatory response involves changes in blood flow and cellular function. The purpose of this stage is to contain, destroy, and dilute unwanted substances in the body.
- Hemorrhage occurs when the vascular system is damaged or its permeability increases and allows blood to escape into the surrounding tissues.
- The debris and temporary tissue formed during acute inflammation are removed during the proliferation phase and are followed by revascularization, wound contraction, and wound remodeling.
- The replacement tissues are organized and strengthened during the maturation phase of injury response.
- Edema forms when the inflow to the area is greater than the outflow. This results in a clogging of the vasculature and decreased range of motion. If the blood supply is decreased, further cells die from a lack of oxygen (hypoxia).
- The fluid component of edema is removed through the venous system. The solid (protein) component of edema is removed via the lymphatic system.
- Pressure on nerve endings can cause muscle spasm and lead to a cycle of pain-spasm-pain.
- Muscles begin to atrophy in as little as 24 hours of disuse or immobilization.

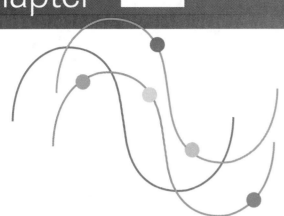

Chapter 2

The Physiology and Psychology of Pain

Robert W. Sikes, PhD

Of all the components of the injury response, none is less consistent or less understood than an individual's response to pain. The perception of pain is a primal property of the nervous system and inherent to all people. Created by nerves and neurons like all sensations, pain may transcend the physiological response, producing a deeply personal experience that all humans must endure. Acute pain is the primary reason why people seek medical attention and the major complaint that they describe on initial evaluation. Chronic pain may be more debilitating than the trauma itself and, in many instances, is so emotionally and physically debilitating that it is a leading cause of suicide.[47-49]

Perhaps the most important function of the body's sensory systems is self-protection. The human body is fragile and easily damaged or destroyed by any of the numerous threats found in our environment. Some of our sensory systems act as early warning systems. We look both ways before crossing the street and freeze at the sound of a rattlesnake thanks to input from our visual and auditory systems. Our somatosensory system provides information regarding temperature and informs us when our body contacts an object so that we do not freeze or burn ourselves and avoid serious collisions.

Pain sensation serves as the body's final line of self-defense. It warns us that our tissues are in immediate jeopardy or have already been damaged. It activates protective reflexes and motivates behaviors that help to avoid—or at least decrease—physical trauma. Although we may not like pain, it is crucial to our survival. Loss of pain sensation leaves the body, or a portion of the body, unprotected against serious damage.[50]

Although pain is a physiological response produced by activation of specific types of nerve fibers, our overall pain response is a complex phenomenon involving sensory, behavioral (motor), emotional, components that are influenced by cultural and social factors as well as our own past experiences. Once the painful impulse has been initiated and received by the brain, our interpretation of pain is influenced by interrelated physiological, psychological, and social factors.[51] When certain nerve fibers, **nociceptors** ■, are stimulated, pain impulses are sent to the brain as a warning that the body's integrity is at risk. The evaluative portion of the brain interprets these signals as pain. The emotional response may be expressed by screaming, crying, fainting, or just thinking, "That hurts!"

The cultural components of pain response are almost too complex to define. However, pain perception has been linked to ethnicity and socioeconomic status.[52–55] For example, Italian patients are less inhibited in the expression of pain than are Irish or Anglo-Saxon patients.[53, 54] Ultimately, cultural components can be viewed as any variable that relates to the environment in which a person was raised and how that environment deals with pain and responses to pain.

Stimuli that activate nociceptors are called **noxious** stimuli. Intense pressure, extremes of cold or heat, and certain chemicals when applied to the body generate action potentials in the nociceptors that are transmitted to the central nervous system (CNS). Behavioral responses to this input can be separated into unconscious defensive reflexes and conscious behaviors.

When a noxious stimulus is intense or unexpected, the **withdrawal reflex** ■ is activated. Activity from the nociceptors is transmitted from the afferent nerves to motor neurons in the spinal cord through interconnected spinal cord **interneurons** ■. These interneurons excite or inhibit motor neurons so that the appropriate muscles are activated to remove the body part from the noxious stimulus. An example of this is accidentally sticking your finger with a pin (Fig. 2–1). In this case, the pin activates nociceptors, which generate action potentials in afferent nerves of the finger that travel back to the spinal cord, where the fibers may either terminate immediately or travel up or down the spinal cord for several levels. Motor neurons are activated that extend the finger and wrist away from the pin. If the stimulus is intense, motor neurons at other levels of the spinal cord that can generate movements at the elbow and shoulder to move the hand away are also activated. Motor neurons that would normally produce opposing movements are inhibited. Thus, the finger and hand are

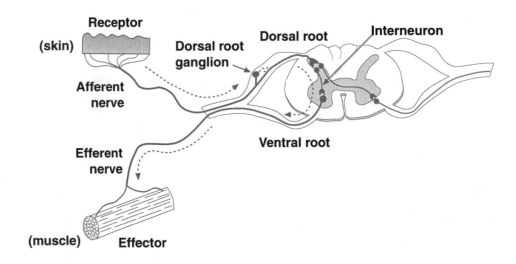

Figure 2–1. **The Withdrawal Reflex.** Stimulation of superficial pain receptors in the skin produces action potentials that travel along the afferent nerve fiber to the spinal cord. This fiber forms synapses with interneurons that project to motor neurons in the ventral horn. These motor neurons project back to muscle and generate protective movements that withdraw the limb from further damage. The interneurons also activate tract neurons that project to higher levels of the nervous system and produce the sensation of pain. Thus, activation of pain receptors normally produces both a reflexive and cognitive response.

Interneuron: A CNS neuron that forms an intermediate synaptic connection between other neurons.

Nociceptors: Specialized receptors on nerves that transmit pain impulses.

Withdrawal reflex: A multisynaptic spinal reflex that is normally elicited by a noxious stimulus. Muscle groups are activated so that the body is moved away from the damaging stimulus.

rapidly and unconsciously removed from danger through these spinal reflexes.

The afferent fibers also activate spinal cord neurons called **tract cells ▪** (T cells). The axons of tract cells cross the midline of the spinal cord and ascend to higher levels of the spinal cord, brainstem, and brain. Some of these fibers activate motor neurons on the opposite side of the spinal cord, but the activity is also relayed to the cerebral cortex, forming a cognitive pathway. As a result, your finger is not only unconsciously removed from the pin but also you become conscious of its penetration. You respond by saying, "Ouch!," and you find the experience rather unpleasant. Thus, the cognitive pathway transforms pain sensation into pain perception.

▪ Pain Perception

Like all sensations, pain is both a physiological and psychological entity. Although they are complex, the physiological components can be identified and traced from their origin in the tissues to their termination in the cerebral cortex. This provides us with important diagnostic information about the source of pain or reasons for its absence, and suggests plans for effective therapy.

However, individuals do perceive pain differently, and in fact, a person can have varying interpretations and reactions to the same source of pain at different times. This indicates that some form of processing must occur in the cerebral cortex that alters our perception of the location, type, and intensity of the pain and how we will react to the stimulus (Table 2–1).[56—58]

Influences on Pain Perception

Several intrinsic factors influence an individual's perception of pain. For example, extroverts express pain more

TABLE 2–1	Dimensions of Pain Perception	
Component	*Description*
Sensory—Discriminative	Localizes the area (source) and type of pain.
Cognitive—Evaluative	Interprets sensations based on past experiences, expected outcomes, etc.
Affective—Motivational	Influenced by the limbic system, affects internal (e.g., fear, anxiety) and outward response (e.g., crying) to the stimulus.

freely than introverts, but introverts are more sensitive to pain.[59] Cognitive-evaluative influences include the activities in which the person is involved, the perceived impact that the injury may have, and past experiences.

Perhaps the largest social and cultural influence on pain perception in the United States is that of gender role stereotypes. As young children, we often heard, "Big boys don't cry." Children often have engraved into their minds that boys are not supposed to cry, but it is appropriate for girls to cry. Although social consciousness has helped decrease this and other types of stereotyping, its influences are still with us.

When comparing pain response between genders, the literature indicates that women have lower **pain thresholds ▪** and pain tolerances than men as reported in epidemiological, experimental, and clinical studies. Further research indicates that women are more likely than men to experience a variety of types of recurrent pain and have more severe levels of pain, more frequent pain, and pain of longer duration than men.[60] In some clinical studies, female subjects reported greater pain than male subjects at high levels of stimulation, greater pupil dilation with noxious stimuli,[61] shorter time to ischemic pain tolerance,[62] and lower threshold to esophageal pain.[63] Male college students have a statistically significant higher pain tolerance than their female counterparts, and the female subjects had significantly higher scores of fearful thoughts related to the experience of pain.[64]

Gender differences have also been noted in pain response in their relationship to expenditures for healthcare services. Women use more specific health-care services based on psychological need and screening than men.[65] Female patients described significantly more pain than male patients and were perceived by their caregivers to experience more pain, resulting in more and stronger pain medications being prescribed for women than for men. Likewise, female patients were less likely than male patients to receive no medication for their pain.

Although these studies seemingly indicate significant gender differences in pain tolerance and pain threshold, it is unclear whether these differences are biologically, psychologically, or socially generated. It is uncertain whether women are simply more willing to report and express pain than men.[66] Although the root of these differences is unclear, clinicians should consider that possible differences in pain threshold and pain tolerance may exist between men and women.

In young athletes, pain perception may be influenced by the presence of peers. Children tend to "tolerate" more pain when they are observed by their peers than when alone.[67] The perception of pain is also negatively correlated with anxiety levels about pain.[68] Patients who are

---

Pain threshold: The level of noxious stimulus required to alert the individual to possible tissue damage.

Tract cells: Second-order neurons of the pain and temperature pathways. The axons of these cells cross the midline of the spinal cord and ascend in the anterior lateral fasciculus. Tract cells are sometimes called T cells, but this should not be confused with the T cells of the immune system.

anxious or fearful about pain may have a lower tolerance to pain than their less anxious counterparts.

Differences in the definition and expression of pain based on culture and ethnicity can affect the perception and expression of pain.[59, 60] A person's past experience influences the pain perception of a current injury. The experience may be recalling a previous injury that required surgery, or even the image of a similar injury on television. A fear of doctors or hospitals may cause increased anxiety because the person is afraid of being exposed to these stressors when an injury occurs. Likewise, if an injury is potentially career-threatening, the reaction may be increased.

Athletic participation and the type of sport played also appear to influence an individual's response to pain.[70–74] Athletes who participate in contact sports are able to tolerate significantly higher levels of pain than athletes who participate in noncontact sports or nonathletes, although no significant differences in the pain threshold between athletes and nonathletes were found.[75] Professional ballet dancers were found to have significantly higher pain thresholds and pain tolerances than a group of nonathletes of the same age.[76] Likewise, competitive swimmers had significantly higher tolerances of ischemic pain than did a comparable group of club swimmers.[77]

Sometimes other events override the processing of pain because the brain is preoccupied with more urgent matters. Immediate processing of information not related to pain may push the processing of the pain response to the background. A good example of this is the typical movie portrayal of British soldiers just after a fierce battle:

> "I say, old chap, that was a nasty one, wasn't it? Too bad about your leg."
> "My leg?"
> "Your leg. You've been hit."
> "Oh, bloody 'ell. Cup of tea, then?"

In this case, the soldier was so happy to make it out of combat alive, and his brain was so focused on analyzing the situation that he did not realize an injury had occurred. This same type of processing occurs in athletics. An athlete may be so focused on the competition that, when an injury occurs, its magnitude may not be immediately recognized.

Based on this integrative process, the perception of pain is subjective and variable in nature. Notwithstanding, it does consist of several measurable objective parameters. When you ask a patient how he or she feels today, the response is usually "better," "worse," or "the same." By asking, you are requiring the person to measure the pain and compare it to the way it felt yesterday. Several standardized methods are available to measure the amount of pain in relatively objective terms. Through the use of these tools, the location, intensity, and duration of the pain may be ascertained. Other methods exist that assess activities, emotions, and/or personality traits that influence the perception of pain.

Pain Threshold and Pain Tolerance

Pain perception can be broken down into two distinct categories: (1) pain threshold and (2) pain tolerance. **Pain threshold** is the level of noxious stimulus required to alert the individual to a potential threat to tissue. The pain threshold can be measured experimentally by introducing a painful stimulus (e.g., cold water, pressure, or heat) to tissue to a point at which the individual reports "pain." In experimental pain models, researchers use water cooled to 1° to 3°C (cold pressor test), **radiant heat ■**, or mechanical pressure created by placing dull metal spikes inside a blood pressure cuff to measure pain threshold and tolerance. You can perform a simple experiment on yourself by squeezing your fingernail. The point at which you subjectively first experience pain could be quantitatively measured as your pain threshold by recording the amount of foot-pounds of pressure used.

Pain tolerance, on the other hand, is a measure of how much pain a person can or will withstand. In an experimental model, pain tolerance is measured by the amount of pain or "quantity" of exposure (cold water, pressure, heat) that an individual can or will endure. Clinically, pain tolerance can be related to a person losing consciousness because of pain or declaring in a half-lucid state, "I can't take this any more." In assessing the physiological model of pain transmission, pain tolerance is associated with the **limbic system ■** and the cortex. Within these structures, many synaptic interactions occur, and various levels of cognition can help the individual to determine the maximum level of noxious stimulation that can be tolerated. Examination of the physiology of noxious transmission and experimental research indicate that pain threshold and pain tolerance are not correlated.[77] Therefore, an athlete who reports feeling excessive pain immediately after an injury may be able to endure the pain and continue to participate because of a high level of pain tolerance. An athlete having a low pain tolerance may declare that an otherwise minor injury is prohibiting normal activity.

■ Assessment of Pain

The nebulous nature of pain makes it difficult to assess and quantify. The perceived pain level is a personal expression of what one person feels. The feeling is based on a discriminative, affective, and evaluative process. Assessment of pain should encompass both the subjective and objective evaluations to properly document the level and amount of pain that the patient is experiencing.

Limbic system: System in the brain that controls emotion.

Radiant heat: Heat that is gained or lost through the indirect transmission of energy.

TABLE 2-2	Subjective Assessment of Pain

Where is your pain?
When did your pain begin?
What is the duration of your pain?
Have you ever experienced this pain before?
Can you describe how the pain feels?
Is the pain getting better or worse?
Does your pain increase with activity?
Do you have more pain after activity?
Do you have pain at night?

A subjective assessment of pain is commonplace in all evaluations. The patient is queried about the location, duration, and type of pain being experienced (Table 2–2). The responses to these questions allow the clinician to chart a subjective baseline of the patient's present pain status. In turn, these responses can also help in further evaluation of the underlying pathology.

Once the subjective evaluation is made, determine the patient's pain should be objectively evaluated. This allows decreases or increases in the levels or types of pain experienced by the patient to be measured and documented. Several types of objective pain scales are available for use. The **Visual Analog Scale** (VAS) is one of the most common and reliable pain assessment tools (Box 2–1).[78] Variations of the visual analog scale include the **numeric rating scale** (NRS), a system that uses numbers from 0 to 10 to rate the pain.

Another tool that is used to assess pain is the **McGill pain questionnaire** (MPQ) (Box 2–2).[79] This instrument usually consists of three parts: Part A localizes the area of pain and identifies whether the perceived source of the pain is superficial (external), internal, or both. Part B identifies the type of pain sensation and the intensity of the pain. Part C is a visual analog scale or numeric pain rating scale.

The MPQ takes longer (approximately 10 minutes) to complete and score than the VAS, but it can be a use- ful tool in the objective assessment of pain. It is primarily used during the first visit to a clinic and upon discharge.[80]

The **submaximal effort tourniquet test** (SETT) is used clinically to "match" a patient's pain or experimentally to standardize pain threshold (Box 2–3).[81] Clinically, the SETT procedure is repeated until the patient experiences pain that resembles ("matches") the pain of the original pathology. Experimentally, the amount of time between the start of the text to the point where pain is experienced provides data for research purposes.

■ Temporal Dimension of Pain

Although the intensity and quality of pain is important and should be carefully assessed, the duration of pain is possibly the most significant dimension of pain to the patient and therapist. Pain, even intense pain, can be endured if it does not last very long. In contrast, a dull, low intensity pain that continues for months or even years can lead to complete disablement, depression, and even suicide. Pain is often categorized according to duration as acute or chronic pain.

Acute Pain

Acute pain is caused by the activation of nociceptors. External sources, such as a burn or a cut, or internal sources, such as a muscle strain or a ligament sprain, can generate this stimulus. Common to all these stimuli is trauma—destruction of the tissue cells. As a result of this trauma, substances such as bradykinin, prostaglandins, substance P, and other chemicals are released by the damaged cells.[82] As we describe in more detail later, these chemicals directly activate the nociceptors until the damaged tissue has been repaired.

Once the tissue has healed, acute pain ends. Because the duration of healing varies, the duration of acute pain will also vary, but the presence or absence of pain is tightly linked to the healing process.

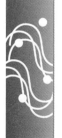

Box 2–1. The Visual Analog Scale

Pain as
bad as it ——————————————————————————————— No pain
could be

Using a 10-cm line labeled as above, the patient places a mark on the line at the point that best represents the current pain intensity. The distance from the right side of the line to the "mark" is measured in centimeters and represents the pain "score." A new VAS should be used for every assessment, and the patient should not see or be allowed to use prior responses for reference. The VAS is consistent, reliable, and easy to use. It can be used before and after treatments to measure the effectiveness of treatment or day to day to measure a patient's progress.

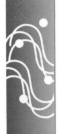

Box 2-2. McGill Pain Questionnaire

A. Where is your pain?

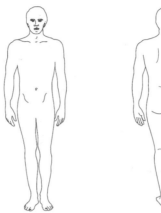

Using the above drawing, please mark the area(s) where you feel pain. Mark an "E" if the source of the pain is external or "I" if it is internal. If the source of the pain is both internal and external, please mark "B".

B. Pain rating index

Many different words can be used to describe pain. From the list below, please circle those words that best describe the pain you are currently experiencing. Use only one word from each category. You do not need to mark a word in every category -- **Only mark those words that most accurately describe your pain.**

1.	**2.**	**3.**	**4.**
Flickering	Jumping	Pricking	Sharp
Quivering	Flashing	Boring	Cutting
Pulsing	Shooting	Drilling	Lacerating
Throbbing		Stabbing	
Beating			
Pounding			

5.	**6.**	**7.**	**8.**
Pinching	Tugging	Hot	Tingling
Pressing	Pulling	Burning	Itchy
Gnawing	Wrenching	Scalding	Smarting
Cramping		Searing	Stinging
Crushing			

9.	**10.**	**11.**	**12.**
Dull	Tender	Tiring	Sickening
Sore	Taut	Exhausting	Suffocating
Hurting	Rasping		
Aching			
Heavy			

13.	**14.**	**15.**	**16.**
Fearful	Punishing	Wretched	Annoying
Frightful	Grueling	Blinding	Troublesome
Terrifying	Cruel		Miserable
	Vicious		Intense
	Killing		Unbearable

17.	**18.**	**19.**	**20.**
Spreading	Tight	Cool	Nagging
Radiating	Numb	Cold	Nauseating
Penetrating	Drawing	Freezing	Agonizing
Piercing	Squeezing		Dreadful
	Tearing		Torturing

The McGill Pain Questionnaire is used during the patient's first visit to identify painful areas and quantify the intensity of the pain. In part A the patient is asked to localize the area(s) of pain and indicate if the source of the discomfort is superficial (external) or deep (internal). The pain rating index, Part B, consists of 76 words grouped into 20 categories and is used to assess the level and nature of the patient's pain. The patient is instructed to circle or underline the words in each group that best describe the sensation of pain being experienced. The patient may pick only one word in each category, but each category does not have to be used. These words are categorized as somatic (groups 1 to 10), affective (11 to 15), evaluative (16), and miscellaneous words that are only used for scoring purposes (17 to 20). Many versions of the McGill Pain Questionnaire also contain a visual analogue scale similar to that presented in Box 2-1.

To score the Pain Rating Index, add up the total number of words chosen, up to the maximum of 20 words (one for each category). The level of the pain intensity is determined by assigning a value to each word by its order (first word equals 1, second word equals 2, and so on). Therefore, a patient could have a high MPQ score of 20 (selecting a word in each group), but have a low-intensity score by selecting the first word in every group.

Chronic Pain

Acute pain is useful indication that something is wrong within the body. It forces us to do something to fix the problem—let go of the hot pan, stay off the sprained ankle, or seek medical advice. This is ultimately beneficial to our health. But sometimes pain persists long after the healing process has completed, or the amount of pain perceived is much greater than the detectable tissue damage would seem to produce. This is chronic pain—pain that extends beyond the normal course of injury or illness.

Chronic pain is difficult to treat and takes a serious toll on the lives of sufferers. It can be incapacitating and lead the afflicted person to take increasingly drastic actions to obtain even temporary relief. Depression is a common consequence and depression itself may increase the level of perceived pain in a vicious cycle that produces great anguish for patients and their families. Chronic pain becomes integrated into the person's life and affects behavior and mood (Table 2–3).

Although chronic pain is categorized in many different and sometimes conflicting ways, we will divide it into two categories—nociceptive chronic pain and neuropathic chronic pain.

TABLE 2–3	Characteristics of Chronic Pain

Symptoms last longer than 6 months
Few objective medical findings
Medication abuse
Difficulty in sleeping
Depression
Manipulative behavior
Somatic preoccupation

Nociceptive Chronic Pain

Chronic pain may reflect an ongoing disease that continually activates nociceptors. The pain is produced by activation of nociceptors by the mechanisms discussed in the *Mechanisms of Nociceptive Transduction* section. The pain persists because the disease persists. For example, arthritis produces chronic inflammation of the joints resulting in increasingly severe pain when the affected joints are moved. Although cancerous tumors may initially grow painlessly, when they begin to compress nerve fibers considerable pain is produced. Other chronic diseases produce pain because tissue is destroyed as the disease progresses.

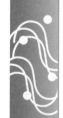

Box 2–3. The Submaximal Effort Tourniquet Test

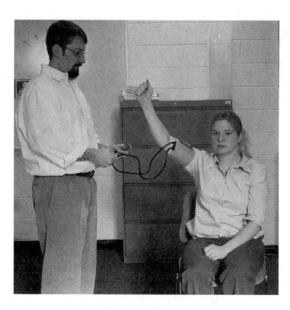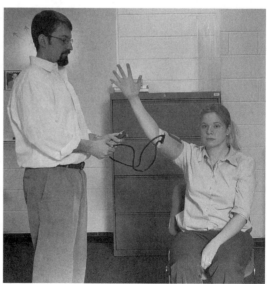

The SETT is performed by inflating a sphygmomanometer cuff to above the systolic blood pressure on the patient's elevated arm. Once the cuff is inflated, the patient is instructed to open and close the hand or fist rhythmically. A handgrip dynamometer and a metronome can be used for standardization. The patient should continue opening and closing the hand or fist until the cramping sensation that he or she feels "matches" the pain from the original pathology. The amount of time that elapses from onset to fruition of matched pain is the recorded objective measure. The SETT can be repeated at every treatment session to gauge treatment progress and is effective in "matching" all types of pain.[80]

In cases of nociceptive chronic pain, the primary goal of treatment is to stop the underlying disease process. If the disease can be stopped, the pain should be resolved. Unfortunately, treatment of chronic, progressing diseases is often difficult or unsuccessful. Too much attention to treatment of the disease with inadequate treatment of pain symptoms can lead to considerable unnecessary suffering by the patient.

Neuropathic Chronic Pain

If no persistent disease can be identified as the source of chronic pain, the problem is likely to be an abnormality in the neurons of the pain system. The problem may be in the peripheral nerves or in neurons within the CNS. We have only a very minimal understanding of the changes that occur to produce neuropathic chronic pain. And because there is no identifiable disease to treat, providing effective therapy is challenging. Even the development of a consistent way of naming the different clinical syndromes has proved difficult.[83] Successful treatment of neuropathic chronic pain requires more research into the neuroscience of pain.

■ Neuroscience of Pain

Neuroscience research into the anatomy, physiology, and pharmacology of pain has provided us with considerable insight into the mechanisms of pain. As we shall see, the identity of specialized pain receptor nerve fibers and many details of the anatomy and pharmacology of the pain pathways are well known.

This information helps in the development of better treatments for managing pain. Understanding the specific neurotransmitter molecules and their actions has allowed the development of more effective **analgesic** ■ drugs. Research into the physiology of the pain system has improved our understanding of how therapies such as **transcutaneous** ■ electrical nerve stimulation (TENS), exercise, and even acupuncture affect the pain process. Nevertheless, the cognitive aspects of pain perception are poorly known, particularly those that relate to chronic pain.

This section describes the basic anatomy and physiology of the touch and pain systems to provide a clear understanding of the production of acute pain and how damage to the nervous systems can lead to loss of acute pain sensation. Furthermore, we will see how abnormalities of these pain pathways may lead to certain forms of chronic pain.

■ Somatosensory Transduction– Environmental Energy into Action Potentials

Before you can detect any stimulus in your environment, the energy that produces the stimulus must be converted into the one and only type of energy that the nervous system can process—action potentials. This process is called **transduction** and is accomplished by specialized neurons in the peripheral nervous system. For instance, light energy activates specialized neurons in the retina called photoreceptors; sound vibrations in the air act on auditory receptor cells in the inner ear. To detect the contact of mechanical, thermal, or chemical stimuli with the body, the skin, connective tissues, muscles, and **visceral** ■ organs contain specialized sensory neurons called **first-order neurons**.

Sensory first-order neurons have large cell bodies located in the sensory **ganglia** ■ of the peripheral nervous system (Fig. 2–2). At the spinal cord levels, these neurons are called the **dorsal root ganglia**. A single process exits the cell body and splits into a peripheral process and central process. The peripheral processes are specialized to allow for transduction. At the ends of the peripheral process are the sensory receptor organs. These organs differ both structurally and physiologically and tune the first-order neuron to specific qualities of the mechanical, thermal, or chemical energy applied to the tissue. The central process of the first-order neuron travels into the CNS, where it makes synaptic contact with **second-order neurons** located in the **nuclei** ■ of the spinal cord or brain stem. The entire sensory process of first-order neurons—peripheral process and central process combined—is called **primary afferent fiber**.

The axons of second-order neurons normally cross the midline of the nervous system and ascend to contact higher order neurons (Table 2–4). Thus, an ascending chain of progressively higher order neurons extends from the sensory receptor organ all the way to the cerebral cortex. This chain must be intact for **somatic** ■ sensation to reach conscious awareness.

Sensory first-order neurons are divided into three functional classes—mechanoreceptors that detect pressure, thermal receptors that detect temperature, and nociceptors that detect painful stimuli. The response differences between these neurons are a product of the structure and physiology of their receptor organs.

Analgesic: A pain-reducing substance.

Ganglia: A cluster of neurons in the peripheral nervous system.

Nucleus (Nuclei): A cluster of neurons in the CNS.

Somatic: Pertaining to the body.

Transcutaneous: Through the skin.

Visceral: Pertaining to organs of the body.

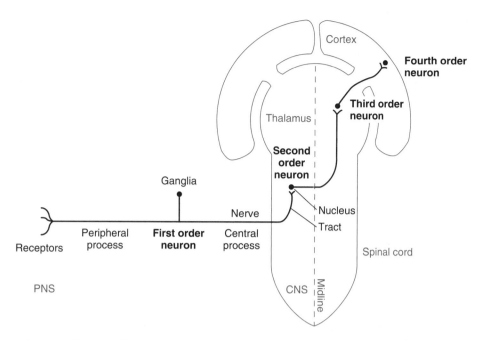

Figure 2–2. **Sensory Neurons, Nerves, and Tracts**. Primary afferent fibers connect the sensory receptor to second-order neurons in the CNS. The cell bodies of the primary afferent fibers are located in ganglia within the vertebra or skull but outside the CNS. Second-order neurons are located in nuclei within the spinal cord or brain stem and project across the midline to reach higher order neurons.

Mechanoreceptors

At the cellular level, the receptor organs that detect pressure often have a microscopically visible connective tissue capsule that surrounds the end of the peripheral process. These **encapsulated receptor** ■ organs are further characterized by their location as superficial or deep. Superficial receptor organs are located in or just beneath the skin and are responsible for detecting stimuli that contact the body.

Deep receptor organs are located in muscle and tendons and normally provide proprioceptive information about the state of muscle contraction and limb position. Deep receptor organs in the viscera provide sensations such as fullness of the bladder and hunger.

Several distinct types of superficial receptor organs have been identified in the skin (Fig. 2–3). These receptor organs are classified by their location, structure, and sensitivity. They activate peripheral processes that are large-

TABLE 2–4	**Sensory Neuronal Levels**
Level	*Function*
First-order neuron	A neuron that connects the sensory receptor in the PNS to neurons in the CNS. The cell bodies are found in the dorsal root ganglia or cranial nerve ganglia.
Second-order neuron	The neuron that receives sensory input from first-order neurons and projects to neurons at higher levels of the CNS. The cell bodies are located in the dorsal horn of the spinal cord or trigeminal nuclei of the brain stem.
Third-order neuron	The neuron that receives sensory input from second-order neurons and projects to still higher levels of the CNS – possibly the cerebral cortex. The cell bodies are located in many locations in the CNS, but primarily in the **thalamus** ■.

CNS = central nervous system; PNS = peripheral nervous system.

Encapsulated receptor: A sensory receptor formed by a nerve fiber and surrounding connective tissue cells.

Thalamus: Gray matter in the center of the brain.

diameter well-myelinated **A-beta** fibers. Varying levels of pressure (touch), movement, and vibration of the skin and texture (rough versus smooth) are detected by these receptor organs.

The most superficial of the receptor organs are **Merkel's disks**. These disks are located in the epidermis and consist of several small disks of connective tissue cells that surround the end of A-beta fibers. Merkel's disks have a low threshold to mechanical pressure and slowly adapt to stimuli applied to the skin. Within the epidermal hair follicles, the peripheral processes wrap around the base of the hair to form **hair follicle receptors**. The low threshold of these receptors and the lever action of the attached skin make these receptors exquisitely sensitive to bending of the hair. Together these receptors function to detect very light touch of the skin.

Within the dermis are a variety of receptor organs that are somewhat less sensitive to mechanical pressure, but are specialized to detect moving or vibrating stimuli on the skin. The small oval **Meissner's corpuscles** have low thresholds like Merkel's disks, but rapidly adapt to constant pressure. If you placed a coin on the skin, initially both Merkel's disks and Meissner's corpuscles would activate. Within a few milliseconds, Meissner's corpuscle would adapt to the pressure

and deactivate while Merkel's disks would stay active. If the stimulus is moving or vibrating back and forth over the receptor, however, Meissner's corpuscles remain activated and are able to transduce the velocity of the movement better than sluggish Merkel's disks.[84] The larger and deeper **Pacinian corpuscles** ■ also detect moving stimuli well, though more pressure is required to activate them. Pacinian corpuscles show rapid adaptation to constant pressure, responding best to varying pressure levels.

Mechanisms of Mechanoreceptor Transduction

Although the mechanisms mechanoreceptors use to convert pressure applied to the skin into action potentials are complex, the presence of mechanically gated ion channels in the nerve membrane at least partially explains the process.[85]

Mechanically gated ion channels are large protein molecules that pass through the neuronal membrane of the receptor. As shown in Figure 2–4, these channels are mechanically coupled to Merkel's disk through extensions of the molecules at the surface of the membrane. This extension acts like a lever so that when the disk is

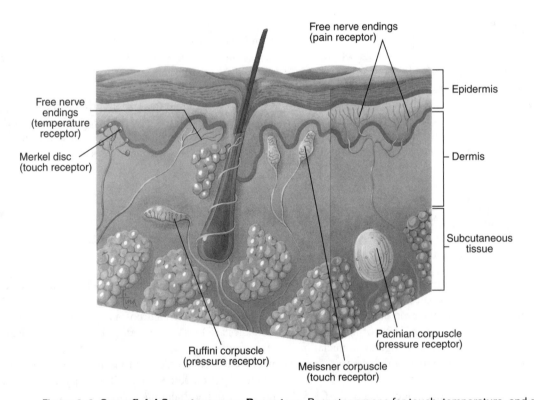

Figure 2–3. Superficial Somatosensory Receptors. Receptor organs for touch, temperature, and pain in the skin and the peripheral fibers that connect the receptor organs to the central nervous system.

Pacinian corpuscles: Large encapsulated receptor organs found in the skin and deeper tissues. These rapid adapting receptors are best activated by an alternating stimulus, for example, a tuning fork. Within the joints, they assist in relaying proprioceptive information.

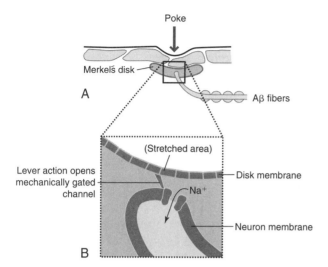

Figure 2–4. Mechanically Gated Channels. (A) Pressure of a sharp object is transferred to a mechanoreceptor through the skin by compression. (B) The pressure stretches mechanically gated channels open, allowing sodium ions to enter and depolarize the receptor. This depolarization produces action potentials in the primary afferent fiber.

compressed, the channel is stretched open allowing sodium ions to flow into the receptor (Fig. 2–4B). This depolarizes the receptor and generates action potentials in the primary afferent fiber. As more pressure is applied, the frequency of action potentials increases proportionately. The amount of pressure applied to the skin is thereby converted into the frequency that action potentials are transmitted along the primary afferent fiber.

Thermal Receptors

The second class of first-order neurons, the thermal receptors, detects temperature. They distinguish cold from hot and allow us to make very fine assessments of thermal energy. There is still some disagreement about the anatomical identification of the receptor organs that detect temperature. Early research suggested that thermal receptors were encapsulated, but it now seems more likely that no capsule is present.[83] Such receptor fibers are called **free nerve endings**. Temperature-gated ion channels in free nerve ending membranes would provide a mechanism for this transduction, but such molecules have not been identified experimentally.

Nociceptors

The identity and mechanism of the final type of first-order neurons, the **nociceptor** (from the Latin word *nocere,* to harm) has been the most elusive of all. No anatomically distinct receptor organ has been associated with pain sensation. Like thermal receptors, nociceptors are located on unencapsulated free nerve endings. This lack of structural identity led to a theory that pain was transmitted by

the same first-order neurons that transmitted temperature and touch sensations. The difference in sensation was a result of differing frequencies or patterns of action potentials traveling along these fibers. A simple experiment shows the motivation for this theory.

If you squeeze a fold of skin between your fingernails, at first you feel a little pressure, then much pressure and then—as you begin to harm your tissue—the touch sensation quickly changes to the distinctly unpleasant sensation of pain. Similarly, if you place your hand on an iron that is slowly heating up, you first feel warmth, then hot, then very hot and suddenly "ouch!" Such experiences make it tempting to think that pain is just an extreme state of mechanical or thermal receptor activation. Figure 2–5 shows that this is clearly not the case.

When the skin is contacted by a heated object, thermal receptors and nociceptors show markedly different activity in their afferent fibers (see Fig. 2–5). At 95°F, a temperature that we normally describe as warm, nociceptor fibers are silent, and non-nociceptive thermal receptor fibers are active. As the temperature increases, the frequency of action potentials in the thermal receptor fibers increases until the temperature reaches about 115°F, a temperature that is very hot, but not quite painful. At this point, the maximum action potential frequency of thermal receptors is reached. Nociceptors, however, show little, if any, response to this temperature. These fibers are not activated until the temperature reaches the pain threshold of about 120°F. Furthermore, the frequency of the action potentials increases with higher temperatures right up to the point when the fiber is destroyed. This is the response of a nociceptor. It detects and distinguishes dangerous levels of temperature well outside the range of thermal receptors. Although no structurally distinct nociceptor has been identified, physiological evidence like this, as well as pharmacological and clinical evidence, strongly supports the presence of separate receptors for pain.

Types of Nociceptors

Nociceptors are classified as mechanical, thermal or polymodal. First-order neurons with lightly myelinated primary afferent fibers (A-delta fibers—see Table 1–3 for additional information on fiber types) are activated by either very high levels of mechanical pressure or extremes of temperature.[86] The sensation from these nociceptors is described as rapid and sharp, and is normally well localized to a specific spot on the body.[83]

First-order neurons with unmyelinated primary afferent fibers (C fibers) often respond to both intense pressure and extreme temperature. Furthermore, they are activated by several chemicals that are released when the body tissue is damaged as described in the next section. Because a variety of stimuli activate these receptors, they are called **polymodal nociceptors**. Activation of the polymodal nociceptors generates pain sensation that is slower in onset, duller in intensity, and diffusely localized.

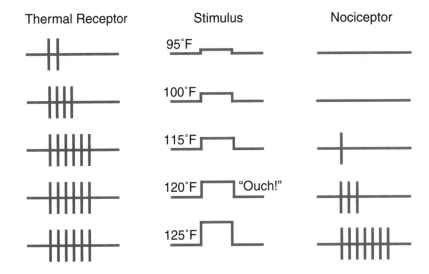

Figure 2–5. **Nociceptive Versus Non-nociceptive Thermoreceptor Fiber Response.** Non-nociceptive thermal receptors respond to innocuous levels of heat, increasing activity proportionately to the temperature until a maximal response is reached. Nociceptors show little or no response to thermal stimuli until the temperature reaches noxious levels (above 120°F).

Mechanisms of Nociceptive Transduction

The mechanical and thermal activation of A-delta and C fibers may depend on mechanically or thermally gated ion channels in the receptor membrane. Although similar to channels found in low-threshold mechanoreceptors, these channels have much higher thresholds and open only when free nerve endings are subjected to extreme pressure or temperature.

The chemical activation of polymodal nociceptors is produced by interaction of certain molecules with chemical receptors on the surface of these nociceptors.[86] Normally sequestered inside connective tissue and blood cells, histamine, bradykinin, and potassium ions leak into the intercellular space if these cells are ruptured (Fig. 2–6). These chemicals directly activate polymodal nociceptors and produce pain in human subjects when injected into the skin.[83] Damage to tissue cells also results in the production of prostaglandins—chemicals that do not directly activate nociceptors but do cause nociceptors to become more sensitive to mechanical, thermal, or chemical stimuli. Once these chemicals are released from the damaged cells, they can diffuse through the tissue for considerable distances, activating nociceptors outside the area of direct tissue damage and stimulating inflammatory reactions such as edema and vasodilation (see Chapter 1).

■ Transmission of Somatosensory Information to the Cerebral Cortex

Although transduction is the first step in detecting somatic sensation, the action potentials produced by transduction must be transmitted from the periphery all the way to the cerebral cortex before stimulus can be experienced. This involves at least three synapses and a crossing of fibers from one side of the nervous system to the other (Fig. 2–7). If the nervous system is damaged, this transmission may be disrupted, producing sensory loss in patterns that can be very complex. Fortunately, by understanding the anatomy of the ascending pathways, these patterns of sensory loss become more predictable. The evaluation of these patterns of sensory loss is an important component of the neurological examination as the patterns help to identify the location and extent of damage to the nervous system.

The most common pattern of sensory loss occurs when peripheral nerves are damaged. Damage to a peripheral nerve normally destroys all fibers in the nerve—sensory and motor—producing a complete loss of function distal to the site of damage. The affected area is confined to the region of the body innervated by the damaged nerve.

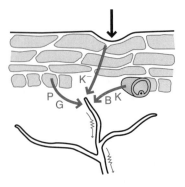

Figure 2–6. Damage to tissue produced by mechanical or thermal stimuli releases chemicals from tissue cells. These chemicals (K—potassium; BK—bradykinin; PG—prostaglandin) activate nociceptors, producing action potentials in primary afferent fibers.

For example, damage to the musculocutaneous nerve results in loss of motor and sensory function in the peripheral distribution shown in Figure 2–7.

If damage occurs more centrally, affecting spinal nerves or dorsal roots, the pattern of sensory loss changes to a **dermatome** ■ pattern (see Fig. 2–7). For example, damage to the sixth cervical dorsal root (C6) produces loss of all sensation in a narrow region of skin that includes innervation patterns of three peripheral nerves: the radial, median, and musculocutaneous nerves.

When the spinal cord itself is damaged, a much more complex pattern of sensory loss occurs (Box 2–4). For instance, a patient who suffers spinal cord damage at the C6 level may lose sensation of touch and proprioception in the C6 dermatome and all the lower dermatomes on the **ipsilateral** ■ side of the body. From the patient's perspective, it would seem that the ipsilateral side of the body was "missing" from the C6 dermatome inferiorly with one notable exception. The patient would still experience pain when stuck with a sharp needle. Pain would still be processed but with no apparent source of the stimulus. While touch and proprioception are intact on the **contralateral** ■ side of the body, pain sensation on that side of the body would be absent below the C6 dermatome.

To understand the last example, we need to know more about the somatosensory pathways inside the CNS. We need to learn what fibers cross from one side to the other and where they cross. Only then will we be able to understand why spinal cord injured patients often have such complex symptoms.

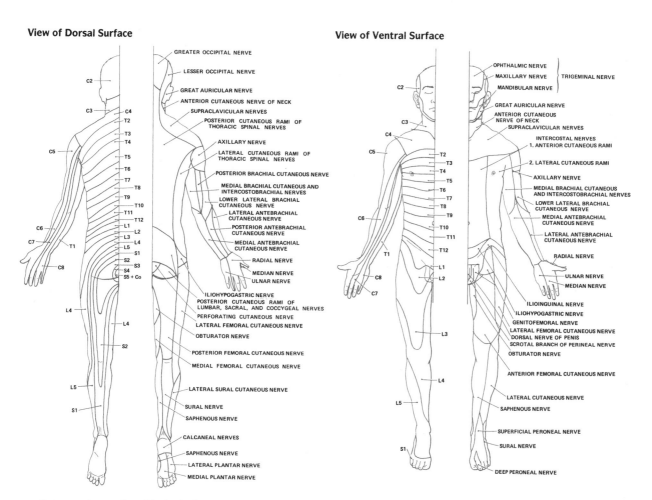

Cutaneous innervation of the back of the body. Dermatomes are on the left, and peripheral nerves are on the right.

Cutaneous innervation of the front of the body. Dermatomes are on the left, and peripheral nerves are on the right.

Figure 2–7. **Peripheral Nerves and Dermatomes.** The right side of the body shows the innervation patterns of peripheral nerves. Spinal nerve and root patterns are shown on the left side of the body. (From Gilman S, Newman SW: Manter and Gatz's Essentials of Clinical Neuroanatomy and Neurophysiology, ed 10. FA Davis, Philadelphia, 2003, pp 43–44.)

Contralateral: Pertaining to the opposite side of the body. The left side is contralateral to the right.
Dermatome: A segmental skin area supplied by a spinal nerve root.
Ipsilateral: On the same side of the body.

Spinal Cord Somatosensory Pathways

Although touch and pain fibers travel together in peripheral nerves and dorsal roots, the fibers diverge within the spinal cord, forming two distinct systems of connected nuclei and tracts that conduct somatic sensation from the spinal cord to the cerebral cortex. Touch and proprioception sensation travels in the **dorsal columns/medial lem-**

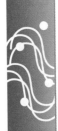

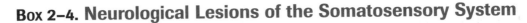

Box 2–4. Neurological Lesions of the Somatosensory System

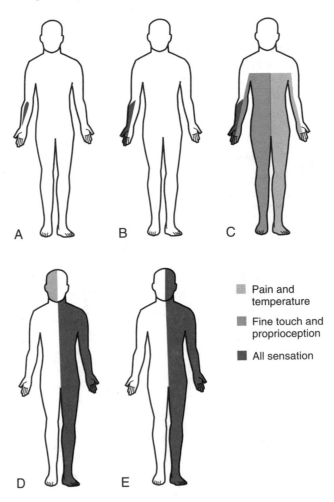

Pain and temperature

Fine touch and proprioception

All sensation

When the somatosensory system is damaged, the pattern of sensory loss helps neurologists to identify the location of the damage. The results of damage to neural structures on the right side of the body are shown. When peripheral nerves are damaged (A–right musculocutaneous nerve) sensory loss is confined to the region of the body that the nerve innervates. Damage to spinal nerves or roots (B–right C6 root) affects a larger area of the body and produces sensory loss that follows the dermatome patterns (Fig. 2-7). Damage to a single spinal root always produces ipsilateral sensory loss that is confined to a single dermatome. When the spinal cord itself is damaged (C–right spinal cord at C6 level) sensory loss occurs at the level of the damage but also at lower levels. Fine touch and proprioception are lost on the ipsilateral side at and below the damaged level of the spinal cord. Pain and temperature, however, are lost on the contralateral side below the damaged level. Damage to the medulla (D–right medulla) produces loss of all sensation in the contralateral limbs and trunk. The face, however, often shows loss of pain and temperature sensation on the ipsilateral side due to trigeminal tract damage. When the damage occurs rostral to the brain stem (E–right cerebral cortex) complete loss of somatic sensation in the contralateral face and body is likely.

niscus (DC/ML) system, whereas pain and temperature sensation ascends in the **anterior lateral system ▪** (ALS).

Fine Touch and Proprioception Spinal Pathways

The path of the fibers carrying fine touch and proprioceptive information through the spinal cord is straight forward. The large myelinated type A and B primary afferent fibers from the encapsulated receptors pass through the medial side of the dorsal root and enter a massive bundle of fibers called the **dorsal columns** (Fig. 2–8). This large group of fibers in the posterior spinal cord ascends all the way to the **medulla ▪** without interruption.

Thus, the nerve fiber that began as a Merkel disk or Pacinian corpuscle in the left toe travels without forming a synapse all the way to the brain stem. As a rule, primary afferent fibers do not cross the midline, so damage to the dorsal columns always produces loss of touch and proprioceptive sensation on the same side as the lesion. Because the dorsal columns contain fibers from all lower levels, a dorsal column lesion at a single spinal cord level blocks touch and proprioception from all ipsilateral dermatomes at and below the site of injury.

When the dorsal columns reach the medulla, the primary afferent fibers finally end in a pair of nuclei named **nucleus gracilis ▪** and **nucleus cuneatus ▪** (see Fig. 2–8). Fibers from the lower body terminate in nucleus gracilis, those from the upper body end in nucleus cuneatus. Notice that this is the first synapse of the DC/ML pathway. The second-order neurons in these two nuclei are activated and their axons form the next link in the ascent to the cerebral cortex. But before ascending, the axons cross to the opposite side of the nervous system. This is a common feature of somatosensory pathways—the crossing of secondary afferent fibers. After the crossing, the fibers that form the **medial lemniscus** continue through the brain stem to a nucleus in the posterior thalamus.

Because the fibers of the DC/ML system cross the midline in the caudal medulla, damage to this system above the crossing causes the loss of fine touch and proprioception contralateral to the lesion. For instance, if a patient has a stroke that damages the medial lemniscus in the left **midbrain ▪**, the patient will lose all sensation of touch and limb position on the right side of the body.

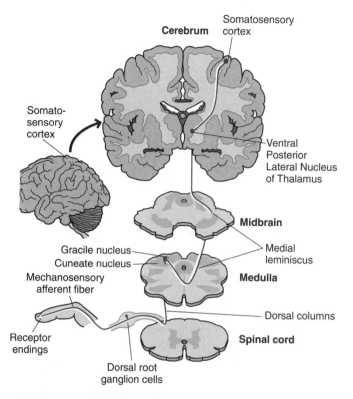

Figure 2-8. **Discriminative Touch and Proprioceptive Pathways.** The fibers of the dorsal columns/medial lemniscal system.

Pain and Temperature Spinal Pathways

The path of fibers of the ALS through the spinal cord and brain stem is complex. This is primarily due to the fact that these fibers *do* synapse in the spinal cord, and the ascending projection of pain and temperature information is accomplished by the axons of neurons in the dorsal horns. Therefore, these axons are secondary afferent fibers, and cross the midline within the spinal cord.

The A-delta and C fibers enter the cord on the lateral side of the dorsal roots. Although some fibers immediately synapse on neurons in the dorsal horn, many fibers travel up or down several spinal levels before forming synapses with neurons in the dorsal horn. This presynaptic fiber bundle, called the **dorsolateral fasciculus ▪** (or by its older name of

---

Anterior lateral system: The ascending fiber system that conveys pain and temperature sensation from spinal cord to the cerebral cortex. A major fiber bundle in this system of connections is the anterior lateral fasciculus.

Dorsolateral fasciculus ("Lissauer's tract"): The small bundle of fibers in the dorsolateral spinal cord formed by ascending or descending primary afferent fibers that carry pain and temperature sensation.

Medulla: The most caudal region of the brain stem. The medulla contains many cranial nerve nuclei and is also important in visceral control.

Midbrain: The most rostral region of the brain stem. Involved in muscle control and modulation of pain. Also processes visual and auditory information.

Nucleus cuneatus: A nucleus in the caudal medulla that relays fine touch and proprioceptive information from the upper body to the thalamus.

Nucleus gracilis: A nucleus in the caudal medulla that relays fine touch and proprioceptive information from the lower body to the thalamus.

Lissauer's tract), plays a key role in multisegmental spinal reflexes such as the withdrawal reflex (see Fig. 2–1).

When the primary afferent fibers reach their final spinal level, they exit the dorsolateral fasciculus and enter the dorsal horn. The dorsal horn contains cells that are organized into layers called **lamina**, which are numbered from posterior to anterior. Some lamina have additional names. In particular, lamina I is often called the marginal nucleus, and lamina II is called the substantia gelatinosa.

The C fibers from polymodal nociceptors primarily synapse on neurons lamina I and lamina II (Fig. 2–9), and many fibers from thermal receptors synapse here as well. Fibers from the mechanical nociceptors, the A-delta fibers, end primarily in lamina V at the base of the dorsal horn. Physiological studies show that cells in these deep lamina do indeed respond to noxious stimuli but they also respond to gentle touch. Such cells are called **wide dynamic range ■** (WDR) neurons because of the wide range of skin pressures that activate them. In addition to this direct input, the deep lamina cells receive input relayed from lamina I and II cells. The importance of this relayed input on pain modulation is discussed in a later section.

The axons of dorsal horn cells carry the pain and temperature sensation to nuclei in the brain stem and thalamus. Because these axons are secondary afferent fibers, they cross the midline before ascending. They sweep medially through the spinal gray matter and cross in a bundle of fibers called the **ventral white commissure**. The fibers

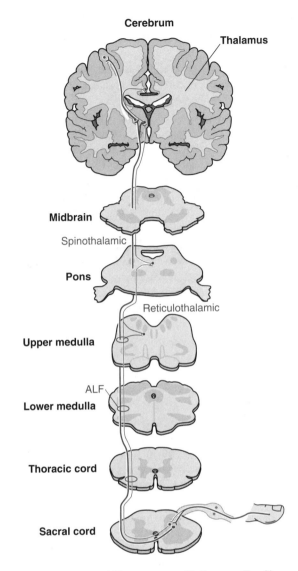

Figure 2–10. **Pain and Temperature Pathways.** The fibers of the anterior lateral fasciculus divide into two pathways to the cerebral cortex—the spinothalamic and reticulothalamic pathways. Both pathways connect to medial and lateral thalamic nuclei.

then continue to the lateral edge of the spinal cord and finally begin their ascent in a fiber bundle called the **anterior lateral fasciculus ■** (ALF), or **spinothalamic tract** (Fig. 2–10). However, not all of the ascending fibers reach the thalamus (and are therefore not technically in the spinothalamic tract). A significant portion of the fibers terminate in a series of brain stem nuclei called the **reticular nuclei**. These nuclei are important in maintaining level of alertness and regulating visceral responses. The reticular nuclei also project to thalamic nuclei, providing an alternate route to the thalamus.

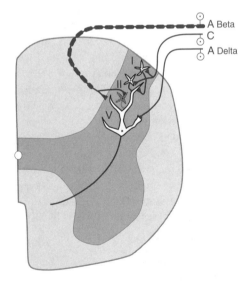

Figure 2–9. **The First Synapse.** Primary afferent fibers of the anterior lateral system terminate in the dorsal horn lamina, particularly lamina I and lamina II (the substantia gelatinosa) and lamina V. The fibers either terminate directly on tract cells or on interneurons.

Anterior lateral fasciculus: The large bundle of fibers in the anterolateral spinal cord and brain stem that carry second-order pain fibers to the brain stem and thalamus. This bundle includes fibers that are often called the spinothalamic tract.

Wide dynamic range cells (neurons): Neurons in the spinal cord and thalamus that respond to a broad range of mechanical pressures. They respond to both touch and pain.

The crossing of pain and temperature fibers in the spinal cord and the fact that touch and proprioceptive fibers do not cross explain the confusing clinical picture that often occurs when the spinal cord is damaged on one side. For example, if the left side of the spinal cord is damaged, loss of the sensation of touch and limb position is expected on the left side below the level of the lesion due to damage to the dorsal column. Damage to the ALF results in loss of pain and temperature sensation below the lesion level, but on the right side.

The Thalamus and Thalamocortical Projections

The final target of ascending secondary afferent fibers is the thalamus, a large mass of nuclei in the center of the **forebrain** ■. Although pain and touch fiber systems in the spinal cord and brain stem traveled in separate pathways, they partially converge in the thalamus.

Touch and Proprioceptive Thalamocortical Pathways

Secondary touch and proprioceptive afferent fibers from the body terminate in nuclei located in the ventral aspect of the posterior thalamus, specifically the **ventral posterior lateral nucleus** (VPL).

The VPL provides the third and final link from the peripheral receptors to the cerebral cortex. Third-order touch and proprioceptive afferent fibers exit the VPL and pass though the **internal capsule** ■ to reach the anterior edge of the parietal lobe, adjacent to a deep groove called the central sulcus, in a region of the cerebral cortex called the postcentral gyrus.

The fibers from different regions of the body are systematically distributed along the surface of this gyrus forming a "map" of the body spread across the cortex called the **homunculus** (Fig. 2–11). Fibers that originated in the feet and legs lie very medially, those from the body and back of the head take an intermediate position, and fibers from the hand lie laterally. Fibers that originated in the face reach the extreme lateral edge of this gyrus. The amount of cortex that is devoted to each body region is not uniform. Areas with high discriminative ability such as the tips of the fingers have a proportionally large representation in the cortex.

Pain and Temperature Thalamocortical Pathways

The classic description of pain pathways from thalamus to cerebral cortex parallels that of fine touch and propriocep-

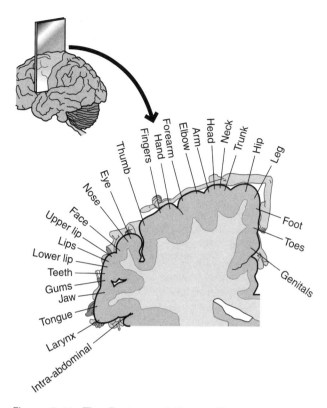

Figure 2–11. **The Postcentral Gyrus.** The somatosensory pathways terminate in the postcentral gyrus of the cerebral cortex in an orderly fashion, forming a map of the body called the somatosensory homunculus.

tive fibers. Many secondary pain and temperature fibers within the ALF also terminate in the VPL, and pain and temperature information is then relayed to the postcentral gyrus through the internal capsule. This lateral pain system is thought to provide the ability to localize pain sensation to a specific part of the body and determine how intense the painful stimulus is. This discriminative pain sensation is sometimes called **epicritic pain** ■.

Although localization of the site of tissue damage and intensity of the pain are important, pain has another key quality. It is very unpleasant. Most people do not like pain. Pain is something we are motivated to avoid. This emotional or affective quality of pain is conveyed to the cerebral cortex by a different route, the medial pain system.[87]

Many fibers in the ALF enter the **midline** and **intralaminar nuclei** of the thalamus. Third-order fibers from these nuclei travel anteriorly in the internal capsule but do not terminate in the postcentral gyrus. Instead they reach a midline area of cortex called the **cingulate gyrus**. The cingulate gyrus is part of the **limbic system** ■.

Epicritic pain: Pain that is well localized.

Forebrain: The cerebral hemispheres and thalamic region of the brain.

Internal capsule: A massive band of ascending and descending fibers in the forebrain that connect the cerebral cortex to thalamus, brain stem, and spinal cord.

Limbic system: System in the brain that controls emotion.

Magnetic resonance image (MRI) ■ studies sugggest that this area of cortex is important in producing the affective quality of pain. This poorly localized but unpleasant pain sensation may be called **protopathic pain** ■. Conversely, damage to the cingulate gyrus alters pain perception by removing the unpleasantness of the pain. Patients with **bilateral** ■ cingulate cortex damage, but with an intact **somatosensory cortex** ■, report that they still feel the pain, but it no longer bothers them.

In summary, the ascending pathways carrying touch and proprioceptive information terminate in the primary somatosensory cortex of the postcentral gyrus. However, pain and temperature pathways, divide at the thalamic level into the medial and lateral pain systems. The medial pain system travels to the midline and intralaminar nuclei, then to the cingulate cortex. The lateral pain system enters the VPL nucleus and then is relayed to the primary somatosensory cortex. This separation of the pain pathways into a medial and lateral component with different cortical terminations seems to explain a classic clinical misperception regarding the cortical representation of pain.

A common clinical observation is that somatosensory cortex damage abolishes contralateral touch sensation but spares pain sensation. Because both touch and pain sensation travel to the somatosensory cortex, the persistence of pain sensation is puzzling. An early explanation was that unlike touch and proprioception, pain is experienced at the thalamus.[88] This explanation, however, ignores the fact that pain information also reaches the cingulate cortex. With the loss of the somatosensory cortex, pain sensation is certainly altered. The patients cannot determine the intensity of pain sensation, and they cannot localize the injured part of the body accurately. Their response to pain is purely affective—they do not know where it hurts, but they do not like it—and it is likely that this is due to the medial pain system and its termination in the cingulate cortex.

■ Modulation of Pain Sensation

In the preceding sections, we saw that as long as the pain pathways to the cortex are undamaged, activation of A-delta and C fibers produce a sensation of pain that is localized to a specific region of the body and is very unpleasant. Also we saw that damage to these pathways produces a predictable reduction in pain sensation. But as described earlier, some aspects of pain perception cannot be easily explained by basic knowledge of the transduction mecha-

nisms and pathways. Our perception of pain is strongly influenced by complex factors through mechanisms that are largely unknown. Because the patient's perception of his or her pain has serious impact on treatment, we will identify some of these mechanisms by looking again at the transduction process and some of the finer details of the somatosensory pathways.

Peripheral Pain Modulation

Nociceptors are normally activated as the result of the destruction of tissue cells. Following tissue damage, normally innocuous stimuli such as light touch or warmth will easily activate these receptors, especially the C fiber polymodal nociceptors. This is called **hyperesthesia**, pain produced by normally nonpainful stimuli. Furthermore, a pin prick that would normally be described as mildly painful can generate considerable pain, **hyperalgesia**. In both instances, damage to tissue not only activates nociceptors, it also makes the nociceptors more sensitive to all other forms of stimulation. At the site of the damage, this change in threshold is called **primary hyperalgesia**. Over time, the hyperalgesia may spread to adjacent tissues, producing **secondary hyperalgesia**—pain experienced when adjacent, undamaged tissue is lightly touched or exposed to innocuous heat. Hyperesthesia and hyperalgesia are chemically mediated responses initiated by tissue damage (Fig. 2–12 and Table 2–5).

When skin tissue cells are damaged, potassium, prostaglandin, and bradykinin are released, and polymodal nociceptors are activated. This activation also produces release of the peptide substance-P from the nociceptors, and this peptide has a variety of actions. First, additional bradykinin, histamine, and serotonin are released from skin and vascular cells. These chemicals further activate the nociceptors (hyperalgesia) and may decrease the mechanical and thermal thresholds as well (hyperesthesia). Next, these chemicals diffuse through the skin tissues to adjacent undamaged tissue, **sensitizing** ■ nociceptors producing secondary hyperesthesia and hyperalgesia. Finally, dilation of the blood vessels and edema is produced (Box 2–5).

Spinal Cord Pain Modulation

Although hyperalgesia and hyperesthesia result in decreased thresholds of pain receptors after damage to the skin or underlying tissues, the first thing we tend to do

---

Bilateral: On both sides of the body.

Magnetic resonance image (MRI): A view of the body's internal structures obtained through the use of magnetic and radio fields.

Protopathic pain: Poorly localized pain sensation.

Sensitized: The process of being made sensitive to a specific substance.

Somatosensory cortex: An area in the cerebral cortex, located in the postcentral gyrus of the parietal lobe, that is important in the perception of touch and proprioception and in the localization of pain sensation.

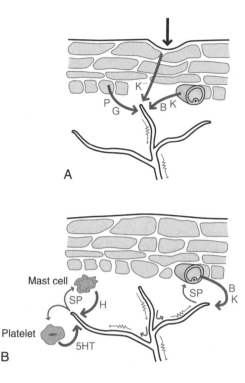

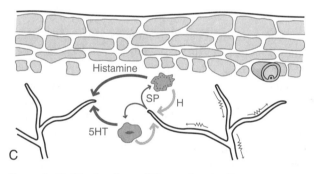

Figure 2-12. **Mechanism of Hyperalgesia.** Damage to tissue releases chemicals that activate nociceptors and also affects adjacent tissue. (A) The initial damage activated the nociceptor. (B) The branches of the primary afferent fibers stimulate adjacent connective tissue and vasculature. (C) The threshold of nociceptors in undamaged tissue is altered. (K—potassium; PG—prostaglandin; BK—bradykinin; SP—substance P; H—histamine; SHT—serotonin)

TABLE 2–5	Inflammatory Integration of Pain Response
Mediator	*Action*
Bradykinins	Directly stimulates nociceptors
Prostaglandin	Sensitization of the nerve fibers so that other mediators can enhance nociception
Substance P	Neurotransmitter released centrally to produce the pain response and peripherally producing hyperalgesia and inflammatory responses
Histamine	Released by mast cells to directly stimulate nociceptors

inhibit the dorsal horn interneurons. By activating an inhibitory interneuron, the I cell is disinhibited. That is, it increases its response more than produced by just the direct activation. This allows the C fibers to produce strong activation of the tract cells of the ALF, when activated alone.

As the large myelinated A-beta fibers enter the dorsal columns, branches from the fibers enter the spinal gray matter. A-beta fibers synapse on tract cells and dorsal horn interneurons. It is this second synapse that gives the gate-control theory its name. By activating these inhibitory interneurons, the tract cells are inhibited. The interneurons act like gate-keepers—either opening or closing down activation of the tract cells by the primary afferent fibers. If only the A-beta fibers are activated, the interneurons close the gate, inhibiting the tract cells and blocking their activation by the A-beta fibers or C fibers. If only C fibers are activated, the gate-keepers are inhibited and the gate to the tract cells opens.

Now consider what happens if both afferent fiber types are activated together. A tug-of-war of sorts ensues—with the A-beta fiber attempting to close the gate while the C fibers attempt to open the gate wide. If you can activate enough A-beta fibers by rubbing the area around a wound, the A-beta fibers win the battle. They succeed in turning on the interneurons and therefore decreasing activation of tract cells by the C fibers. This results in a decrease in the pain we feel from the wound. This illustrates the basis of the gate-control theory: Nonpainful stimulus can override the transmission of painful stimuli.

Experimental studies over the years have supported some aspects of the gate-control theory while raising questions about other aspects. The importance is that it provides a testable hypothesis to explain not only the effect of rubbing the area of a wound but also the effects of clinical treatments such as TENS, moist heat packs, cryotherapy, or whirlpools. It suggests a possible site for interaction between the touch and pain systems.

following injury is to rub the affected area. Rubbing the area does reduce the pain for some injuries. It makes it feel better. Thus, the touch and pain systems must interact; although interactions may well occur at multiple levels—dorsal horn, thalamus, or cerebral cortex—the most developed theories have focused on interactions in the dorsal horn. Much of this work has been conceptualized into what has been called the **gate-control theory** of spinal pain control of Melzack and Wall. This theory holds that the A-beta fibers form indirect connections with cells of the ALS in the dorsal horn.[57, 89, 90–92]

Figure 2–13 summarizes the gate-control theory. C fibers enter the dorsal horn and synapse directly on the second-order afferent neurons (T cells) of the ALS and

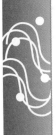

Box 2–5. Peripheral Anesthetics and Analgesics

Although acute pain is a useful signal that tissue has been damaged and that we need to let the limb rest, many therapies have been developed to decrease this signal as much as possible. Ideally, we would like to block the pain sensation while preserving the touch and proprioception sensations. But this goal has proved difficult.

Applying ice packs to a bee sting or painful joint has many effects on tissue, but one effect is to decrease the activity of nerve fibers. This produces **anesthesia ▪** in the cooled area of skin. The sensations of both touch and pain are decreased.

A medical approach to blocking activity in peripheral nerves is the application of a local anesthetic drug, such as lidocaine. Lidocaine blocks the action of voltage-gated sodium channels and very effectively shuts down action potential production in nerve fibers. As anyone who has had a tooth drilled knows, lidocaine blocks both pain fibers and touch fibers. Most drugs that produce pain relief, analgesia, without complete anesthesia act on the CNS, but one very popular analgesic works directly on the nociceptor.

For centuries, the bark of the willow tree has been used to relieve pain. By chewing the bark, or by producing extracts of its chemicals, pain can be significantly reduced although not fully blocked as with topical anesthetics. We now know that the active ingredient is acetylsalicylic acid—commonly known as aspirin.

Aspirin's primary action is to block the action of prostaglandin. Because prostaglandin sensitizes polymodal nociceptors, aspirin counteracts this effect and thereby reduces pain.

Descending Pain Modulation

Although peripheral and spinal mechanisms alter the amount of pain sensation traveling in the ascending pain pathways, the amount of pain we perceive is also strongly affected by cognitive factors. When in danger, or during the excitement of athletic competition, we often can ignore the pain produced by even severe injury. If we can get a nervous child to think about *anything* else, the pain of an injection might go unnoticed. Pain tolerance varies widely among people and is influenced strongly by gender, culture, and other sociological factors. Astonishing feats of

pain tolerance have been shown by people who are under hypnosis or are in an altered cognitive states. It seems clear that the mind, or at least its physiological representative, the cerebral cortex, can alter how we respond to activation of pain receptors.

The mechanisms of this action is certainly complex and poorly understood, but research has shown that a series of descending connections from the cerebral cortex may block pain at the level of the first synapse. Furthermore, this system is highly influenced by opiate drugs, such as morphine, and helps to explain the action of these pain-blocking analgesic drugs. Three brain stem reticular nuclei—the periaqueductal gray, the locus ceruleus, and the raphe nucleus—relay cortical activity to the dorsal horn to block, or at least decrease, pain transmission.

Located in the midbrain, the **periaqueductal gray (PAG) nuclei** receive descending fibers from the cingulate cortex and several other regions of the cerebral cortex that play a role in emotional control. The PAG connects the emotional centers of the cortex to pain centers in the spinal cord, and indeed in animals, direct stimulation of the PAG blocks responses to painful stimuli.[83]

The PAG does not project directly to the spinal cord; instead it projects to the medulla, activating neurons in the raphe nucleus (Fig. 2–14A). The raphe neurons then project to the dorsal horn, activating interneurons that inhibit the activity of tract cells through the action of the endogenous opiate neurotransmitter **enkephalin ▪**. Additional

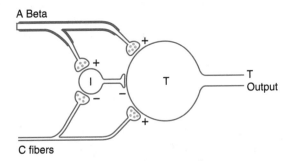

Figure 2–13. **Opening and Closing the Gate.** The gate-control theory models the interaction of A-beta and C fibers at their synapse with the secondary afferent neurons. T: tract cell; I: inhibitory interneuron.

Anesthesia: A loss of, or decrease in, sensation.

Enkephalin: A substance released by the body that reduces the perception of pain by bonding to pain receptor sites.

descending fibers originate in the locus ceruleus nucleus in the pontine region of the brain stem.

These fibers either act directly on the primary afferent pain fibers or the tract cells of the ascending pain systems (Fig. 2–14B). Fibers from the raphe nuclei release the neurotransmitter serotonin, which directly inhibits tract cells and also activates inhibitory interneurons. Descending fibers from the locus ceruleus release norepinephrine, which activates inhibitory interneurons.

An additional important route for cortical **modulation** ■ of ascending pain systems exerts its influence systemically through the circulatory system rather than through the descending fibers of the CNS. Nuclei within the hypothalamic region of the forebrain control the hormones released by the pituitary gland—in particular, the hormone **beta-endorphin**. By activating these hypothalamic nuclei, regions of the cerebral cortex can increase

the level of beta-endorphin circulating in the blood system. Beta-endorphin acts on opiate receptors throughout the nervous system and inhibits activity in pain systems (Box 2–6).

Through these descending connections, the cerebral cortex acquires a remarkable potential. The very region of the brain that is most responsible for providing conscious awareness of noxious stimuli, the cerebral cortex, may be able to block the ascending transmission of pain information to the cerebral cortex—in essence deciding whether or not it will receive the message that tissue is damaged. This may underlie several curious clinical observations about the perception of pain—observations that were sometimes said to be psychological with the implication that there was no underlying physiological basis.

One such observation is the reduction of pain by the placebo effect. In experiments to determine a drug's **efficacy** ■ as an analgesic, two control groups are often used to compare results with the experimental group of patients who receive the tested drug. One group receives no treatment at all, whereas a "**sham** ■ control" group is given a placebo—a pill that contains sugar or some other inactive substance cleverly disguised as to be indistinguishable from the pills containing the active substances (Box 2–7). Experimenters take particular care to make sure that the participants do not know if the medicine they receive is the actual drug or the placebo. In such experiments, the

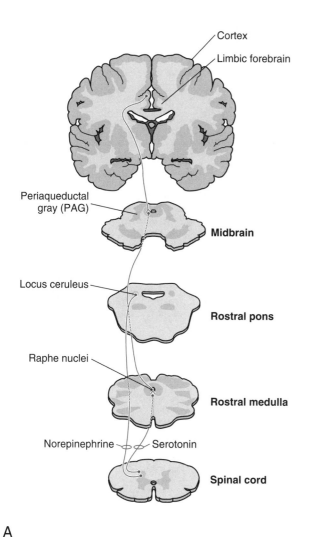

A

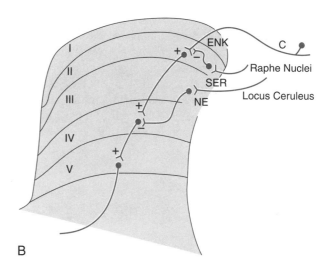

B

Figure 2–14. **Descending Modulation Pathways of Pain.** (A) The cerebral cortex can modulate transmission in the ascending pain pathways through a series of descending connections with brain stem nuclei. (B) Descending modulation of dorsal horn neurons. Descending fibers from the raphe nucleus and locus ceruleus modulate the activation of dorsal horn neurons by C fibers.

Efficacy: The ability of a modality or treatment regimen to produce the intended effects.

Modulate (Modulation): To regulate or adjust.

Sham: A device or "drug" that has no physiological effect on the body (e.g, an ultrasound unit with the output intensity set to zero).

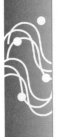

Box 2–6. Opium and the Opioids

Although much maligned because of its many negative physiological, psychological, social, and political attributes, opium and its chemical derivatives, opioids, are certainly one of the best pure analgesics. Opioids block the affective component of pain–the unpleasantness–with little effect on touch or proprioception.

Like many drugs derived from plants, the opioids act by interacting with neurotransmitter receptors on cells in the nervous system. These cells are normally regulated by a family of neurotransmitters sometimes called the endogenous opioids or collectively endorphins. These include small peptide molecules–enkephalin and dynorphin or larger protein molecules such as beta-endorphin.

The endorphins act on many neurons of the pain system (Fig. 2–14). As described in the text, enkephalin acts to inhibit the tract cells in the dorsal horn. This inhibition occurs both presynaptically, by blocking the release of neurotransmitter from the primary afferent fibers, and postsynaptically, acting directly on the neurons in the dorsal horn. It also activates the cells of the PAG, initiating their descending pain control. Neurons in the hypothalamus and cingulate cortex are also under control of the endorphins.

Because opium and opioid drugs like heroin, Percocet, and other narcotics simulate the action of the endorphins, these drugs are important in providing pain relief.

placebo results in a surprisingly significant reduction in pain compared with the sham control group. In some cases, the placebo's effect exceeded the medication being tested—no doubt to the dismay of the experimenters.

Although some would assume that the reported pain reduction was not real, that it was just "in their heads" or possibly mystical, the descending pain control projections of the cerebral cortex offer a plausible explanation of this seemingly impossible observation. Knowing that you have received treatment for your pain, the areas of the cerebral cortex become activated and send signals to the PAG that "help is on the way." The PAG then activates the descending pain modulation centers and blocks the activity within the spinal cord, thus reducing the pain experienced by the subject. Pain would be reduced not by some internal psychological process of the cerebral cortex but due to active blocking of sensory pathways. Further research into this system may provide insight into a wide array of psychological aspects of pain reduction ranging from hypnosis to the power of those comforting words "it will be okay."

■ Pathology of Pain

Pain provides us with an important signal that tissue has been damaged. It lets us know where the damage is located

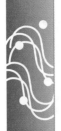

Box 2–7. The Placebo Effect

Placebo, stemming from the Latin word for *I shall please,* is the term used to describe pain reduction obtained through mechanisms other than those related to the physiological effects of the treatment. The placebo effect is linked to a psychological mechanism whereby, if the patient thinks that the treatment is beneficial, then a degree of pain reduction occurs. The physiological mechanisms of the placebo effect are not well understood.

All therapeutic modalities have some degree of placebo effect. This effect may be increased when the modality is applied with a sense of enthusiasm and faith. Indeed, most studies comparing pain reduction between a sham therapeutic modality and an actual treatment have shown decreased levels of pain in both groups. The placebo effect is so powerful that, in one instance, patients who receive placebo pills may even display some side effects of the presumed medication.[59]

The placebo effect can be exploited in the application of therapeutic modalities. Changing modalities and new approaches in the treatment of an injury can positively influence the patient's perception and result in decreased pain.

so we can act to remove ourselves from the cause of the damage and can protect the damaged area so that it can heal. When a muscle is torn or a ligament is sprained, the pain system insists, in no uncertain terms, that we should stop exercising and give the damaged limb some rest. Although we never enjoy pain, we should realize that pain normally helps us to heal.

Unfortunately, pain sometimes misinforms us about the location of the damage especially when the actual damage is to a visceral organ. Pathology in the muscle of the heart might be felt in the shoulder or arm instead of the chest and lead to failure to understand the seriousness of the felt pain. And pain sometimes persists for weeks, months, or even years after healing should have taken place. Treatment of such pathological pain symptoms can be difficult, and the effects can be severely incapacitating.

Referred Pain

Pain is normally well localized to the site of injury. If we take a pin and poke the skin, we know exactly where the pin prick occurred. This is the result of the precise topography of the ascending pain system from the surface of the body all the way to the homunculus in the cerebral cortex. However, pain originating from the visceral organs is difficult to localize. Imagine taking a drink of very hot coffee. We can distinguish clearly if the coffee burns the lips, tongue, or cheeks. But if we ignore these warning signals and hastily swallow the burning brew, we feel pain on the inside but will have a difficult time localizing this internal pain to the esophagus versus trachea or stomach. Even damage to deeper muscles may sometimes seem to originate from the skin or muscles at some distance from the actual damage. Frequently, pain originating from visceral organs is perceived as originating from an area of the skin far removed from the organ. For example, damage to the diaphragm is normally not felt as pain at the base of the thorax but rather an ache in the skin and muscles of the neck and shoulder. Pain from angina may be felt in the chest but also may seem to radiate down the arm. Pain originating in a small region of the appendix organ is normally felt as originating diffusely from the abdominal region (McBurney's point) or trauma to the spleen causing pain in the upper left shoulder (Kerr's sign). This is referred pain—pain originating from damage to the visceral organ is referred to the surface of the body.

Not only does the sensation of pain seem to originate from the surface of the body, but referred pain produces hyperalgesia in the affected skin area. Careful evaluation shows that the patterns of hyperalgesia after damage to different organs were fairly consistent across patients. By mapping the area of hyperalgesia, the neurologist gains insight into the identity of the damaged organ. Also, these patterns suggest a possible explanation of referred pain (Fig. 2–15). During development, the visceral organs migrate from their original location in the embryo. For instance, the diaphragm originates at cervical levels in the neck, but then relocates to its adult position in the lower thorax. Owing to this migration, the branches of the primary afferent fibers innervate both organ and skin (Fig. 2–15A). Because the skin area is more exposed, we learn to associate pain due to damage to the skin with activation of the cutaneous branch. Later, if the visceral organ is damaged, the same afferent fibers are activated and we misinterpret the origin of the pain.

Patients who are suffering from pain of unknown origin may be experiencing referred pain. A careful, thorough history and evaluation is required to identify the actual cause of the patient's discomfort. Ultimately, the underlying pathology of the pain should be clear before treatment is prescribed. In cases in which the true cause of the pain is suspect, or if there is uncertainty of the nature of the pain, the patient should be referred to a physician for further evaluation.

Phantom Limb

Perhaps the most extreme form of pain mislocalization is phantom limb pain. Following amputation of a limb, pain is often reported as originating from the missing appendage. The pain can be quite severe and can be very specifically localized to a missing arm, hand, or finger.

Various causes of phantom limb pain may exist, but in many cases, the pain originates in the cut ends of the primary afferent fibers near the surface of the stump. Ideally, the cut afferent fibers cease to function after an amputation. In some cases, however, the ends of the fibers form a **neuroma ■**. Owing to instability of the neuronal membrane in the neuroma, the fiber becomes spontaneously active (called **ectopic ■** activation) and can produce a constant barrage of action potentials heading down the primary afferent fiber. The pain produced by these action potentials seems to originate at the location of the skin that originally activated the fibers before the amputation. And this happens to be a part of the body that no longer exists.

This hypothesis is supported by the fact that injections of local anesthetics into the stump can block this activity and provide pain relief. Some phantom limb cases, however, do not respond well to local anesthetics, and this suggests that other changes in the circuitry within the dorsal horn or even within the cerebral cortex itself may also play a role in generating phantom pain.

Ectopic: Outside or away from its normal position; in an abnormal position or sequence.

Neuroma: Swelling or other mass formation around a nerve (*Neuro* = nerve; *oma* = tumor). Normally formed by connective cells instead of neurons.

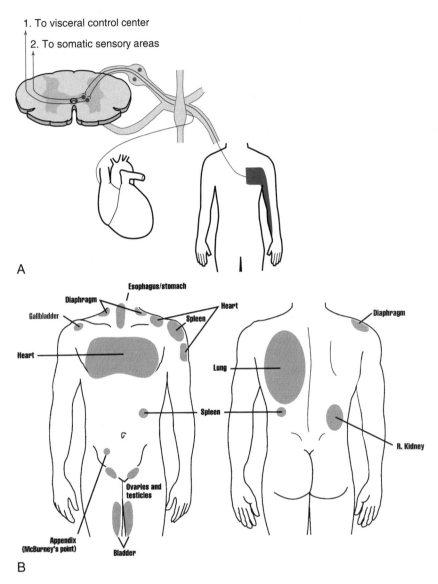

Figure 2–15. **Referred Pain.** Pain originating from visceral organs is poorly localized and may seem to originate from the surface of the body some distance from the site of injury. (A) Possible mechanism of referred pain. (B) Common patterns of experienced pain after damage to different organs.

Chronic Pain Syndromes

The least understood, but most troublesome, form of pain is chronic pain. As we saw earlier, the most difficult form of chronic pain to treat is neuropathic chronic pain. We will examine three different examples of neuropathic chronic pain—partial neuropathies, myofascial pain syndrome, and sympathetically maintained pain syndrome. Although similar in that each produces long-lasting pain, each of these syndromes has unique characteristics that suggest different mechanisms of production.

Neuropathy

Complete severance of a peripheral nerve, a **neuropathy ■**, normally abolishes all somatic sensation the nerve

provides. If nerves are partially damaged, however, neuropathic pain can develop. The initial damage can be caused by trauma that compresses the nerve, damaging some of the nerve fibers inside. Entrapment of the nerve or repetitive small injuries over time, as in carpal tunnel syndrome, may also produce this syndrome. The key distinction between this and nociceptive chronic pain is that the pain persists after the damaged tissue has completely healed. There is no ongoing disease which is activating the nociceptors. Instead, the nociceptors are spontaneously active.

Similar to phantom limb pain, this spontaneous activity may result from ectopic activation of the primary pain afferent fibers in the periphery. Neuroma may form at the

---

Neuropathy: Destruction, trauma, or inhibition of a nerve.

site of damage to the nerve and generate action potentials. If so, injection of local anesthetics into the nerve proximal to the damage blocks the neuropathic pain.

If nerve blocks do not stop the pain, or in the case of avulsion of the dorsal roots when the roots are pulled free from the spinal cord, the generation of neuropathic chronic pain must be due to changes in the CNS. Exactly what changes occur and where the nervous system is abnormally active is poorly understood.

One plausible hypothesis derived from the gate-control theory focuses on the synapse with the secondary afferent neurons in the dorsal horn. Compressive nerve damage often affects the larger diameter fibers more than the thin fibers. A disproportionate loss of the A-beta fibers would lower the level of activation of inhibitory interneurons in the dorsal horn and produce a disinhibition of the tract cells (see Fig. 2–13). Alternately, loss of synaptic input to tract cells may stimulate the surviving fibers to form abnormal connections to these neurons. Some research suggests that synaptic reorganization at higher levels, even in the cerebral cortex, may play a role in neuropathic chronic pain.[93]

Myofascial Pain Syndrome

Muscle aches and pains are certainly a common occurrence and normally are self-resolving. Pain emanating from muscle and connective tissues that is persistent and shows no indication of being caused by arthritis or other nociceptive process may result from **myofascial pain syndrome** or trigger point pain. Muscles in the painful area often have very high tone—the muscles feel very tense and are quite sore. A key sign of this syndrome is the presence of trigger points. Even though the pain is felt over a large area, the trigger point may be confined to a small part of just one of the affected muscles.

The anatomical and physiological identification of trigger points and the mechanism of the pain generation is unknown, but one hypothesis holds that trigger points exist in many muscles but are inactive. If the muscle is damaged, even slightly, in the area of a trigger point, the trigger point produces a reflexive muscle contraction that further activates the trigger point. The process becomes self-sustaining. This hypothesis is supported by treatment approaches which relax the muscle by stretching or directly inactivate the trigger point by injection of anesthetic. This breaks the self-sustaining loop, and can produce permanent relief (see Treatment Strategies: Muscle Spasm and Trigger Points, p 27).

Sympathetically Maintained Pain Syndrome

Perhaps the most disabling of all chronic pain syndromes is pain that is produced by action of the sympathetic nervous system, also known by other names such as complex regional pain syndrome or reflex sympathetic dystrophy. This syndrome often starts with trauma, possibly minor trauma, to the soft tissues or bones. Despite appropriate treatment for the trauma, the wound or broken bone does not heal well. The affected area reddens and may sweat profusely—signs of sympathetic activation. Nerve blocks provide temporary relief, but the pain continues to increase over time and can reach severe levels. Even cutting the sensory nerve proximal to the affected area may provide only temporary relief.

The key sign is that blockade of sympathetic innervation to the affected area provides profound and even permanent pain relief. This may be done by injecting local anesthetic into the sympathetic ganglia or by infusing the affected area with drugs that block sympathetic activity. Furthermore, this blockade allows healing of the damaged area to progress. The mechanisms of this syndrome are unknown, but it does appear to be due in part to the development of sensitivity of nociceptors to norepinephrine—the neurotransmitter released by sympathetic nerves.[83]

It is important to note that sympathetically maintained pain is best treated early. Poorly healing injuries that show signs of increased sympathetic activation in the damaged area should be carefully evaluated for signs of this syndrome and treatment should be started before the pain becomes severe. In some cases, once the pain reaches severe levels, no treatment is effective.

● Chapter Highlights

- Pain is a sensation with attitude that informs us of damage to our bodies and then strongly insists that we protect ourselves from further damage.
- Neuroscience has provided a growing understanding of the pathways of pain sensation.
- The destruction of tissue creates action potentials that are conducted to multiple areas of the cerebral cortex that produces the sensation of pain, the physiological response of the body to noxious stimuli.
- The pain response is more than just the sum of activity in sensory pathways. Pain perception is influenced by psychological, cognitive, emotional, social, and cultural factors through neural mechanisms that are poorly understood.
- Although pain is inherently subjective in nature, it can be quantitatively and qualitatively measured with a reasonable degree of accuracy. The visual analog scale, McGill Pain Questionnaire, and other tests provide a unique view of an individual's perception of pain, although caution should be used when attempting to correlate one person's pain with another's.
- Acute pain can be controlled through one of two mechanisms using therapeutic modalities. The better of these is to restore the body's homeostasis and provide the optimal environment for healing to occur. Once the inflammatory process subsides and the mechanical and chemical stimulation of the nociceptors has ceased, pain should be eliminated. Modalities may also be used to affect

the transmission of the painful impulses. Heat, cold, electrical stimulation, and other therapeutic techniques can be used to disrupt the pain process.

- We are only beginning to understand the mechanisms of chronic pain—pain that persists after healing is complete. It is clear only that chronic pain has multiple causes. It can be produced in the peripheral nervous system at the site of injured nerves or within the CNS by neural pathologies that are largely unknown.

- In chronic pain, the pain experienced by the patient is not related to underlying tissue trauma, or the location of the pain is not associated with the area of tissue trauma. These cases require keen evaluative skills and atypical treatment protocols.

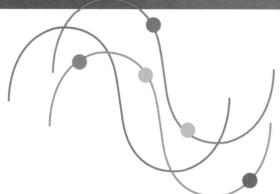

Chapter 3

Development and Delivery of Treatment Protocol

Jeff Ryan, PT, ATC

This chapter presents an overview of the decision-making process used in developing treatment plans and modality selection. A case study is used to help reinforce the problem-solving approach presented in this chapter.

The problem-solving approach (PSA) is a logic-based technique that uses the patient's long-term goals to develop a treatment plan. Although "logical thinking" is something that we usually do not do consciously, we practice it as a part of our daily routine. It may involve such basic skills as getting dressed in the morning or more complicated tasks such as finding your way around an unfamiliar city for a job interview. The PSA extends this logical thinking into the treatment of the patient.

This text began by explaining that therapeutic modalities are used to create the proper environment for healing to occur. The components of the injury response process are interrelated. For example, edema causes pain, pain causes spasm, and spasm causes pain (Fig. 3–1). Although pain may be the patient's primary complaint, simply focusing your treatments on pain relief does little to resolve the underlying cause of the discomfort and the associated dysfunction. Approaching the patient's problems on a purely symptomatic basis often produces unsatisfactory results.

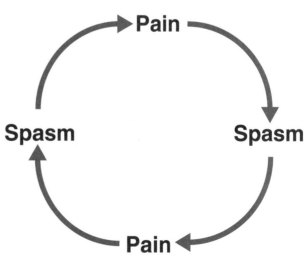

Figure 3–1. **The Pain-Spasm-Pain Cycle.** This represents a self-perpetuating process in which pain causes muscle spasm and muscle spasm produces pain. This cycle continues until either pain or muscle spasm is resolved.

The ability to plan a treatment and rehabilitation program is among the most complex skills that must be mastered. This process integrates clinical evaluation skills and knowledge of pathology with knowledge of therapeutic techniques and principles, goal setting, and patient motivation and education. The body of knowledge is continuously progressing and the efficacy of treatments are being established or refuted. Treatment planning is as much an art as it is a science, and your ability in this area will grow and be perfected with experience.

■ The Problem-Solving Approach

Individuals respond to trauma differently, necessitating individualized treatment plans. When based on **normative data** ■, generalized treatment protocols provide a reference point for determining where the patient "should be" and what treatment approaches should be considered. Preestablished treatment protocols should not be viewed as unyielding individual treatment plans. Individual treatment plans differentiate the specifics of each patient's case and lead to a more efficient and successful outcome.

The PSA is an ongoing process of evaluation, analysis, and planning that comprises five steps: (1) recognition of the patient's problems, (2) prioritization of the problems, (3) goal setting, (4) treatment planning, (5) and reevaluation (Table 3–1). To illustrate each of these

components, an ongoing case study is presented throughout this chapter and continued in each of the following sections of this text. Case studies also appear at the end of each section. Although the focus of this text is on therapeutic modalities, the role of these interventions is to prepare the patient for therapeutic exercise, manual techniques, and functional activities. Modalities are also used after these treatments as a way of controlling exercise-induced inflammation.

Problem Recognition

To provide proper care, the pathology being treated must be identified. The problem recognition stage is designed to identify the type of tissues involved, the nature and effects of the pathology, and the stage of the healing process (Table 3–2).

Different types of tissue respond differently to various modalities. The biological properties and functions of the traumatized tissues, their depth below the skin, and their stage in the inflammation and healing process dictate which modalities can effectively stimulate them. The use of a superficial modality to treat structures that are located deep within the tissues will produce little or no benefit. When we start to develop the treatment plan, the type of modality (e.g., heat, cold, electrical) must be appropriate for the patient's stage of healing and treatment goals.

Recognition of the problems begins by reviewing

TABLE 3–1	Components of the Problem-Solving Approach
Component	*Purpose*
Recognition of the problem	Identify the type and depth of the involved tissues
	Identify the nature of the pathology
	Determine the stage of healing
	Recognize the indications for the use of modalities and exercise
	Recognize any contraindications to the use of modalities or exercises
	Recognize the demands a patient's activity level places upon the tissues
Prioritization of the problem	Develop the logical treatment order based on a cause-and-effect relationship between the pathology and the signs and symptoms
Goal setting	Develop structure and sequence in the treatment plan
	Establish benchmarks to determine efficacy of the treatment plan
Treatment planning	Determine the modalities and exercises to be used and their sequence based on the patient's problems and treatment goals
Reevaluation	Evaluation of the patient's current physical status:
	Reassessment of previously identified problems
	Evaluation techniques that are no longer **contraindicated** ■
	New problems that have developed since the previous examination
	The findings are used to:
	Assess the effectiveness of the current treatment protocol
	Reassess the short and long term goals
	Determine changes that are needed in the treatment plan

Contraindicate: To make inadvisable.

Normative data: Information that can be used to describe a specific population.

Case Study Part 1: The Patient's Medical History

A 22-year-old woman diagnosed with patellofemoral pain syndrome of the right knee has been referred by an orthopedic surgeon. The following information has been obtained:

Report: Intermittent pain "under the right kneecap" that increases when she goes up or down stairs and occasionally after long periods of sitting. The pain and intermittent "giving way" prohibit the patient from participating in strenuous activity.

History: While participating in soccer, the patient twisted her knee with her foot planted, resulting in a tear of the anterior cruciate ligament (ACL) and medial meniscus. She underwent ACL reconstruction with a bone–patellar tendon–bone autograft and a partial medial meniscectomy. She returned to play soccer 6 months after the surgery. One month later, she developed her present symptoms that have persisted for 6 months.

Diagnostic tests: Radiographic studies were negative.

Activity: Unable to participate in strenuous activity .

General medical conditions: No significant illnesses.

Medications: Nonsteroidal anti-inflammatory drugs.

Contraindications to modality use: None.

Contraindications to therapeutic exercise: Painful arc of motion.

Patient goals: Pain-free activities of daily living (ADLs). To return to recreational soccer.

Evaluation findings:

Function:	The patient cannot play soccer because of anterior knee pain. The patient cannot climb or descend stairs without pain. The patient cannot sit for more than 30 minutes without developing knee pain.
Observation:	Healed incision over the patellar tendon. **Keloid** ∎ formation is present.
Patellar mobility:	The patella is hypomobile superiorly and medially.
Patellar tracking:	Increased lateral tracking relative to the opposite side.
Range of Motion:	Involved: 2 degrees of extension to 135 degrees of flexion (0 − 2 − 135 degrees) Uninvolved:

	5 degrees of hyperextension to 145 degrees of flexion (5 − 0 − 145 degrees)
Girth:	Girth is 1 cm greater than that of the uninvolved knee as measured over the joint line. Mild effusion is present.
Tone:	The patient displays poor control of the quadriceps muscle group. The vastus medius oblique (VMO) lacks tone and mass compared with that on the uninvolved side.
Strength:	Hip muscle groups are 5/5. Quadriceps are 5/5, with pain elicited at the patellofemoral joint Hamstring groups are 5/5. Ankle groups are 5/5.
Flexibility:	All hip muscles are within normal limits. The quadriceps muscle is tight, demonstrating prone knee flexion to 120 degrees. Hamstrings are tight. The knee lacks 10 degrees of extension with the hip at 90 degrees. Gastrocnemius and soleus muscles are tight. The ankle can be dorsiflexed only to 10 degrees while the knee is extended.
Pain rating:	Patient describes pain as 5/10 when she is descending stairs, 1/10 while sitting.
Special tests:	All demonstrate negative results.
Biomechanical analysis:	Feet excessively pronate (bilaterally) during walking gait.
Palpation:	Pain is produced during palpation along the medial **retinaculum** ∎ and at the inferior patellar pole.

This introduces the patient, her relative medical history, and reports from which we can build our problem list. The problem recognition uses this patient history to identify functional deficits and those conditions that should be the focus of the patient's treatment goals.

Keloid: A nodular, firm, movable, and tender mass of dense, irregularly distributed collagen scar tissue in the dermis and subcutaneous tissue. Common in the African-American population, keloid scarring tends to occur after trauma or surgery.

Retinaculum: A fibrous membrane that holds an organ or body part in place.

TABLE 3–2   Information Gained During the Patient Evaluation

Segment	*Examples*
Patient's complaints	The patient's description of the problems
Medical history	Any significant medical condition that may affect the current course of treatment
Medications	Current use of prescription, nonprescription, or recreational medication that may alter the findings of the evaluation or present a contraindication to the use of therapeutic modalities or therapeutic exercise
Mechanism of injury	The description of how the injury occurred or the onset of symptoms
Normal level of activity	Identifies the patient's activity lifestyle
Type of tissues involved	Anatomy, function, size, depth of trauma
Nature of the trauma	For example, sprain, strain, fracture, contusion, improper biomechanics
Stage of injury response	Acute inflammation, proliferation, maturation, chronic inflammation
Limitations	Pain, decreased range of motion, decreased strength
Patient goals	Long-term, short-term
Contraindications	Modalities, exercises, and manual techniques that cannot be used

existing medical records of the patient's condition. Diagnostic test reports, operative reports, the physician's prescription, and referral notes are all good sources. Prior treatment notes describe modalities that have been used, the parameters used in their application, and how effective they were. Other sources of information include preparticipation medical examinations and notes pertaining to prior evaluation and treatment of unrelated conditions. Medical contraindications to the use of specific therapeutic modalities must also be identified during the patient interview (Box 3–1).

Subjective ▪ information can be obtained during both the formal patient interview and informal discussion (Fig. 3–2). Good clinical skills require keen listening skills and the ability to identify and solicit pertinent information from the patient. For instance, a patient's comment such as "My knee feels as if it is going to give out" may identify quadriceps muscle weakness. Complaints of feeling "worse" after therapy may indicate that the exercise and/or treatment protocol was too intense. Remarks indicating improvements may help determine the best patterns of modality use or parameters applied to optimize the effects of the modality. When applicable, these remarks should be noted in the patient's medical file.

It is easy to focus your attention solely on observable signs such as swelling, discoloration, decreased range of motion, and the reported symptoms of pain, numbness, and so on. Although the short-term objective of any given treatment session is to provide symptomatic relief or objective improvement in one of these parameters, the long-term goal of proper healing and return to a normal lifestyle will not be met until the underlying pathology is identified and managed (Fig. 3–3). If we consider the case of the patient who complains of pain during internal shoulder rotation, permanent pain relief not will be obtained until the underlying biomechanical dysfunction of tissue tightness is remedied. As we will see in the following sections, symptomatic treatments may be required in the early treatment phases but only as a transition to curative treatments.

Many different pathologies may be identified during the evaluation process. Using valid and reliable tools, correct measurement techniques, consistency during reevaluation, and proper documentation of the results contribute to the accumulation of documented evidence of the patient's progress (Table 3–3). These tools are not appropriate for every condition, and the patient may have one or more contraindications to their use.

Formal patient evaluations and reevaluations should be conducted at regular intervals. Before each treatment session, interview the patient to evaluate the effectiveness of the prior treatments and home treatments and evaluate the patient's physical and mental/emotional status.

The patient's mental and emotional states must be considered in treatment planning. To maximize participation, educate the patient about the nature of the injury, the treatment plan, the treatment goals, and the expectations for recovery. Ultimately, the pace of the recovery is based on the patient's motivational level. Some patients need to be held back because of their high motivation. Other patients have to be continuously motivated to reach their treatment goals. Patients who consistently lack motivation or display behavioral signs of disinterest in their recovery may need the assistance of a mental health-care provider.

The information collected during evaluation and the treatment sessions should be identified and recorded in the patient's file using measurable and objective terms.

Subjective: Symptoms stated by the patient that are not externally apparent, such as pain. Personal beliefs and attitudes may alter subjective symptoms.

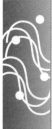

Box 3–1. Medical Contraindications to Therapeutic Modality Use

Certain therapeutic modalities or therapeutic exercises may be contraindicated based on the patient's current stage of healing, application over specific body areas or organs, or because of unrelated medical conditions. Identifying regional contraindications requires knowledge of the modality being used. The clinical evaluation and reevaluation tends to focus on identifying conditions that are immediate, but changing, indications and contraindications to modality use. However, underlying medical contraindications against the use of certain therapeutic modalities must be identified prior to beginning any treatments.

Contraindications are either absolute or relative. An **absolute contraindication** means that the modality or protocol must not be used under any circumstance. **Relative contraindications** mean that the treatment can be modified to accommodate the patient's condition, decreasing the temperature of a warm whirlpool for example. **Precautions** identify how misuse of the modality can cause harm to the patient.

Many medical contraindications can be identified through a comprehensive medical questionnaire and be confirmed during the history taking/patient interview process. The medical questionnaire should be administered at the start of the academic year in the case of institutional sports medicine facilities or at the time of the first visit for other outpatient facilities.

The following is a partial list of common medical contraindications and methods to identify them. Health-care providers are legally, morally, and ethically responsible to be familiar with the contraindications of the device, technique, or procedure being administered. In the case of therapeutic modalities, the manufacturer's user's guide lists the precise contraindications and precautions for that device.

Contraindication	Identified By	Example
Acute injury/	Written Questionnaire	"When did this injury occur?"
inflammation	Clinical Evaluation	Assess the cardinal signs of inflammation
Implanted metal	Written Questionnaire	"Have you had a fracture that required surgery?"
		"Do you have implants such as plates or screws?"
	Clinical Evaluation	Observe the area to be treated for surgical scars
High blood pressure	Written Questionnaire	"Are you currently taking medication for high blood pressure?"
	Clinical Evaluation	Assess blood pressure
Circulatory impairment	Written Questionnaire	"Have you been diagnosed as having circulatory problems such as peripheral vascular disease, blood clots, or Raynaud's phenomenon?"
		"Are your hands or feet sensitive to heat or cold?"
		"Have you been diagnosed as having a heart condition?"
	Clinical Evaluation	Assess capillary refill
		Observe the feet and ankles for edema
Cardiorespiratory insufficiency	Written Questionnaire	In addition to findings for high blood pressure and circulatory impairment:
		"Are you taking medication for your heart?"
		"Have you ever suffered a heart attack or stroke?"
		"Do you ever suffer from chest pain?"
		"Do you regularly suffer from shortness of breath or have difficulty breathing?"
	Clinical Evaluation	Inspect the nail beds for cyanosis or enlargement
Thrombophlebitis ■	Written Questionnaire	"Have you been diagnosed as having blood clots?"
		"Do you suffer from unexplained swelling in the feet and ankles?"
	Clinical Evaluation	Homans' sign for deep vein thrombosis
Sensory impairment	Written Questionnaire	"Do you suffer from tingling, burning, or numbness in your arms or legs?"
	Clinical Evaluation	Perform a sensory (dermatome) screen
Infection	Written Examination	"Are you currently taking prescription antibiotic medications?"
	Clinical Evaluation	Inspect the area for signs of infection including pustules, increased temperature, and red streaks
Cancer	Written Questionnaire	"Have you ever been diagnosed with cancer?"
		"Do you have constant unexplained pain at night?"
Pregnancy	Written Questionnaire	"Are you pregnant or is there the chance that you are pregnant?"

Thrombophlebitis: Inflammation of the veins.

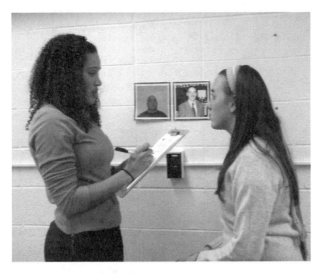

Figure 3–2. **The Patient Interview.** Much of the success in treatment planning lies in effective communication between the patient and the clinician.

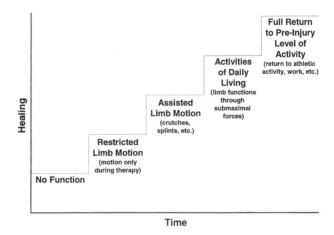

Figure 3–3. **Return to Function After Injury.** The return to the preinjury level of activity follows a progressive sequence in which one level of function must be obtained before progressing to the next level.

Although each treatment session should begin with a patient interview, a full reevaluation of the patient's condition should be conducted at regular intervals (e.g., at the end of a goal period). Ongoing reevaluation allows the patient's current state to be compared with baseline information. A determination can then be made as to whether the patient has improved as expected or if the treatment plan must be modified because of a lack of patient progress.

Prioritization of the Problems

Prioritizing the patient's problems assists in developing the logical treatment progression. This step requires an understanding of pathophysiology, the events associated with each stage of the healing process, and the beneficial effects (and the potentially hazardous effects) that each modality has on the injury response process. Prioritizing the problems based on their cause-and-effect relationship to the patient's chief complaints gives rise to an orderly treatment sequence, defining the focus of **self-treatment ■**, and maximizing the use of available treatment time.

The key to resolving the patient's functional deficit is to identify the problem or problems that trigger the other signs and symptoms. A question that can be used in prioritizing the treatment plan is "What other signs and symptoms will be reduced if this problem is resolved?"

Consider a patient who cannot bear weight secondary to pain, decreased range of motion (ROM), and swelling in the left ankle. Which one of these problems should receive the highest treatment priority? If our treatment approach focused solely on pain, the patient would still be unable to walk properly because of the swelling, decreased joint ROM, and a lack of strength. Indeed, a treatment approach of this nature would more than likely aggravate the remaining problems. The ROM exercises could not be adequately conducted because of the patient's pain and joint swelling, leaving swelling reduction as our highest treatment priority.

Recall that swelling places mechanical pressure on the nerve endings, inhibits blood flow to and from the area, and expands the tissues in the area. A treatment plan that emphasized edema reduction would decrease pain and increase ROM, enabling the return of normal gait. Because pain itself is so debilitating, reducing symptomatic pain must be emphasized. The treatments used to reduce swelling (e.g., ice, compression, and elevation) are likely to have a direct effect on suppressing pain transmission by lessening the pressure on nerve endings (compression and elevation) and slowing nerve conduction velocity (ice). The physician may also prescribe prescription or over-the-counter anti-inflammatory or pain medication.

Once inflammation has been controlled, swelling reduced, and limited pain-free motion restored, functional exercises can be initiated. The ROM exercises, stretching, balancing, proprioception, and strengthening protocols would be introduced into the treatment plan, followed by functional exercises leading to normal gait and a return to the preinjury activity level.

Goal Setting

Clear, concise, and measurable goals translate the prioritized problem list into a well-structured treatment plan (Box 3–2). Short-term and long-term goals guide the rehabilitation program by establishing timelines, identifying outcomes, and providing a benchmark to measure the effectiveness of the treatment protocol. The patient meeting the established goals indicates that the program may advance to the next stage. A lack of progress may indicate

---

Self-treatment: Treatment or rehabilitation performed by the patient without direct supervision including home treatment programs.

TABLE 3–3   Tools Used in the Evaluation of Orthopedic Injuries

Tool	How Measured	Information Gained	Contraindications to Use
Subjective information	Active listening and note taking on the subjective information offered by the athlete, coach, teammates, and others.	(1) Injury mechanism, (2) inflammation stage, (3) functional limitations, and (4) treatment considerations based on outcomes of prior treatment.	None.
Active range of motion	Goniometric measurement or a percentage of full movement in the case of the spine.	Ability to move actively or passively with reference to specific motions.	Acute unstable musculoskeletal injuries. Orthopedic tests that would over stress unstable or recently repaired structures.
Resisted range of motion (strength)	Measurement by manual muscle test using a grading scale, a hand-held **dynamometer ■**, or an isokinetic device. May also use descriptors of the neuromuscular function and integrity of the involved tissues: strong and pain-free (normal), strong and painful (tendinitis), weak and painful (musculotendinous tear), or weak and pain-free (musculotendinous tear or neurological involvement).	Indication of muscular strength deficits. Can also determine injury to a muscle or tendon by eliciting pain and/or weakness associated with contraction of the muscle or muscle group.	Acute unstable injuries to ligaments, tendons, or bones. Any orthopedic test that would directly stress unstable or recently repaired structures. Recent repairs of ligaments or tendons.
Edema/effusion	Circumferential measurement with a tape measure around specific landmarks or **volumetric measurements ■**.	Indication of the presence of swelling or edema relative to the opposite extremity.	None.
Weight-bearing status	Measurement as full, partial, or non–weight bearing. Can also be described as a percentage of full weight bearing.	Ability of the patient to bear weight in the presence of pain, swelling, weakness, and/or decreased range of motion.	None.
Atrophy or **hypertrophy ■**	Circumferential measurement with a tape measure and result compared with that for opposite extremity.	Determination of the decrease or increase of tissue mass. Note that there is little correlation between limb girth and strength.	None.
Pain	Pain rating scale of 0 to 10, with 0 being no pain and 10 being the worst pain imaginable.	Presence of pain with a specific functional activity (squatting), movement (shoulder flexion), special test (valgus stress to the elbow), or at rest.	Caution should be exercised not to use a functional activity to assess pain that may compromise unstable or recently repaired tissues.
Deep tendon reflex	Grading system in an orthopedic population: 0 = absent, 1 = **hyporeflexia ■**, 2 = normal.	Determination of the functional level of the reflex arc.	Recently repaired tendon.

(Continued on following page)

Dynamometer: A device used for measuring muscular strength.
Hypertrophy: To develop an increase in bulk, for example, in the cross-sectional area of muscle.
Hyporeflexia: Diminished function of the reflexes.
Volumetric measurement: Determination of the size of a body part by measuring the amount of water it displaces.

TABLE 3–3　Tools Used in the Evaluation of Orthopedic Injuries (Continued)

Tool	How Measured	Information Gained	Contraindications to Use
Sensation	Light touch to bilateral areas of the body having the same dermatomal or specific nerve distributions.	Assessment of the sensory nervous system. Note that dermatomal distributions may vary greatly from person to person.	**Dementia** ■ or disorientation.
Joint mobilization	Evaluation of the accessory motions found in joints. Graded as **hypomobile** ■ , normal, and **hypermobile** ■ .	Determination of the presence of adequate accessory motion needed to produce normal physiological motion.	Acute unstable injuries to ligaments, tendons, or bones. Recent repairs of ligaments or tendons, moderate to severe **osteoporosis** ■ .
Balance and proprioception	Test of the ability to balance or successfully determine joint position compared to the contralateral limb or normative data. Can be a simple stance test, replication of joint position test, or use of a balance assessment system.	Determination of the function of the proprioceptive receptors in a joint.	Any contraindication to weight bearing on one leg. Any test that would directly stress unstable or recently repaired structures.
Flexibility	Assessment of muscle length by fixing one end of the muscle and moving the other end until maximum length is reached. Can sometimes be measured goniometrically or assessed as normal or tight compared with the uninvolved limb.	Determination of whether a muscle or muscle group is functioning at a normal length or if it is producing abnormal stresses because of tightness.	Acute injuries to musculotendinous tissues. Any test that would directly stress unstable or recently repaired structures.
Posture	Inspection and observation of posture and comparison with normative information.	Assessment of abnormal tissue stress caused by poor postural control or habits.	None.
Special tests	Use of tests designed to (1) elicit pain in the presence of pathology, (2) measure ligament laxity, or (3) evaluate the integrity of structures, etc.	Determination of clinical function and degree of pathology.	Acute unstable injuries to ligaments, tendons, or bones. Recent repairs of ligaments or tendons.
Biomechanical assessment	Observation and measurement of biomechanical problems that can alter function. It may be performed as a specific measurement (leg length) or observed as a part of a functional activity (gait analysis).	Determination of the causes of abnormal stresses placed on the body by inherent biomechanical problems. Some-times the effects of these problems can be decreased or eliminated with exercise or the use of **orthotics** ■ .	Any analysis that would directly stress unstable or recently repaired structures.
Function	Measurement as the capability of a patient to perform **activities of daily living** ■ at work or home as well as sport-specific function.	Determination of the amount of function the patient has with regard to a specific injury.	Any functional task that would directly stress unstable or recently repaired structures.

Activities of daily living (ADLs): Fundamental skills that are required for a certain lifestyle, including mobility, self-care, and grooming.
Dementia: The progressive loss of cognitive and intellectual functions without impairment of perception or consciousness. Symptoms include disorientation, memory impairment, impaired judgment, and impaired intellectual ability.
Hypermobile: An abnormally large amount of motion.
Hypomobile: An abnormal limitation of normal motion.
Orthotics: Orthopedic devices for correcting deformity or malalignment.
Osteoporosis: A porous condition resulting in thinning of bone. Most commonly seen (but not exclusively) in postmenopausal women.

Case Study Part 2: Problem Recognition

The following problems have been identified based on the information presented in the case study scenario:

1. Decreased ability to function without pain
2. Poor patellar mobility and tracking secondary to muscular weakness and soft tissue adhesions, including the presence of a keloid
3. Increased swelling of the right knee as compared with the uninvolved knee
4. Decreased range of motion of the right knee
5. Decreased flexibility of the quadriceps, hamstrings, and calf muscles on the involved side
6. Improper biomechanics of the right foot (pathological subtalar **pronation** ■)

Commentary

- The pain ratings are important because pain indicates pathology and affects the individual's quality of life. Even though this patient is active, attention must be paid to the functional limitations affecting her daily life and work. Her relatively sedentary occupation contributes to her discomfort. Certainly she spends more time per week sitting at her desk, sitting in meetings, and going up and down stairs than she does exercising. Pain experienced during palpation should not be used to determine improvement in the patient because the amount of pressure applied to the area is not well controlled.
- The finding of joint effusion is significant. Accumulation of 20 to 30 mL of fluid within the knee joint capsule may cause inhibition of the vastus medialis, suggesting alteration of patellofemoral biomechanics leading to chronic inflammation.
- The ability to restore ROM this long after surgery may appear to be futile, but scar and tissue remodeling can remain active for 12 to 24 months. The chronic pain and swelling could indicate that the

inflammation and remodeling phase is still active, increasing the possibility of restoring the tissue. Keep in mind that scarring, decreased patellar mobility, and muscle tightness negatively affect ROM. The loss of even a few degrees of ROM is problematic because of the biomechanical changes at the patellofemoral joint. This can lead to other biomechanical changes in both lower extremities caused by a length discrepancy that is created when the patient is weight bearing.

- Findings of a hypomobile patella, decreased ROM, and chronic swelling may be indicative of **hypertrophic** ■ scarring of the **infrapatellar** ■ area. Abnormal patellofemoral joint biomechanics and patellofemoral pain are the most common complications after an ACL reconstruction. Normal tissue biomechanics must be restored before normal joint biomechanics can return and pain be decreased.
- Decreased flexibility of the quadriceps and hamstrings may cause increased stress on the knee joint capsule, retinaculum, and patellofemoral joint. The most common compensatory motion caused by tightness of the gastrocnemius and soleus is foot pronation, leading to increased tibial rotation and increased lateral forces on the patellofemoral joint.

Even though the patient mentions that her knee "gives out," it is not listed as a problem because the results of all special tests were negative. In this case, the "giving out" sensation is most probably indicative of pain, quadriceps inhibition, or muscle weakness and will be resolved as these individual problems are addressed. If the patient continues to report this problem after strength has returned and swelling has decreased, ligamentous stability should be reevaluated and/or the patient referred back to the physician.

that the treatment approach needs to be modified. Properly written and documented goals are also used for insurance and legal purposes and demonstrate the criteria used to decide when to discharge the patient from care.[94] When based on **outcome measures** ■, treatment goals can be used as the basis for research on treatment efficacy.[95]

Treatment goals are estimates of the patient's

progress at a specific points in time and should be consistent with the patient's priorities, lifestyle, and expectations.[96] The patient and, when applicable, the patient's family should be encouraged to participate in setting the treatment goals.[97] Patient compliance with the protocol and the program's effectiveness are increased when the goals are understood and agreed on by all involved.[98-100]

Hypertrophic: Increased size.

Infrapatellar: The distal portion of the patella including the patellar tendon.

Outcome measure(s): Data used to evaluate the efficacy of a treatment program or protocol.

Pronation: An inward flattening and tilting of the foot, resulting in the lowering of the medial longitudinal arch.

Case Study Part 3: Prioritization of the Problem

The patient's problems ranked in terms of treatment priority are:

1. Improper foot biomechanics
2. Decreased flexibility and range of motion of the quadriceps, hamstrings, and calf muscles
3. Swelling of the right knee
4. Poor patellar tracking
5. Pain during stair climbing, sitting, and contraction of the right quadriceps
6. Inability to play soccer

Commentary

Correcting the biomechanical causes for the patient's pain and dysfunction takes the highest priority in this treatment program. The patient may excessively pronate to compensate for the lack of dorsiflexion arising from tightness of the calf muscles. This will place increased stress on the patellofemoral joint and contribute to decreased ROM of the knee and ankle. To prevent further compensation in the kinetic chain, the gastrocnemius and soleus flexibility must be increased.

- If, after normal gastrocnemius-soleus flexibility is restored, hyperpronation of the feet is still believed to be contributing to the pathology, a trial use of orthotics would be warranted. Treating the symptoms of pain and swelling without addressing the possible causes will provide only temporary relief of the symptoms. The plan must contain therapeutic exercises and the correction of biomechanical problems in the patient.

- The patient's effusion causes pain and inhibition of the quadriceps. Eliminating the swelling will improve the quadriceps tone, ability to improve strength, and the ability to control patellar tracking within the femoral groove. If the treatment does not eliminate the swelling, the patient should be referred back to the physician.
- The hypomobile peripatellar tissues are important in the overall health of the patellofemoral joint. Before the quadriceps can properly track the patella through active muscle contraction, the patella must be able to move freely. Hypomobility of the peripatellar tissues hinders normal tracking and places pathological stresses on the joint. Along with restoring normal movement, the clinician must emphasize neuromuscular reeducation of the muscle group to provide active control.
- The pain and dysfunction caused by tendinitis are primary contributors to the patient's problems, and some clinicians may rank these as the highest priority. In this case, we chose to focus on eliminating the stresses that cause the inflammation and will purposefully avoid strengthening exercises through painful arcs of motion; strengthening will occur only within the patient's pain-free ROM.
- The functional problems of this patient have not been given the highest treatment priority. The treatment is prioritized to eliminate and correct those problems that contribute to the symptoms. We would expect to see improved function as the patient's symptoms are decreased.

Perhaps the most important function of treatment goals is to motivate the patient. Motivated patients will most likely be more compliant in actively participating in their recovery.

The treatment goals and outcomes are relative to the pathology being treated. Ideally, the optimal goal is a full recovery or "100%." In some cases, "98%" may be the highest possible outcome but would be sufficient for a full return to activity. Clinically, full function may never be restored, but the final outcomes may still be sufficient to meet the patient's specific needs.

Consider the two goals presented in Table 3–4: a loosely defined goal, "To increase active dorsiflexion," and a more measurably stated goal, "To increase active dorsiflexion to 10 degrees." In the first example, the patient may show improvement by increasing active dorsiflexion from 0 to 8 degrees, but because 10 degrees of dorsiflexion is required for a normal gait, the patient probably will not demonstrate a normal walking gait. Noting that the patient

has increased active dorsiflexion to 8 degrees documents improvement in the ROM and the fact that the patient must still gain 2 degrees of dorsiflexion to achieve the treatment goal.

Long-Term Goals

Long-term goals provide direction to the treatment plan by identifying and quantifying the final outcomes of the program. In most cases, the long-term goal is to return the patient to the preinjury level of function, but this is not always feasible (Table 3–5). Although long-term goals are subject to modification throughout the treatment process, they are revised less often than short-term goals. Long-term goals are also fewer in number than short-term goals. Most important, long-term goals identify the patient's needs as the focus of the treatment rather than the individual pathologies afflicting the person.

Although every attempt should be made to make long-

Box 3-2. Developing Written Goals

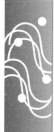

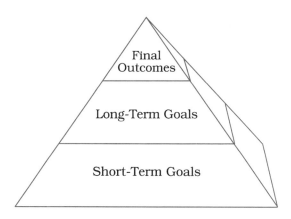

Short-term (1 to 14 days) and long-term (more than 14 days) goals should be stated in objective, measurable terms that describe the quality and quantity of the desired outcome. Not only should the question "Has this goal been met?" be answered with a "Yes" or "No" response; they should also describe the magnitude of the performance. Suppose you must obtain a score of 73 to pass an examination on your ability to write patient goals. A qualitative measure of your success would be a grade of "Pass" or "Fail" when your examination was returned. Although this scoring system informs you (and your instructor) if you scored above or below the passing point, it does not indicate by how much. If the examination is returned with a grade of 99 or 66, you can base your performance relative to the passing point.

Start the goal writing process by taking all of the prioritized problems, and in an orderly fashion, formulate the final treatment outcome, a list of long-term goals, and the list of short-term goals. Some short-term goals may apply to more than one long-term goal. The final step is to determine a reasonable time frame for the accomplishment of each goal.

Goals can be written using the ABCD format and should be stated in terms of what will be accomplished rather than what limitations will still be present (e.g., "Shoulder elevation = 140 degrees" versus "Shoulder elevation limited 30 degrees"). This serves to motivate the patient and also keep the clinician focused on how the plan must be altered to facilitate the patient's progress. Goals should be written in precise versus general terms for each problem. For example, a general short-term goal stating that "All ROM will increase 50 degrees" may not be clear if some motions are increased by only 30 degrees, whereas others are increased greater than 50 degrees.

The ABCD Goal Writing Structure

Segment	Purpose	Example
Audience	Person who will perform the task	"The patient will." "The patient and coach will modify practice to ..." "The patient and employer will alter..."
Behavior	Description of task to be performed using action verbs	"The patient will demonstrate 90 degrees of knee flexion."
Condition	Definition of tools, devices or techniques used in obtaining the goal	"The patient will balance for 30 seconds using one hand for support."
Degree	Quality with which the task will be performed, usually described in numerical terms	"The patient will demonstrate 90 degrees of knee flexion."

Adapted from Kettenbach, G: Writing SOAP Notes, ed 2. FA Davis, Philadelphia, 1996.

TABLE 3-4	Measurable Goals
Problem	The patient has an inversion ankle sprain.
	Active range of motion produces 2 degrees of dorsiflexion and the patient cannot ambulate with a normal gait.
Nonobjective goal	To increase active dorsiflexion.
Objective goal	To increase active dorsiflexion to 10 degrees.
Reevaluation	The patient has 8 degrees of active dorsiflexion.
Assessment	The patient has met the nonobjective goal of increasing active dorsiflexion but has not met the objectively stated goal. Because a minimum of 10 degrees of dorsiflexion is accepted as the requirement for normal gait, we can assume that the patient has an altered gait.

term goals measurable, they should also be functional. Goals such as "To return to full competition in college football" or "To return to the preinjury level of activity at work" define the final outcome of the patient's therapy, and successful completion of the activity is measurable.

Short-Term Goals

Short-term goals describe the patient's projected progress in a specific time frame. The short-term goals focus on the specific problems identified during the evaluation that, if met, will achieve the long-term goals. The length of time set to achieve the short-term goals depends on the specific condition at the time of the evaluation. In general, the time established for meeting the short-term goals is the time that the clinician feels is needed to produce a measurable change in the patient's condition. These typically are in terms of 2 weeks or less.

The short-term goals serve as measuring sticks for the treatment plan. Subsequent patient reevaluations will determine if the patient is meeting the goals. If the short-term goals are not being met, the treatment program should be reevaluated and appropriate changes made.

Treatment Planning

Once the patient's problems have been identified, prioritized, and the appropriate goals have been established, the planning of the treatment naturally follows. Treatment planning is the application of your knowledge of the physiological effects of the therapeutic modalities and exercise to resolve the problems and to achieve the goals established for the patient's rehabilitation. The stage of the healing process and the choice of therapeutic techniques largely determines what types of modalities will resolve the pathology (Fig. 3–4).

The decision process regarding the type of modality to use (e.g., heat, cold, electrical) is based on the tissue characteristics, their **conductive properties** ■, the stage of the healing process, the depth to which the particular modality penetrates, and the desired physiological responses for the stage of inflammation (Fig. 3–5). Once the type of modality to use has been determined, the optimum method of application is determined based on physical characteristics such as the size and shape of the surface area being treated. For example, if a chronic lateral ankle sprain is being treated and there is little or no swelling, the

TABLE 3-5	Feasible Goals
Problem	The patient has degenerative disk disease of the lumbar spine.
Nonfeasible goal	The patient will be pain-free.
Feasible goal	The patient's symptoms will be controlled with therapeutic exercise so that he or she is able to return to full function.
Assessment	With a chronic condition such as degenerative disk disease, the patient will most likely have a continuation of the symptoms or have intermittent symptoms. A feasible goal is to control the patient's symptoms to the point at which the individual can function within the limits of pain.

Conductive properties: The ability of a tissue to transfer heat (from a high temperature to a low temperature) or electrical energy.

Case Study Part 4: Long-Term Goals

At the time of discharge, the following long-term goals will be achieved:

1. The patient will be able to perform normal ADLs (e.g., climbing stairs, prolonged sitting) without pain.
2. The patient will be able to fully return to soccer and other recreational activities.
3. The patient will display normal strength in the right leg.
4. The patient will display normal ROM in the right leg.

Commentary

Long-term goals 1 and 2 reflect the patient's expected treatment outcomes as derived from the patient interview. The remaining goals describe the functional behaviors that would be necessary for the patient to return to full athletic activity (goal 2). Each of these long-term goals will be addressed by one or more short-term goals. Notice that not all of the patient's problems are specifically cited in the long-term goal list. These issues, such as swelling, are addressed by the short-term goals.

Case Study Part 5: Short-Term Goals

The following short-term goals have initially been established for this patient:

1. The patient's hyperpronation will be controlled through stretching the calf muscles.
2. The patient's edema will be decreased by 0.5 cm around the joint line.
3. Medial patellar glide will improve to two out of four patellar quadrants.
4. The patient's flexibility will increase to:

   Quadriceps: Knee flexion will increase to 140 degrees.

   Hamstrings: Knee extension will increase to 0 degrees.

   Calf Muscles: Dorsiflexion will increase to 15 degrees.
5. The ROM of the knee will be from 0 to 140 degrees.
6. Quadriceps can contract during exercise without pain.
7. The patient will be compliant and independent in a home exercise program.
8. The patient will not participate in soccer at this time.

Commentary

A 2-week period of short-term goals is initially set because it will take this long to appreciate changes in the condition of this patient. Goals have been set that can either be measured or easily answered as met or not met. The goals are a reasonable expectation of what the patient's condition should be after 2 weeks. All the goals represent progress in the condition and, if met, will signify that the plan is working.

- The patient's hyperpronation must be controlled to obtain a normal gait pattern. The physical evaluation findings indicate tightness of the calf muscles that prohibits an appropriate amount of dorsiflexion. Orthotics can be used to assist in restoring normal biomechanics. Decreasing the amount of swelling within the joint capsule can prevent inhibition of the vastus medialis oblique, further improving biomechanics by assisting in terminal knee extension and patellar tracking. Flexibility and ROM for the entire lower extremity will be emphasized.
- Decreasing the adhesions associated with functional shortening of the lateral patellar retinaculum will increase medial patellar glide. This goal will probably not be achieved during the 2-week time frame, and we would expect to see improvements in patellar mobility as the amount of swelling is decreased and the strength of the VMO increases. Exercises will have to be conducted to improve patellar tracking. The pain associated with contraction of the quadriceps should be decreased as patellar tracking is improved.
- Goal 8, "The patient will not participate in soccer at this time," is different from the others in that it describes a behavior the patient must avoid. In this case, the rest from the aggravating activity is important for the rest of the treatment plan to be effective. With this in mind, the patient must remain compliant with her home treatment program and stay within her prescribed limits of physical activity.

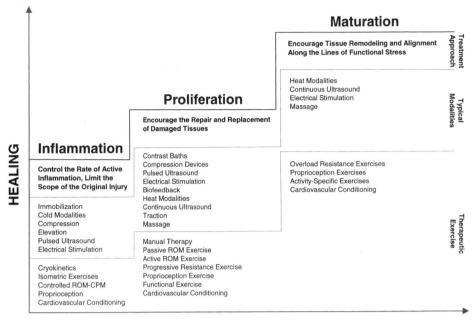

Figure 3–4. **Modality Boilerplate.** Each stage of the injury response has specific treatment goals that best respond to certain modalities or therapies. When the patient is in the "overlap" phase between two plateaus, the modalities and therapeutic exercises from the advanced stage on the right are commonly followed by the modalities of the lesser stage on the left. For example, a patient may use a hot whirlpool and perform active range-of-motion exercises followed by the use of an ice pack. CPM = continuous passive motion. (Adapted from Buxton, BP: Physiological considerations of healing. In Anderson, MK and Martin, M [eds]: Quick Reference Guide in Athletic Training. Williams & Wilkins, Baltimore, 1998, p 57.)

modality of choice would probably be heat. In this scenario, the physical characteristics of the lateral ankle (an irregular surface) would most likely call for the use of a warm whirlpool rather than a moist heat pack because a heat pack would not fit the contour of the area being treated.

A common frustration is that in many cases there is no one "best" choice of modality. Often the final decision of what modality to use is based on personal comfort, past experience with the modality, and patient input. However, this situation can also work to your advantage. If satisfactory results are not being obtained from one modality, the treatment protocol can easily be modified to incorporate an alternate modality.

Considerations of the Healing Stage

Each stage of the injury response process has special needs that must be addressed during treatment. Although the time needed to reach each stage of the healing process differs from case to case, the process of healing and the associated treatment strategy follow an orderly, predictable sequence (see Fig. 3–4).

A common trait among these treatment approaches is the need to maintain, and in some cases improve, the patient's cardiovascular level. Except in conditions in which cardiovascular exercise is impractical or medically contraindicated, some form of cardiovascular endurance exercise should be incorporated into the patient's treatment plan. Patients who are suffering from lower extremity injuries may be able to exercise with an upper body **ergometer** ■ or perform pool or wheelchair exercises (Fig. 3–6). In cases in which the upper extremity is injured, stationary bike exercises, pool exercise, or jogging may be used for cardiovascular maintenance.

Active Inflammatory Stage

Initially following the onset of acute trauma or after surgery, the treatment approach should attempt to reduce the amount of active inflammation and to contain the scope of the original injury by reducing secondary hypoxic injury and controlling edema and spasm. The inflammatory response is necessary, but controlling its secondary effects is critical to restoring the patient back to activity as quickly as possible. Cold modalities are used to reduce the amount of secondary hypoxic injury, reduce pain, and

---

Ergometer: A device used to measure the amount of work performed by the legs or arms.

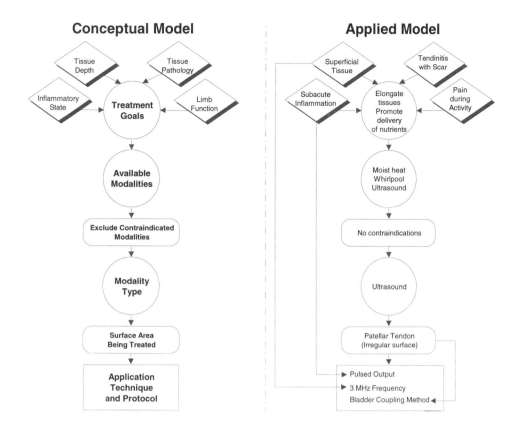

Figure 3–5. **Decision-Making Scheme for the Selection of Therapeutic Modalities.** The model on the left shows the factors used when deciding what therapeutic modality to use. First, the treatment goals are considered, along with the types of tissues that are injured and the current inflammatory state. Contraindicated modalities are excluded from the modalities available to the clinician and the most appropriate modality type is selected. The contour and size of the body area are then considered in deciding the best application technique. Note that often more than one modality can be considered the best to use. The applied model demonstrates the decision making for a patient with subacute patellar inflammation.

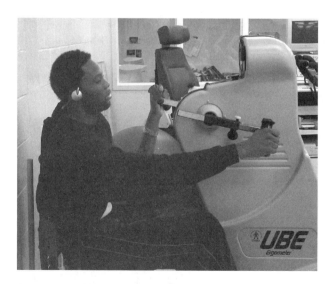

Figure 3–6. **Upper Body Ergometer.** Used to maintain cardiovascular endurance in patients suffering from lower extremity injury or other conditions that would prohibit running.

eliminate spasm. Compression devices and elevation are used to encourage venous and lymphatic return, and immobilization devices are used to limit the limb's ROM. Electrical stimulation may be used to help to reduce pain.

Exercise may take the form of gentle, pain-free ROM and possibly **isometric** ■ exercises within the patient's pain tolerance. In some acute injuries or postsurgical conditions, a physician may prescribe continuous passive motion exercises to maintain joint mobility. Obtaining this motion should not come at the expense of compromising tissue integrity. Cardiovascular maintenance programs should be implemented as soon as possible into the rehabilitation program.

Proliferation Phase
The proliferation stage overlaps portions of the inflammatory and maturation stages (see Fig. 1–5). During the proliferation stage, the treatment goal is to assist the body in delivering oxygen and nutrients necessary to repair the injured tissues and to remove the inflammatory waste

---

Isometric: Muscle contraction without appreciable joint motion.

products. This goal is met by increasing blood flow to and from the injured tissues.

ROM is needed to stretch the tissues, to prevent functional shortening of the fibers, and to encourage the alignment of collagen along the lines of stress. Low-intensity tension is placed on the structures to slowly increase their tensile strength and to assist in the formation of proprioceptive receptors. Proprioceptive activities and muscle reeducation exercises are begun to help protect the limb during ADLs. Newly formed capillary buds are fragile, and care must be taken not to damage them through excessive joint movement or increased tissue tension.

Early in the proliferation stage, these needs may still conflict with the residual effects of acute inflammation. As the signs and symptoms of acute inflammation are resolved, the patient should report decreased pain. Edema may continue to congest the delivery of fresh blood and the modalities used during this stage may tend to increase edema, so a balance must be maintained among the treatment approaches. A common example of this is the use of heat before rehabilitation exercises, followed by ice application afterward.

Maturation Phase

Therapeutic modalities are used during the maturation phase to increase tissue extensibility and to control postexercise inflammation because the tissue is still remodeling to form a strong, permanent repair. Usually, this scar tissue does not have the same functionality as the tissue it replaces, so the fibers must be arranged along the lines of functional stress to prevent the scar from creating limitations in ROM or strength.

Proprioceptive activities and muscle strengthening are used to protect the limb during exertion. These exercises should follow a functional progression from that of ADLs to sport- or work-specific activities (e.g., walking, jogging, running in a straight line, running in all forms, and cutting).

Patient Self-Treatment

The patient's compliance with the program determines the return to full, unaltered activity in the least possible time. The time spent between treatment visits is the most important factor in determining the return-to-activity time frame. A kind of "protective custody" is formed when the clinician is working directly with the patient. In this situation, the clinician ensures that the patient complies with the prescribed routines. However, once the patient leaves this structured care, his or her behavior will either reinforce or hinder the healing process.

Most rehabilitation plans contain home treatment components with which the patient self-administers treatments (e.g., an ice pack), performs exercise routines (e.g., straight-leg raises), and adheres to modified activity (e.g., the use of crutches). Noncompliant patients reduce their

actual therapeutic activities to the time spent with the clinician and may cause harm to their condition by not following the prescribed protocol (e.g., not using crutches as prescribed, going dancing 2 weeks after anterior cruciate ligament reconstruction). Compliance with the full scheme of the rehabilitation program can be increased by educating the patient about the nature of the injury being treated, the benefits of complying with the home treatment program, and the potential consequences of straying from the plan.

To help maintain compliance, self-treatment plans should include no more than three treatments or exercises at any one time. The patient should be instructed on how to perform the self-treatments and exercises before being allowed to leave the treatment facility. These instructions should be given to the patient in writing, and illustrations that depict the exercises to be performed are also helpful.

Reevaluation

Reevaluation determines the patient's progress toward meeting the short- and long-term goals. If the short-term goals are met, new short-term goals are established, and any necessary adjustments to the plan are made. If the goals are not met, identify the reason or reasons for the deficiency. After identifying why the goals were not met, reestablish short-term goals and develop a new treatment plan based on the reevaluation of the patient (Table 3–6).

This portion of the problem-solving approach should assess the initial decision-making and planning process. Asking yourself questions such as "were the original goals too aggressive or too conservative," "what other factors that I didn't anticipate affect the patient" helps build proficiency in treatment planning. Making notations of your strengths, weaknesses, and common errors (and everybody makes them) in treatment planning serves as a good self-assessment tool. Once you notice trends, you can build on your strengths and correct your weaknesses.

■ Influences on Patient Care

The physical setting where the treatment is provided influences the patient's treatment plan. Possible clinical settings include acute care hospitals, subacute settings, home care, outpatient rehabilitation, and athletic training rooms. The focus of treatment and the criteria for discharge vary from setting to setting. In many instances, a patient is discharged from one rehabilitation setting to enter a different setting. For example, an athlete who receives hospital-based therapy after surgery is then discharged to the college's athletic training staff. An industrial worker who has suffered a back injury would receive outpatient therapy and then participate in a **work hardening** ■ program before returning to work.

Work hardening: Job-specific exercises used to prevent work-related injuries or to rehabilitate injured workers.

Case Study Part 6: Treatment Planning

The following treatment approaches have been selected to meet the short-term goals:

1. Orthotics to Control Hyperpronation

Theory

Permanent control of foot motion is needed to decrease recurrent stress on the patellofemoral joint.

2. Thermal Ultrasound Application to the Lateral Retinaculum

Output of 3 MHz; 6 minutes; high intensity.

Theory

Ultrasound is applied over the lateral retinaculum while patellar mobilization is being performed. Stretching the tissues during heating is more effective than mobilization alone.

3. Patellar Mobilization

Theory

Increase patellar motion through stretching of peripatellar tissues before performing ROM and neuromuscular reeducation techniques.

4. Electrical Stimulation

Motor-level stimulation targeting the quadriceps femoris muscle group.

Theory

Electrical stimulation will help restore normal neuromuscular innervation. The patient would be encouraged to voluntarily contract the muscle during stimulation to maximize motor unit recruitment. Once the patient can voluntarily contract the muscles, biofeedback can be used to further develop muscle strength during functional exercise.

5. Flexibility Exercises: Quadriceps, Hamstrings, and Gastrocnemius-Soleus Muscle Group

Minimum of 30 seconds, five repetitions each.

Theory

Increasing flexibility will improve the joint mechanics and decrease abnormal stress on the joint capsule. Flexibility techniques should produce a gentle stretch in the involved muscle but not cause pain in the patellofemoral joint. A 10-minute warm-up on a stationary bicycle could be used to physiologically elevate tissue temperatures before stretching as long as the patient did not have symptoms while on the bike.

6. Strengthening of the Hip, Hamstring, and Gastrocnemius-Soleus Muscle Group

Theory

Strengthening exercises can be performed immediately as long as the exercises do not create pain at the patellofemoral joint.

7. Cardiovascular Exercise

Theory

The patient is very active and must maintain her cardiovascular fitness. An upper body ergometer could be used. The patient could also attempt freestyle swimming for cardiovascular endurance as well as for strengthening of the lower extremity.

8. Ice

Theory

The patient's program may create inflammation in the patellofemoral joint. Application of ice would be effective because the affected tissues are superficial.

9. Home Exercise Program: Patella Mobilization, Flexibility Exercises, and Ice

Theory

When increasing the home program beyond three exercises or modalities, the clinician should use the best judgment based on the time available to the patient to perform the exercises, the motivation of the patient, and the activity level of the patient.

The treatment plan is affected by both internal and external factors. Internal factors include the experience and expertise of the staff and the type of equipment available. External influences include time and financial constraints imposed by insurance companies, the time the patient is able to dedicate to the supervised and home therapeutic program, the support the patient receives from friends and family, and the patient's motivation.

Treatment plans for patients hospitalized in acute care settings will focus on stabilizing the patient and preparing him or her for discharge to subacute care, home, or outpatient rehabilitation. The goals of treatment are more immediate, focusing on short-term goals such as wound healing, restoration of ROM, and maximal independence in **transfers** ■ and mobility.

Patients who can be discharged from hospital care but

Transfers: Assisted patient mobility, such as moving from a wheelchair to a bed.

TABLE 3-6	Reasons for Not Obtaining Goals
Unrealistic goals	Initial patient goals were too ambitious given the time established.
Unobtainable goals	Established goal was not physically possible.
A plan that is too conservative	Protocol used did not evoke the physiological responses required for healing to occur in an appropriate timeframe.
A plan that is too aggressive	Protocol increased unwanted inflammatory reactions or otherwise delayed the healing process.
Incorrect treatment used	Treatment used was not appropriate for the patient's healing stage or was inappropriately applied.
Problem missed during the evaluation	Treatment plan cannot address problems that were not identified.
Problem not addressed in the plan	Treatment plan did not adequately address all of the patient's problems or were incorrectly prioritized during the treatment plan.
Lack of patient compliance	Patient did not follow the home care program, did not give full effort during rehabilitation sessions, or did not follow activity recommendations.
Unexpected and unavoidable setbacks	Uncontrollable events in the patient's life (e.g., illness, accident, family matters) delay the patient's progress and prevent a regular treatment schedule.

require further rehabilitation may be discharged to a subacute care facility, such as a skilled nursing facility or rehabilitation hospital. The treatment goals focus on attaining maximal functional independence so the patient may return home. The focus of the plan will be developing the ROM, strength, and mobility required to allow the patient to perform ADLs with the least amount of assistance at home.

Because it is more cost-effective than inpatient care, home rehabilitation is becoming increasingly popular. This is an ideal alternative for patients who no longer require inpatient care but cannot attend outpatient rehabilitation. Patients may lack the resources to get to the outpatient setting or may lack the physical mobility required to travel to and from the clinic. The goals and plan for the home care are more long-term in their scope, similar to those of outpatient settings, focusing on the maximum relief of symptoms and restoration of function. If the patient will eventually attend outpatient rehabilitation, the home rehabilitation plan will focus on permitting the patient to travel to the clinic.

Outpatient rehabilitation focuses on obtaining maximum patient independence. Areas that enter into the treatment plan are relief of symptoms, restoration of range of motion, strength, balance, and return to ADLs. Although the goals and plan focus on these areas, the ultimate goal is the restoration of function.

Historically, patients may have received outpatient rehabilitation until all aspects of their condition had been alleviated or they had reached a plateau. With restrictions placed on the amount of outpatient rehabilitation by the insurance industry, new factors have entered into the planning process for a patient's condition. Time constraints may affect the patient's treatment planning. For example, an insurance company may establish a limit of 60 consecutive days of treatment, regardless of the severity of the

Case Study Part 7: Changes in the Program

Changes in the program are based on the patient reevaluation. These findings indicate which treatment goals have been met. If goals have not been met then the treatment program must be modified accordingly.

1. Ultrasound can be used before patellar mobilization until the tissue extensibility is restored and patellar mobilization are discharged from the program.
2. Modalities other than ice may be used to treat the patellar tendinitis. Phonophoresis and iontophoresis are two options.
3. Electrical stimulation and biofeedback may be discharged as the patient demonstrates control of the patella during functional activity.

4. Strengthening exercises are progressed based on the clinician's judgment. Using pain-free exercise as a guide, any strengthening exercise may be performed throughout the rehabilitation.
5. ROM exercises would be eliminated as full motion is restored. The patient would be encouraged to continue active-assisted ROM.
6. As soon as the patient could tolerate standing on one leg without symptoms, proprioception exercises would be added to improve function in the surgically reconstructed leg. The patient would be taken through a functional progression of running, agility training, and sport-specific skills to return to full activity.

injury. With less serious injuries, the treatment goal is to return the patient to normal activity, but in instances of greater pathology, the focus may be for the patient to recover to the point at which self-treatment could be conducted in a safe manner.

The athletic training room presents some unique circumstances for treatment planning. The patients are a specific group of athletes who are the sole responsibility of the clinicians. The patients in this case tend to be in better physical condition, younger, and oriented to intense exercise. Patients may be available for multiple treatment sessions per day. All of these factors allow for more aggressive goal setting and planning. Because the circumstances are unique, clinicians must keep in mind that the expectations for return to activity are also unique. The patients in this setting will be returning to activities that place them under great physical stress and require psychological confidence, and these factors must be considered when formulating a treatment program.

● Chapter Highlights

The PSA consists of five segments: Recognition of the patient's problems, prioritization of the problems, goal setting, treatment planning, and reevaluation.

- Recognition of the problem: Identifies the patient's pathology and possible contraindications to treatment techniques.
- Prioritization of the problem: Determines the logical treatment progression.
- Goal setting: Identifies the treatment outcomes and provides benchmarks for gauging patient progress.
- Treatment planning: Selection of therapeutic modalities and exercises based on the patient's pathology and treatment goals.
- Reevaluation: Determines if the treatment plan has been successful in meeting the patient's goals and subsequently adjusts the treatment plan.

4

Administrative Considerations

This chapter discusses administrative concerns as they relate to the delivery to treatment and rehabilitation programs, maintaining a safe facility, and the role of medical records. Issues relating to billing and third-party reimbursement are also discussed.

The actual application of therapeutic modalities is only part of the treatment and rehabilitation process. Health care is bound by governmental regulations and fraught with areas of potential liability. Federal, state, and institutional regulations are meant to ensure safe, effective, and efficient patient care. Further administrative needs are required when the services provided are billed to a third party for **reimbursement** ∎

■ Legal Considerations in Patient Care

The legal issues associated with patient care are a constant concern. During treatment and rehabilitation, the caregiver's minimum legal duty is to prevent further injury or harm to the patient by performing the tasks at hand in a professionally accepted manner. Professional ethics and responsibility mandate that the care provided be in the best interest of the patient and be effective in meeting the patient's goals in a safe and efficient manner. Courts have ruled that reasonable facilities and equipment, as well as qualified personnel, are necessary to provide proper medical coverage.[101]

Before using a therapeutic modality, the operator must be familiar with the effects and side effects of the device or protocol being used and be able to recognize contraindications that prohibit their use (see Box 3–1). Proper application also requires knowledge of the characteristics, maintenance requirements, and safety considerations of the devices being used.

This section primarily addresses legal considerations pertaining to patient treatment and rehabilitation. It does not represent all aspects of liability that the clinician may be exposed to in the daily routine of professional practice.

Scope of Practice

The legal boundaries that define the manner in which clinicians may practice, or the **scope of practice**, are established on a state-by-state basis through regulation such as licensure, registration, or certification (Table 4–1). Such regulation exists to protect the public from unqualified health-care providers. There are differences in the scope of practice from one profession to another and discrepancies in the scope of practice for a single profession from state to state.[102] The scope of practice also defines the **standard of care** used in liability cases.

Reimbursement: Payment for services rendered.

Professional practice statements such as the National Athletic Trainers' Association Position Statements or the American Physical Therapy Association Guide to Physical Therapy Practice also serve to define appropriate professional behavior, although state legislation may override these documents. The institutional or facility **Policies and Procedures Manual** should reflect both state practice acts and professional **standards of practice ■**.

Generally, state practice acts make provisions for students to practice those skills that they have been taught, as long as these techniques are delivered under the direct, on-site supervision of a licensed practitioner. The services that students render cannot generally be billed for services to an insurance carrier.

Knowledge of the legislation that regulates professional practice in your state is a part of your professional responsibility. This information can be obtained through the state board overseeing your field of practice.

Medical Prescriptions

State regulation may require that a physician directly refer all patients or require a physician's supervision of the care given. Professions granted **direct access ■** by state regulation do not require a physician's referral. However, third-party payors will often not provide reimbursement for services unless the care is prescribed (and in some instances, preauthorized) by a physician. In cases in which the patient is prescribed a specific protocol for treatment, the clinician is bound to abide by the prescription unless a verbal or written change is granted by the physician.

In states where direct access is not granted, the use of some therapeutic modalities such as electrical stimulation, ultrasound, and traction may also require a physician's prescription. Cold packs, moist heat packs, and whirlpools typically do not require a physician's prescription.

Phonophoresis ■ (Chapter 7) and **iontophoresis** (Chapter 13) that use prescription medications required that each patient being treated have a prescription for the medication being used. State pharmacy practice can further restrict the use of these protocols. "Blanket prescriptions" in which the medication is prescribed to the health-care facility and then administered at the practitioner's discretion may be common practice, but its legality is precarious.

Informed Consent

Except in cases of emergency care and treatment, patients must grant their consent to be treated. Otherwise, an act of criminal **battery ■ or professional negligence** may have been committed. A patient seeking care is a form of implied consent, so simply treating someone without formal consent being granted is normally not sufficient to determine professional negligence in this area. For negligence to be determined for a lack of inform consent, the patient must suffer **harm** from the care rendered (see Negligence, p 76).[103, 104]

Before beginning the treatment, patients should be educated about the modality or exercise, the sensations to be expected during the treatment, and any adverse signs or symptoms that indicate that the treatment should be modified or discontinued. The patient should also be fully informed about any potential hazards associated with the use of the device and any residual side effects (Table 4–2). Informed consent is not a waiver of the patient's right to pursue claims of negligence or liability against the facility or clinician.

All facilities should have an informed consent form signed by the patient on file or documentation of verbal consent. If the patient is younger than the age of 18 years,

---

TABLE 4–1	Types of Professional State Regulation
Type	*Description*
Licensure	Most restrictive form of regulation. Establishes the scope of professional practice, sets the minimal education standards for licensure eligibility, and protects professional titles.
Certification	A state-based certification test is often required; defines the scope of professional practice, but does not protect professional titles.
Registration	A person must register with the state Board prior to practicing the profession. Registration has minimal (if any) prerequisites. Only registered professionals can use the given title.
Exemption	Allows one profession to perform some of the skills and roles of another profession without infringement.

Battery: The unwanted touching of one person by another.

Direct access: Health-care services can be provided without physician referral. Note that a physician referral is often required for third-party reimbursement.

Phonophoresis: The introduction of medication into the body through the use of ultrasonic energy.

Standards of practice: The criteria against which an individual's performance is measured.

TABLE 4-2	Elements of Informed Consent for Treatment

Description of the modality or exercise
An overview of how the device works
Benefits provided by the device (physiological responses)
Expected normal sensations
Adverse sensations to be reported
Potential hazards associated with the device
Residual effects

this document (and all other consent forms) must be signed by the patient's parent or **legal guardian ■**. This document notwithstanding, patients have the right to refuse any particular form of treatment or modality.

Patient Confidentiality

All medical records are confidential documents. The patient must grant written permission before these records are released to an outside individual (e.g., physicians, college recruiters, employers). The authorization to release medical information should explicitly state to whom the information is being released and for what purpose it will be used (Table 4–3). Additionally, if this information will be used to assist in determining the patient's medical clearance for an athletic college scholarship or employment, the release form should include a disclaimer noting that the information found in the medical records will be used as a part of the decision-making process and may either aid or hinder the patient's cause.[94]

The unauthorized release of medical information, including treatment and rehabilitation records, not only breaks the bond of patient-caregiver confidentiality but may also be outside the parameters of state and professional codes of conduct. Liability may be found through **defamation of character**. When this occurs by the spoken word, it is termed **slander**; when it occurs through print it is termed **libel**.

Individuals who are in the public eye, athletes for example, have a lesser right to privacy than "private" figures. However, health-care providers must maintain a high standard of ethical and moral conduct to protect the patient's right to confidentiality from being breached.

The patient should be allowed to review his or her medical records on request.[95] Whenever the patient's medical records are removed from the facility, the date the records were sent, the purpose of the release, and the date of the return should be documented.

The duration of time that medical records must be kept is established by each state. The records of current and past patients must be stored in a manner conducive to maintaining their confidentiality.

The **Health Insurance Portability and Accountability Act** (HIPAA), originally created by the US Health and Human Services Department to ensure that workers have continual health-care coverage while changing jobs, has affected the maintenance and communication of patient records and information.[105] The HIPAA regulations affect past, present, and future medical records. Health-care facilities must be in compliance with these regulations by April 14, 2003, but state regulation can override the HIPAA requirements.

In addition to standardizing the electronic exchange of medical information, HIPAA also seeks to ensure patient confidentiality and control the security of this information. HIPAA also increases the importance of informed consent and release of information documents, which must be written using understandable terms. HIPAA is currently undergoing significant changes that can potentially affect the manner in which health-care providers manage medical records and other forms of patient information.

Negligence

Patients have the right to receive safe and proper treatment without exposure to undue hazards. This implies that care is provided in a professionally competent and accepted manner. This standard covers not only the physical act of applying therapeutic modalities and implementing rehabil-

TABLE 4-3	Medical Information Release Authorization

Description of the information to be released
The individual or individuals who will receive the information
For what purpose or purposes the information will be used
The date that the authorization will expire
The person granting the authorization's signature. If someone other than the patient authorizes the release, the relationship between the two (e.g., parent, guardian) must be documented.
The release of information form should also note that the patient has the right to revoke the authorization, consequences of failing to sign the authorization, and that the potential exists that the recipient of the information may be redisclosed.

Legal guardian: An individual who is legally responsible for the care of a minor.

itation routines, but also means that the devices being used must be in safe operating condition and the facility free of foreseeable hazards (Box 4–1).

Professional negligence is loosely defined as providing care that falls below the minimally accepted standard (substandard care), although there are many factors and influences leading into the final determination.[104]

Professional standards of practice, the facility policies and procedure manuals, and state practice acts form the benchmark for determining if the care provided was standard or substandard.

Not all negligence that occurs in the patient-care setting is professional negligence. Hazards that are not pertinent to the care being rendered, tripping on an upturned

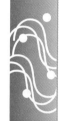

Box 4–1. Negligence

Negligence implies the lack of malice and forethought that results in harm. Ordinary negligence is the failure to act as a reasonable and prudent person would in the same situation. Gross negligence is the complete failure to foresee and act upon a situation to prevent harm from occurring (e.g., not having a fence around a swimming pool). Professional negligence occurs when the individual provides substandard care or acts outside of the professional norms or acts out of carelessness, thus breaching the duty of care (see below).

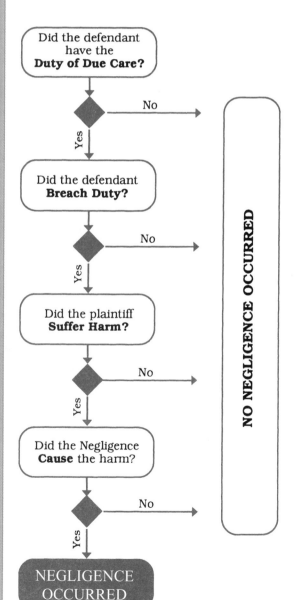

For the courts to find a person guilty of negligence, a clear relationship between the alleged act of negligence and the harm suffered by the individual must be established. A court must first establish if the defendant had a **duty** to act on behalf of the plaintiff. Then, if a duty exists, the court asks, "Did the defendant **breach this obligation?"** The breach of duty is determined by comparing the actions that the defendant did (or did not) take with those that a reasonable and prudent person having a similar level of education and experience would have taken under similar circumstances (see Box 4-2). If the defendant had no duty to respond or was determined to have acted in a reasonable and prudent manner, no negligence can be found.

If the defendant was obliged to respond but failed to act in a reasonable and prudent manner, the court must determine if plaintiff actually suffered physical or **financial harm.** The final link in determining negligence is that of **causation.** A direct relationship between the actions of the defendant and the harm suffered by the plaintiff must be established.

Ordinary torts can be classified as:

Malfeasance: The performance of an unlawful or improper act.

Misfeasance: The improper performance of an otherwise lawful act. (commission)

Nonfeasance: The failure to act when there is a duty to act. (omission)

Malpractice: Negligence on the part of a professional serving in the line of duty.

carpet in a clinic for example, could be determined as being ordinary negligence, but because this event has no bearing on patient care, professional negligence would not be considered.[104]

A supervisor can be held liable for ordinary or professionally negligent acts performed by employees or students, or their failure to supervise, under the **doctrine ■** of **vicarious liability** (sometimes called "**respondeat superior,**" Latin for "let the master answer").[104, 106] In cases in which physician supervision is required, the physician can be liable for the acts of the health-care provider, especially when Food and Drug Administration (FDA)–regulated modalities or medications are involved.

Negligent Delivery of Treatment

Negligent professional behavior occurs when a health-care practitioner departs from the standard of care imposed by society.[107] If a clinician, or a student serving under the direction of the professional staff, performs unnecessary or detrimental acts, liability for failure to use **due care ■**, or is reckless or careless in treatment, professional negligence could be found.[101] Negligence may be classified into two types on the basis of behavior: (1) omission and (2) commission.

Omission occurs when an individual fails to respond to a given situation when a response is necessary to limit or reduce harm. Consider the following example: a patient goes to the physician with complaints of an injury. If the physician fails to evaluate, treat, or refer the injury, an act of omission may have occurred. In this case, the negligent act stems from the physician's failure to properly respond to a medical condition.

Commission occurs when an individual acts on a situation but does not perform at the level that a reasonable and prudent person would (Box 4–2). In the rehabilitation process, an act of commission could occur if a clinician treats a stress fracture with ultrasound. In this example, negligence occurred because the individual acted, but with an improper technique.

The relationship between the patient's treatment goals and professional negligence is remarkably ambiguous. Goals could be construed as a "professional promise" to the patient. However, goal setting is generally considered to be professional judgment rather than a contractual obligation between the caregiver and the patient, especially when the patient is made a part of the goal-setting process. What is of concern is the manner in which the goals are communicated to the patient. Presenting the goals as "… to obtain 90 degrees of knee flexion" is much different than the clinician stating "I will be able to make you walk again." If miscommunicated or overstated, therapeutic promises can be interpreted to be a binding legal contract that could result in a breach of contract or fraud if they are not met.[104]

Negligent Care of Facilities

The design of the rehabilitation facilities must guarantee that patients receive treatment in the safest environment possible. The facility should also conform to state codes governing health-care facilities.

Ensuring safety is an ongoing process involving thorough planning, evaluation, and maintenance. Injury sustained through improper or unsafe facilities can result in charges of negligence being brought against the staff, the facility, or the institution. The hydrotherapy area and areas where electrical modalities are used are of special concern regarding the facility's physical design (Table 4–4).

Knowingly using an unsafe therapeutic modality or other equipment reflects negligence on the part of the clinician or facility administrator. All therapeutic equipment must be inspected and calibrated by a qualified service technician yearly, although more frequent service should be performed on intensive-use equipment. Manufacturer and/or local regulation pertaining to equipment in a health-care facility may also mandate shorter inspection and maintenance cycles. The inspection or service date, the technician, and the services performed should be documented and kept on file.

Proper daily care is needed to help maintain the equipment in safe working order. Wear and tear through normal use is to be expected, and proper care of the equipment will keep this to a minimum. Logical precautions, such as avoiding liquid spilling into the equipment, proper positioning of electrical cords, and regular inspection of plugs assist in maintaining the longevity of equipment.

Food and Drug Administration Oversight

The United States Congress established the US Food and Drug Administration (FDA) to provide oversight to ensure that medical devices (and medications) are reasonably safe and effective. The FDA's **Center for Devices and Radiologic Health** regulates a wide range of therapeutic devices to ensure patient safety, to evaluate claims regarding their efficacy, and to eliminate unnecessary exposure to **radiation ■** emitted from the device. Other FDA regulations relate to those devices that produce electrical interference or are controlled by microprocessors. The FDA also is the major regulator of over-the-counter and prescription medications. A discussion of this process is beyond the scope of this text.

Doctrine: A statement of fundamental government policy.

Due care: An established responsibility for an individual to respond to a given situation in a certain manner.

Radiation: The transfer of electromagnetic energy that does not require the presence of a medium (see Chapter 5).

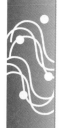

Box 4–2. So Who Is This Reasonable and Prudent Person?

When an individual is charged with negligence, the person's actions are measured against those that a reasonable and prudent person would have taken in the same situation. So who is this reasonable and prudent person?

The reasonable and prudent person is a fictitious individual who is created by the courts. Variables such as the defendant's age, physical condition, education, professional experience, and mental capacity are factored together to determine what actions would be considered reasonable.[107] Because the criteria for determining reasonable and prudent change from situation to situation, and because juries are not qualified to determine what the proper standard of care would be in a given situation, a mechanism exists that identifies what is "reasonable and prudent" for any given type of situation.

Through the testimony of expert witnesses, professional position statements, and other accepted (documented) protocols, a standard of care is established that describes what actions should be expected of an individual in a given situation. The standard of care is determined by the professional standards of practice, state practice acts, and the testimony of experts. Profession-specific documents such as the Guide to Physical Therapist Practice can also be used to judge or to determine the appropriateness of the individual's actions.

If a practitioner exceeds his or her scope of practice and enters another field, for example a health-care professional who performs a task that falls within a physician's domain, that practitioner would be held to the standard of that profession.

Although the FDA's definition of a medical device is quite lengthy, it can be summarized as relying on a mechanism other than chemical action to diagnose, treat, or prevent conditions in humans and animals.[108] Medical devices are assigned to one of three classifications based on their potential harm to the individual in the event of their failure with a class I device carrying little risk to the patient and class III presenting the greatest risk. The device may also be restricted to sale to, or under the orders of, a licensed physician or health-care practitioner.

Before being marketed, devices controlled by the FDA, such as electrical stimulators, and therapeutic ultrasound must undergo a rigorous Premarket Review Process (PMA) that evaluates the product's inherent safety, efficacy, and manufacturing processes.[108]

Devices having the investigational status designation are not eligible for reimbursement and a strict clinical protocol must be used. Devices in the PMA must be granted an Investigational Device Exception by the **Institutional Review Board** ■ before being applied to humans.

The FDA also regulates product labeling, information, and instruction manuals.[109] Regulated therapeutic modalities must minimally include the information presented in Table 4–5 and, when possible, the device description, indications, and contraindications should appear together on the first page of the product information. If the device is being marketed on the basis of clinical data, the information presented is expanded to include supporting clinical studies. Depending on the

TABLE 4–4   Considerations for Safe Facilities

- All electrical modalities should be connected to a ground-fault interrupter. Whirlpools and jacuzzis must be connected to these devices (see Box 4–5).
- Patients must not be permitted to turn whirlpools or jacuzzis on or off while they are in the water. Ideally, the switches should be located so that they cannot be reached from these tubs.
- Hydrotherapy areas must have an adequate line of sight to monitor patients.
- All modalities should be inspected and calibrated by a licensed professional at intervals prescribed by the manufacturer.
- Flooring should be made of a nonslip material.
- A policies and procedure manual for describing the use, inspection, and maintenance of the equipment should be maintained.

Institutional Review Board: An institutional agency that oversees medical investigations involving humans or animals by assuring compliance with federal regulations. In research involving humans, the IRB functions to protect the rights and health of the subjects.

TABLE 4–5   US Food and Drug Administration (FDA) Device-Labeling Minimal Requirements

Information	Description
Description	A brief description of how the device functions, physical characteristics, and performance characteristics.
Indications	Describes the intended use and the specific types of conditions (e.g., injuries, diseases) that warrant the use of the device.
Contraindications	Describes conditions where the risk of use outweighs the anticipated benefits.
Warnings	Warnings describe hazards (serious effects or death) to use other than those described in the contraindications. An example of this would be a device such as diathermy that also emits radiation.
Boxed warning	The FDA may require that especially concerning or hazardous warnings be placed in a box close to the device description. Warning boxes are generally issued when clinical human data, or in some instances animal data, show a high probability of adverse effects.
Precautions	Alert the user to special care necessary for safe and effective use of the device. Precautions is used as the plural of "Caution."
Adverse effects	An undesirable side effect stemming from the use of the device that is not presented in the Contraindications, Warnings, or Precautions sections.
Conformance to standards	If applicable, this section refers to the FDA medical device, materials, or standards used in the evaluation and/or manufacture of the device.
Operator's manual	A brief description of the contents of the unit's operator's manual.
Patient's manual	A brief description of the contents of the unit's instruction/informational packet for use by the patient.

complexity of the device, an operator's manual, patient's manual, and references may also have to be included with the device.[109]

Occupational Safety & Health Administration Regulations

The Occupational Safety & Health Administration (OSHA) is a division of the US Department of Labor that is charged with protecting the health of most of the United States workforce. OSHA both develops codes—safety standards and regulations—to prevent work-related injuries and illnesses and, through an enforcement branch, fines or prosecutes employers who do not comply with the standards. Many states also have departments that work cooperatively with OSHA.

OSHA has developed a series of rules that require institutions to protect workers from blood-borne pathogens such as the hepatitis B virus (HBV). These rules apply to all employees who may, as a part of their job requirements, be exposed to biological hazards (biohazards) including blood, synovial fluid, and saliva.

The **Universal Precautions** ■ are a set of standards that help prevent against accidental contact with biohazards. Exposure control plans focus on personal protection

(and when applicable, protective equipment), proper disposal of medical wastes including hypodermic needles and scalpels ("sharps"), and proper handling of soiled laundry. Institutions must develop an exposure control plan to protect its employees and conduct an annual in-service that describes these policies and procedures.

■ Medical Documentation

Medical records serve several functions (Table 4–6). Within the context of this text, treatment documentation serves a valuable purpose in the planning and evaluation of the treatment protocol. Documentation provides a method to determine the effectiveness of the protocol and records describe the quantity and quality of the services provided by the facility. Not only could failure to maintain accurate, legible medical records result in professional negligence, the absence of these records places the caregiver in an indefensible position.

The length of time that medical records should be kept after the patient is no longer receiving care is based on the state's **statute of limitations** ■, but the computerization of these records allow them to be stored indefinitely.

Medical records document the course of the patient's

Statute of limitations: A legal time limit allowed for the filing of a lawsuit.
Universal Precautions: A series of steps, established by OSHA, that individuals should take to avoid accidental exposure to bloodborne pathogens. Universal precautions are also referred to as "Standard Precautions."

TABLE 4–6	Purpose of Medical Records

Serve as a communication tool among health-care providers

Document treatment or rehabilitation progression

Assist in the continuity of care given

Provide a basis for developing future treatment and/or rehabilitation plans

Documents informed consent

Serve as a legal document to show that the medical staff provided reasonable care

Memory aid in legal cases

Meets professional requirement and standards

Serve as a basis for reimbursement decisions

Basis for discharge/discontinuation of care

Provide a database for research

care from the initial visit to discharge or return to activity. As described in Chapter 3, specifically stated treatment goals and objective measurements should be used. From both a legal and third-party reimbursement perspective, remember that "If it wasn't documented, it wasn't done."

Several different record-keeping systems are used for clinical documentation (e.g., SOAP, HOPS) and desktop computers and Personal Digital Assistants (PDAs) are playing an increasing role in this area (Table 4–7). Third-party reimbursement places unique and increased demands on the documentation process. The following sections describe the role and purpose of medical records.

Continuity of Care

The evaluation findings and the treatment plan should be documented as specifically and clearly as possible so that continuity of care can be maintained when more than one clinician is involved in the patient's care. The medical record should include all communication to and from other health-care providers, the patient, and the patient's family members as well as referral forms.

Treatment Rendered and Patient Progress

Treatments provided to a patient on a daily basis must help meet the goals documented in the patient's plan. Daily treatment sessions should begin with an interview and reevaluation to determine the patient's current status. That is, did the prior treatment improve the patient's condition, worsen it, or was there no appreciable change? (see Chapter 3).

Documentation of the day's treatments should describe the date, time, individual or individuals providing the care, the pathology being treated, the therapeutic modalities and exercises that were used, and the parameters used.

Following the conclusion of the treatment, reinterview the patient and note any necessary adjustments to the patient's medical record. Even seemingly minor changes in a modality's application parameters can produce drastically different physiological effects. A lack of continuity of treatment is a pitfall that may delay the patient's rehabilitation progress. Well-documented evaluation and treatment records help to ensure that all caregivers—and the patient—understand the patient's current **disposition ■**.

TABLE 4–7	Types of Medical Records

Document	Purpose
Medical history	Details prior medical conditions. Identifies conditions that contraindicate the use of certain modalities, although the patient should be specifically questioned before applying any device (e.g., a person with a history of cardiovascular disease requiring medication would be excluded from full-body warm whirlpools).
Preparticipation examination	Used with athletes to identify the status of any existing condition physical examination and to determine the current status of preexisting conditions.
Consent forms	Indicates that the patient (or the parent[s] if the patient is under the age of 18 years) has granted permission to be treated. Consent forms do not protect the clinician from liability stemming from acts of negligence.
Injury reports	Used in athletics to document the onset of an acute injury or the aggravation of a chronic condition.
Referral forms	Allows for feedback from the physician regarding the level of activity and prescribed course of rehabilitation.
Prescription record	For modality use (if required) and medications (e.g., phonophoresis, iontophoresis) if indicated.
Treatment record	Provides an ongoing record of the patient's treatment plan and rehabilitation notes.

Disposition: The patient's current physical status and projected course of recovery.

A facility treatment log is a beneficial administrative tool. Documentation of facility usage and the demands placed on the staff and equipment can be used to justify the need for more clinicians or the purchase of new equipment.

Legal Record

Medical records protect both the caregiver and the patient. Well-documented records can assist in proving that the staff exercised reasonable care in the management of an injury. If a liability case were to come to trial, the medical staff may use these records to refresh their memories when testifying about the case, and the documents themselves may be admitted as evidence.[107]

Professional Standards of Practice and most state practice acts require that complete and accurate medical records be maintained. Medical records correlate the care given with that prescribed by the physician. Different work settings such as high schools, colleges, for-profit clinics, and hospitals may also have additional record keeping requirements.

Reimbursement Documentation

Although the primary role of documentation is to improve patient care by ensuring treatment continuity among caregivers, when seeking third-party reimbursement medical records are business documents. Insurance companies require the use of goal-based treatment plans for reimbursement. Therapeutic modalities and therapeutic exercises billed for this purpose will be reimbursed only if they meet the patient's treatment goals.

Third-party payors, insurance companies, may review these documents to determine if reimbursement for the services is warranted. When the bill for service appears excessive or the amount of care provided seems prolonged, the documentation may undergo peer review for determination of reimbursement.

In the case of possible excessive billing, the documentation is compared with the billing during the treatment session. The documentation must be clearly and concisely written so that someone reviewing the chart can gain a full understanding of the care provided in order to make a fair determination of the reimbursement.

The claim reviewer will evaluate the objective measures such as range of motion, pain rating scales, and strength in the patient's record. If the patient appears to continue to show no improvement or if the treatment protocol does not appear to match the patient's goals, payment for services can be declined. Further investigation may be initiated to determine if care was truly needed or if it was unnecessarily extended.

■ Third-Party Reimbursement

The **Centers for Medicare and Medicaid Services (CMS)**, formerly the Health Care Finance Administration (HCFA), oversees the two largest medical payors, Medicare and Medicaid. Other third-party insurance companies use the Medicare and Medicaid standards for establishing their own guidelines in determining what services are reimbursable and the reimbursement rate.

The rate of reimbursement, the amount paid, is frequently based on the usual, customary, and reasonable (UCR) system. Changes in health-care financing and insurance coverage are resulting in the increased use of capitation methods (fixed payment rate per patient) and the resource based relative value scale (RBRVS) system.

Receiving reimbursement for services rendered requires documentation of the condition being treated and documentation of the treatment services that are being billed. The individual or individuals rendering the treatment must be state licensed in their area of practice and the treatment provided must meet the patient's treatment goals. The decision to provide reimbursement for a claim is ultimately left to the individual insurance company.[110]

Billing Codes

Receiving third-party reimbursement for services rendered requires the submission of two forms of documentation: Diagnostic codes using the **International Classification of Diseases (ICD)** and the **Current Procedural Terminology (CPT) codes.**

The ICD codes describe the patient's pathology. The CPT codes describe the care provided to the patient. For billing purposes, the CPT codes must correlate with the ICD codes to be reimbursed. Medicare has established treatment and rehabilitation protocol for most ICD conditions.[105]

Improper coding can result in a claim being rejected. In the worst case, improper coding can result in facility audits, loss of provider status, or fines.[105]

International Classification of Diseases Codes

The International Classification of Diseases codes were developed by the American Hospital Association (AHA) to describe pathology and surgical procedures and arrange them into relevant groups. The National Center for Health Statistics developed the Clinical Modification (CM) of the ICD codes; most relevant to this text is the addition of a classification system for surgical, diagnostic, and therapeutic procedures (Box 4–3). The coding scheme is regularly updated and is now in its ninth edition, carrying the name ICD-9-CM (ICD: International Classification of Disease; 9: Ninth edition; CM: Clinical Modification). The ICD codes are currently undergoing revision and will soon be at version ICD-10 (CM).[111]

Current Procedural Terminology Codes

The CPT codes were established by the AMA Department of Coding and Nomenclature to define those treatments rendered by health-care providers who are licensed by the state to perform the service.[110] The AMA uses the term "therapist" generically, but certain codes, such as evaluation and reevaluation are specific as to the type of professional providing the service.

Physical medicine codes include both therapeutic modalities and therapeutic exercise. Although therapeutic modalities are reasonably well defined, therapeutic exercise is not. Between 1979 and 2001, the definition of "therapeutic exercise" has been changed by Medicare and insurance companies 10 different times and 3 times in an 18-month period.[105]

Therapeutic modalities fall under the CPT's **Physical Medicine Codes** category. The reimbursement rate for most of these procedures is based on 15-minute **time units** that are rounded up or down from the halfway point. Each procedure has a unique CPT code, although on first glance there may appear to be overlap between them. For this reason, CPT coding is usually performed by someone with expertise in this area.

Most therapeutic modalities and therapeutic procedures are covered by the CPT physical medicine code (Box 4–4). However, cold packs and moist heat packs are not eligible for reimbursement unless they are used in conjunc-

tion with another therapeutic procedure (e.g., range-of-motion exercises). Phonophoresis, another technique described in this text, is not billable as well. However, the application of ultrasound is billable or the treatment could be coded as 97039 (unlisted modality), although there is the potential of having the claim denied.

■ Evidence-Based Practice

Changes in the health-care system have caused third-party payors to reexamine those services that are performed for reimbursement. As a consequence, to control costs, third-party payors are requiring documentation and evidence that the treatments being rendered are beneficial to meeting the patient's treatment goals.[112] Treatments rendered must conform with the patient's treatment plan and the devices used must be beneficial to the patient's condition. Proof that therapeutic treatments and, by extension, therapeutic modalities produce the effects that we believe is termed **evidence-based practice**.

The concept of evidence-based practice is not new. Governmental agencies from the Consumer Protection Agency to the FDA have been investigating manufactur-

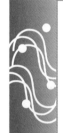

Box 4–3. ICD-9-CM Coding System Examples

ICD-9-CM Description

Knee Bursitis

726.60	**Enthesopathy ■** of knee, unspecified
844.20	Pes anserinus tendinitis or bursitis
844.21	**Prepatellar ■** bursitis

Knee Sprains

844.20	Old disruption of the lateral collateral ligament
844.21	Old disruption of the medial collateral ligament
844.22	Old disruption of the anterior cruciate ligament
844.23	Old disruption of the posterior cruciate ligament
844.00	Acute lateral collateral ligament sprain
844.20	Acute medial collateral ligament sprain
844.21	Acute anterior cruciate ligament sprain/tear
844.30	Acute posterior cruciate ligament sprain/tear

The ICD-9-CM code is a five-digit string (trailing zeros are often dropped) that describes the pathology and structure involved. The evolution of this system has, at times, made the codes relatively disjointed. The first three digits identify the body area, although the progression is not always sequential. The second two digits describe the pathology. In addition to reimbursement purposes, these data are used for record keeping, **epidemiology ■**, and other research purposes. ICD codes change regularly.

The information above is presented for informational purposes only.

Enthesopathy: Pathology of the bony attachment of tendon, ligament, or joint capsule.

Epidemiology: The study of the distribution, rates, and causes of injuries and illness within a specified population. This information may then be used to prevent future occurrence.

Prepatellar: Around the patella.

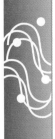

Box 4–4. CPT Coding System (Selected Entries)

CODE	PROCEDURE	TIME UNIT	COMMENT
Evaluation			
97001	Physical Therapy Evaluation	Per-service	For use by a licensed physical therapist with a new patient
97002	Physical Therapy Re-evaluation	Per-service	Follow-up evaluation by a physical therapist
97003	Occupational Therapy Evaluation	Per-service	For use by a licensed occupational therapist with a new patient
97004	Occupational Therapy Re-evaluation	Per-service	Follow-up evaluation by an occupational therapist
97005	Athletic Training Evaluation	Per-service	For use by a licensed athletic trainer with a new patient
97006	Athletic Training Re-evaluation	Per-service	Follow-up evaluation by an athletic trainer
Therapeutic Modalities			
97010	Moist heat pack	Per-visit	For payment, must be used in conjunction with another procedure
97010	Ice bag/ice massage	Per-visit	For payment, must be used in conjunction with another procedure
97014	Electrical stimulation (unattended)	Per-visit	For those treatments which do not require constant clinician involvement (e.g., sensory-level pain control, edema reduction)
97016	Vasopneumatic therapy	Per-visit	Compression for edema reduction
97018	Paraffin bath	Service-based	
97022	Whirlpool therapy	Per-visit	For restoration of range of motion
97022	Fluidotherapy	Service-based	Sterile application for wound debridement
97024	Diathermy	Service-based	Only shortwave diathermy is approved for clinical use
64550	TENS application	Service-based	For pain reduction
97032	Electrical stimulation (manual)	Time-based	Requires constant clinician-patient contact (e.g., trigger point therapy)
97033	Iontophoresis	Time-based	Covers the cost of the technique, medication, and electrodes
97034	Contrast baths	Time-based	
97035	Ultrasound	Time-based	Minimum of 8 minutes billable time required
97039	Unlisted therapeutic modality	Time-based	Requires constant attendance
Manual Techniques			
97012	Manual traction	Per-visit	
97124	Massage therapy	Time-based	
97140	Manual therapy, one or more regions	Time-based	Used to code myofascial release and edema reduction
Therapeutic Exercise			
90901	Biofeedback	Service-based	Used for neuromuscular re-education or relaxation
97110	Therapeutic exercise	Time-based	Used for establishing range of motion, strength, and endurance for one or more joints. Requires one-on-one clinician/patient interaction
97112	Neuromuscular re-education	Time-based	Used for re-education of function, motion, proprioception, balance, etc.
97113	Aquatic therapy	Time-based	
97150	Group therapeutic procedure	Service-based	Clinician constantly oversees two or more patients
97750	Physical performance test	Time-based	Functional evaluations

The above represents common Current Procedural Terminology evaluation and Physical Medicine codes. Evaluation codes are service-based and are not included in time-based treatment services.

These codes change regularly and are presented as an example and, as presented here, should not be used for billing purposes. Refer to the current CPT coding documents for an up-to-date reference on these codes and their interpretation.

ers' claims that products actually perform as claimed and protect the public from fraud, ensuring that devices and techniques perform as claimed. Just as we question the accuracy of the claim that we can lose 50 pounds overnight, we also need to question the benefits of the therapeutic devices and techniques that we use. It is important to distinguish what works from that which does not work.

Although the concept is straightforward, the process of identifying the efficacy of treatment devices is not. Controlled research studies are the key to identifying those techniques that are effective from those that are not effective. The research questions are often along the lines of "How effective is the technique?" or "What is the end result of the protocol?"

Although we may feel that various treatment protocols are effective, the real "evidence" of evidence-based practice is found in professional, peer-reviewed journals. However, a review of the literature often reaches confusing and contradictory conclusions.

Outcomes measures determine the end result of medical care. The determination is made based on the procedures used in patient care and the resulting patient satisfaction and quality of life. Much of the research that has been performed is limited by a small number of patients, a narrow range of physical pathologies or too broad a spectrum of pathologies, and methodological flaws. Because of this, many studies cannot be viewed as being clinically relevant. Additionally, many therapeutic devices and techniques have not been thoroughly investigated.

Each therapeutic modality or classification of modalities (e.g., cold agents, heating agents) presented in this text includes a section titled **Controversies in Treatment**. This section is intended to provide a brief overview of questions and concerns regarding the general efficacy of the device or specific concerns with individual application techniques.

■ Facilities

The physical facility where care is given must be free of potential hazards and be conducive to patient care, including access by disabled patients or clinicians. The hydrotherapy area, treatment area, plumbing, and electrical systems are of particular concern when addressing the use of therapeutic modalities. Hospital-based clinics and some outpatient clinics are accredited by outside agencies such as the Joint Commission on Accreditation of Healthcare Organizations (JCAHO) or state regulatory boards. These organizations may have specific safety guidelines that must be met and the facility may be subject to inspection.

Electrical Systems

The health-care facility's electrical system deserves special scrutiny. The presence of water and the potential for accidental patient contact with electrical sources are potential hazards. Many therapeutic modalities operate on 110-v "household" current (some equipment may operate on rechargeable or replaceable batteries). Other equipment, such as large icemakers, may require 220 volts. Some equipment, such as isokinetic devices, whirlpools, or electrodiagnostic equipment, may require a dedicated circuit, where there is only one outlet. Extension cords should never be used to operate therapeutic equipment.

Electrical outlets leading to whirlpools and other modalities where water is a concern must be served by a ground-fault interrupter (GFI), although GFIs are recommended for all outlets that will serve patients (Box 4–5). Outlets in the treatment area should be located 2 to 3 feet above the floor; in the hydrotherapy area, 4 feet or higher (and out of the reach of patients using the tub). Microprocessor-controlled modalities, such as electrical stimulators, may also require a surge protector. State building and/or health codes may also prescribe other requirements.

Treatment Area

The patient treatment area should be spacious and well lighted. Treatment tables should be approximately 30 inches high, although adjustable tables are useful for certain types of treatments and meet **Americans with Disabilities Act** ■ (ADA) specifications for access by patients or clinicians with disabilities. Split-leg tables allow for the body part to be elevated during the treatment (Fig. 4–1). If shortwave diathermy treatments are to be used in the facility, all-wood tables are required.

Tables should be no less than 30 in. apart from each other. Even using this minimum figure, one or two treatment tables should have more space on the side to allow for range-of-motion exercises, massage, myofascial release, and other procedures.

Fixtures should provide a lighting power of 50 to 75 **footcandles** ■ at a height of 4 feet above the floor. In other areas of the facility, the power of the lighting can be reduced to 30 to 50 footcandles at a height of 4 feet above the floor.[115]

Hydrotherapy Area

The hydrotherapy area possesses unique safety concerns. Here, perhaps more than in any other portion of the health-care facility, the greatest potential for hazards exists. The

---

Americans with Disabilities Act: Legislation passed in 1990 (Public Law 101-336) that protects the right of disabled individuals by creating standards to ensure access and prohibit discrimination in transportation, accommodation, public services, and so on.

Footcandle: A measure of light equal to 1 lumen per square foot. One lumen is the amount of light emitted by one international candle.

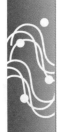

Box 4–5. Ground-Fault Circuit Interrupters

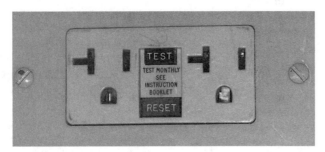

Ground-fault interrupters (GFIs, or GFCIs for ground-fault circuit interrupters) are used to guard against hazardous currents by continuously monitoring the amount of current entering a circuit compared with the amount of current leaving it. If there is a discrepancy of more than 5 mA, current leakage has been detected, and the GFI will stop the flow of electricity to the unit in as little as 1/40 of a second.[113]

Always seeking the course of least resistance, electrical currents tend to stay within the insulation of the path formed by the circuit, but because of condensation, microscopic imperfections in the circuitry, or even dust, some current leakage inevitably occurs. Only two leads are required to complete an electrical circuit; however, most outlets contain a third conductor that leads to the ground. As this name implies, the grounded wire literally leads to a pipe or other conductor that is buried in the ground. Normally, when current leaks into the **chassis ■**, it will follow the ground wire back to the earth. This leakage is termed a "ground fault" and occurs to some degree in all electrical equipment.

Any leaked current must find an alternate path back to the ground. Ideally, this route is through a grounded circuit, but if the circuit is not properly grounded or the leakage is too great, the current must find an alternate route back to the ground. A person who is in contact with an ungrounded device while touching a grounded source (e.g., a whirlpool and a pipe) can easily form this alternate route for the current to take. In this case, the current would leak from the chassis of the ungrounded device and flow through the person to the ground, producing potentially fatal results.

Ground-fault interrupters must be distinguished from standard circuit breakers. Although GFIs stop the current flow at very low amperages, standard circuit breakers require a much larger discrepancy (up to 25 A) to be activated. Circuit breakers are not adequate for use in athletic training rooms, physical therapy clinics, or hospitals, especially in hydrotherapy areas. The 1991 National Electric Code requires the use of GFIs in all health-care facilities that use therapeutic pools.[114] A GFI may be housed in either the wall outlet or in the circuit breaker box. In either case, GFIs are easily recognizable by their TEST and RESET buttons. Each GFI should be tested at regular intervals, with monthly intervals being considered ideal. Each testing date should be documented.

In the event that the GFI trips, disconnect the patient from the unit, and turn off the power to the unit. Check all connections, depress the RESET button on the GFI, restart the equipment without the patient being in contact with it, and ensure that a ground fault does not reoccur. If the GFI trips again, disconnect the unit, label the unit and the outlet "Out of Order," and call for service.

hydrotherapy area typically houses whirlpools, rehabilitation "swim tanks," ice machines, hot and cold water supply (for whirlpools, immersion tubs, and coolers), sinks, refrigerator, freezer, and ice machine.

Ideally, the ON-OFF switches controlling the whirlpool motors should be located so that the patient who is in the tub cannot reach them. If the whirlpool has this switch mounted on the motor, patients are not to turn the unit on or off while in the water. It is a good practice to post

signs stating rules for the use of these devices in the hydrotherapy area.

The hydrotherapy area itself should be in full view of the staff. Because of the noise associated with this modality, this area is normally "glassed off" from the rest of the rehabilitation facility (Fig. 4–2). A closed door will help reduce the noise in the rest of the treatment facility.

Enclosing the hydrotherapy area increases the amount of humidity; ice machines, refrigerators, freezers, and other

---

Chassis: The framework to which electrical components are attached.

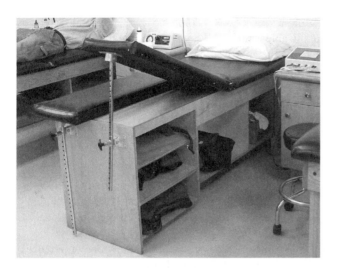

Figure 4-1. **Split-leg Table.** These tables assist in venous return from the lower extremity by being elevated during treatment.

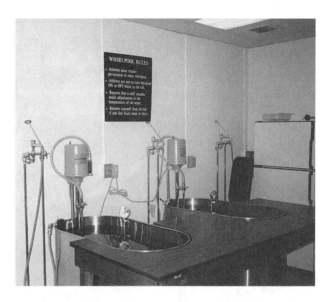

Figure 4-2. **The Hydrotherapy Area.** The hydrotherapy room is a high-risk area. This room should be in full view of the staff and is therefore usually enclosed in glass to prevent humidity and noise from affecting the rest of the facility.

appliances produce heat. The combination of heat and humidity encourages the growth of fungi, bacteria, and viruses. To thwart this problem, the hydrotherapy area should be well ventilated and air conditioned to maintain 40% to 50% humidity and recycle the air 8 to 10 times per hour.[116]

Ideally, each whirlpool should have its own fill faucets, although a hose may be used to fill multiple tubs. Each tub should have a hot and cold control or a mixing valve that regulates the temperature of the water entering the tub (Fig. 4–3). Whirlpool temperature gauges must be annually calibrated. A large swan neck faucet should be available for filling immersion tubs, coolers, and so on.

The floor should be covered with a nonslip surface and should be gently sloped toward one or more floor drains. Each whirlpool should have a dedicated drain.

■ Product Maintenance

Knowingly using an unsafe therapeutic modality can be considered negligent professional behavior. All therapeutic equipment must be kept in its optimum working condition. This requires regular inspection for defects or hazards, periodic cleaning, and professional calibration according to the manufacturer's recommendations.

Electrically operated modalities such as electrical stimulators, therapeutic ultrasound, and shortwave diathermy are required to be regularly (e.g., annually or biannually) inspected and calibrated by a qualified service technician. The date of these inspections must be documented on the unit and the type of work performed should be documented in an equipment maintenance logbook.

Wear and tear of equipment through normal use is expected. Proper treatment of the equipment will help to reduce the long-term toll of use. Logical precautions such as avoiding spills into the equipment, keeping electrical

cords neatly stored, and regular inspection of electrical plugs and leads will assist in maintaining the longevity of the equipment.

If a defect is found in the plug or cord, the GFI continues to trip, or the unit fails to function properly, unplug it, label it as being inoperative, and remove it from the treatment area. A qualified technician should then service the unit. Operators must not attempt to perform maintenance or repairs beyond those that are described in the operator's manual.

■ Policies and Procedure Manual

A policies and procedure manual (manual) delineates the facility's scope of service, operational plans, and standard operating procedures. Policies are used to guide administrative decision making. Procedures describe the processes used to carry out the policies. The standards and procedures described in the policies and procedures manual can be used to determine if professional negligence has occurred. The depth and breadth of policies and procedure manuals cannot be covered here, but there are implications to treatment and rehabilitation that must be discussed.

One of the primary purposes of a policies and procedure manual is to define the roles and lines of reporting amongst administrators and the clinical staff. **Job descriptions** define the roles, responsibility, and minimum expectations for each profession. An **organizational chart** describes the relationships between all of the individuals involved in the delivery of health care.

Standard operating procedures describe the procedures that are to be followed in various situations and may

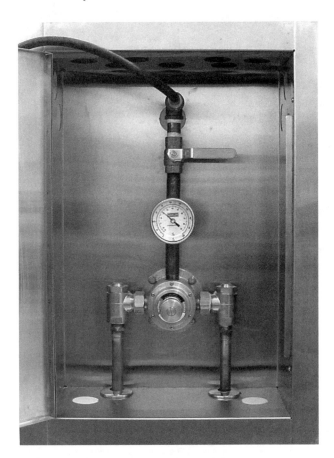

Figure 4-3. **Hot/Cold Water Mixing Valve.** A mixing valve helps prevent scalding by safely controlling the flow of water (bottom control). A thermostat indicates the temperature of the water flow (middle dial) that is controlled by the handle on the top. The thermometer must be calibrated annually. The hose to the whirlpool has been moved out of the way.

include **standing orders** ▪. Standing operating procedures or standing orders are not prescriptive "cookbooks" that dictate the patient's treatment. Rather, they present a conceptual framework for the procedures to be implemented. Procedures for medical emergencies should also be described in this section.

Another portion of the reporting structure that should be covered in the policies and procedures manual are the medical documentation procedures, including annotated examples of how to complete each document and any applicable routing. An appendix of the manual should also include the approved medical shorthand and abbreviations for the facility.

Sections of the manual should be dedicated to how the facility meets the compliance requirements of governmental regulations (including OSHA) and educational or facility accreditation requirements agencies.

● Chapter Highlights

- Engaging in patient health care carries with it an inherent risk of personal and professional legal liability.
- State practice acts establish the scope of practice for each profession, defining the legal boundaries of the care provided.
- Patients must grant consent before being treated, and the treatments should be documented. All medical records are confidential documents.
- Negligence may be ordinary, gross, or professional and is established by duty, breach of duty, harm, and causation.
- In addition to state governments, several other agencies oversee health care, including the FDA and OSHA.
- Patient documentation serves as a communication tool to measure patient progress, ensure continuity of care, a legal record, and is used for third party reimbursement.
- Billing documentation is based on the ICD codes which describe the pathology and the CPT codes that describe the treatment rendered.
- Increased awareness is being placed on the efficacy of modalities and techniques, evidence-based practice.
- Health-care facilities are subject to specific codes and have unique design needs.
- Many therapeutic modalities have special maintenance needs and must be regularly inspected and calibrated by a qualified technician.
- The facility's policies and procedure manual serves as the operational guide for the services rendered.

Standing orders: A "blanket prescription" from a physician describing how injuries are to be managed
   when the physician is not present.

The scenario, recognition, and prioritization of problems and the short- and long-term goals of the patient in this case study are introduced here. Each of the sections in this book concludes with a discussion regarding how the various modalities could be incorporated into the patient's treatment and rehabilitation plan, although not all of the modalities described in this text would be applicable to these cases.

Case Study: Case Study 1

The Patient's Medical History

A 62-year-old man sprained his left ankle 2 days ago while participating in a tennis tournament. He was evaluated by his primary physician and was diagnosed with a grade 1 lateral ankle sprain. He has been referred to you for evaluation and treatment of his injury. The following information has been obtained from the patient and the patient's medical records.

Complaint: He reports that he has pain on weight-bearing, located along the lateral aspect of the left ankle.

History: The patient reports that he "rolled" on his left foot while playing tennis. He was able to continue playing, but the pain increased and the ankle began to swell later in the day. The patient has a history of bilateral ankle sprains.

Diagnostic tests: X-ray studies showed a previous avulsion fracture of the lateral malleolus.

Activity: The patient desires to participate in a tennis tournament 5 days from now.

General medical: The patient has a history of peptic ulcers and has insulin-dependent diabetes.

Contraindications to modality use: The patient has diabetes. Caution must be used with heat modalities if sensory exam of feet is not normal.

Medications: Insulin. The doctor prescribed acetaminophen for the pain because the patient does not tolerate nonsteroidal anti-inflammatory drugs as a result of his peptic ulcer.

Patient goals: To play in the tennis tournament in 5 days. Pain-free ADLs.

Evaluation Findings:

Function: The patient cannot walk without pain. The patient cannot play tennis.

Observation: The patient ambulates with an **antalgic gait** ◾.
Swelling is present along the distal aspect of the lateral malleolus.

The rest of the foot and ankle, including the skin, is in good condition with no signs of ulceration.

Weight-bearing status: Full weight bearing

ROM:	Left	Right
Dorsiflexion (knee extended)	7°	15°
Dorsiflexion (knee flexed)	10°	15°
Plantarflexion	32°	37°
Inversion	5°	15°
Eversion	3°	5°

Swelling:

	Left	Right
Figure eight technique	21.25 in.	19.5 in.
Base of the fifth metatarsal	12.25 in.	12.0 in.

Strength:
Dorsiflexors: 5/5, but painful
Plantarflexors: 5/5
Invertors: 5/5
Evertors: 5/5, but painful

Balance:

	Left	Right
One-leg stance for 20 seconds	2 deviations	0 deviations

Pain rating: 2/10 with level walking

Special tests: All tests for laxity negative

Palpation: Pain over the anterior talofibular ligament

Sensation: Intact for light touch and hot and cold discrimination throughout both feet

This patient is an active senior citizen. Although his age may be a concern, his history of regular participation in competitive tennis indicates that he is a good candidate for relatively aggressive rehabilitation. His history of diabetes could be an influence on the selection of therapeutic modalities and exercises, but this condition appears to be well controlled. Because he is sensitive to nonsteroidal anti-inflammatory medications, his level of discomfort and swelling may be beyond that expected.

Antalgic gait: A gait resulting from pain on weight bearing. The stance phase of gait is shortened on the affected side.

There is noticeable swelling and range-of-motion restrictions in the left ankle, but strength is within normal limits. Balance is a problem, but the fact that the patient is within normal limits for the right leg indicates that this disruption is probably related to the pathology. Pain is slight and there are no other significant findings.

Problem Recognition

The following problems have been identified based on the information presented in the case study scenario:

1. Decreased function secondary to pain, including the ability to participate in tennis.
2. Decreased ROM of the left ankle.
3. Swelling of the left ankle.
4. Decreased balance and proprioception of the left ankle.

Commentary

- The pain rating given by the patient is consistent with an acute grade I lateral ankle sprain. It is significant that he does have pain with weight bearing and must compete again in 5 days. In many instances the course of treatment for this injury would consist of rest, but because he desires to play in a tournament, it is prudent to attempt to return him to safe activity. The ramifications and risks with an aggressive treatment approach must be explained to the patient so that he may make a reasonable, informed decision as to continuing to participate.
- The ROM deficits are probably related to pain and swelling. Running requires a minimum of 15 degrees of dorsiflexion to maintain a normal biomechanical pattern.
- Although swelling is minimal, it may reduce the overall motion in the ankle. The patient's balance difficulties may be affected by swelling disrupting the joint receptors responsible for proprioception.
- The dorsiflexors and evertors evoke strong contractions, but pain is experienced. The pain does not arise from the muscles; therefore, a strength rating of 5/5 is given.
- The patient's balance deficit is a key factor in his return to activity in a safe and timely manner. Balance and proprioception during functional activities related to tennis must be obtained prior to clearing him to play.
- The patient's diabetes and ulcer could have an influence on the course of care, but the diabetes appears to be well controlled. If present, decreased

sensation or ulceration associated with diabetes would affect the modalities used.

Prioritization of the Problem

The patient's problems ranked in terms of treatment priority are:

1. Swelling of the left ankle.
2. Decreased ROM of the left ankle.
3. Decreased balance and proprioception of the left ankle.
4. Decreased function secondary to pain, including the ability to participate in tennis.

Commentary

- Most of the patient's problems are related to swelling within the ankle joint, increasing pain, decreasing ROM, and decreasing weight-bearing ability. The treatment goals should address edema removal as the highest priority while being cautious about causing more swelling.
- The decreased ROM is a significant deterrent to the patient's ability to play tennis in 5 days. To return to safe activity, ROM must be restored to provide an adequate amount of ankle plantarflexion and dorsiflexion. Strength and flexibility will most likely be restored to normal as the swelling and pain are reduced.
- Balance and proprioception are essential to most activities. In the case of this patient, balance is required because he will be called on to quickly stop, start, and change direction. Proper proprioception is needed for the patient's muscles to protect the joint from potentially injurious forces.
- Balance is essential to any activity, either walking or running. This patient's balance is even more essential because he will be called on to stop and start quickly as well as to change directions. The clinician must be careful to respect any pain that the patient has while performing balance exercises. These exercises cannot be performed at the expense of any harm they may do to the injury.
- The inability to function in a safe, pain-free manner is the biggest problem facing the patient and clinician because of the time constraints in this scenario. By addressing these problems, the rehabilitation will lead to a return to safe function.

Long-Term Goals

At the time of discharge, the following long-term goals will be achieved:

1. Regain a normal gait pattern within 5 days.
2. Be able to play in a tennis match using a protective support in 5 days.

Commentary

- The goals are reasonable and obtainable within the 5-day time frame. However, the clinician must carefully evaluate the patient at the end of 5 days to verify that it is safe for him to compete. The patient must be withheld from competition if these goals are not met.
- The ability to return to competition does not imply that the patient is totally healed. After the match, the patient will need to resume therapy so that the rehabilitation program can be completed.

Short-Term Goals

The following short-term goals have initially been established for this patient:

1. Swelling will decrease to within 1/4 inch relative to the right ankle within 3 days.
2. The patient will be able to walk without pain (0 to 1/10) within 3 days.
3. The patient's ROM in the left ankle will be 10° of dorsiflexion, 35° of plantarflexion, 8° of inversion, and 4° of eversion within 4 days.
4. The patient will be able to display equal balance between the left and right ankle within 4 days.
5. The patient will not participate in tennis at this time.

Commentary

- A 3-day period was established for reaching the first short-term goal. Referring back to the commentary for prioritizing the problems, note that swelling must be reduced before any improvement can be seen in the remaining problem areas. If the first goal is met early, the remaining time frames can be accelerated. The fifth goal is different from the rest in that it describes a behavior that is to be avoided. In this situation, the patient must avoid placing harmful stresses on the involved joint.

Treatment Planning

The following treatment approaches have been selected to meet the short-term goals:

1. Intermittent Compression with Elevation

Sixty minutes. Pressure setting of 60 mm Hg with an on-off cycle of 30 seconds "on" to 15 seconds "off."

Theory

Intermittent compression and elevation assists in the venous and lymphatic return of edema. Edema reduction will decongest the area and allow nutrients

and oxygen to reach the damaged tissues. As the edema becomes stabilized, this intermittent compression may be used post-treatment to control the edema.

2. Retrograde Massage

Effleurage strokes from the toes to the lower leg to "milk" edema proximally. "Uncorking" the leg proximal to the ankle precedes the effleurage strokes.

Theory

Effleurage massage will aid the venous and lymphatic system in transporting edema proximally. Movement of this material out of the injured area will decrease pain and help to improve ROM.

3. Range of Motion and Flexibility Exercises

Theory

The patient will need specific exercises to promote increased ROM to achieve functional limits. Cryokinetics may initially be used to speed the reacquisition of motion.

4. Resistance Exercises

Theory

The patient will need to maintain strength in the injured area and return the surrounding musculature to proper function. He may start out with isometric contractions and progress to isotonic contractions or resistance tubing as tolerated.

5. Balance Exercises

Theory

The patient demonstrated balance deficits during the initial evaluation that will decrease optimal function. The patient can use a balance system or one-leg stance exercises, progressing from stable to less stable surfaces as tolerated.

6. Maintain Cardiovascular Conditioning

Theory

Cardiovascular and musculoskeletal endurance must be maintained so that the patient is ready to return to strenuous physical activity.

7. Progressive Return to Activity

Theory

The capability of the injured ankle to withstand progressively more difficult stresses must be addressed to allow the patient to return to activity in a safe manner. The functional progression would include jogging, running, and progressively harder agility, as well as sport-specific drills to tax the injured area.

8. Ice, Compression, and Elevation

Twenty minutes after exercise and during home treatments.

Theory

Cold will decrease the metabolic rate in the treated tissues, helping to limit further damage secondary to anoxia and will assist in decreasing pain. The patient will be educated about how to apply a compression wrap and instructed to keep his leg elevated as much as possible, including at work, at rest, and during sleep.

9. Home Exercise Program: ROM, Strengthening, Balancing Exercises, and Ice with Elevation

Theory

To achieve the goals in a short time, the patient must have an inclusive home program addressing the areas of deficits. Patient compliance is imperative because of the goal of return to activity in 5 days.

Case Study: Case Study 2

The Patient's Medical History

A 16-year-old basketball player has been referred to you by his primary care physician for evaluation, treatment, and rehabilitation. The patient was involved in a motor vehicle accident and has been given a diagnosis of a cervical strain and sprain. The following information has been obtained from the patient and the patient's medical records.

Complaint: The patient reports pain and muscle spasm in his cervical musculature that limits his motion. Basketball practice is scheduled to begin in 1 week.

History: While driving with his father 4 days ago, they were "rear-ended" by another driver. He was in the passenger seat and was wearing his seat belt. He was taken to the emergency room from the accident scene and released home that night. The next day he followed up with his family physician and was referred to you.

Diagnostic tests: X-ray studies taken at the emergency room were negative.

Activity: The patient is a student at the local high school and a point guard on the school's basketball team. He should start for the varsity team this year.

General medical: The patient suffers from asthma; otherwise, he is healthy.

Contraindications to modality use: None.

Medications: The patient uses an inhaler for his asthma. Muscle relaxants have been prescribed for his cervical injury.

Patient goals: To be able to sleep through the night and begin basketball practice as soon as possible.

Evaluation Findings

Function:	The patient cannot play basketball because of pain and spasm.
	The patient cannot sleep through the night undisturbed by pain.
Observation:	The patient wears a soft cervical collar for comfort.
	The patient has a guarded posture.
Active ROM :	Flexion: 50%
(C-spine)	Extension: 40%
	Right rotation: 50%
	Left rotation: 50%
	Right-side bending: 25%
	Left-side bending: 50%
Strength:	Testing of all cervical musculature elicits pain—no grades given because of pain.
Passive ROM:	Flexibility of cervical musculature cannot be assessed due to pain and guarding.
Pain rating:	Pain with right-side bending is 7/10.
	Patient reports constant pain of varying intensity with all ADLs.

Upper quarter screen:	Deep tendon reflexes are 2/2 bilaterally.
	Sensations are intact to light touch bilaterally.
	Result of manual muscle test is 5/5 throughout.
Special tests:	Cervical compression: No radicular pain; increased cervical pain.
	Cervical distraction: No radicular pain; increased cervical pain.
Palpation:	Increased tone is present in the left upper trapezius due to muscle spasm.

Trigger points are palpated in both upper trapezius muscles, with the left more tender than the right.

This patient suffered a "whiplash"-type injury and now has significant deficits in cervical mobility. Cervical fracture, dislocation, and trauma to the spinal cord have been ruled out. The patient's primary complaints are related to muscle spasm that is most likely related to cervical nerve root impingement.

Note that the patient's physical examination could not be completed because of pain and range of motion restrictions. These should be performed as permitted during subsequent re-evaluations.

Problem Recognition

The following problems have been identified based on the information presented in the case study scenario:

1. Inability to play basketball.
2. Inability to sleep undisturbed secondary to pain.
3. Decreased cervical ROM.
4. Inability to assess strength and flexibility of the cervical musculature because of pain.
5. Pain is rated 7/10 during right-side bending.
6. Increased tone because of muscle spasm of the left upper trapezius.
7. Patient wears a soft cervical collar for comfort.

Commentary

- The inability to function is the result of the pain, spasm, and loss of ROM of the cervical muscles. Although all of these are significant problems, the primary reason why someone seeks and needs rehabilitation is to reduce pain and restore function.
- The decreased cervical ROM is most likely a result of pain and spasm versus true joint restriction of the connective tissues about the joint. In an otherwise healthy 16-year-old patient, you would not see changes in the joint structures so quickly after an injury of this type.
- The inability to complete any portion of the patient assessment should be noted, and the reason for the omission should be explained. This documentation serves as a reminder to assess these at a future

date and informs other clinicians who are not familiar with the patient's history that these tests were not performed. By noting that these examinations were not conducted, other clinicians will not assume that areas were not assessed or were assessed and were normal.
- The increased muscle tone of the trapezius is caused by the pain-spasm-pain cycle and is typical after acute musculoskeletal injury, secondary to a reflexive protective mechanism. Although this mechanism is protective during the acute stages of an injury, the clinician must work to relieve the pain-spasm-pain cycle so that healing may take place. The spasm will restrict blood flow and the delivery of nutrients and oxygen to the injured tissues and surrounding areas.
- The soft cervical collar is not a problem itself; it is a reasonable treatment option at this time. Although this collar serves an important protective purpose, it does not allow normal function.

Prioritization of the Problem

The patient's problems ranked in terms of treatment priority are:

1. Pain is rated 7/10 during right-sided bending.
2. Increased muscle tone secondary to muscle spasm of the left upper trapezius.
3. Decreased cervical ROM.
4. Inability to assess strength and flexibility of the cervical musculature because of pain.
5. Inability to play basketball.
6. Inability to sleep undisturbed because of pain.
7. Patient wears a soft cervical collar for comfort.

Commentary

- This patient's pain and spasm are given the highest priority because they cause the patient's restricted motion. The pain-spasm cycle is a protective response that, when prolonged, can delay the return of the patient to full activity. The decreased cervical ROM will limit the ability of the patient to perform ADLs, will prohibit him from competing in basketball, and will hinder rehabilitation exercises. The clinician must use modalities and exercise to reduce the pain-spasm cycle and increase blood flow to the area.
- Assigning a low priority to the functional problems should not be interpreted as indicating that these concerns are trivial. These functional problems are a result of the patient's other problems. By correcting the problems of pain, spasm, ROM, and any inadequacies of strength and flexibility, the clinician will be able to return the patient to functional activity.
- The wearing of the soft cervical collar is not of great concern at this time. Although a patient should not be allowed to rely on this orthosis, it is prudent to

allow him to wear it for comfort. He should be weaned from it as tolerated.

Long-Term Goals

At the time of discharge, the following long-term goals will be achieved:

1. The patient will return to full activity playing basketball.
2. The patient will be able to sleep undisturbed without use of the cervical collar.
3. The patient will have normal ROM, flexibility, and strength.
4. The patient will be symptom-free.

Commentary

- The long-term goals have been established for a 3-week period. The goals address basic ADLs such as sleep as well as more strenuous activities (e.g., sports, fitness, and work). Note that the patient will have normal ROM, flexibility, and strength. This goal is certainly feasible in this period and essential if this patient is to return to activity, predisposing himself to further injury.

Short-Term Goals

The following short-term goals have initially been established for this patient:

1. The patient's pain with right-side bending will be reported as 3/10 or less.
2. The patient's muscle spasm will decrease to the point at which the cervical collar will be worn only at night.
3. The patient's cervical ROM will improve to:

Flexion:	75%
Extension:	60%
Right rotation:	75%
Left rotation:	75%
Right-side bending:	50%
Left-side bending:	75%

4. The clinician will be able to assess the strength and flexibility of the patient's cervical musculature.
5. The patient will be able to sleep throughout the night undisturbed by pain.
6. Patient will not participate in basketball at this time.
7. Patient will be compliant and independent in a home exercise program.

Commentary

- A 1-week period for attaining the short-term goals is initially set. In a young, active, otherwise healthy person this period should be adequate to note changes in the patient's condition. Because this

patient has a short time frame before the start of basketball season, the clinician will want to evaluate the patient more frequently so that changes can be expediently made to the rehabilitation program.
- The first three goals are set to measure the efficacy of the program in relieving the patient's pain and spasm. Goal 4 is information that could not be determined during the initial evaluation because of the patient's pain.
- The goals concerning sleep and the use of the collar are reasonable. If they are met, the patient will be less dependent on the collar and function better. The patient should not be participating in basketball because he is likely to aggravate the injury and may be at risk for reinjury.
- The final goal is always important because we should always strive to make our patients independent through compliance with their home program, which will expedite the rehabilitation process.

Treatment Planning

The treatment plan for this case study is presented at the end of Sections 2 through 5. The plan outlined in each chapter focuses on modalities discussed in that chapter. Although the various chapters present a wide range of treatment strategies, this is not to imply that all of these modalities would be used during the same treatment session. Care must be taken to avoid overtreating the patient, especially when the patient is billed per modality used. All of the possible treatment approaches are not necessarily presented, and your instructor may describe other treatment plans or challenge you to devise your own strategy. The following would also be incorporated into the patient's treatment plan:

1. Cardiovascular Exercise

Stationary bicycle riding for 30 minutes, maintaining the patient's heart rate at 122 to 163 beats per minute.

Theory

Cardiovascular exercise would be incorporated early to maintain the patient at a high level of conditioning. The patient must maintain his heart rate in the target range to achieve aerobic conditioning. The patient could progress to other forms of cardiovascular conditioning as his healing permits.

2. Weaning from the Cervical Collar

Theory

The patient should be allowed to wear the cervical collar as needed as long as he does not become dependent on it. He should be encouraged to wean himself from its use, wearing it less during waking hours, only at night for sleep, and then not at all as long as he can sleep undisturbed and perform normal ADLs without increasing his symptoms.

3. Strengthening Exercises

Progressive resistance exercises (PREs) for the lower extremities, upper extremities, and spinal musculature as the patient's cervical ROM becomes normal and there is no pain with ADLs.

Theory

Strengthening of the injured area and maintaining peak muscular strength are needed so that the patient may return to full activity in the shortest possible time. Exercise for the lower extremities could be started almost immediately; PREs for the upper extremities and spine should be started after the pain begins to subside and the ROM begins to increase.

4. Progressive Return to Basketball

The patient would first progress through individual basketball drills and then to one-on-one drills. After successful completion of these, he could progress to scrimmaging and then full competition.

● ● ● Section One Quiz

1. An example of an injury caused by macrotrauma is:
   A. Stress fracture
   B. Sprain
   C. Tendinitis
   D. Pes planus

2. This phagocyte is released immediately following trauma to contain bacteria, but in the process destroys viable tissues:
   A. Serotonin
   B. Kinin
   C. Neutrophil
   D. Leukotriene

3. Which of the following cell types is anaerobic and therefore is able to withstand a low-oxygen environment?
   A. Fibrocyte
   B. Granuloma
   C. Macrophage
   D. Anerocyte

4. After depolarization of the nerve, the period during which a stronger-than-normal stimulus is required to initiate another action potential is the:
   A. Absolute refractory period
   B. Relative refractory period
   C. Silent refractory period
   D. Latent refractory period

5. The rate of atrophy is accelerated through the stimulation of:
   A. Golgi's tendon organs
   B. Phasic stretch receptors
   C. Actin and myosin filaments
   D. Blood flow

6. The healing process begins with:
   A. Inflammation
   B. Coagulation
   C. Phagocytosis
   D. Repair phase

7. All of the following aid in venous return except:
   A. Gravity
   B. Muscular contractions
   C. The sodium-potassium pump
   D. One-way valves

8. Which of the following structures has the poorest blood supply?
   A. Muscle
   B. Fascia
   C. Meniscal cartilage
   D. Bone

9. According to the gate-control theory of pain modulation, what structure monitors the activity of the incoming nerves and subsequently opens or closes the gate?
   A. T cell
   B. Dorsal horn
   C. Paleospinothalamic tract
   D. Substantia gelatinosa

10. The transformation of a chemical stimulus into action potential is called:
    A. Nociception
    B. Saltatory conduction
    C. Binding
    D. Transduction

11. The fibers that start as Merkel's disks in the periphery cross the midline in the:
    A. Spinal cord
    B. Medulla
    C. Thalamus
    D. Cerebral cortex

12. Moist heat packs, whirlpools, cryotherapy and electrical nerve stimulation all can be effective at reducing perceived pain. The mechanism through which these modalities work is called:
    A. Descending pain modulation
    B. Hyperalgesia
    C. Gate-control theory
    D. Referred pain

13. Pain produced by irritation of the brachial plexus due to entrapment of its roots will be felt in the arm or hand instead of the arm pit. This mislocalization is closely related to a phenomenon called:
    A. Phantom limb pain
    B. Referred pain
    C. Chronic pain
    D. Epicritic pain

14. Damage to the anterior lateral fasciculus usually results in:
    A. Ipsilateral loss of fine touch
    B. Contralateral loss of fine touch
    C. Ipsilateral loss of pain
    D. Contralateral loss of pain

15. Which type of state regulation establishes the scope of profession practice, sets the minimal education standards, and protects professional roles and titles?
    A. Certification
    B. Exemption
    C. Licensure
    D. Registration

16. Whirlpools and other electrical devices that may be used in the presence of water must be connected to a:
    A. Hospital-grade plug
    B. Three-pronged outlet
    C. Circuit breaker
    D. Ground-fault circuit interrupter

17. Employers or clinical instructors can be held liable for negligent acts of their employees or students through the doctrine of:
    A. Contributory negligence
    B. Vicarious liability
    C. Gross negligence
    D. Omission

18. The intentional and unwanted touching of one person by another is termed:
    A. Nonfeasance
    B. Slander
    C. Battery
    D. Assault

19. _____ is the coding system used to identify the type and nature of care provided to the patient.
    A. CPT
    B. ICD
    C. OSHA
    D. PMC

20. Which of the following would be considered when determining the actions that a "reasonable and prudent person" would have taken under similar circumstances?
    A. Testimony of expert witnesses
    B. The defendant's age, education, and mental capacity
    C. State practice regulations
    D. All of the above

References

1. Knight, KL: Cryotherapy in Sport Injury Management. Human Kinetics, Champaign, IL, 1995.
2. Allen, RJ: Human Stress: Its Nature and Control. Burgess Publishing, Minneapolis, 1983.
3. Bryan, JM, et al: Altered load history affects periprosthetic bone loss following cementless total hip arthroplasty. J Orthop Res 14:762, 1996.
4. Lamme, EN, et al: Allogenic fibroblasts in dermal substitutes induce inflammation and scar formation. Wound Repair Regen 10:152, 2002.
5. Enwemeka, CS: Inflammation, cellularity, and fibrillogenesis in regenerating tendon: Implications for tendon rehabilitation. Phys Ther 69:816, 1989.
6. Gross, MT: Chronic tendinitis: Pathomechanics of injury, factors affecting the healing response, and treatment. J Orthop Sports Phys Ther 16:248, 1992.
7. Wilkerson, GB: Inflammation in connective tissue: Etiology and management. Athletic Training 20:298, 1985.
8. Kloth, LC and Miller, KH: The inflammatory response to wounding. In Kloth, LC, McCulloch, JM and Feedar, JA (eds): Wound Healing: Alternatives in Management. FA Davis, Philadelphia, 1990, pp 1–13.
9. Starkey, C and Ryan, J: Evaluation of Orthopedic and Athletic Injuries, ed 2. FA Davis, Philadelphia, 2002.
10. Ward, PA and Lentsch, AB: The acute inflammatory response and its regulation. Arch Surg 134:666, 1999.
11. Hopkins, JT and Ingersoll, CD: Arthrogenic muscle inhibition: A limiting factor in joint rehabilitation. J Sport Rehabil 9:135, 2000.
12. Salter, RB, et al: The biological effect of continuous passive motion on the healing of full thickness defects in articular cartilage. J Bone Joint Surg 62:A1232, 1980.

13. Denegar, CR, et al: Influence of transcutaneous electrical nerve stimulation on pain, range of motion, and serum cortisol concentration in females experiencing delayed onset muscle soreness. J Orthop Sports Phys Ther 11:100, 1989.

14. Voight, ML: Reduction of post-traumatic ankle edema with high-voltage pulsed galvanic stimulation. Athletic Training 19:278, 1984.

15. Vander, AJ, et al: Human Physiology: The Mechanisms of Body Function, ed 3. McGraw-Hill, New York, 1980.

16. Houglum, PA: Soft tissue healing and its impact on rehabilitation. J Sports Rehabil 1:19, 1992.

17. Hebda, PA, et al: Mast cell and myofibroblast in wound healing. Dermatol Clin 11:685, 1993.

18. Tranquillo, RT and Murray, JD: Mechanistic model of wound contraction. J Surg Res 55:233, 1993.

19. Daly, TJ: The repair phase of wound healing: Re-epithelialization and contraction. In Kloth, LC, McCulloch, JM and Feedar, JA (eds): Wound Healing: Alternatives in Management. FA Davis, Philadelphia, 1990, pp 14–30.

20. Dickinson, A and Bennett, KM: Therapeutic exercise. Clin Sports Med 4:417, 1985.

21. Garrett, WE: Muscle strain injuries: Clinical and basic aspects. Med Sci Sports Exerc 22:436, 1990.

22. Lechner, CT and Dahners, LE: Healing of the medial collateral ligament in unstable rat knees. Am J Sports Med 19:508, 1991.

23. Russell, B, et al: Repair of injured skeletal muscle: A molecular approach. Med Sci Sports Exerc 24:189, 1992.

24. Vanudevan, SV and Melvin, JL: Upper extremity edema control: Rationale of the techniques. Am J Occup Ther 33:520, 1980.

25. Rucinski, TJ, et al: The effects of intermittent compression on edema in postacute ankle sprains. J Orthop Sports Phys Ther 14:65, 1991.

26. Gilbart, MK, et al: Anterior tibial compartment pressures during intermittent sequential pneumatic compression therapy. Am J Sports Med 23:769, 1995.

27. Halvorson, GA: Therapeutic heat and cold for athletic injuries. Phys Sports Med 18:87, 1990.

28. Kolb, P and Denegar, C: Traumatic edema and the lymphatic system. J Athletic Training 18:339, 1983.

29. Stöckle, U, et al: Fastest reduction of posttraumatic edema: Continuous cryotherapy or intermittent impulse compression? Foot Ankle Int 18:432, 1997.

30. Myrer, WJ, et al: Cold- and hot-pack contrast therapy: Subcutaneous and intramuscular temperature change. J Athletic Training 32:238, 1997.

31. Shoemaker, JK, et al: Failure of manual massage to alter limb blood flow: Measures by Doppler ultrasound. Med Sci Sports Exerc 29:610, 1997.

32. Silverberg, SM: Trouble in the vascular periphery. Emerg Med 19:22, 1987.

33. McCulloch, J and Boyd, VB: The effects of whirlpool and the dependent position on lower extremity volume. J Orthop Sports Phys Ther 16:169, 1992.

34. Von Schroeder, et al: The changes in intramuscular pressure and femoral vein flow with continuous passive motion, pneumatic compressive stockings, and leg manipulations. Clin Orthop 218, May, 1991.

35. Merrick, MA, et al: A preliminary examination of cryotherapy and secondary injury in skeletal muscle. Med Sci Sports Exerc 31:1516, 1999.

36. Kisner, C and Colby, LA: Therapeutic Exercise: Foundations and Techniques, ed 4. FA Davis, Philadelphia, 2002.

37. McCray RE and Patton NJ: Pain relief at trigger points: A comparison of moist heat and shortwave diathermy. J Orthop Sports Phys Ther 5:175, 1984.

38. Alvarez, DJ and Rockwell, PG: Trigger points: Diagnosis and management. Am Fam Physician 65:653, 2002.

39. Fomby, EW and Mellion, MB: Identifying and treating myofascial pain syndrome. Phys Sports Med 25:67, 1997.

40. Cailliet, R: Soft Tissue Pain and Disability. FA Davis, Philadelphia, 1977.

41. Urbancova, H, et al: Bone fracture influences reflex muscle atrophy which is sex-dependent. Physiol Res 42:35, 1993.

42. DeVahl, J: Neuromuscular electrical stimulation (NMES) in rehabilitation. In Gersh, MR (ed): Electrotherapy in Rehabilitation. FA Davis, Philadelphia, 1992, pp 218–268.

43. Spence, AP and Mason, EB: Human Anatomy and Physiology, ed 3. Benjamin/Cummings, Menlo Park, CA, 1987.

44. Hopkins, JT, et al: Cryotherapy and transcutaneous electric neuromuscular stimulation decrease arthrogenic muscle inhibition of the vastus medialis after knee joint effusion. J Athletic Training 37:25, 2001.

45. Shaw SR, et al: Mechanical, morphological and biochemical adaptations of bone and muscle to hindlimb suspension and exercise. J Biomech 20:225, 1987.

46. Lieher, RL and Kelly, MJ: Factors influencing quadriceps femoris muscle torque using transcutaneous neuromuscular stimulation. Phys Ther 71:715, 1991.

47. Lester, D and Yang, B: An approach for examining the rationality of suicide. Psychol Rep 79:405, 1996.

48. Orbach, I: Dissociation, physical pain, and suicide: A hypothesis. Suicide Life-Threatening Behav 24:68, 1994.

49. Fishbain, DA: Completed suicide in chronic pain. Clin J Pain 7:29, 1991.

50. Biswal N, et al: Congenital indifference to pain. Indian J Pediatr 65:755, 1998.

51. Monks, R and Taenzer, P: A comprehensive pain questionnaire. In Melzack, R (ed): Pain Measurement and Assessment. Raven Press, New York, 1983, pp 233–237.

52. Garron, D and Leavitt, F: Demographic and affective covariates of pain. Psychosom Med 41:525, 1979.

53. Zombroski, M: Cultural components in response to pain. J Soc Issues 8:15, 1952.

54. Zola, I: Culture and symptoms: An analysis of patients presenting complaints. Am Soc Rev 31:615, 1966.

55. Edwards CL, et al: Race, ethnicity and pain. Pain 94:133, 2001.

56. Guyton, AC: Textbook of Medical Physiology, ed 6. WB Saunders, Philadelphia, 1980.

57. Melzack, R and Wall, PD: The gate control theory of pain. In Soulairac, A, Cahn, J and Carpentier, J (eds): Pain: Proceedings of the International Symposium on Pain. Academic Press, London, 1968.

58. Fulbright RK, et al: Functional MR imaging of regional brain activation associated with the affective experience of pain. AJR Am J Roentgenol 2001;177:1205.

59. French, S: Pain: Some physiological and sociological aspects. Physiotherapy 75:255, 1989.

60. Unruh, AM: Gender variations in clinical pain experience. Pain 65:2, 1996.

61. Ellermeier, W and Westphal, W: Gender differences in pain ratings and pupil reactions to painful pressure stimuli. Pain 61:435, 1995.

62. Fillingim, RB and Maixner, W: The influence of resting blood pressure and gender on pain response. Psychosom Med 58:326, 1996.

63. Nguyen, P, et al: Evidence of gender differences in esophageal pain threshold. Am J Gastroenterol 90:901, 1995.

64. Karchnick, KL, et al: Gender differences in pain threshold, tolerance and anxiety. J Athletic Training 32:S44, 1997.

65. Weir, R, et al: Gender differences in psychosocial

adjustment to chronic pain and expenditures for health care services used. Clin J Pain 12:277, 1996.

66. Vallerand, AH: Gender differences in pain. Image J Nurs Sch 27:235, 1995.

67. Lord, RH and Kozar, B: Pain tolerance in the presence of others: Implications for youth sports. Phys Sports Med 17:71, 1989.

68. Solsona, AM, et al: Relationship between acute pain and pain anxiety. J Athletic Training 32:S43, 1997.

69. Buxton, BP, et al: Pain and ethnicity in athletes. J Sports Rehabil 2:13, 1993.

70. Hall, EG and Davies, S: Gender differences in perceived intensity and affect of pain between athletes and non-athletes. Percept Mot Skills 73:779, 1991.

71. Jarmenko, ME, et al: The differential ability of athletes and non-athletes to cope with two types of pain: A radical behavioral model. Psychological Rec 31:265, 1981.

72. Newman, S: Dealing with pain. Coaching Rev 6:25, 1983.

73. Walker, J: Pain distraction in athletes and non-athletes. Percept Mot Skills 33:1187, 1971.

74. Yamaguchi, AY, et al: Difference in pain response and anxiety between athletes and non-athletes. J Athletic Training 32:S45, 1997.

75. Ryan, ED and Kovacic, CR: Pain tolerance and athletic participation. Percept Mot Skills 22:383, 1966.

76. Tajet-Foxell, B and Rose, FD: Pain and pain tolerance in professional ballet dancers. Br J Sports Med 29:31, 1995.

77. Scott, V and Gijsbers, K: Pain perception in competitive swimmers. BMJ 282:91, 1981.

78. Hussisson, EC: Visual analogue scales. In Melzack, R (ed): Pain Management and Assessment. Raven Press, New York, 1983.

79. Melzack, R: The McGill pain questionnaire: Major properties and scoring methods. Pain 1:277, 1975.

80. Bowsher, D: Acute and chronic pain and assessment. In Wells, PE, Frampton, V and Bowsher, D (eds): Pain Management in Physical Therapy. Appleton & Lange, Norwalk, CT, 1988, pp 39–44.

81. Smith, GM, et al: An experimental pain method sensitive to morphine in man: The submaximal tourniquet technique. J Pharmacol Exp Ther 154:324, 1966.

82. Bonica, JJ, et al: Biochemistry and the modulation of nociception and pain. In Bonica, JJ (ed): The Management of Pain, ed 2. Lea & Febiger, Philadelphia, 1990, pp 95–121.

83. Fields, HL: Pain. McGraw-Hill, New York, 1987.

84. Macefield, VG: The signaling of touch, finger movements and manipulation forces by mechanoreceptors in human skin. In Morley, JW: Neural Aspects of Tactile Sensation. Elsevier, Amsterdam, 1998.

85. Takahashi, A and Gotoh, H: Mechanosensitive whole-cell currents in cultured rat somatosensory neurons. Brain Res 869:225, 2000.

86. Taylor, DCM and Pierau, F-K: Nociceptive afferent neurons. In Winlow, W (ed): Studies in Neuroscience, vol 14. Manchester University Press, Manchester, 1991.

87. Vogt, BA, et al: Anterior cingulate cortex and the medial pain system. In Vogt, BA and Gabriel, M: Neurobiology of Cingulate Cortex and Limbic Thalamus. Birkhäuser, Boston, 1993.

88. Head, H and Holmes, G: Sensory disturbances from cerebral lesions. Brain 34:102, 1911.

89. Melzack, R and Wall, PD: Pain mechanisms: A new theory. Science 150:971, 1965.

90. Melzack, R: Neurophysiology foundations of pain. In

91. Melzack, R: The Puzzle of Pain. Basic Books, New York, 1973.

92. Melzack, R and Wall, PD: The Challenge of Pain, Basic Books, New York, 1983.

93. Juottonen, K, et al: Altered central sensorimotor processing in patients with complex regional pain syndrome. Pain 98:315, 2002.

94. Menard, MR and Hoens, AM: Objective evaluation of functional capacity: Medical, occupational, and legal settings. J Orthop Sports Phys Ther 19:249, 1994.

95. Deyo, RA and Carter, WB: Strategies for improving and expanding the application of health status measures in clinical settings: A researcher-developer viewpoint. Med Care 30:176, 1992.

96. Wilson, BM: Promoting compliance: The patient-provider relationship. Adv Ren Replace Ther 2:199, 1995.

97. Baker, SM, et al: Patient participation in physical therapy goal setting. Phys Ther 81:1118, 2001.

98. Northern, JG, et al: Involvement of adult rehabilitation patients in setting occupational therapy goals. Am J Occup Ther 49:214, 1995.

99. Nelson, CE and Payton, OD: A system for involving patients in program planning. Am J Occup Ther 45:753, 1991.

100. Randall, KE and McEwen, IR: Writing patient-centered functional goals. Phys Ther 80:1197, 2000.

101. Drowatzky, JN: Legal duties and liability in athletic training. Athletic Training 20:10, 1985.

102. Morin, GE: An overview of selected state licensure athletic training laws. J Athletic Training 27:162, 1992.

103. Gallup, EM: Law and the Team Physician. Human Kinetics Publishers, Champaign, IL, 1995.

104. Scott, RW: Legal Aspects of Documenting Patient Care, ed 2. Aspen Publishers, Gaithersburg, MD, 2000.

105. National Athletic Trainers' Association: Understanding and Initiating the Reimbursement Process. NATA, Inc., Dallas, 2002.

106. Gieck, J, et al: Trainer malpractice: A sleeping giant. Athletic Training 19:41, 1984.

107. Pozgar, GD: Legal Aspects of Health Care Administration, ed 3. Aspen Publications, Rockville, MD, 1987.

108. Park, J, et al: Premarket approval (PMA) manual. HHS Publication, FDA, 1997.

109. Food and Drug Administration: Medical device labeling—Suggested format and content. Center for Devices and Radiological Health, http://www.fda.gov/cdrh/ode/labeling.pdf. Last accessed 28 February 2003.

110. Albohm, MJ, et al: Reimbursement for Athletic Trainers. Slack, Inc, Thorofare, NJ, 2001.

111. Brown, F: ICD-9-CM Coding Handbook, with Answers: 2002. American Hospital Association, Chicago, 2002.

112. Streator, S and Buckley, WE: Clinical outcomes in sports medicine. Athletic Therapy Today 5:57, 2000.

113. Porter, MM and Porter, JW: Electrical safety in the training room. Athletic Training 16:263, 1981.

114. Therapeutic pools and tubs in health care facilities. In National Electric Code. National Fire Protection Association, Quincy, MA, 1996.

115. Penman, KA and Penman, TM: Training rooms aren't just for colleges. Athletic Purchasing Facilities 6:34, 1982.

116. Ray, R: Where athletic trainers work: Facility design and planning. In Ray, R: Management Strategies in Athletic Training, ed 2. Human Kinetics Publishers, Champaign, IL, 2000, pp 130–157.

Sternbach, RA (ed): The Psychology of Pain. Raven Press, New York, 1986, pp 1–24.

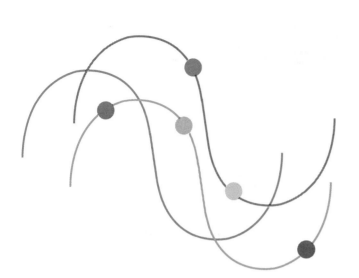

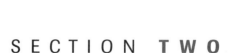

Therapeutic Cold and Superficial Heating Agents

This section describes the physics and biophysical effects (Chapter 5) and the clinical application of cold modalities and superficial heating agents (Chapter 6). Deep heating modalities, those that penetrate deeper than 2 cm, are presented in Section Three.

Chapter 5

Thermal Modalities

This chapter presents information regarding those modalities that rely on thermal properties to elicit various responses in the body's systems. The chapter is broken down into two sections, cold and heat. Use of specific modalities and their various local effects are described in the next chapter.

Thermal agents transfer energy to or from the tissues. This exchange of energy is based on a temperature gradient, as with ice or heat, or the conversion of electromagnetic energy, as with the diathermies (see Appendix B). Compared with the extreme range of temperatures found throughout the universe, there is relatively little difference between the upper and lower temperature limits of thermal treatments. Within our tissues, the 65°F (18.3°C) that span the upper limits of heat modalities and the lower limits of cold modalities elicit a wide range of cellular and vascular events (Box 5–1).

"Heat" is not an actual form of energy; rather, it is a term used to describe a specific type of energy transfer. Within the range of thermal therapeutic modalities, heat transfer involves the exchange of **kinetic energy** ■ between two or more objects (e.g., a hot pack and the skin). For this exchange to occur, one fundamental condition must be met: one object must have a higher temperature than the other object. Energy carriers then transmit energy from the high temperature area to the cooler object.[3] Heat is added to or removed from the body by one of five mechanisms: conduction, convection, radiation, evaporation, or conversion, although multiple mechanisms may occur at the same time (Box 5–2).

The skin contains thermoreceptors, some that are responsive to heat and others that are responsive to cold. In total, there are more cold receptors than heat receptors. Many thermoreceptors are wide dynamic range neurons that trigger a pain response when the temperature becomes too hot or too cold. Although the sensation of heat or cold is the most outwardly noticeable effect, the primary benefit of these modalities occurs by altering cell metabolism. The rate of the body's chemical and, therefore, physiological processes are affected by changes in temperature. Each 1.8°F (1°C) change in tissue temperature results in a 13 percent increase (heat) or decrease (cold) in the tissues' metabolic rate.[4]

Each type of tissue conducts heat at a different rate (Table 5–1).[5] This means that changes in skin temperature do not immediately reflect the changes in underlying temperatures (see Box 5–2).[6] Skin temperature is approximately 91°F (33°C), although there is a great deal of variability in this temperature, especially when compared with the fairly constant core temperature. Skin temperature is easily influenced by such factors as ambient temperature, humidity, exercise, time of day, and food and alcohol consumption. The deeper the tissue is within the body, the higher the temperature. Skin tempera-

Kinetic energy: The energy an object possesses by virtue of its motion.

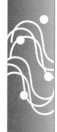

Box 5-1. Heat as a Physical Entity

Temperatures and their effects are relative. If the temperature outside is 60°, but it was 80° yesterday, you might think, "It's cold." If it was 40° yesterday, you might think "It's warming up." or "I wish the weather would change" if the previous day's temperature was also 60°. This concept holds true for the application of thermal modalities. The classifications of "heat" and "cold" are based on the physiological response elicited by the temperature. When the temperature of an object is measured, the speed of molecular movement is being quantified. An increased rate of molecular motion is measured as an increase in temperature. Temperature is used to describe the amount of kinetic energy, heat, in an object. Heat, infrared energy, is emitted from any object having a temperature greater than **absolute zero** ■.

The basic principle behind any thermal modality is to transfer heat across a temperature gradient (that is, one object is hotter than the other). Heat, a form of energy exchange, is lost from the warmer object and moved into the cooler object. The greater the temperature gradient, the more quickly energy is transferred.[1] When a moist heat pack is placed on a patient, energy is transferred away from the pack and absorbed by the tissues. Likewise, when a cold pack is used, the heat is drawn away from the tissues and delivered to the pack.

Heat is measured in **calories.** The common definition of a calorie is the amount of energy needed to raise the temperature of 1 gram of water by 1°C (note that this calorie is different from the k-calories used to describe food energy). Scientists, however, changed this definition to be 1.0 calorie equals 4.1860 Joules of energy.[2]

Different materials require different amounts of energy to increase their temperature. **Specific heat capacity** (often simply shortened to "specific heat") is the amount of energy needed to increase the temperature of a unit of mass by 1 unit of temperature, usually Celsius. A substance's specific heat varies with its temperature. **Thermal conductivity** is the quantity of heat (in calories per-second) passing though a substance 1 cm thick by 1 cm wide separating a temperature gradient of 1°C. As it relates to therapeutic modalities, thermal conductivity is used to describe how well different tissues do (or do not) transfer thermal energy.

ture is cooler than adipose tissue, which is cooler than muscular tissue. As such, the temperature changes of deeper tissues are always less than those of the overlying tissues.

Energy that is absorbed by one tissue layer cannot be transmitted to deeper layers: the **law of Grotthus-Draper** (see Appendix B). As more energy is absorbed by the superficial layers, there is less energy to be transmitted to the deeper layers. This means that the energy being used must be able to affect the target tissues to be effective as a treatment modality. Using a superficial heating or cooling agent for a deep injury affects the superficial sensory nerves but does not produce the needed metabolic changes in the traumatized tissues.

Cold application is indicated under three conditions: (1) in the acute stages of the inflammatory response, (2)

before range-of-motion exercises (i.e., cryokinetics), and (3) after physical activity. When cold is applied as a form of immediate treatment or in the active inflammation stage, some form of ice pack should be used. When cold is being administered before rehabilitation exercises, a cold whirlpool or immersion should be used because of the latent cooling effects of these modalities.[7] Athletes and other highly motivated persons often return to physical activity before full healing of the tissues, thus perpetuating the inflammatory process. As a result, cold application is often used over an extended time frame in these persons as compared with the general population.

Heat application is indicated under these five conditions: (1) to control the inflammatory reaction in its subacute or chronic stages, (2) to encourage tissue healing, (3) to reduce edema and ecchymosis, (4) to improve range of motion (ROM) before physical activity (e.g., participation in the sport) or rehabilitation, and (5) to promote drainage from an infected site.

■ Cold Modalities

Cold modalities are perhaps the most versatile of therapeutic modalities. The body's response to cold elicits a wide range of cellular, vascular, and nervous system responses that regulate the inflammatory response, limit

TABLE 5-1	**Tissue Thermal Conductivity**
Tissue	*Thermal Conductivity (W/m °C)*
Skin	0.96
Adipose Tissue	0.19
Muscle	0.64

Absolute zero: Theoretically, the lowest possible temperature, equal to –273°C or –460°F. At this point, all atomic and molecular motion ceases.

Box 5–2. The Transfer of Thermal Energy

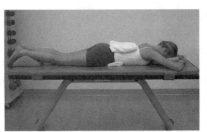
Conduction (e.g., ice pack, moist heat pack)

Conduction is the transfer of heat between two objects that are touching each other. Examples of therapeutic modalities that operate by way of conduction include moist heat packs and ice application. Within the body, the transfer of energy from one tissue layer to another occurs by way of conduction.

Some materials are better conductors of heat than others. Consider wooden and metal picnic tables that have been sitting in direct sunlight and have the same temperature. If you placed one hand on the wooden table and the other hand on the metal table, the metal table would feel "hotter" more rapidly. Even though you are touching two objects with equal temperatures, the greater ability of metal to conduct heat (compared to wood) warms your hand more rapidly (see Box 5–1).

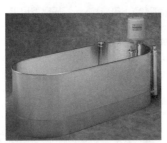
Convection (e.g., warm or cold whirlpool)

Convection is the transfer of heat by the movement of a **medium** ■, usually air or water. Of the three **states of matter** ■, gases are poor conductors of heat. Liquids are better conductors and solids, generally speaking, are the best conductors. Circulating air or water increases their ability to transport heat. The actual transfer of energy from the medium to the body still occurs through conduction; the delivery of the energy occurs by movement of the medium. The circulation of the medium results in the cooling of one object and the subsequent heating of another object. Whirlpools are the most common example of therapeutic modalities that use convection.

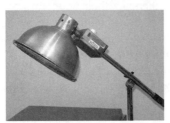
Radiation (e.g., infrared lamp)

Radiation is the transfer of energy without the use of a medium, and the heat gained or lost through radiation is termed radiant energy. Radiant energy **diverges** ■ as it travels, resulting in a reduction of the energy received at different distances along its path. All thermal therapeutic modalities provide radiant energy. For some, such as ultraviolet light, LASER, and shortwave diathermy, this is how the energy is transmitted. Even conductive modalities, such as moist heat packs, lose some of their energy through radiation. This effect can be illustrated by placing your hand just above a moist heat pack. The heat you feel is being lost from the pack via radiation.

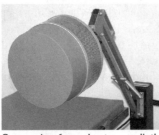
Conversion (e.g., short wave diathermy, ultrasound)

Some forms of energy must be changed to another form to have a thermal effect on the body. This process, **conversion,** is seen in modalities such as short wave diathermy where electrical energy is converted into heat and therapeutic ultrasound where acoustical energy is converted into heat.

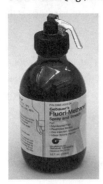
Evaporation (e.g., vapocoolant spray)

Heat loss can also occur through **evaporation.** The change from the liquid state to the gaseous state requires that thermal energy be removed from the body. The heat absorbed by the liquid cools the tissue as the liquid changes its state into gas via conversion. Vapocoolant sprays are an example of a modality that operates by evaporation.

Divergence: The spreading of a beam or wave.

Medium: A material used to promote the transfer of energy. An object or substance that permits the transmission of energy through it.

States of matter: Physical matter can take three forms: solid, liquid, and gas. Using H_2O as example, we see the three states of matter as ice, water, and steam.

TABLE 5-2 Effects of Cold Application	
Local Effects	*Systemic Effects**
Vasoconstriction	General vasoconstriction in response to cooling of the
Decreased rate of cell metabolism resulting in a decreased	posterior hypothalamus
need for oxygen	Decreased respiratory and heart rates
Decreased production of cellular wastes	Shivering and increased muscle tone
Reduction in inflammation	
Decreased nerve conduction velocity	
Decreased pain	
Decreased muscle spasm	
Decreased muscular force production	

* These systemic effects primarily occur when the entire body is exposed to cold temperatures. Therefore, we would expect them to occur during a full-body cold immersion rather than during the application of an ice pack.

the scope of the original injury, decrease pain, and decrease muscle spasm. Cold may be safely applied to most orthopedic injuries and other conditions throughout the healing process. The primary benefit of cold application, especially in the treatment of acute injuries, is the reduction of cell metabolism.

The term "cold" is used to describe a relative temperature state characterized by decreased molecular motion and the relative absence of heat (see Box 5–1). Because of this, "cold" cannot be transferred because thermal energy always moves from a high energy concentration ("heat") to a lower concentration ("cold"). When a cold modality is placed on the skin, the heat transfer is from the skin to the cold modality.

Cryotherapy is the application of cold modalities that have a temperature range between 32°F and 65°F (0°C and 18°C). During cryotherapy, heat is removed from the body and absorbed by the cold modality until the temperatures are equal. The body responds to the loss of heat with a series of local and systemic responses. The local effects of cold application include vasoconstriction, decreased metabolic rate, decreased inflammation, and decreased pain (Table 5–2). Indications for the use of cold include acute injury or inflammation, pain, muscle spasm, and restoration of ROM (Table 5–3).

Magnitude and Duration of Temperature Decrease

The depth, magnitude, and duration of the effects of cryotherapy are based on the modality being used and the anatomical and physiological properties of the tissues being treated (Table 5–4).[5, 10–19] The rate of heat exchange between the cold modality and the tissues is determined by the temperature difference between the two. The greater the temperature difference between the modality and the skin, the **temperature gradient**, the more rapid the energy

exchange and the deeper the effects of the treatment because more energy is transferred. The cold modality will continue to remove heat from the body until the temperature of the modality and the skin are equal. During this process, the modality also gains heat from the atmosphere (Fig. 5–1).

Tissue Cooling

The depth of cooling is related to the treatment duration: the longer the treatment, the greater the depth of cooling and the greater the temperature decrease. Because the skin is in direct contact with the modality, it is the first tissue to lose heat. As the skin cools, it draws heat from the underlying tissues, most commonly adipose tissue, fascia, and muscle in that order. The adipose tissue layer is the limiting factor in the effective depth of penetration of thermal modalities (with the exception being therapeutic ultrasound) (Box 5–3).

A moderate correlation (r = 0.65) exists between skin temperature and **intra-articular** ■ temperature.[3, 22] As the temperature of the skin overlying a joint decreases, the temperature within the joint decreases proportionally (e.g., decreasing the skin temperature 10°F [5.6°C] would result in a 6.5°F [3.6°C] decrease in the intra-articular temperature).[11, 23] Intra-articular temperatures may decrease as much as 16.9°F (9.4°C) during the application of an ice pack to the knee.[24] This principle can also be related to the application of heat modalities: Increased skin temperature results in increased joint space temperature (although, as we will see, the effects of heat do not penetrate as deeply as those of cold).

Local metabolic factors also affect cooling. Acting similarly to a car radiator, venous flow carries cold blood away from the area while the arteries deliver blood that warms the area, a form of convection. A normally functioning sympathetic nervous system will better regulate cooling than a dysfunctional one. Desensitized or dener-

---

Intra-articular: Within a joint.

TABLE 5–3 General Indications and Contraindications for Cold Treatments

Indications	Contraindications
Acute injury or inflammation	Cardiac or respiratory involvement
Acute or chronic pain	Uncovered open wounds
Small, superficial, first-degree burns	Circulatory insufficiency
Postsurgical pain and edema	Cold allergy/Cold-induced **urticaria**■
Use in conjunction with rehabilitation exercises	Anesthetic skin
Spasticity accompanying central nervous system disorders	Advanced diabetes
	Peripheral vascular disease■
Acute or chronic muscle spasm	**Raynaud's phenomenon**■: Although this is usually a benign condition, Raynaud's phenomenon may be a symptom of an underlying disease state, most commonly systemic sclerosis.[9]
Neuralgia■[8]	**Lupus**■ or other conditions where cryoglobulins are present: May result in the aggregation of serum proteins, **cryoglobulinemia**■.
	Cold-induced myocardial ischemia (when large areas are treated)

TABLE 5–4 Factors Influencing the Depth, Magnitude, and Duration of Cold Treatments

Factor	Influence
Modality	
Treatment temperature	Lower treatment temperatures result in deeper cooling and longer-lasting effects. Larger temperature gradients between the modality and the skin increase the rate of exchange. The treatment temperature is often directly related to the type of cold modality used.
Specific heat	The modality's ability to transfer heat from the skin. The use of insulating materials (e.g., terry cloth towel) must also be considered.
Insulating medium between the modality and skin	Insulating medium slows the heat exchange from the skin to the modality (needed for reusable cold packs or patients who have precautions to cryotherapy).
Treatment duration	Longer treatment durations result in greater decreases in skin, subcutaneous, and intramuscular temperature and a longer rewarming time.
Area (size) of skin affected	Cooling larger areas of skin results in deeper tissue cooling relative to smaller areas.
Use of a compression wrap	The use of a compression wrap improves the conduction of energy, thus increasing the depth of cooling.
Post-treatment activity	Muscular exertion in the treated area increases the rate of rewarming.
Anatomical/Physiological	
Subcutaneous adipose tissue	An increased amount of adipose tissue reduces the effective depth of temperature decrease. The treatment duration should be increased as the amount of adipose tissue increases.
Depth of target tissues	Deeper tissues require longer treatment durations.
Vascularity of target tissues	Increased blood flow to and from the area decreases the rate of cooling. Arterial flow delivers warm blood to the area; venous blood carries away cool blood.
Cell metabolism	Active cell metabolism produces heat.
Sympathetic nervous system	An intact sympathetic nervous system is needed to maintain local temperature.

Cryoglobulinemia: A condition in which abnormal blood proteins, cryoglobulins, group together when exposed to cold. This can lead to skin color changes, hives, subcutaneous hemorrhage, and other disorders.

Lupus: A chronic disorder of the body's immune system that affects the skin, joints, internal organs, and neurological system.

Neuralgia: Pain following the path of a nerve; a hypersensitive nerve.

Peripheral vascular disease: Actually, a syndrome describing an insufficiency of arteries or veins for maintaining proper circulation (also known as PVD).

Raynaud's phenomenon: A vascular reaction to cold application or stress that results in a white, red, or blue discoloration of the extremities. The fingers and toes are the first to be affected.

Urticaria: Skin vascular reaction to an irritant characterized by red, itchy areas; wheals; or papules. Commonly referred to as "hives."

Box 5–3. Nature's Insulator: Adipose Tissue

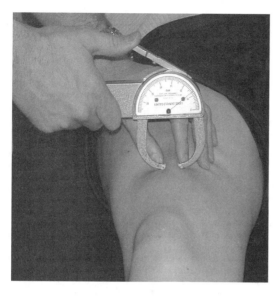

The thickness of the patient's adipose tissue layer can be calculated by determining the skinfold overlying the treatment area and then dividing that number by two (skinfold/2).[12]

Most mammals have a subcutaneous layer of adipose tissue. Those that live in cold climates have a thick layer of adipose tissue that serves as insulation, retaining body temperature by reducing the loss of heat to the surrounding environment. This principle also applies to cryotherapy.

Thick insulating layers of adipose tissue reduce the rate and depth of intramuscular cooling and require longer treatment durations to reach therapeutic treatment temperatures.[5, 13, 14, 20] With less than 8 mm of subcutaneous adipose tissue, intramuscular cooling occurs at a rate of 1.30°F (0.72°C) per/minute 1 cm within the muscle. At 10 mm to 18 mm of adipose tissue, the rate of cooling decreases to 0.81°F (0.45°C)/min. When the amount of adipose tissue increases to over 20 mm in thickness, the rate of cooling slows to 0.45°F (0.25°C)/min.[13] Each of these rates decreases as the depth within the muscle increases.

Skin-fold measurements can be used as a guide for determining treatment duration for intramuscular tissues located 1 cm below the adipose tissue:[20]

Skin-Fold Measurement	Treatment Duration
20 mm or less	25 min
20 to 30 mm	40 min
30 to 40 mm	60 min

If the facilities, time, or equipment are not available to measure the subcutaneous tissue thickness, such as the immediate management of an injury, treatment durations can be estimated based on the patient's body build and estimation of body fat: thin patients would be treated for 25 minutes; patients with a large amount of adipose tissue (i.e., obese patients) would be treated for 60 minutes.

Although it may take longer for intramuscular cooling to occur, adipose tissue also slows the rewarming process. If the patient remains still following the treatment, thicker layers of adipose tissues will result in longer rewarming times than thinner layers.[12–14, 21]

Although most of the research has examined the relationship between adipose tissue and intramuscular cooling, this tissue layer will also influence the effectiveness of superficial heating.

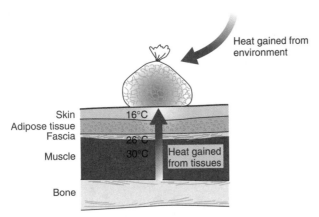

Heat gained from environment

Skin
Adipose tissue   16°C
Fascia   26°C
Muscle   30°C   Heat gained from tissues

Bone

Figure 5–1. Conductive Cooling of the Skin and Subcutaneous Tissues. The deeper the tissues, the less cooling that occurs. The subcutaneous adipose tissue layer is the greatest barrier to deeper cooling.

vated areas or areas lacking normal **vasomotor** ■ function may be overcooled (and the risk of cold injury increased) by lacking the blood regulation needed to maintain tissue temperatures.[13, 14]

The type of cold modality being used also influences the amount of cooling. When applied directly to the skin, ice packs and ice massage produce the greatest temperature gradient. Although the temperature gradient is not as great, cold immersion treatments (including cold whirlpools) affect a larger surface area than cold packs. An ice pack results in a greater decrease in skin and subcutaneous tissue temperature than a 50°F (10°C) whirlpool, but each method is equally effective in reducing intramuscular temperature.[14]

Using a compression wrap to secure the ice bag to the body part causes a significant reduction in subcutaneous tissue temperatures when compared with the use of an ice bag alone, as long as the wrap is not placed between the ice pack and the skin.[12, 21] The compression improves the contact between the ice pack and the skin and compresses the subcutaneous tissues, aiding in the exchange of heat. Tight compression, greater than 30 to 40 mm Hg, may reduce blood flow and keeps the area from being rewarmed. Covering the ice pack also reduces the amount of heat lost to the surrounding environment and enhances the effectiveness of the treatment.[5, 12] Unneeded insulation, such as an elastic wrap or terry cloth towel between the cold pack and the skin, decreases the temperature gradient and slows the transfer of heat, often rendering the treatment ineffective

Tissue Rewarming

In the outpatient orthopedic and sports medicine setting, it is unusual to have a patient remain sedentary following

treatment. Moderate activity such as walking or rehabilitation exercises increases the rate of intramuscular rewarming by increasing local cell metabolism and blood flow,[16] but does not appear to affect the rewarming of capsular or ligamentous tissues.[25]

If the patient remains sedentary following the treatment, intramuscular temperatures will continue to decrease for another 5 to 10 minutes and the effects of cooling will last for approximately 20 to 60 minutes.[12, 13] The continued cooling of the intramuscular tissues is caused by a delayed hormonal response that triggers vasodilation and the thermal conductivity of the target and overlying tissues.[5] Deeper tissues require a longer rewarming period than do superficial ones. Just as adipose tissue insulates deeper structures from the effects of the cold, adipose tissue also slows the rewarming process as its thickness increases.[12–14, 21] Increasing the surface area being treated results in a longer rewarming period.

Therapeutic Temperature Benchmarks

The application of cold to the skin activates a mechanism that is thought to conserve heat in the body's core, triggering a series of metabolic and vascular events that produce the beneficial effects of cryotherapy. During treatment, the most rapid and significant temperature changes occur in the skin and **synovium** ■. The magnitude of this temperature change varies according to the method of cold application. However, the skin is rarely the target of the treatment and we must deduce the effects on the underlying tissue based on changes in skin temperature (Fig. 5–2).[5] The thresholds of these events are discussed here, with more specific information being described in the following sections.

Superficial blood flow begins to decrease shortly after a cold modality is applied and continues a relatively steady decrease for the next 13 minutes. At approximately 13 minutes into the treatment, the rate of blood flow decrease begins to level out and small fluctuations in blood flow begin to occur.[26] When the skin temperature decreases to approximately 57°F (13.9°C), the maximal decrease in local blood flow is obtained. Changes in the lymphatic system are slower to occur. Lymphatic vessels are relatively unaffected by cold treatment until the temperature reaches 59°F (15.0°C), at which point their cross-sectional area begins to decrease.

Neurological changes begin to occur when the skin temperature decreases 9.0°F (5°C). At this point, the sensitivity of muscle spindles is decreased. A 13.3°F (7.4°C) decrease in skin temperature results in motor nerve conduction velocity being reduced by 14 percent and sensory nerve conduction velocity by 33 percent.[27] Tissue

Synovium: Membrane lining the capsule of a joint.

Vasomotor: Muscles and their associated nerves acting on arteries and veins that cause constriction or dilation.

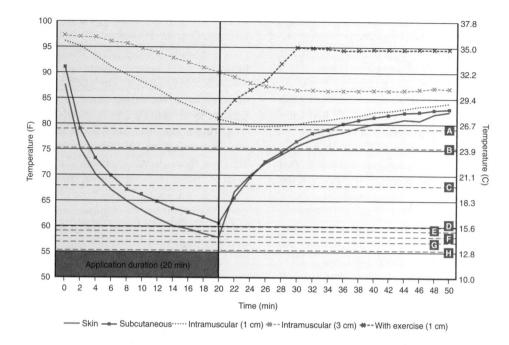

Figure 5–2. **Tissue Cooling During a 20-Minute Ice Pack Application.** (A) 9°F skin temperature decrease: Sensitivity of muscle spindles is decreased. (B) 13°F skin temperature decrease: Motor nerve conduction velocity decreased by 14 percent; sensory nerve conduction velocity decreased by 33 percent. (C) 20°F tissue temperature decrease: Acetylcholine concentrations decrease 20 percent. (D) 60°F skin temperature: Previously inhibited sensory nerve transmission begins to return during rewarming from maximum cooling. (E) 59°F skin temperature: Permeability of lymph vessels is decreased. (F) 58°F skin temperature: Maximum analgesia occurs. (G) 57°F skin temperature: Maximum decrease in blood flow. (H) 55°F skin temperature: risk of cold-related injury increases.

temperatures of 68°F (20°C) result in a 60 percent decrease in **acetylcholine ■** levels.[28]

Maximum analgesia is obtained when skin temperature is decreased to approximately 58°F (14.4°C) and sensation returns when skin temperature reaches 60°F (15.6°C).[10, 29, 30] These temperatures are reached after approximately 20 minutes of treatment time using ice packs. Tissues begin to lose their viscoelastic properties when their temperatures reach 64°F (18°C).[31]

If the temperature of circulating blood is decreased by 0.2°F (0.1°C), the **hypothalamus ■** responds by initiating several systemic events (see Table 5–2). A systemic vasoconstriction occurs, and the heart rate is decreased in an attempt to localize the cold. If the proportion of the body area being cooled is sufficient, the heart rate is reduced in an attempt to maintain the body's core temperature by limiting the rate at which cool blood is circulated. If the core temperature continues to decrease toward the point of **hypothermia ■**, shivering and increased muscle tone assist in keeping the body heat inward. This severe response is normal when the human body is exposed to extremely cold environments (e.g., falling into a near-frozen lake). It is not a common response in therapeutic cold application.

The risk of cold-related injury increases once skin temperature reaches 55°F (12.8°C). If the skin temperature reaches 32°F (0°C) **intracellular ■** fluids begin to freeze and result in **frostbite** (see the Frostbite section in this chapter).

● E F F E C T S   O N

The Injury Response Process

The cellular and hemodynamic effects of cold application can be beneficial in the treatment of acute, subacute, and chronic conditions. Unlike heat modalities, cold can normally be safely used throughout the course of tissue healing.

During the treatment of acute injuries, the primary physiological effect of cold application is the reduction of cell metabolism. Reducing cell metabolism limits the amount of secondary injury by reducing the cell's need for oxygen. Immediate care of musculoskeletal injuries is augmented by the use of compression and elevation. These three elements together prevent secondary injury (see the Effects of Immediate Treatment section in this chapter).

Acetylcholine: Neurotransmitter responsible for transmitting motor nerve impulses.
Hypothalamus: The body's thermoregulatory center.
Hypothermia: Decreased core temperature.
Intracellular: Within the membrane of a cell.

Cellular Response

The most beneficial effect of cold application for an acute injury is the decreased need for oxygen in the area being treated, thus limiting the scope of secondary injury.[1, 32, 33] Cold application decreases cell metabolism and reduces the rate of damaging cellular reactions, thus decreasing the amount of oxygen the cells require to survive.[33] Reducing the cells' metabolic load also lessens the amount of cellular mitochondrial damage.[33]

During a 20-minute crushed ice pack treatment, cell metabolism decreases by 19 percent.[10, 17] By reducing the number of cells killed by a lack of oxygen, the amount of secondary hypoxic injury is limited. Because fewer cells are damaged from secondary hypoxic injury, reduced amounts of inflammatory mediators are released into the area, containing the scope of the injury (see Chapter 1).

The depth and magnitude of decreased cellular response is related to the subcutaneous tissues' temperature decrease, not the change in skin temperature. Traditional treatment durations of 20 to 30 minutes may not be sufficient to adequately cool deep target tissues, even with average amounts of overlying adipose tissues.[13, 33]

Inflammation

Changes in cellular function and blood dynamics serve to control the effects of acute inflammation. Cold application suppresses the inflammatory response by:

- Reducing the release of inflammatory mediators[32]
- Decreasing prostaglandin synthesis[32]
- Decreasing capillary permeability[32]
- Decreasing leukocyte/endothelial interaction[34]
- Decreasing creatine kinase activity[35]

The secondary formation of edema and hemorrhage is reduced because of an inhibitory effect on the mediators and decreased capillary permeability.

As we saw in the injury response cycle (see Fig. 1–4), limiting the amount of inflammation inhibits the effects of the remaining components. Limiting inflammatory mediators reduces the degree of hemorrhage and edema; lessening the mechanical pressure on nerves decreases pain. As muscle spasm and edema are reduced, there is less congestion in the area, and the amount of secondary hypoxic cell death is limited.

Blood and Fluid Dynamics

The primary hemodynamic effects of cold application are local arteriole vasoconstriction (capillaries cannot constrict because their walls do not contain smooth muscle), increased blood viscosity, and reduced blood flow. Because cold application decreases the rate of cell metabolism and reduces the tissue's need for oxygen, it would seem

to follow that blood flow to the treatment area would be reduced. Despite this seemingly sound logic, the effect of cold application on blood flow still is a topic of investigation.

Vasoconstriction is mediated by the autonomic nervous system. Decreasing tissue temperatures stimulates thermoreceptors in the blood vessels and local soft tissues, triggering a response from the sympathetic nervous system instructing the vessels to constrict. The body then attempts to maintain intramuscular temperatures by releasing hormonal mediators from the hypothalamus and adrenal medulla.[5] Vasoconstriction is also influenced by a reduction in the release of histamine and prostaglandin, two inflammatory mediators that produce vasodilation.

As the molecular motion of the blood and tissue fluids slows, viscosity increases, increasing resistance to flow. The reduction in blood flow occurs too late in the injury response process to affect the hemorrhaging process, but it may prevent hematoma formation.[1]

The effect of cold application on blood flow has been measured using **impedance plethysmography** ■, with most studies concluding that cold application causes decreased blood flow,[10, 17, 36, 37] but the results are not universally conclusive.[10, 38] Current research suggests that blood flow decrease begins to occur soon after the application of cold and continues to steadily decrease for the next 13 minutes and begins to oscillate between 13 and 17 minutes of treatment (Table 5–5).[5, 10, 17, 34, 37] Because capillaries do not constrict, blood flow reduction at this level results from vasoconstriction and reduced perfusion of the arterioles, reducing local **perfusion** ■ .[39]

One school of thought suggests that the body will increase blood flow through local vasodilation in an attempt to warm the treated area, but researchers generally no longer consider this to occur (Box 5–4). The treated skin does turn red during treatment (erythema), an event that could be related to increased blood flow, but is more

TABLE 5–5	Blood Flow Changes Following a 20-Minute Cold Pack Application

Vasculature	*Blood Flow Decrease (% reduction)*
Arterial	38
Capillary	25
Soft tissue blood flow	26
Skeletal blood flow	19

Impedance plethysmography: A determination of blood flow based on the amount of electrical resistance in the area.

Perfusion: Local blood flow that supplies tissues and organs with oxygen and nutrients.

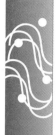

Box 5–4. Hunting for Proof of Cold-Induced Vasodilation

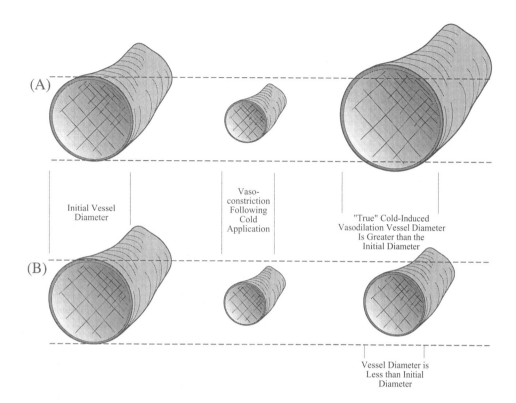

Vascular Response to Cold Application. (A) The concept of cold-induced vasodilation. After the application of therapeutic cold there is an immediate vasoconstriction. This is followed by vasodilation, resulting in a larger diameter than before the ice application. This event has not been substantiated. (B) Vascular reaction as suggested by Knight. After the initial vasoconstriction there is a dilation of the vessel, but its diameter is still reduced in comparison to the original diameter.

What effect does cold application have on local blood flow? In the early 1930s, Lewis[40] performed studies on skin temperature changes during cold treatments. When the fingers were immersed in cold water, alternating periods of cooling and warming were seen in the skin. Terming it the "hunting response," Lewis deduced that blood vessels underwent a series of vasoconstrictions and vasodilations in an attempt to adapt to the temperature (A). The magnitude and frequency of the hunting response varies with the body's core temperature. Cooler body temperatures lead to a reduced frequency and magnitude of this response.[41] However, the hunting response has been identified only in selected areas of the body (e.g., fingers, nose) and most often is associated with exposure to extreme cold environments.[36]

The concept of the hunting response influenced the manner in which cold was used clinically for several decades following Lewis' discovery (and still may be an influence today). Clinicians worked under the incorrect assumption that using too long a treatment duration (e.g., more than 20 minutes) would result in cold-induced vasodilation.

Many of the misconceptions of the hunting response were clarified by Knight.[1, 30] His work suggested that the degree of vasodilation only lessened the amount of initial vasoconstriction. Despite the vasodilation, there was still a net vasoconstriction when compared with the vessel diameter before treatment (B).[19]

Contemporary thought suggests that cold-induced vasodilation does not occur during standard cryotherapy sessions. However, certain diseases and/or neurological deficits that affect the sympathetic nervous system or local thermal regulation could result in vasodilation.

likely the result of local histamine release and an increased concentration of **oxyhemoglobin** ■.

Contemporary research using relatively healthy subjects and therapeutic temperature ranges and durations agrees that reactive vasodilation does not occur during cold application in healthy subjects. Any increase in blood flow is transitory, remains significantly below the pretreatment level, and is probably related to another mechanism, such as increased heart rate or stroke volume, because the vessel diameter does not appear to increase.[36]

Edema Formation and Reduction

A distinction must be made between the role of cold application in the control of edema formation and its role in edema reduction. The use of cryotherapy can substantially reduce the formation of edema and reduce the effects of arthrogenic muscle inhibition (see arthrogenic muscle inhibition, p 26).[42] The use of cryotherapy in and of itself does not encourage the removal of edema that has already collected and, in some instances, could hinder the venous and lymphatic return mechanism.

Cryotherapy limits the formation of edema by reducing cell metabolism, thereby decreasing metabolic activity and limiting the amount of secondary hypoxic injury. The subsequent vasoconstriction decreases the permeability of the post-capillary venules and the reduced blood flow decreases the intravascular pressure. Both events discourage fluids from escaping into the tissues.[43] Although the use of cryotherapy does substantially reduce edema formation following musculoskeletal trauma, cold application does not prevent edema formation associated with disease states such as venous insufficiency.

Because lymphatic and venous return are not influenced by arterial blood flow, the hemodynamic changes associated with cold application have little, if any, effect on edema reduction. The mechanisms of compression, elevation (gravity), muscle contractions, and muscle milking must still be incorporated into the treatment plan to reduce edema.

It stands to reason that the vasoconstriction described for arteries would apply to both the venous and lymphatic vessels. However, whereas cold application results in constriction of the arterioles and venules, the amount of arteriole vasoconstriction is greater than that for venules. This effect occurs until tissue temperatures decrease more than 27°F (15°C). After this, the permeability of lymph vessels begins to decrease. The surface area of the venules relative to the arterioles increases the area for reabsorption and limits the formation of edema (Fig. 5–3).[39, 44] This effect has also been substantiated in clinical studies.[37]

Overcooling the tissues can hinder the control of edema formation.[43, 45] Prolonged, inappropriate cooling can increase the permeability of superficial lymphatic vessels and result in the lymph contents spilling back into the tissues.[45] This effect is increased when the limb is

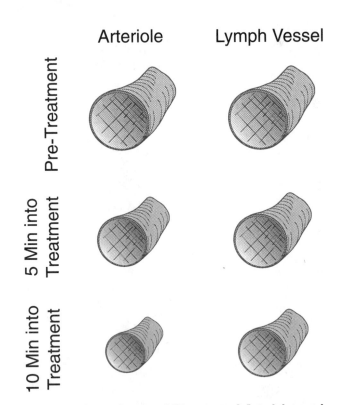

Figure 5–3. **Cross-Sectional Diameter of Arterioles and Lymph Vessels During Treatment.** As the tissue temperatures decrease, the cross-sectional diameter of both vessels decreases, but the change is greatest in arterioles, making the relative surface area of the lymph vessels larger.

placed in a gravity-dependent position and no form of external compression is used.[43] Prolonged cold application can increase the viscosity of fluids in the area, increasing the fluid's resistance to flow and potentially hindering the venous return process.

Nerve Conduction

During cold application, the rate that nerves can transmit impulses is decreased and the depolarization threshold of the impulses is increased. Because tissues cool at different rates and different depths have their own cooling rate, changes in nerve depolarization and nerve conduction velocity do not occur simultaneously. Longer cooling times are required to effect changes in nerves located at different depths. Superficial nerves will be affected before those nerves that are located deeper within the tissues.

Nerve conduction velocity is decreased by reducing the rate of synaptic transmission and increasing the time required for the nerve to depolarize and repolarize. As the temperature of the nerve decreases, its depolarization threshold increases. The nerve's resting potential is decreased, increasing the duration of the action potential and the refractory period. The time required for nerves to depolarize and repolarize is lengthened, decreasing the overall frequency of transmission.[46]

Oxyhemoglobin: Hemoglobin that is carrying oxygen found in the arterial system.

TABLE 5–6	Decrease in Muscular Afferent Nerve Transmission During Cryotherapy

Nerve	Percent Decrease*
Ia receptor	56
Ib receptor	42
Golgi's tendon organs	50

Per 18°F (10°C) decrease in intramuscular temperature

All types of nerves are affected by cold application. A 13.3°F (7.4°C) reduction in skin temperature reduces motor nerve conduction velocity by approximately 14 percent and sensory nerve conduction velocity by 33 percent. Each 1.8°F (1°C) drop in intramuscular temperature results in a 1.1- to 2.4-m/sec reduction in nerve conduction velocity.[27] Based on the type of nerve, the reduction of afferent impulses from muscles is proportionate to the amount of cooling that occurs (Table 5–6).[47] Cryotherapy reduces the amount of edema-induced arthrogenic muscle inhibition by facilitating motoneuron pool recruitment.[42]

Cold also reduces the speed of nerve conduction by slowing communication at the synapse. Acetylcholine concentrations decrease approximately 60 percent as neuromuscular temperatures decrease by 36°F (20°C), further slowing the rate of transmission.[28] In certain cases, this can lead to **neurapraxia** ■ and **axonotmesis** ■.[48, 49]

During normal treatment duration and intensity, nerve conduction velocity displays the greatest decrease immediately after the application of ice.[50] If the tissue temperature continues to decrease (i.e., a constant cold temperature is used) or if the treatment continues for extended periods, the nerve conduction rate will drop to a point at which nerves can no longer transmit impulses. Cold-induced nerve palsy has been reported after the treatment of injuries to the anterior compartment of the lower leg.[51, 52]

Pain Control
Cold application affects pain perception and transmission by interrupting nerve transmission, decreasing nerve condition velocity, reducing muscle spasm, and reducing or limiting edema. By stimulating the large-diameter neurons, cold inhibits pain transmission, acting as a **counterirritant** ■ in terms of the gate-control theory.[53] The sensory events associated with the application of a cold modality stimulate the large-diameter nerves to decrease the transmission and perception of pain.

Physiologically, the transmission of noxious impulses is reduced by lowering the excitability of free nerve endings, resulting in an increased pain threshold. Small-diameter, myelinated nerves are the first to exhibit a change in their conduction velocities. The last to respond to cold temperatures are unmyelinated, small-diameter nerves. This sequence of nerve fiber activation can provide an explanation for the sequence of sensations that accompany cryotherapy.

Proprioception
Despite its ability to interrupt the transmission and perception of pain and decrease the afferent conduction velocity of cutaneous sensory nerves, cold application does not appear to significantly inhibit joint proprioception.[15, 54] Cryotherapy does not significantly decrease lower leg proprioception, balance, agility, or joint position sense.[54–56]

Several factors have been proposed to account for the lack of effect on proprioception (Fig. 5–4). Proprioceptive nerves are low-threshold mechanoreceptors that have thick, myelinated axons. Their deep location within the tissues and myelin layer insulate these nerves from the full effects of cold therapy and, therefore, they may be less affected than superficial nerves.[15] Secondary spindles are possibly less affected by cold application than are primary spindles,[54] and different types of stretch receptors are activated at different points in the ROM.[55]

The loss of sensation does not appear to affect joint position receptors. Other nerve receptors may compensate for those receptors that are affected.[57] When the treatment targets the joint capsule but not the muscle, type II nerves may be inhibited and proprioceptive function is compensated for by other sensory input such as the brain interpreting the amount of effort needed to perform the movement.[15, 54]

Muscle Spasm
Cold reduces muscle spasm by suppressing the stretch reflex by two mechanisms:

1. It decreases pain by reducing the threshold of afferent nerve endings.
2. It decreases the sensitivity of muscle spindles.

A drop of 9°F (5°C) in surface skin temperature reduces the sensitivity of muscle spindles. The decrease in muscle spindle activity, combined with the decreased rate of afferent nerve impulses, inhibits the stretch reflex mechanism and results in decreased muscle spasm.[46, 58] The activity of type Ia fibers decrease with cold, type II fibers become more active, and type Ib fibers are less affected by

---

Axonotmesis: Damage to nerve tissue without physical severing of the nerve.
Counterirritant: A substance causing irritation of superficial sensory nerves so as to reduce the transmission of pain from underlying nerves.
Neurapraxia: A temporary loss of function in a peripheral nerve.

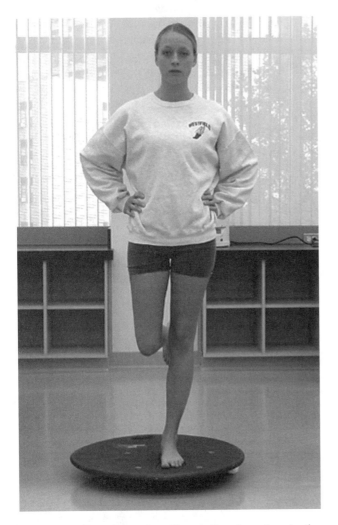

Figure 5–4. **Proprioception Board.** Proprioception is the ability to determine the joint's position and velocity of movement. Despite decreased nerve conduction velocities and increased depolarization thresholds, lower leg cryotherapy does not affect proprioception.

cold.[46] Cold inhibits **gamma-motoneurons** ■ and facilitates **alpha-motoneurons** ■ . To reduce spasticity, gamma inhibition must exceed alpha facilitation.[46]

Because cold disrupts muscle spasm, pain is reduced by alleviating the mechanical stimulation placed on the nerve receptors in the area of spasm. A short-term break in the pain-spasm-pain cycle may result in long-term relief of muscle spasms secondary to decreasing the amount of mechanical pressure placed on the nerves and other tissues. A brief disruption in pain may also break the injury response cycle and allow tissue healing and repair to proceed unhindered.[32]

Muscle Function

Decreased nerve conduction velocity and the neurophysiological effects that result in decreased muscle spasm also affect the limb's muscular ability. Decreased nerve conduction velocity, decreased sensitivity of muscle spindles, and increased fluid viscosity may lead to a decreased ability to perform rapid muscle movements. The latency of H-reflexes decreases by approximately 5.3 milliseconds (μsec), indicating decreased conduction velocity of muscle spindles.[45]

Changes in temperature increase motoneuron pool excitability. During a 20-minute cold application, the H-reflex is negatively correlated with temperature. As the temperature decreases, the motoneuron pool excitability increases, making more motor units available. During the rewarming phase, the reverse effect occurs and the two variables become positively correlated: As temperature increases the motoneuron pool excitability continues to increase.[59]

After a 20-minute cold application, the quadriceps femoris muscle group produces decreased concentric and eccentric strength and decreased isokinetic strength, power,[60–64] and endurance[60–63] for up to 30 minutes after the termination of treatment. For this reason, patients should be provided with adequate rewarming time before beginning intense work or athletic activities. A 3-minute ice application between exercise bouts has demonstrated the ability to increase exercise work, velocity, and power, possibly the result of slowing the increase of intramuscular temperatures.[65]

Sensations Associated with Cold Application

The terms traditionally used to describe the sensations accompanying cold application are cold, burning, aching, and analgesia (the absence of pain).[66] Numbness—anesthesia—is a result of decreasing the nerve conduction velocity and increasing the threshold required to fire the nerves.[32] Eighteen to 21 minutes of cold application are needed before analgesia occurs. True anesthesia is seldom achieved.[67]

Although these reactions are most pronounced during ice immersion, they may also occur during other methods of cold application, and the affective response during the initial treatment period may deter patient compliance. Not all people experience the same sensations during cold application, but educating the patient about the sensations to be expected during the treatment tends to make cold application, especially cold immersion, more tolerable.[68, 69] Also, repeated exposures to cold treatments can decrease the sensory and affective response to cold application.[70]

Effects of Immediate Treatment

Immediate treatment—rest, ice, compression, and elevation (RICE)—serves to counteract the body's initial response to an injury, including postsurgical care (Fig. 5–5). Rest limits the scope of the original injury by preventing further trauma. In acute trauma, "rest" may take

---

Alpha-motoneurons: Efferent motor neurons that innervate muscle fibers.

Gamma-motoneurons: Efferent motor nerves that innervate the intrafusal fibers of a muscle spindle.

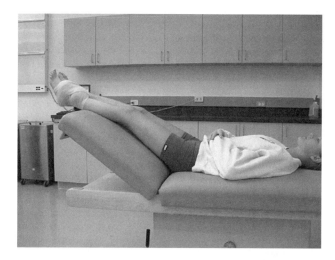

Figure 5–5. Ice, Compression, and Elevation. An ice bag is secured in place with an elastic wrap and the body part is elevated. This technique decreases the pressure gradient, lessening the amount of fluids that escape into the tissues and encourages venous and lymphatic return. See Clinical Techniques: Compression Wraps on the next page.

the form of immobilizing the body part, the use of crutches, or other methods of avoiding additional insult to the injured tissues. Crushed ice is the ideal form of cold application during immediate treatment because it produces the most rapid and significant temperature decrease relative to other forms of cold application, while conforming to the body part being treated.[7, 71]

The function of ice application during immediate treatment is to decrease the cell's metabolism, therefore decreasing the need for oxygen in the injured area. This effect reduces the amount of secondary hypoxic injury and secondary enzymatic injury by enabling the tissues in the injured area to survive on the limited amount of oxygen they are receiving. Larger amounts of adipose tissue require a longer treatment duration than the "traditional" 20 to 30 minutes to obtain the desired cooling (see Box 5–3).[33]

Ice application also provides secondary benefits in the immediate treatment of an injury by reducing pain. Because of the other factors surrounding the injury (e.g., the severity of the injury or the person's emotional state), the effects of ice on limiting pain cannot be accurately predicted for every case.

Compression decreases the pressure gradient between the blood vessels and tissues. This discourages further leakage from the capillary beds into the interstitial tissues while also encouraging increased lymphatic drainage. Compression wraps must be applied so that a pressure gradient is formed between the distal end of the wrap and the proximal end (see Clinical Techniques: Compression Wraps, p 114).

Using an elastic wrap to secure the ice bag to the body part produces a significant reduction in subcutaneous tissue temperatures as compared with simply placing the ice pack on the skin.[21] However, placing the wrap

between the pack and the skin reduces the amount of skin temperature drop because the wrap acts as an insulator.[12, 21]

The combination of ice and compression results in reduced cell metabolism deeper within the tissues, helping to limit the scope and severity of secondary injury. An additional benefit of using an elastic wrap is increased joint proprioception secondary to stimulating the afferent receptors in the skin and superficial subcutaneous tissues.[72] This effect can serve to protect injured joints by assisting the body's awareness of the joint's position. The compression wrap also helps to decrease pain by stimulating sensory and proprioceptive nerve endings that override noxious stimulus.

Compression and **elevation** decrease the vascular hydrostatic pressure within the capillary beds, reducing capillary outflow to the tissue. The difference in pressures encourages absorption of edema by the lymphatic system. The force of gravity acting on the elevated extremity encourages venous and lymphatic return. This effect is greatest when the extremity is at 90 degrees perpendicular to the ground; however, this position is not necessarily practical. The limb should be elevated as high as possible while still maintaining a comfortable position. Mechanical implements such as split-leg tables can effectively raise the lower extremity to a 45-degree angle, at which point the effect of gravity is 71 percent of that in the vertical position (see Fig. 1–13). The effects of elevation in reducing edema are short-lived. Edema returns to pretreatment volumes within 5 minutes of returning the limb to the gravity-dependent position.[42]

Cryokinetics

Cryokinetics involves the use of cold therapy in conjunction with movement (*cryo* = cold; *kinetic* = motion) and is used to improve ROM by eliminating or reducing the element of pain. Early, safe, pain-free motion through the normal range results in a more pronounced macrophage reaction, quicker hematoma resolution, increased vascular growth, faster regeneration of muscle and scar tissue, and increased tensile strength of healed muscle.[24]

Cryokinetics may be initiated in cases in which the underlying soft tissue and bone are intact and in which pain is limiting the amount of functional movement. Although cryokinetics is useful in increasing ROM, care must be taken to prevent masking pain that would otherwise alert the individual to further tissue damage.

Cold-Related Injury

Two factors associated with cryotherapy can increase the risk of cold-related injury during treatment: the skin temperature decrease and the amount of pressure used to secure the cold pack. Extreme temperatures, those not normally reached during properly applied treatments can result in frostbite. Cold and the pressure associated with a compression wrap can traumatize superficial nerves.

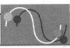

CLINICAL TECHNIQUES: COMPRESSION WRAPS

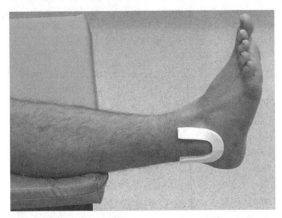
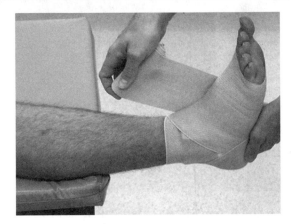
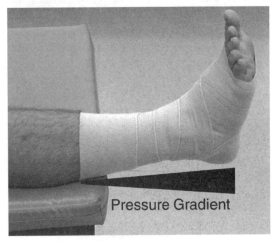

Pressure Gradient

Focal Compression to the Lateral Ankle Ligaments. (A) A U-shaped "horseshoe" pad is placed around the lateral malleolus. (B) Starting at the metatarsophalangeal joints, apply the compression wrap and work proximally. (C) More pressure is applied at the distal end than the proximal end, creating a pressure gradient.

Apply the compression wrap starting at the distal extremity and working proximally, gradually decreasing the pressure with each turn. Wraps applied with even pressure throughout their length are often counterproductive because they form a kind of tourniquet, inhibiting flow both to and from the area. Too much compression over superficial veins, such as the popliteal vein in the posterior knee, can elevate peripheral venous pressure and increase the risk of deep vein **thrombosis ■** .[12, 45]

Compression may be applied to an injured area through three different techniques[73]:

1. **Circumferential compression** provides an even pressure around the entire circumference of the body part. The cross-sectional area remains circular, but the diameter of the body part decreases. This type of compression is used for evenly shaped body areas, such as the knee or thigh. Elastic wraps and pneumatic or water-filled sleeves are common forms of circumferential compression.
2. **Collateral compression** produces pressure on only two sides of the body part, so that the cross-sectional area deforms elliptically. The soft tissues are compressed

between the device and the bone. A common form of collateral compression is found in air-filled stirrup braces.
3. **Focal compression**, applied with U-shaped "horseshoe" pads, provides direct pressure to soft tissue surrounded by prominent bony structures (e.g., the lateral ligaments of the ankle or the acromioclavicular joint). The pad is placed over the area so that it is in contact with the injured soft tissue while avoiding the bone. A circumferential or collateral compression wrap is then used to apply pressure (see illustration above).

Check capillary refill in the distal extremity (fingers, toes) to ensure that adequate circulation is maintained.

Compression should be applied up to 30 to 40 mm Hg of pressure.[5] To develop a feel for how much pressure is being applied during a compression wrap, inflate a blood pressure cuff to 20 mm Hg and place it on the skin. Then apply an elastic wrap over top of the cuff. When you are finished, observe the value on the sphygmomanometer. Subtract the original value (e.g., 20 mm Hg) from the final value to determine how much pressure was applied.

See Chapter 14 for more information on the effects of compression.

Thrombosis: The formation or presence of a blood clot within the vascular system.

Cold-Induced Neuropathy

Securing a cold pack with an elastic wrap increases the depth and magnitude of the treatment. When too much pressure is applied to an elastic wrap that is securing a cold pack over large, superficial nerves, the resulting overcooling can result in neuropathy, causing the loss of sensory or motor function, or both. The common peroneal nerve (located just superior to the fibular head) and the ulnar nerve (posteromedial aspect of the elbow) are most prone to this condition. Decrease the amount of pressure used when securing a cold pack over any superficial nerve.

Compression wraps should not be used when treating **compartment syndromes ■**. The external pressure from the wrap can significantly increase the amount of pressure within the compartment and result in neurological or vascular insufficiency in the distal extremity. During any treatment, regularly check the patient for signs of nerve dysfunction, such as tingling in the distal extremity and normal blood flow in the fingers or toes, by observing the capillary refill in the nail bed.

Frostbite

Under normal conditions there is little chance of developing frostbite when frozen water is used as the means of cold application.[58] In your mind, picture these forms of ice application: an ice bag, ice massage, and ice immersion. During the course of each of these treatments, water is present. An ice bag fills with water as it melts, ice massage leaves a trail of water with each stroke, and water is the medium used during an ice immersion.

The presence of water indicates that ice is melting and the water is in its **change of state ■**; therefore, the temperature of the ice pack is slightly above 32°F (0°C). Frostbite occurs when the skin temperature falls below freezing. When the subcutaneous temperature falls below 55°F (12.8°C), the risk of cold-related tissue damage increases. During the course of a 20-minute treatment, cold modalities that have water present cause a decrease in skin temperature to 56°F (13.3°C).[58]

The risk of frostbite is present when using reusable cold packs. These devices contain water mixed with antifreeze and are stored at temperatures below freezing. Because the surface temperature of the pack may be below freezing, a medium such as a wet towel must be placed between the pack and the skin in order to reduce the risk of frostbite.

After 5 minutes of cold application, the skin should be marked by erythema, indicating that the circulatory system is continuing to deliver warm blood, even though the skin temperature has dropped substantially. If the area displays signs of **pallor ■**, the circulatory system has been unable to maintain tissue temperatures within normal physiological limits, increasing the risk of frostbite. If the tissues become **cyanotic ■**, the treatment should be discontinued.

If the treatment is applied below the recommended temperature, if the duration of the treatment exceeds the recommended time, or if the patient suffers from severe circulatory insufficiency or decreased sensation, the risk of frostbite (or cold injury) increases (Box 5–5). Prolonged exposure to intense cold decreases circulation throughout the body. Blood traveling through the veins cools the incoming arterial blood and acts to increase the amount of systemic vasoconstriction and to further lower the heart rate. If the treated area is ischemic, warm blood cannot reach the tissues.

Contraindications and Precautions in the Use of Cold Modalities

The primary contraindications to the use of cold modalities are conditions in which the body is unable to cope with the temperature because of allergy, hypersensitivity, or circulatory or nerve insufficiency (see Table 5–3). True cold contraindications must be carefully differentiated from the dislike of cold. Most of the disease states that contraindicate cold application affect the blood or nerve supply.

Recall that arterial blood warms the treated area and venous blood carries cold away. Edema caused by circulatory problems such as peripheral vascular disease can be increased by cold application. Decreased blood flow to or from the treated area can cause the tissues to be overcooled. Nerve inhibition can interfere with local thermoregulation, either producing overcooling of the tissue or, in some instances, increased blood flow. Impaired sensory function will increase the risk of cold-related injury.

Some people do not tolerate cold exposure well. In some instances, this can be related to neurovascular disorders such as Raynaud's phenomenon, which can indicate underlying cold-induced myocardial ischemia.[74] In other cases the individual may have a true allergy to cold. This condition is characterized by urticaria, the outbreak of hives, itching, and in rare cases, anaphylactic shock.

Disease states such as lupus are also contraindications to cold application. Abnormal blood proteins, cryoglobu-

---

Change of state: Transformation from one physical state to another (e.g., ice to water).

Compartment syndrome: Increased pressure within a muscular compartment, causing decreased blood flow to and from the distal extremity, and decreased distal nerve function and decreased local muscular blood profusion and pain.

Cyanosis (cyanotic): A blue-gray discoloration of the skin caused by a lack of oxygen.

Pallor: Lack of color in the skin.

lins, can adhere to each other during cold exposure. Patients suffering from **hypotension** ■, **hypertension** ■, or other cardiovascular or cardiorespiratory diseases may experience increased blood pressure or difficulty breathing if large areas (i.e., immersion) or temperatures that are too cold are used.

Patients who have mild contraindications can be treated by placing a terry cloth towel between the cold pack and the skin to prevent the temperature from becoming too cold. However, this approach can render the treatment ineffective. Adding an insulating barrier or increasing the temperature of cold immersions can prevent a negative reaction to the cold. The patient's physician should always be consulted prior to using apparently contraindicated techniques.

Controversies in Treatment

Researchers and clinicians generally accept the efficacy of cold modalities. Some debate still exists about fluctuations in blood flow and other vascular reactions that occur during treatment. Some researchers have reported a spike in blood flow approximately 10 to 17 minutes into the treatment.[36] However, this appears to be inconsequential to most treatment approaches. Likewise, as we will see with modalities such as contrast baths, the fact that capillaries do not change their size must be considered when determining the effectiveness of various treatment approaches.

Twenty minutes is used as the default treatment duration for ice packs (and to a lesser extent, 15 minutes has become the "standard" for immersion and 10 minutes for ice massage), but this "one size fits all" treatment duration limits the effectiveness of cold application. With the exception of cutaneous sensory nerves that are superficial to the adipose tissue layer, the rate, depth, and magnitude of intramuscular cooling is dependent on the thickness of the adipose tissue layer. Therefore, the appropriate treatment duration is based on the thickness of this insulating layer and the depth of the target tissue.

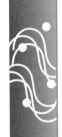

Box 5–5. Signs and Symptoms of Frostbite

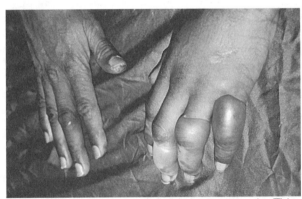

Even the most minor case of frostbite is accompanied by extreme pain. This pain is so severe that patients who have normal sensory function will not allow the treatment to continue. The primary concern is for patients who have sensory and/or circulatory impairment or those on whom reusable ice packs are applied.

The first physical sign of frostbite is the fading of the redness normally associated with cold application. This color is replaced by a waxy white sheen. If frostbite is allowed to continue, the skin will blister or molt and lead to an obvious buildup of edema.

Even though the chance of frostbite is slim, patients with impaired circulation are at a higher risk. The use of elastic wraps and cold further decrease skin temperature and require that the skin reaction be more closely monitored. During any physical procedure, the circulation to the extremities can be checked by monitoring the flow of blood to the nailbeds. Gently squeezing the nail removes the blood, making it turn white or pale. When the force is removed, the original color should return. If it fails to return, circulatory impairment should be suspected.

If frostbite is suspected, immediately remove the patient from the source of the cold. Rewarm the body part by immersing it in water between 100° and 108°F and refer the patient to a physician for follow-up evaluation and treatment.

(From Kozol RA: When to Call the Surgeon: Decision Making for Primary Care Providers. FA Davis, Philadelphia, 1999, with permission.)

Hypotension: Low blood pressure.
Hypertension: High blood pressure.

The method of cold application does apparently affect some treatment outcomes. The use of intermittent cold application appears to result in deeper cooling of the tissues. Allowing some skin rewarming to occur maintains a steeper temperature gradient that allows further cooling of the underlying tissue. This is in contrast to some clinical approaches that call for constant cooling, such as is often applied immediately postsurgery. The cost-effectiveness of cold compression therapy units has also been questioned.[45] The effectiveness of various methods of cold application on reducing intramuscular temperature also depends on the size (area) of the skin being treated. For example, ice massage results in a more rapid decline in intramuscular temperatures, but only when a small (4 × 4 cm) area is treated.[5]

Another common clinical practice, placing an insulating barrier between the skin and cold pack, can render the treatment ineffective by reducing the temperature gradient between the skin and the ice pack. An insulating barrier should only be used when a reusable ice pack is applied or the patient displays sensitivities or contraindications to cold treatment.

■ Heat Modalities

Heat, the increase in molecular vibration and cellular metabolic rate, is commonly classified into three major categories based on its source:

1. Chemical action associated with cell metabolism
2. Mechanical action as found with ultrasound (see Chap. 7)
3. Electrical or magnetic currents as those found in diathermy devices (see Chap. 9)

The application of therapeutic heat, **thermotherapy**, is classified as superficial or deep (Table 5–7). Superficial heating agents must be capable of increasing the skin temperature within the range of 104°F to 113°F to produce therapeutic effects.[75] The transfer of heat to underlying tissues occurs through conduction, but superficial heating agents are limited to depths of less than 2 cm. Deep-heating agents, therapeutic ultrasound, and short-wave diathermy are capable of heating tissues located at depths greater than 2 cm. These devices are presented in the next section.

TABLE 5-7 Classification of Heating Agents

Superficial Heat	Deep Heat
Infrared lamps (see Chapter 19)	Microwave diathermy*
Moist heat packs	Shortwave diathermy (see Chapter 9)
Paraffin baths	Ultrasound (see Chapter 7)
Warm whirlpool and/or immersion	

Approved only for research purposes.

The effects of heat on metabolic rate, blood and fluid dynamics, and inflammation are generally opposite to those of cold (Table 5–8). Both heat and cold applications decrease pain and muscle spasm by altering the threshold of nerve endings. Systemically, local heat application results in increased body temperature, pulse rate, respiratory rate, and decreased blood pressure. The use of heat is indicated in the subacute and chronic inflammatory stages of injury (Table 5–9).

Magnitude and Duration of Temperature Increase

When therapeutic heat is applied to the body, the temperature gradient causes the modality to lose heat and the body to gain heat. Some heat is also lost to the surrounding environment (Fig. 5–6). The larger the temperature gradient, the faster the energy exchange occurs. Some thermal modalities, such as moist heat packs, are too hot to be applied directly to the skin. In this case, an insulating medium must be used to prevent the skin from being burned.

Maximum therapeutic benefits occur when the skin temperature rapidly increases, increasing the excitability

TABLE 5-8 Effects of Heat Application

Local Effects of Heat Application	Some Systemic Effects of Heat Exposure*
Vasodilation	Increased body temperature
Increased rate of cell metabolism	Increased pulse rate
Increased delivery of leukocytes	Increased respiratory rate
Increased capillary permeability	Decreased blood pressure
Increased venous and lymphatic drainage	
Edema formation	
Removal of metabolic wastes	
Increased elasticity of collagen-rich tissues (ligaments, joint capsule, fascia, tendons, skin)	
Analgesia and sedation of nerves	
Decreased muscle tone	
Decreased muscle spasm	
Decreased pain	
Increased nerve conduction velocity	

These systemic effects primarily occur when the entire body is exposed to warm temperatures. Therefore we would expect them to occur during a full-body warm immersion rather than during the application of a moist heat pack.

TABLE 5–9	General Indications and Contraindications for Heat Treatments

Indications	*Contraindications*
Subacute or chronic inflammatory conditions	Acute injuries
Reduction of subacute or chronic pain	Impaired circulation
Subacute or chronic muscle spasm	Advanced arthritis (vigorous heating)
Decreased range of motion	Poor thermal regulation
Hematoma resolution	Anesthetic areas
Reduction of joint contractures	**Neoplasms** ∎
	Thrombophlebitis

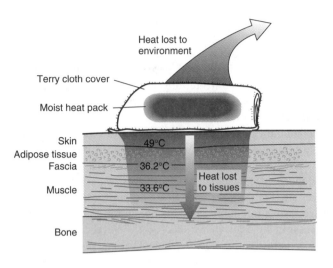

Figure 5–6. **Conductive Heating of the Skin and Subcutaneous Tissues.** When a moist heat pack is placed on the skin, the subcutaneous adipose tissue layer limits deeper penetration of the energy. The maximum treatment depth of moist heat packs is between 2 and 3 cm.

of local temperature receptors, causing a more active release of vasoactive mediators.[76] If the rate of temperature increase is too slow, the associated increased blood flow will keep tissue temperatures low. If the rate is too great, wide dynamic range thermoreceptors will be activated, producing pain, and burns may result. Some heating agents such as moist heat packs require the use of an insulator to protect the skin, thus regulating the temperature gradient to within therapeutic limits.

During the first 5 to 6 minutes of treatment, the body absorbs heat faster than the body can dissipate it. After approximately 7 to 9 minutes of exposure, the temperature gradient begins to even out and slightly decline.[77] At this point, the body is able to counteract the energy being applied by supplying an adequate amount of blood to cool the area, and the tissue temperatures stabilize. The fluctuations in skin temperature (presumably occurring as a defense mechanism to prevent burning) limit the amount of subcutaneous heating that can be obtained.[78]

When a maximal vasodilation has occurred and the intensity of the treatment stays constant (or increases), the vessels begin to constrict. This phenomenon, known as **rebound vasoconstriction**, occurs approximately 20 minutes into the treatment. This is the body's attempt to save underlying tissues by sacrificing the superficial layer. If the intensity of treatment is too great or if the duration of exposure is too long, burns will result. The likelihood of rebound vasoconstriction increases with treatments in which the temperature and intensity are kept constant, such as infrared lamps and paraffin immersion baths. With modalities such as moist heat packs, the intensity of the treatment decreases with time because the modality loses heat during the application. **Mottling** ∎ of the skin is a warning sign that tissue temperatures are rising to a dangerously high level. In this case, ghost-white

areas and beet-red splotches mark the patient's skin. When mottling occurs, the treatment should be discontinued immediately.

Central and local mechanisms and a reflex arc attempt to maintain the core temperature at a "set point" that is monitored by the hypothalamus. The temperature of local areas is permitted to fluctuate more than the core temperature. Blood flow is regulated to prevent excessive heat exchange, with vasodilation occurring to help cool the treated area. The body may (theoretically) decrease blood flow to prevent the increased temperature from affecting the core.[79, 80]

As we saw with cold modalities, the adipose tissue layer is also a primary limiting factor for the effective depth of heat penetration (see Box 5–1). As the thickness of the adipose tissue layer increases, more of the superficial heating agents thermal energy is absorbed in this layer, preventing temperature increase in deeper layers. The increased intramuscular temperature also decreases the temperature gradient, limiting the transfer of energy.

Tissue Rewarming

Skin and subcutaneous adipose tissue temperatures rapidly decrease following the removal of the heating agent. Heat is lost to the surrounding air, and the increased circulation continues to deliver relatively cool blood to the treated area while the venous system removes relatively warm blood. Superficial intramuscular temperatures remain elevated for approximately 30 minutes following the conclusion of the treatment. The magnitude and duration of the latent effects of heat are less pronounced than those demonstrated with cold.

Mottling: A blotchy discoloration of the skin.

Neoplasm: Abnormal tissue, such as a tumor, that grows at the expense of healthy tissue.

Therapeutic Temperature Benchmarks

The magnitude of heating is based on the temperature increase of the target tissues (Table 5–10). Increases in cell metabolism and blood flow occur soon after the application of the heating agent. Increased temperature causes blood hemoglobin to release oxygen, providing more oxygen for the healing process. At 106°F (41.1°C), the release of oxygen is approximately twice as great as at baseline temperatures (Fig. 5–7).

Enzymatic activity begins to increase when temperatures approach 102°F (38.9°C) and continues to be accelerated up to 122°F (50°C). After this point, the rate of enzymatic activity rapidly decreases.

Heating to 104°F to 113°F (40°C to 45°C) more easily allows for plastic deformation of collagen-rich tissues (joint capsule, ligaments, fascia, tendons). However, the structure must be physically stretched to place a load on it for elongation to occur.[6] Protein damage occurs and cells and tissues are destroyed when the tissue temperature is increased to greater than 113°F (45°C). Extreme heating, such as that obtained by lasers used during thermal shrinkage of the joint capsule, heat the tissue to between 140° and 158°F (60°C and 70°C), resulting in contraction of the capsular fibers.[81]

TABLE 5–10	Tissue Temperature Increase from Baseline Required to Achieve Therapeutic Effects*	
Classification of Thermal Effects	*Temperature Increase*	*Used for*
Mild	1.8°F (1°C)	Mild inflammation Accelerates metabolic rate
Moderate	3.6°–5.4°F (2°–3°C)	Decreasing muscle spasm Decreasing pain Increasing blood flow Reducing chronic inflammation
Vigorous	5.4°–9.0°F (3°–4°C)	Tissue elongation, scar tissue reduction Inhibition of sympathetic activity

It is unclear if the relative temperature increase (e.g., 2°C) or absolute temperature for the target tissue (see Controversies in Treatment for heat modalities).

● EFFECTS ON

The Injury Response Process

Despite the fact that heat and cold produce many of the same outcomes, decreased pain for example, the timing of when to begin using heat modalities is much more critical. A primary effect of heat modalities is an increase in cell metabolism and the rate of inflammation. If heat is applied too soon in the injury response process, the increased cell metabolism causes an increase in the number of cells injured or destroyed because of hypoxia. Increasing the inflammatory rate could possibly extend the acute and subacute inflammatory stages.

Cellular Response

The rate of cell metabolism increases in response to the rise in tissue temperature. For each increase of 18°F

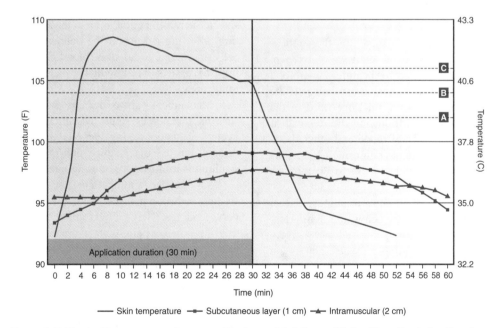

Figure 5–7. **Tissue Temperature Increase During a 30-Minute Moist Heat Pack Application.** (A) 102°F to 109°F: Enzymatic activity increases. (B) 104°F: Plastic deformation of collagen-rich tissue begins to occur. (C) 106°F: Blood hemoglobin release into tissue is twice that of baseline tissue temperature

(10.0°C) in skin temperature, the cell's metabolic rate increases by a factor of two to three, the **Q10 effect**.[82] As the cell's metabolic rate increases, so does its demand for oxygen and nutrients. As with all living organisms that consume energy, the amount of waste such as nitrogen and **lactic acid** ■ excreted from the cell increases as its metabolism increases.

There is a reciprocal relationship between tissue temperature and the rate of cell metabolism. Not only does increased temperature cause an increase in cellular metabolic rate but an increase in cellular metabolic rate also causes tissue temperature to rise. As with all heat applications, increased cellular metabolic rate causes arteriolar dilation and increased capillary flow. This supports the therapeutic properties of exercise.

Effect on Inflammation

The local application of heat accelerates inflammation. Soft tissue repair is facilitated through an accelerated metabolic rate and increased blood supply. Blood flow must be increased to encourage the removal of cellular debris and to increase delivery of the nutrients necessary for the healing of tissues.[83] Increased oxygen delivery stimulates the breakdown and removal of tissue debris and inflammatory **metabolites** ■. Nutrients are delivered to the area to fuel the cells, and there is also an increase in the delivery of leukocytes, encouraging phagocytosis.

Blood and Fluid Dynamics

The body responds to the rise in tissue temperature by dilating local blood vessels. This effect is more pronounced in the superficial vessels than in the deeper vessels. Heat produces vasodilation through the combination of three mechanisms: (1) relaxing the smooth muscle of the arteries, (2) triggering the release of bradykinin, and (3) through a spinal-level reflex.

Blood flow begins to increase soon after the application of the modality, increasing the delivery of oxygen, nutrients, and antibodies required for healing. Peak blood flow, often more than a twofold increase relative to the baseline, usually occurs during the final one third of the treatment or within 10 minutes following the removal of the modality.[77, 84] The viscosity of blood and other fluids decreases as the surrounding temperature increases. This elevated blood flow will continue for up to 60 minutes following the end of the treatment.[84]

In the presence of normal amounts of adipose tissue, this effect occurs in 2 cm or less below the skin. Heat applied to muscles that are normally covered by relatively low amounts of subcutaneous adipose tissue, such as the trapezius, may experience increased blood flow up to 3 cm below the surface of the skin.[85]

Edema Formation and Reduction

Heat application increases the volume of the treated limb, especially when the limb is placed in the gravity-dependent position as is seen during warm whirlpool treatment. During a 20-minute treatment, the limb volume of uninjured lower extremities increases 5 mL for every 1°F (0.6°C) rise in water temperature above 92°F (33.3°C). This increase is greater when pathology is present.[86]

The amount of edema is increased, but the capability of removing it is greater. Increased capillary pressure forces edema and harmful metabolites from the injured area. Increased lymphatic permeability aids in the reabsorption of edema and the dissolution of hematomas. These wastes can drain into the venous and lymphatic systems. If venous and lymphatic return is not encouraged, further edema occurs.

Nerve Conduction

The increased rate of chemical reactions and cell metabolism result in increased nerve conduction velocity. Both sensory and motor nerve function are typically enhanced through heat treatments.

Pain Control

Pain relief is obtained by lessening mechanical pressure on nerve endings, decreasing muscle spasm, reducing ischemia, and a counterirritant effect that increases the pain threshold. Mechanical deformation or chemical irritation of nerve endings stimulates pain transmission. In acute injuries, the primary cause of pain is the mechanical damage done to the tissue in the area. In the subacute and chronic stage of injury, ischemia and irritation cause chemical pain from certain chemical mediators. Mechanical pain is caused by increased tissue pressure (swelling) and the tension placed on nerves by muscle spasm. Increasing circulation to the area decreases congestion, allowing oxygen to be delivered to the suffocating cells. Increased circulation (blood flow to and away from the area) assists in removing the pain-producing chemicals in the area.

Mechanical pain is decreased by reducing the pressure on the nerves, thus lessening the pain-spasm-pain cycle. By encouraging venous and lymphatic return through the use of elevation and muscle contraction, the swelling is removed, decreasing interstitial pressure.

An increase in temperature leads to a state of analgesia and **sedation** ■ in the injured area by acting on free nerve endings. Nerve fibers are stimulated, blocking the transmission of pain with a counterirritant effect. This effect appears to last only as long as the stimulus of heat is applied, and when heat is removed, the pain symptoms quickly return.[48, 87]

Lactic acid: A cellular waste product produced by muscular contraction or cell metabolism. A fatiguing carbohydrate.

Metabolite: A by-product of metabolism.

Sedation: The result of calming nerve endings.

Muscle Spasm and Function

Heat reduces muscle spasm by decreasing the sensitivity of the muscle's secondary gamma afferents (which are more sensitive to tonic tension than phasic tension), which decreases muscle tone and alleviates pressure on the nerve (see Treatment Strategies: Muscle Spasm and Trigger Points, p 27).[88] Increasing blood flow and reducing local muscle metabolites further alleviates spasm.[3] Note that only the most superficial portion of the muscle is directly affected by superficial heating agents.

Decreased fluid viscosity, increased nerve conduction velocity, and the increased rate of Golgi tendon organ firing increases muscle function and strength, as long as the temperature is maintained within therapeutic ranges.[6]

Tissue Elasticity

When collagen-rich tissue such as tendon, muscle, and fascia is heated to 104° to 113°F (40° to 45°C) for 5 minutes, it can be more easily elongated (plastic deformation). ROM is subsequently improved by increasing the extensibility of collagen and the viscosity and plastic deformation of tissues.[89] This effect alone is not sufficient to decrease contractures or increase the elasticity of healthy tissues. Tension, in the form of gentle stretching, is necessary to elongate muscle and capsular tissues while the tissues are still within the therapeutic temperature range.

Unless an adhesion is mechanically restricting ROM, most of the ROM benefits derived from heat application are probably the result of decreasing muscle tone rather than physically elongating tissues. For example, moist heat pack application can increase hamstring flexibility more than three 30-second static stretches. However, this increase is related to muscle relaxation rather than representing an increase in an elongation of the muscle.[90] Neither anterior laxity of the knee or hamstring flexibility has been shown to be affected by heat modalities alone.[91, 92]

Exercise as a Form of Heat

Increased blood flow, increased cell metabolism, and increased intramuscular temperature occur during the application of heat modalities and during active exercise. Moderate to intense exercise increases intramuscular temperatures approximately 4°F (2.2°C) at a depth of 5 cm in the involved muscles, but does not result in a temperature increase in nonexercising muscles.[93]

Although active exercise does not result in vigorous heating of the muscle, moderate heating occurs over a larger cross-sectional area and deeper into the muscle than most other forms of heat. Most important, active exercise is more functional than the use of passive heating modalities. Brief exercise produces a relatively large, short-term increase in blood flow. Heat modalities result in a smaller net increase in blood flow, but the duration of the increase lasts for a longer time.[77, 94]

Contraindications to Heat Application

Because the effects of heat application are essentially the opposite to those of cold, its use in the treatment of acute injuries should be avoided. Applying heat to an active inflammatory cycle increases the rate of cell metabolism and accelerates the amount of hypoxic injury.

Neurovascular deficits can result in overheating of the skin and result in burns. The patient should have normal sensory and vascular function and be able to communicate any abnormal sensations. Heating agents should not be applied to sleeping or unconscious individuals.

High temperatures should not be used on limbs in which thrombophlebitis is present. The vasodilation and increased blood flow related to heat application could cause the clot to become dislodged and enter the circulatory system, potentially blocking blood supply to vital organs such as the heart or brain. The application of therapeutic heat over tumors can increase the rate of tumor growth.

Controversies in Treatment

As with cold modalities, the efficacy of superficial heating agents has been established. Some debate regarding the actual depth of effective penetration of the various forms of superficial heating agents exists, and many forms of moist heat have not been thoroughly investigated. Many of the heating methods described in the next chapter, namely fluidotherapy, paraffin treatment, and whirlpools do not have a strong research base to support or refute their efficacy. Likewise, the reputed effects of contrast therapy have not been established in controlled studies.

The amount of temperature increase required to enhance the plastic properties of collagen-rich tissues is unclear (see Table 5–10). The temperatures of the heating ranges are based on the assumption of an initial temperature of approximately 99°F (37°C); resting muscle is typically less than this. Increasing collagen elasticity is improved when the target tissue temperature is increased to 104° to 113°F (40° to 45°C). Clinically, this is different from obtaining a 5.4° to 9.0°F (3° to 4°C) temperature increase.[95]

The use of certain heating agents over joints affected by rheumatoid arthritis has been questioned. Vigorous heating of arthritic joints may promote the effect of lysosomal enzymes, especially collagenase which degrades articular cartilage. At temperatures greater than 95° to 97°F (35° to 36°C) enzymatic deterioration of articular cartilage markedly increases.[24]

■ Contrast and Comparison of Heat and Cold Application

Cold modalities are more penetrating and their effects longer lasting than those of heat modalities. Heat causes a vasodilation that delivers cool blood to the area while the warmer blood is transported away. In contrast, cold application causes a vasoconstriction, resulting in a decreased amount of blood arriving to warm the area. This causes deeper tissues to be affected more by cold than by superficial heating agents (Table 5–11).

After the modality is removed from the body, the effects of cold are longer lasting than those of heat. This is a result of the same mechanisms that account for the increased depth of the effects of cold. After heat treatment, cool blood continues to flow to the area, decreasing the temperature. In contrast, the cool tissue temperature resulting from cold application causes the vasoconstriction of blood vessels and a decrease in the amount of blood delivered to the area, so that a longer time is needed for rewarming than for recooling.[96]

Both modalities effectively reduce pain perception by increasing the patient's pain threshold. Although patients prefer moist heat modalities, their effectiveness is short-lived after the treatment.[87] Educating the patient about the potentially detrimental effects of using heat too early in the treatment program should help improve patient compliance.

TABLE 5–11	Comparison of Heat and Cold Treatments	
Effect	*Cold*	*Heat*
Effective depth	5 cm	1–2 cm (superficial agents) 2–5 cm (deep-heating agents)
Duration of effects	Hours	Begins to dissipate after the removal of the modality
Blood flow	↓(Vasoconstriction)	↑(Vasodilation)
Rate of cell metabolism	↓	↑
Oxygen consumption	↓	↑
Cell wastes	↓	↑
Fluid viscosity	↓	↓
Capillary permeability	↓	↑
Inflammation	↓	↑
Pain	↓	↑
Muscle spasm	↓(reduced sensitivity of muscle spindles and decreased pain)	↑(reduced ischemia and pain)
Muscle contraction	↓(reduced nerve conduction velocity and increased fluid viscosity)	↑(increased nerve conduction velocity and decreased fluid viscosity)

↓ = *Decrease;* ↑ = *increase.*

The application of cold reduces the amounts of inflammatory mediators and cell by-products released into the area. These cellular wastes, including lactic acid and nitrogen, are insulting to the tissues and increase the amount of tissue damage and pain. When heat is applied during the proliferation stage of inflammation, the vascular response assists in removing cellular waste.

Use of Heat Versus Cold

One of the questions most asked by students is "How do you know when to use heat and when to use cold?" There are no clear-cut answers to this question. Many texts and articles give definitive time frames, such as: "Use ice for the first 24 hours and heat for the next 48." Unfortunately, statements like this are incorrect and unjustified.

One of the first points made in this text was that the body heals an injury at its own rate. Not only does this rate vary from person to person but also it may vary from injury to injury in the same person. The patient's physical and psychological state, as well as the type and amount of tissue damaged, factor into the time frame required for healing.

The decision-making process is similar to the steps involved when a pipe ruptures in the basement of a house. Before bailing out the water and cleaning up the mess, you have to stop the leak. Likewise, before encouraging an increase in the rate of cell metabolism in an injured area, the active process of inflammation must be reduced (Table 5–12).

A distinction should be made between using cold modalities for ROM exercises and using heat modalities before competition. As you will recall, cold increases fluid viscosity and decreases the ability to perform rapid move-

TABLE 5–12	Deciding Whether to Use Heat or Cold

Evaluate the patient to determine the answer to each of the following questions:
1. Does the body area feel warm to the touch?
2. Is the injured area still sensitive to light to moderate touch?
3. Does the amount of swelling continue to increase over time?
4. Does swelling increase during activity (joint motion)?
5. Does pain limit the joint's range of motion?
6. Would you consider the acute inflammation process to still be active?
7. Does the patient continue to display improvement with the use of cold modalities?

If all of the answers to these questions are "no," then heat can be safely used. As the number of "yes" answers increases, so does the indication to use cold.

ments. During participation in a sport, athletes rely on the ability to move the extremities in a rapid, powerful manner. Heat is used for its ability to allow this type of movement. Ice is indicated after the activity to prevent reactivation of the inflammatory process. If motion is limited by pain, then cold should be used; if motion is limited by stiffness, heat would be the modality of choice.

The decision about when to use heat and cold should not be based on any predetermined time frame. This decision should be based on the desired physiological responses at any one point in time. When the desired goal is to limit or reduce the amount of inflammation, cold should be used. When the inflammatory response has subsided to the point at which tissue healing begins, heat is applied. When in doubt, use cold.

To a lesser degree, the patient's preference of modalities may be considered. Some patients prefer cold modalities, but more commonly, they prefer heat. For many, the change from cold to heat is a milestone signaling that their healing process is progressing.

● Chapter Highlights

- Heat exchange is based on a temperature gradient, with energy always moving from a high concentration to a low concentration (from hot to cold).
- Heat exchange occurs by conduction, convection, radiation, and evaporation. Conversion is when heat is produced when one form of energy is changed to another.
- Therapeutic cold decreases cell metabolism; therapeutic heat increases cell metabolism.

Cold Modalities

- Cold modalities can be safely used for acute, subacute, and chronic conditions.
- The magnitude of subcutaneous temperature decrease is based on the temperature of the cold modality, the duration of the treatment, the size of the area being treated, and the amount of subcutaneous adipose tissue.
- Subcutaneous adipose tissue serves as an insulator to both heat and cold modalities. The thicker this layer, the less effect the energy has on intramuscular tissue. The exceptions to this are ultrasound and shortwave diathermy.
- Superficial structures are more significantly affected than deeper tissues.
- Following treatment, intramuscular temperatures return to the pretreatment level more slowly than skin temperature. However, even moderate muscle contractions rapidly increase the rate of rewarming.
- The primary benefit of cold application for the treatment of acute injuries is reducing cell metabolism, which limits the amount of secondary injury.
- Vasoconstriction occurs during cold treatments. Any subsequent vasodilation is still less than the baseline vessel diameter.
- Cold application increases the viscosities of fluids in the treatment area, increasing their resistance to flow.
- Edema formation is prevented by cold application. However, cold application does not cause edema reduction.
- Pain control is achieved two ways: through the gate control mechanism and by slowing nerve conduction velocity.
- Cold application does not affect proprioception.
- Muscle spasm is relieved by desensitizing nerve endings.
- Immediate treatment of musculoskeletal injuries consists of rest, ice, compression, and elevation (RICE). Rest limits the scope of the original injury; ice decreases cell metabolism, compression discourages edema formation and lessens hemorrhage, and elevation promotes venous return.
- Although rare, cold application can cause neuropathy or frostbite. The risk of neuropathy is increased when too cold a temperature and too much compression is applied to a large superficial nerve. The risk of frostbite is primarily present when reusable cold packs are used.

Heat Modalities

- The basic physiological effects of heat are essentially opposite those of cold. Both can be used to achieve similar treatment goals such as decreased pain, decreased muscle spasm, and increased ROM.
- Heat should not be used while the inflammatory response is still in its acute stage.
- Superficial heating agents affect tissues less than 2 cm deep. Deep-heating agents affect tissues 5 cm deep or greater.
- Superficial heating agents primarily affect the skin. The effect of these modalities does not penetrate as deep or last as long as cold modalities.
- Increased temperatures increase cell metabolism, promote muscular relaxation, and can encourage plastic deformation of noncontractile tissues.
- Tissue elongation requires repeated bouts of vigorous heating with concurrent stretching.
- Heat decreases the viscosity of fluids and encourages the resolution of hematoma.
- Exercise can be used as a source of deep heat.

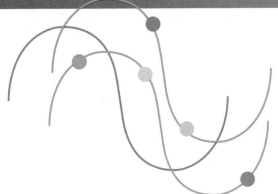

Chapter 6

Clinical Application of Thermal Modalities

This chapter describes the most common methods of applying therapeutic cold and superficial heating agents, any unique physiological effects, the procedures used, and the indications, contraindications, and precautions in their use. The deep-heating agents, therapeutic ultrasound and shortwave diathermy, are discussed in the next section.

Cryotherapy and superficial heating agents can be applied through a wide range of techniques. Although the physiological effects are similar within each classification—cold or heat—each technique has its individual benefits and limitations. The stage of injury, the depth of the target tissues, the uniformity of the surface area being treated, and the treatment goals all factor into selecting the method of application. In many instances more than one technique may be appropriate. Refer to Chapter 5 for a detailed description of the physiological effects of heat and cold modalities.

The various modalities presented in this chapter generally do not require a physician's prescription or supervision (indeed, many may be purchased in drug stores). However, professional responsibility dictates that clinicians become aware of state practice acts and professional standards of practice and work within those boundaries.

COLD PACKS

Cold packs are delivered by one of four techniques: (1) plastic bags filled with crushed or flaked ice, (2) reusable cold gel packs, (3) cold compression therapy (CCT) units, and (4) chemical (or "instant") cold packs. Each method of cold pack application has its own advantages and disadvantages.

The effectiveness of cold packs are based on their ability to safely decrease tissue temperatures to therapeutic levels. Superficial blood flow begins to occur within the first minute of treatment. Subsequent cooling decreases cell metabolism and nerve conduction velocity is eventually decreased. Maximum analgesia is obtained when skin temperature reaches 58°F (14.4°C) (see Therapeutic Temperature Benchmarks, p 106).[10, 29, 30]

Clinicians often place some form of insulation between the cold pack and the skin, often performed with

TABLE 6–1	Skin Temperatures Obtained During Cold Pack Application With and Without Insulators

Ice Pack and Insulator	Minimum Skin Temperature Obtained (°F)
No insulator	37.8
Wet wrap	48.0
Frozen wrap	51.4
Dry wrap	67.1
Synthetic cast	67.5
Plaster cast	65.7
Dry towel	69.6

Sources: Tsang, et al [97] and Metzman, L, et al: Effectiveness of ice packs in reducing skin temperatures under casts. Clin Orthop 330:217, 1996.

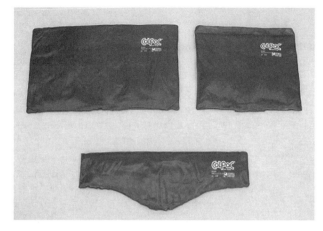

Figure 6-1. **Reusable Cold Packs.** Clockwise from upper left: Oversized (21" x 11"), Standard size (14" x 11"), and Cervical (23" long). Other sizes and shapes are also available. These packs are stored in a refrigeration unit between treatments.

the well-meaning intent of preventing frostbite. With the exception of reusable cold packs, this technique often limits the effects of cold to the point at which little or no therapeutic effects are gained from the treatment (Table 6–1). Cases that indicate the use of an insulating medium include those conditions in which the blood flow to the area is compromised, nerve or cold intolerance, Raynaud's phenomenon, or if reusable cold packs are applied. If the use of an insulating medium is indicated, the treatment duration must be extended beyond the normal treatment time before the skin temperature is decreased to the desired therapeutic range. Ice applied over an elastic wrap would require a treatment duration of approximately 109 minutes to decrease the skin temperature to therapeutic ranges; when applied over a single layer of dry terry cloth toweling, a treatment duration of 151 minutes would be required (assuming that the ice pack does warm up during treatment).[97]

Ice bags are the most commonly used modality in the treatment of acute injuries. They are easy, efficient, and safe to use, requiring only plastic bags and either flaked or cubed ice. A drawback of this method of cold application is that ice machines are expensive and their cost may be prohibitive in some situations.

Reusable cold packs contain a gel consisting of **silica ■**, water, and a form of antifreeze sealed in a plastic pouch (Fig. 6–1). Although they represent a convenient method for cold application in the clinical setting, the effectiveness of reusable cold packs diminishes when they are stored in an ice chest for long periods.

When not in use, these packs are stored in a dedicated cooling unit or freezer at a temperature of approximately 12°F (−11.1°C) and must not be cooled below 0°F (17.8°C) or damage to the pack will result (Fig. 6–2). Some reusable cold packs are also capable of being heated to deliver dry heat. Do not attempt to heat reusable cold packs that are not specifically designed for this purpose.

The risk of frostbite is significantly increased with reusable cold packs. Because this method of cold application does not involve the use of ice (i.e., frozen water), it may lower the skin temperature below the freezing point.

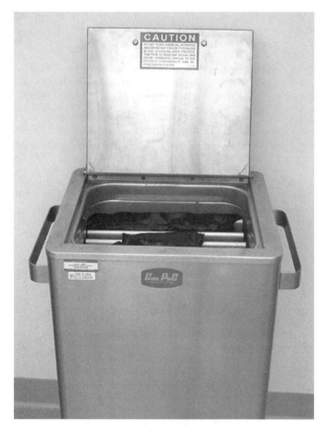

Figure 6-2. **Reusable Cold Pack Storage Unit.** Reusable cold packs are stored at a temperature of approximately 12°F (-11.1°C) when not in use. Allow an appropriate cooling period for the pack to reach its optimum treatment temperature level.

Silica: A finely ground form of sand capable of holding water.

To prevent frostbite, an insulating medium such as one layer of wet toweling or a wet elastic wrap must be placed between the reusable cold pack and the skin. The liquid medium helps to moderate the cold but still provides an effective treatment. Although insulation is needed with reusable cold packs, avoid overinsulating the area. One or two layers of wet toweling or a wet elastic wrap will serve as adequate protection against frostbite. Adding too much insulation will prevent the effects of the cold from reaching the skin. Regardless of the insulating medium being used, the patient's skin should be checked regularly for signs of frostbite (see Box 5–5).

Cold compression therapy (CCT) units combine static external compression and cold application (Fig. 6–3). The CCT's appliances are designed to contour to specific body areas (e.g., the ankle, knee, and shoulder). The appliances are filled with chilled water to provide up to 40 mm Hg of circumferential compression (some units allow the amount of pressure to be preset) that prevents the formation of swelling, decreases the amount of edema, and increases the effective depth of cold penetration (also see Intermittent Compression Devices in Chapter 14).[98] These effects factored together lead to decreased pain, decreased recovery time, and increased range of motion (ROM) after acute injury or surgery.[99–102] Some units have a motorized unit that eliminates the need to manually circulate chilled water into the appliance.

CCTs may not result in significant decreases in pain and edema compared to ice packs, partially because skin surface temperatures do not reach therapeutic levels (newer units may overcome these problems).[45] These units are, however, a convenient method of applying cold and compression. Better CCT knee appliances are designed to prevent placing pressure on the popliteal vein. Compression of this vein can result in edema of the lower extremity.

Instant cold packs contain two chemicals separated from each other by a plastic barrier. When the seal between them ruptures, they are allowed to mix, causing a chemical reaction that produces cold (Fig. 6–4). The degree of cold

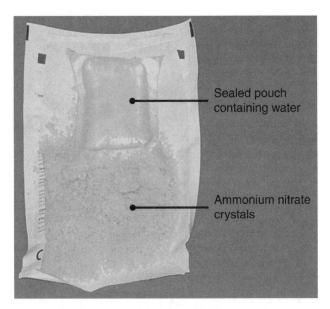

Figure 6–4. **Inside an Instant Cold Pack.** A bag containing water and ammonium nitrate crystals is sealed within a pouch. When the inner bag is ruptured, the water and crystals mix, causing a chemical reaction that produces cold (note that the chemicals may vary). Instant cold packs should not be opened. Torn packs or packs that develop a leak should be immediately discarded.

- Sealed pouch containing water
- Ammonium nitrate crystals

produced and the short duration of the reaction give them a relatively short workable life. Instant cold packs are convenient in that they may be stored in a medical kit for emergency use. These packs can be used only once and must be properly disposed of after use.

When mixed, the chemicals contained in instant cold packs are extremely caustic to the skin. If a pack should develop a leak, discard it immediately and rinse the patient's skin with running water. For this reason, do not use instant cold packs on the face.

● EFFECTS ON
The Injury Response Process

The application of ice packs decreases tissue temperature, resulting in a decrease in cellular metabolic rate. Lowering the transmission rate of nerve impulses and increasing the pain threshold decrease muscle spasm. The decreased release of inflammatory mediators occurs as a result of the reduced rate of cell metabolism and reduced blood flow.

In acute injuries, the most beneficial effect of cold application is to reduce the need for oxygen. More cells are able to survive in the oxygen-starved environment because of their decreased metabolic rate. When coupled with compression and elevation, the edema in the area is reduced, and compression acts to have the effects of cold affect deeper tissues.[12] These factors limit the scope of the original injury and reduce the amount of secondary injury.

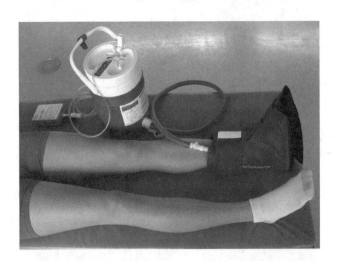

Figure 6–3. **Cold Compression Therapy Unit.** These devices deliver circumferential cold compression. See also Chapter 14.

At a Glance: **Cold Packs**

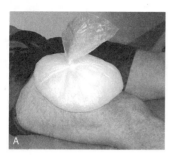

Crushed Ice Pack

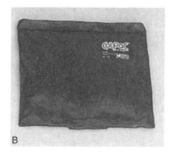

Reusable Cold Pack

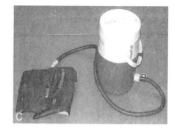

Cold Compression Therapy Unit

Description

Cold packs may be delivered by using crushed, chipped, or flaked ice, reusable cold gel packs consisting of a silica base and an anti-freeze gel, cold compression therapy units that use chilled water to provide cold and compression, and "instant" cold packs that use a chemical reaction to produce cold. Cold packs are used for treating:

- Acute trauma
- Pain
- Muscle spasm
- Postsurgical care

Primary Effects

ACUTE PATHOLOGY

- Decreases cell metabolism, reducing the amount of secondary hypoxic injury
- With compression and elevation, limits the formation of edema

OTHER EFFECTS

- Decreased metabolism reduces the release of inflammatory mediators and cellular byproducts
- Decreases pain by slowing nerve conduction velocity and increasing the threshold of nerve endings
- Causes local vasoconstriction

ICE BAGS, REUSABLE COLD PACKS, AND INSTANT COLD PACKS

- The treatment duration is dependent on the treatment goal, target tissues, and the amount of subcutaneous adipose tissue
- Because of the lasting effects of cold treatments, applications should be no less than 2 hours apart
- In the immediate care of injuries, keep the body part wrapped and elevated between treatments
- When treating deep structures, the treatment duration should be increased as the amount of adipose tissue increases

COLD COMPRESSION THERAPY UNITS

In addition to the preceding protocol, CCTs may be applied continuously for 24 to 72 hours after acute injury or surgery.[99, 101, 102] The periods used to rechill the water provide sufficient time for the body part to rewarm.[104]

Indications

- Acute injury or inflammation
- Acute or chronic pain
- Postsurgical pain and edema

Contraindications

- Cardiac or respiratory involvement
- Uncovered open wounds
- Circulatory insufficiency
- Cold allergy and/or hypersensitivity
- Anesthetized skin

Precautions

- If an elastic wrap is used, avoid applying too much pressure (see Clinical Techniques: Compression Wraps, p 114).
- Application of a CCT unit over an elastic wrap can result in increased pressure being placed on the tissues.
- When reusable cold packs are used or in the presence of vascular insufficiency, check the patient for frostbite.
- Application of ice packs over large superficial nerves (e.g., peroneal or ulnar nerves) could cause neuropathy, especially if an elastic wrap is used to hold the pack in place. Recheck the patient regularly for signs of nerve dysfunction, such as tingling in the distal extremity.
- The content of instant cold packs can produce chemical burns if it comes into contact with the skin. Avoid use around the face, eyes, and other sensitive areas.

■ Set-up and Application

Before the application of each of the following forms of cold application, ensure that the patient is free of contraindications (see At a Glance: Cold Packs).

Ice Bags

1. Ensure the patient is free of contraindications for this treatment technique.
2. Fill the bag with enough ice to last for the duration of the treatment but avoid overfilling. If the bag becomes too full, it cannot be molded to the body part.
3. Remove excess air from the bag to allow the ice to conform to the body part being treated.
4. More than one bag may be required to fully cover the area.
5. In acute injuries, or when compression is desired, wet an elastic wrap and apply one layer around the injured area. This technique results in a further decrease in subcutaneous tissue temperatures.[12] (A tub of cold "wet wraps" can be kept soaking in the refrigerator for this purpose.) Areas such as the acromioclavicular joint are not practical for wet wraps. A moist towel or thin sponge placed over the injured tissues may be substituted. The cold packs may then be held in place with dry wraps. However, ice bags may be (and, arguably, should be) placed directly on the skin for patients who are free of contraindications or precautions to cold therapy. Overinsulating the ice bag will decrease the effectiveness of the treatment.
6. Apply the ice bags over the injured area. Secure in place with an elastic or plastic wrap using approximately 50 to 60 mm Hg of pressure (Fig. 6–5).[103] (Note: Inflating a blood pressure cuff around your arm or leg to 50 to 60 mm Hg will give you a good estimation of the amount of pressure that should be exerted when applying the compression wrap.)

Reusable Cold Packs

1. Ensure the patient is free of contraindications for this treatment technique.
2. Select a pack large enough to cover the injured area, or use multiple packs.
3. Cover the area to be treated with a wet towel or wet elastic wrap. Because of the risk of frostbite, a fully cooled reusable cold pack must not be allowed to come into contact with the skin. Equally important, do not overinsulate the area. Too much toweling may decrease the heat flow from the skin to the point at which the treatment becomes ineffective.
4. Secure the pack in place with an elastic wrap.
5. Check the patient regularly for signs of frostbite (see Box 5–5).

6. The reusable cold pack may lose its effective treatment temperature after 20 minutes of use.[104]

Cold Compression Therapy Units

1. Ensure the patient is free of contraindications for this treatment technique.
2. Fill the cold cooling unit with ice as indicated. Shorter treatment times require less ice than treatments having a longer duration.
3. Add cold water to the depth of the FILL mark.
4. Allow the water to chill for approximately 5 to 10 minutes.
5. Choose the appropriate appliance for the body part and size of the area being treated.
6. Fasten the distal strap snugly, but not tight enough to cut off blood flow.
7. Fasten the proximal strap loosely enough to allow for proper venous drainage. Overtightening the proximal strap can inhibit or block venous and lymphatic drainage.
8. Connect the appliance to the cooler using the hose or hoses provided. If applicable, open the air vent on the top of the cooler to allow the fluid to flow into the appliance.
9. Elevate the cooler above the body part being treated. The height of the cooler determines the amount of pressure within the appliance; consult your unit's user manual.
10. If applicable, remove the air-bleed cap to allow any trapped air to be forced out of the appliance.
11. Disconnect the hose or hoses from the appliance.
12. Draining the appliance or rechilling the fluid: (a) Reconnect the appliance to the hose or hoses. (b) Place the cooler at a level below the cuff. (c) Allow the fluid to drain from the appliance. (d) If the fluid is being rechilled, allow the fluid to remain in the cooler for 15 to 30 minutes; then repeat steps 7 through 10.

Instant Cold Packs

1. Ensure that the patient is free of contraindications for this treatment technique.
2. Shake the bag so that the contents are evenly distributed.
3. Squeeze the bag to break the inner pouch.
4. Shake the bag to thoroughly mix the contents.
5. If indicated on the instructions of the particular brand of chemical cold pack you are using place a wet towel between the pack and the skin.
6. Secure in place with an elastic wrap.
7. If the solution within the bag leaks and makes contact with the skin, immediately remove the pack and thoroughly rise the area with water. Monitor the patient for chemical burns.

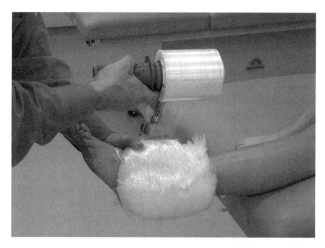

Figure 6–5. Application of a Crushed Ice Pack. Plastic wrapping material (that was originally used for shipping wrap) can be used to secure an ice pack in place. The plastic may help insulate the cold within the pack.

■ Treatment Duration

Historically, cold packs have been administered for 20 to 30 minutes per session. A more precise method of determining the treatment duration is to consider the target tissues, the depth of those tissues, and—in the case of subcutaneous tissues—the amount of overlying adipose tissue. Skin numbness can occur in 10 minutes. Intramuscular cooling is related to the amount of subcutaneous adipose tissue and the depth below this layer (see Box 5–3).

▶ ICE MASSAGE

Ice massage is used to deliver cold treatments to small, evenly shaped areas. It is most effective in cases involving muscle spasm, contusions, and other minor injuries limited to a well-localized area. The patient may be able to administer self-treatment either in the clinical setting or as a part of the home treatment program. This method of cold application is convenient, practical, and time-efficient, providing cold treatments in situations in which there is no ready access to an ice machine.

Ice massage produces a more rapid decline in intramuscular temperature than does an ice pack, but only when it is applied to a small treatment area (e.g., 4 × 4 cm, which is only slightly larger than the face of the ice massage cup). Although ice massage results in a quicker cooling time, following 15 minutes of ice massage and 15 minutes of ice pack application, there are no significant differences in intramuscular temperature or the duration of effects.[5]

● EFFECTS ON
The Injury Response Cycle

In addition to the effects associated with the application of ice packs, the massaging action of this treatment assists in decreasing pain and muscle spasm. The sensation of movement stimulates large-diameter nerves, inhibiting the transmission of pain and, in turn, causing a decrease in muscle spasm. Increasing the amount of pressure used during the ice massage decreases the time required for the skin to become numb.[105]

Ice massage is not always the management of choice for acute injuries because no compression is available during the treatment, potentially increasing the amount of hemorrhage and edema, and because of the relatively small surface area that should be treated with ice massage. Subcutaneous tissue temperatures are not reduced at the same magnitude as other forms of cold application, an effect related to the decreased treatment duration and the movement of ice. There is also the possibility of increased superficial blood flow.[38] In the event that this is the only form of ice treatment available at the time of the injury, additional steps must be taken to limit the amount of swelling. The injured body part should be wrapped with an elastic bandage and elevated to reduce edema after the treatment.

■ Set-up and Application

1. Ensure that the patient is free of contraindications for this treatment technique.
2. Ice cups are made by filling paper cups three-quarters full and storing them in a freezer. Styrofoam cups may also be used for this purpose. However, removal of the excess Styrofoam as the ice melts during treatment can create excess clutter. Because of the insulating effects of Styrofoam, freezing the water may take more time compared to paper cups.
3. The treatment area should be no larger than two to three times the size of the ice cup. Smaller treatment areas will increase the rate of subcutaneous cooling.
4. Surround the body part to be treated with a towel to collect water runoff.
5. Slowly massage the ice over the injured area in overlapping strokes or circles.
6. Increased pressure between the ice and the skin will decrease the amount of time required to obtain skin numbness.[105]
7. The paper (or Styrofoam) must be continually removed from the cup as the ice melts to prevent it from rubbing on the skin.

▶ ICE IMMERSION

Ice immersion (ice slush or ice bath) involves placing the body part into a mixture of ice and water having a temperature range of 50°F to 60°F (10°C to 15.6°C). This treatment is useful for injuries involving an irregular surface.

This can be an uncomfortable method of cold application, especially when the fingers or toes are immersed. Increased pain is experienced because the surface area

At a Glance: Ice Massage

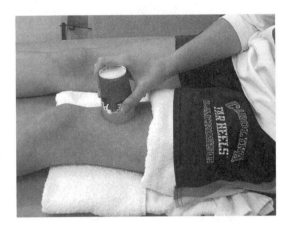

Description

Water frozen in a paper cup that is then massaged over a small area of skin. Ice massage is used for:

- Muscle spasm
- Trigger points
- Prior to ROM exercises
- Rapid cooling of the skin

Primary Effects

- Decreases the sensitivity of cutaneous nerve receptors
- Decreases pain
- Breaks pain-spasm-pain cycle

Treatment Duration

- 5 to 15 minutes (or until the ice runs out). When treating deep structures, the treatment duration should be increased as the amount of adipose tissue increases.
- If the purpose of the ice massage is to produce numbness, the treatment may be discontinued when the patient's skin is insensitive to touch. These treatments may be repeated as necessary (i.e., when sensation returns).

Indications

- Subacute injury or inflammation
- Muscle strains
- Contusions
- Acute or chronic pain

Contraindications

- Cases in which pressure on the injury is contraindicated
- Suspected fractures
- Uncovered open wounds
- Circulatory insufficiency
- Cold allergy and/or hypersensitivity
- Anesthetized skin

Precautions

- In some injuries, the pressure of the massage may be contraindicated.

---

exposed to the cold is increased. When the fingers or toes are immersed, they are exposed to cold across their circumference and at the distal end. Because their diameter is small, the effects of cold penetrate to bone level. Another factor that may account for the increased pain experienced is stimulation of the lumina in the nailbed. This is a hypersensitive area that may be overstimulated by the presence of cold. You can test this hypothesis on yourself by simply applying pressure with your thumbnail on the white crescent in your opposite thumbnail. A **Neoprene** ■ covering ("toe cap") can make ice immersion more tolerable when the fingers or toes are not the target of the treatment (Fig. 6–6).[69, 106]

Repeated exposure to ice immersion increases the patient's tolerance to this treatment.[70] The affective response to the pain associated with this treatment can be decreased by explaining to the patient the sensations to be expected.[68, 69]

Despite the discomfort associated with this treatment, ice immersion allows for circumferential cooling and simultaneous ROM exercise. The use of Neoprene, gradually decreasing the temperature of the immersion, and communicating with the patient can make this treatment more tolerable and maximize its therapeutic potential.

● E F F E C T S   O N

The Injury Response Process

The effects of ice immersion are as described in the general effects of cold application. The intensity of cold is greater with ice immersion because of the large surface area being treated. Therefore, the resultant drop in skin and subcutaneous temperature is more pronounced than with other forms of cold application.[11] As long as a proper rewarming

---

Neoprene: A synthetic rubber material.

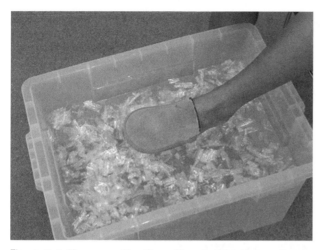

Figure 6-6. **Neoprene Toe Cap.** Covering the toes or fingers with an insulating material such as neoprene makes ice immersion treatment more tolerable.

period is provided, ice immersion does not appear to negatively affect joint proprioception during activity.

The use of ice immersion places the limb in a dependent position, increasing the **hydrostatic** ■ pressure within the capillaries.[86] This encourages the leakage of fluids into the interstitial space, resulting in increased edema. The use of active range-of-motion exercises during the immersion will aid venous return (see the following sections on Whirlpools and Edema Formation and Reduction). After the treatment of acute or subacute injuries, the limb should be wrapped and elevated to encourage venous and lymphatic drainage.

Ice immersion can be used in conjunction with electrical stimulation as a form of immediate treatment. Although the effects of electrical stimulation in acute injuries are debatable (see Chapter 12, p 231) for the electrical stimulation protocol), the limb should be wrapped and elevated after the treatment.

■ Set-up and Application

1. Ensure that the patient is free of contraindications for this treatment technique.
2. Prepare a bucket, tub, or any other container with cold water and ice. The temperature used will depend somewhat on the person's ability to tolerate the cold. Generally, patients who have had repeated exposure to this treatment can tolerate a lower temperature. Another approach is to start the patient at a tolerable temperature and to add ice as the treatment progresses.
3. The temperature of the treatment is related to the size of the body area being treated (Fig. 6–7). To prevent hypothermia, as the size of the area being treated (the proportion of the total body area) is increased, the temperature of the water is increased.

4. Colder treatment temperatures may be tolerated if the fingers or toes are insulated from the water by Neoprene covering.
5. Avoid having the patient continually immerse and withdraw the body part from the immersion. Initially, the cold will cause a burning or aching sensation. To lessen discomfort, explain to the patient that the treatment will be uncomfortable only for a few minutes, but numbness will soon follow. If the limb is repeatedly removed and then reimmersed, it only increases the duration of pain.
6. Continue to monitor the patient. The discomfort, sensation, and possible change in blood pressure associated with ice immersion may result in unconsciousness.
7. Following the treatment, active ROM exercises should be performed if they are not contraindicated.
8. Because the limb is placed in a gravity-dependent position, it should be wrapped and elevated after the treatment.

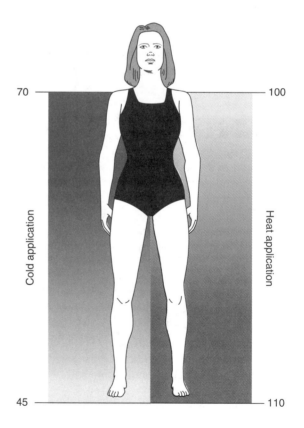

Figure 6–7. **Relationship Between Treatment Temperature and the Percentage of the Body Immersed.** During cold immersion, the temperature of the water should be increased as the percentage of the body immersed increases. During hot immersion, the temperature of the water decreases as the percentage of the body immersed increases.

Hydrostatic: Relating to the pressure of liquids in equilibrium or to the pressure they exert.

At a Glance: Ice Immersion

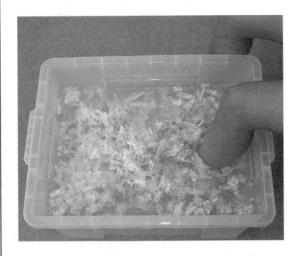

Description

A tub or bucket is filled with ice and water and is used for cooling large and/or irregularly shaped areas. The body part, usually the foot and ankle or elbow, wrist, and hand is then immersed in the solution.

Primary Effects

- Decreases cell metabolism, reducing the amount of secondary hypoxic injury
- Decreased metabolism reduces the release of inflammatory mediators and cellular by-products
- Decreases pain by slowing nerve conduction velocity and increasing the threshold of nerve endings
- Causes local vasoconstriction.

Temperature Range

- 50°F to 60°F (10°C to 15.6°C)
- The temperature should be increased as the proportion of the body area immersed increases.

Treatment Duration

- 10 to 15 minutes. When treating deep structures, the treatment duration should be increased as the amount of adipose tissue increases.
- Lower treatment temperatures may require shorter treatment durations.
- Treatments may be repeated as needed.

Indications

- Acute injury or inflammation
- Acute, chronic, or postsurgical pain
- Prior to ROM exercise

Contraindications

- Cardiac or respiratory involvement
- Uncovered open wounds
- Circulatory insufficiency
- Cold allergy and/or hypersensitivity
- Anesthetized skin
- Absolute inability to tolerate the cold temperature

Precautions

- Ice immersion is the most uncomfortable of all the cold treatments. Neoprene "toe caps" may be used to decrease discomfort.
- Avoid having the patient continually immerse and withdraw the body part from the immersion. If the limb is repeatedly removed and then reimmersed, it only increases the duration of pain.
- The limb's gravity-dependent position increases the risk of swelling.
- Care should be taken when relatively subcutaneous nerves (e.g., ulnar nerve as it crosses the elbow) are immersed. Because of the chance of cold-induced nerve palsy, slightly increase the temperature of the immersion, and check the patient regularly.

► CRYOSTRETCH

The effects of cold application and passive stretching are combined in the cryostretch technique, leading to its alternate name, "spray and stretch." A vapocoolant spray is used to rapidly decrease the temperature of the skin and decrease pain transmission. This is combined with simultaneous passive stretching to relieve local muscle spasm to effectively reduce the amount of pain and spasm associated with strains and trigger points (Fig. 6–8). A chart of trigger point pain patterns is presented in Appendix A.

Cryostretch has traditionally been performed with ethyl chloride because of its ability to evaporate quickly and cool the superficial tissue. However, ethyl chloride possesses many inherent dangers: It is highly flammable; it acts as a general anesthetic if inhaled; and because it

At a Glance: **Cryostretch**

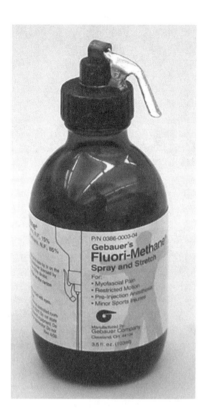

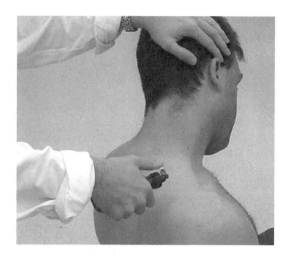

■ See the text for a complete description of the procedure.

Indications

- Trigger points
- Muscle spasm
- Decreased ROM

Contraindications

- Allergy to the spray
- Acute and/or postsurgical injury
- Open wounds
- Contraindications relating to cold applications
- Contraindications relating to passive stretching
- Use around the eyes. When treating the upper extremity, torso, or neck, protect the patient's eyes from the spray.

Description

A vapocoolant spray, a liquid that quickly evaporates and cools the skin, is applied to the skin while the underlying muscles and fascia are simultaneously stretched. Cryostretch is used for treating trigger points, local muscle spasm, and other myofascial conditions.

Primary Effects

VAPOCOOLANT SPRAY
The rapid evaporation of the spray cools the skin and desensitizes nerve endings.
STRETCHING
Elongates muscle fibers and other soft tissues, breaking muscle spasm and releasing adhesions.

Treatment Duration

- The treatment proceeds through three or four sweeps, with sufficient time for the tissue to rewarm between sprays. Treatments are given once a day. When treating deep structures, the treatment duration should be increased as the amount of adipose tissue increases.

Precautions

- Cold sprays are capable of causing frostbite if improperly used.
- If ethyl chloride is used, be aware that:
  - It is extremely flammable. Avoid using it around possible sources of ignition, including smoking and electrical sparks.
  - Ethyl chloride is a local anesthetic. However, if the fumes are inhaled, it very quickly becomes a general anesthetic.[108]
- Fluoromethane contains ozone-depleting chemicals but has been granted an exception for use by the Environmental Protection Agency.
- Vapocoolant sprays are not an effective means of providing immediate treatment for acute injuries.

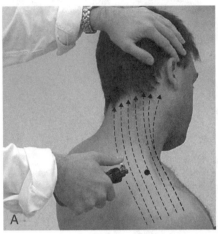
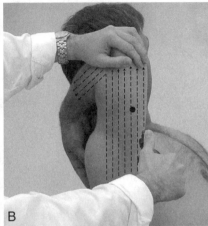
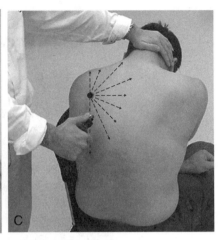

Figure 6–8. **Cryostretch Techniques.** The muscle and skin are placed on stretch and passively elongated as they are cooled (see Set-up and Application). Treatment technique for the (A) upper trapezius, (B) triceps brachii, and (C) lower, middle, and upper trapezius.

decreases the skin temperature so drastically, there is a high potential for frostbite. Because of these risks, ethyl chloride has been replaced by fluoromethane spray, which is less volatile and has a safer cooling effect.[107] Ice massage may also be used instead of fluoromethane.

● E FFECTS ON

The Injury Response Process

The evaporation of the coolant on the skin causes cooling in a manner that stimulates cutaneous sensory nerves and a reduction in motor neuron activity. This stimulus "masks" the previous pain by reducing the intensity and speed of pain transmission. The passive stretching assists in breaking the pain-spasm-pain cycle by lengthening the muscle fibers. This combination of pain reduction and soft tissue stretching makes this a particularly effective method of trigger point therapy. The rewarming period following application is relatively brief, so the analgesic effects are short-lived.

The effect of cold sprays is limited to that of a counterirritant. Vapocoolant sprays do not cause the cellular and vascular responses associated with other forms of cold application. The use of vapocoolant sprays in the treatment of acute injuries is generally based on tradition rather than on fact. Although the evaporation of the liquid rapidly cools the skin and produces temporary pain relief, the other physiological effects of cold application are not achieved.

■ Set-up and Application

1. Ensure that the patient is free of contraindications for this treatment technique.
2. Position the patient so that the muscle group being treated may be easily stretched.
3. If the treatment is being applied to the upper extremities, cervical spine, or upper chest, position the patient's face to avoid being caught in the stream.

4. The nozzle of the bottle should be approximately 12 inches from the skin. The spray should strike the skin at a 30- to 45-degree angle. The closer to the body that the bottle is held, the warmer the coolant stream feels.
5. Spray the entire muscle length in a sweeping manner. The spray should be in one direction only. The speed of the sweep should allow the tissue to become covered, but not frosted because this creates the risk of frostbite.
6. Apply pressure to passively stretch the muscle group. Come to, but do not exceed, the point of pain.
7. Allow the tissue to rewarm.
8. Encourage the patient to take deep, relaxing breaths before stretching the muscle.
9. Continue for two or three more sweeps with increasing stretch on the muscle. Allow the tissue to rewarm between each sweep.
10. Repeat until the desired amount of stretch has occurred.
11. The cryostretch treatment may be followed by a moist heat treatment or massage.

⊞ WHIRLPOOLS

Whirlpools are an effective method of applying heat or cold to irregularly shaped areas. Large immersion tanks make it possible to perform ROM activities and exercise while also receiving the thermal benefits of the treatment by taking advantage of the physical characteristics of water. Energy is transferred to or from the body by means of convection. In a hot whirlpool, heat is transmitted to the body. In a cold whirlpool, heat is transmitted away.

A turbine is used to regulate the water flow and the amount of air introduced into the flow (aeration). Water enters through an inlet on the turbine's stem, where the motor forces it back into the tub, causing agitation of the water (the "whirlpool" effect). Air is also introduced into the stream, causing bubbles to circulate in the tank. The

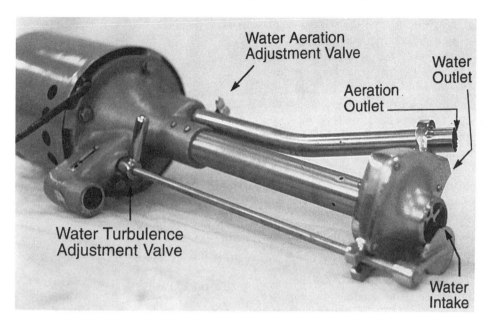

Figure 6-9. **A Whirlpool Turbine.** Note the position of the turbulence and aeration valves, and the water intake port. The water is driven through the turbine and returned to the tub under pressure. The aeration outlet is in front of the water nozzle, forcing bubbles to flow in the water.

agitation and aeration are controlled by separate valves and can be adjusted to produce a wide range of effects, providing a massaging effect that produces sedation, analgesia, and increased circulation (Fig. 6–9).

For both hot and cold whirlpools, the temperature of the immersion depends on the proportion of the total body area that will be immersed. In cold whirlpool treatments, the temperature of the water is increased as the body area being treated increases. In this case, the body may be placed in a state of hypothermia if too large a body area is cooled too rapidly.

During hot whirlpool treatments, the temperature of the water is decreased as the total body area immersed increases (see Fig. 6–7). When the temperature of the water is equal to or greater than the body temperature, heat loss can occur only through evaporation and respiration. If the patient's core temperature is increased too greatly, **hyperthermia** ■ may result. During a full-body immersion the patient can lose heat only through the head and through breathing, increasing the risk of heat stress. Moderate to strenuous exercise while in the immersion will further increase the core temperature.

■ Physical Effects of Water Immersion

The physical characteristics of water, buoyancy, resistance, and hydrostatic pressure, create a good supportive medium for active ROM exercises. These benefits can be obtained

by the extremities in clinical-sized whirlpools or body wide in deeper immersion tanks such as spas, exercise therapy pools, and swimming pools (Fig. 6–10). The temperature of the water is the most important property of immersion treatments.

Buoyancy describes the lifting force (thrust) provided by water and is explained by Archimedes' principle. If the body's **specific gravity** ■ is equal to that of the water (1.0

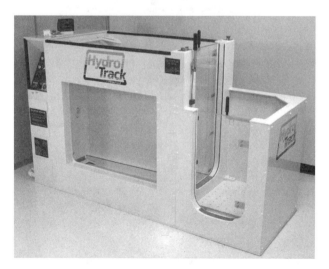

Figure 6-10. **Exercise Therapy Pool.** These water-filled tanks have a treadmill on the bottom, allowing the patient to walk or run during treatment. The water provides buoyancy and resistance during exercise. (The Hydro Track, courtesy of Ferno Performance Pools, Wilmington, OH.)

Hyperthermia: Increased core temperature.
Specific gravity: The ratio of the density of a substance to the density of pure water taken as a standard when both densities are obtained by weighing in air.

for pure water), it floats just beneath the surface. If the body's specific gravity is greater than water, it sinks; if it is less, it floats. Therapeutically, the property of buoyancy is used to reduce compressive forces on weight-bearing joints and assist in anti-gravity motions.

Resistance to movement is produced by the water's viscosity. The amount of resistance depends on the speed of the motion and the proportion of the body (or limb) that is immersed. Faster motions produce more resistance than slower motions; it is easier to walk than run through water 4 feet deep. Resistance also increases as the surface area increases; it is easier to run through ankle-deep water than through waist-deep water.

Hydrostatic pressure describes the force exerted on a body part that is immersed in a nonmoving fluid. As described by Pascal's law, the fluid will conform to the irregular surface area and exert an equal pressure across the circumference. The amount of pressure increases with depth, exerting 0.73 mm Hg per centimeter of immersion. When standing in an immersion, a pressure gradient is formed between the amount of pressure exerted on the skin at the surface of the water (low pressure) and the pressure exerted at the distal extremity (high pressure) (Fig. 6–11). This pressure gradient can help force fluids in the distal extremity proximally, especially when combined with walking. The combination of hydrostatic pressure and buoyancy helps provide the patient with balance and stability.

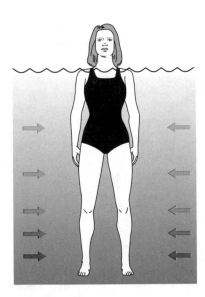

Figure 6–11. **Hydrostatic Pressure During Water Immersion.** As the depth of the body part in the water increases, the pressure exerted on the body increases by 0.73 mm Hg for each centimeter of depth. The resulting pressure gradient can encourage venous return from the lower extremity, but only when the patient is immersed at least to the mid-chest.

● EFFECTS ON
The Injury Response Process

The thermal effects of cold and heat are described in the relevant sections of Chapter 5. Hot whirlpools promote muscle relaxation, and cold whirlpools decrease muscle spasm and muscle spasticity. Cold whirlpools administered at a temperature of 50°F (10°C) for 20 minutes result in the same amount of intramuscular cooling as found with ice packs. Because of the large treatment area, the effects of post-treatment cooling are more pronounced following a whirlpool treatment.[7, 14] This effect is beneficial when used before rehabilitation exercises.[7] An additional effect of the turbulence from the flowing water is the creation of a **sedative** ■ and analgesic effect on sensory nerves.

Blood Flow

The increase or decrease in blood flow is proportional to the temperature of the bath. Hot whirlpool treatments above 101.5°F (38.6°C) cause a 21-percent increase in blood flow and a 50-percent increase when the temperature is increased to 108.5°F (42.5°C).[109] Although agitation of the water is thought to provide a "massaging" effect, agitation in and of itself does not significantly increase blood flow.[109]

Edema Formation and Reduction

The relationship between whirlpool baths and the formation or reduction of edema is complex. Except for cases where the patient is supine in the tank, the limb is placed in a gravity-dependent position that would encourage the formation of edema.

When a patient is standing in a neutral-temperature immersion, the hydrostatic pressure gradient formed by the water pressure at the feet being greater than the water pressure at the surface will encourage venous return. Slow walking or other exercise will cause the deep venous pressure within the calf to increase to 200 mm Hg, further increasing the venous return pressure gradient, thus encouraging venous return.[68] This effect is similar to an air-filled balloon in a swimming pool. The balloon will maintain its shape when it is near the surface of the water. If you grab the balloon and try to swim to the bottom of the pool with it, its shape elongates with the top being wider than the bottom.

Recall that the amount of hydrostatic pressure depends on the depth of the water exerting a force of 0.73 mm Hg/cm of immersion. A mid-calf immersion, approximately 25 cm (10 in.) deep would exert 18.25 mm Hg of pressure at the foot. Increasing this distance to 50 cm (20 in.) would exert 36.5 mm Hg at the feet. Normal **diastolic blood pressure** ■ is approximately 80 mm Hg (see Fig. 6–11). Therefore, an immersion of approximately 110 cm (43.3 in; 3 feet, 7 in) is

---

Diastolic blood pressure: The lowest level of pressure in the arteries. For example, when a blood pressure
   reading is given as 120/80, 80 represents the diastolic value.

Sedative: An agent that causes sedation.

required to exceed diastolic blood pressure and prevent the formation of distal edema.

Increase in limb volume is directly related to the temperature of the water. As the temperature increases, so does the blood volume in the lower extremity, increasing by 44 to 64 mL.[68] The total accumulation of blood associated with hot whirlpools is based on the hydrostatic pressure and exercise acting to reduce the total accumulation. If edema formation is a concern during hot whirlpool treatments, reduce the temperature of the immersion.

Cold whirlpool treatments are not recommended for the care of acute injuries in which edema is still forming. If this method of acute injury management is unavoidable, the turbine should be set on "low" or not be turned on during treatment. A compression wrap should be applied and the body part should be elevated after the treatment.

Pain Control

The temperature of the immersion and the circulation and aeration of the water decrease pain by stimulating A-beta nerve fibers and activating the gate-control mechanism. Increased blood flow, the reduction of edema, and improved ROM also assist in reducing the mechanical and chemical pain triggers. The buoyancy of the water helps to reduce compressive stresses on joint surfaces and provide short-term pain reduction.

Range of Motion

Increased blood flow, reduced pain, and reduced edema all contribute to increasing the joint's ROM. Gravity-assisted motion is aided by the buoyancy of the water. During dry-land exercise, the effect of gravity on the rotational movement of joints is greatest when the limb reaches parallel to the ground. When this motion is performed in water, the buoyancy of the limb helps to counteract the force of gravity, making slow motion through the ROM possible.

Wound Cleansing

Lavage—using water to cleanse wounds—has the ability to reach all portions of irregular shaped surface areas and into open wounds. Water and the associated water pressure encourage the hydration, softening, and subsequent débridement of tissues.[109] Hydrotherapy is often used in the management of open wounds, diabetic ulcers, pressure wounds, thermal burns, and **"turf burns ■ ."**

For wound cleansing, the water is heated to 96°F to 98°F (35.6°C to 36.7°C) and antibiotic agents or other chemicals are added to reduce the bacterial load of the skin.[110] In most cases, the turbine's stream should not directly strike the wound. Doing so may damage the fragile granulation tissue, force bacteria deeper into the tissue, or otherwise cause further damage to the wound.

The presence of open wounds mandates that appropriate sterilization procedures be used both before and after the treatment. Only stainless steel tubs should be used for wound cleansing or débridement, because tile tubs or spa-type whirlpools may harbor germs and are much more difficult to clean properly.[111] The tank should be cleaned with an appropriate disinfectant before and after the treatment (see Cleaning the Whirlpool, p 143). The tank is filled with water, and a disinfectant is added. After the treatment, the tank should be drained and cleaned again. A culture kit can be used to check the whirlpool for contaminants.

■ Hubbard Tanks

The butterfly-shaped Hubbard tank is designed to allow a supine, partially submerged patient to abduct the arms and legs through their full ROM (Fig. 6–12). Although these devices were originally designed for orthopedic patients, their use has evolved to include the treatment of burns and spinal cord–injured patients. Because the extremities and torso are often immersed in a Hubbard tank, the standard treatment temperatures for this device are decreased to the range of 90° to 102°F (32.2° to 38.8°C).

■ Set-up and Application

1. Ensure that the patient is free of contraindications to whirlpool immersion and the temperature of water used.
2. Instruct the patient not to turn the whirlpool on or off or touch any electrical connections while in the whirlpool or while the body is wet.
3. Fill the whirlpool to a depth sufficient to cover the area being treated, keeping in mind the effects of hydrostatic pressure. Be sure the amount of water is enough to run the motor safely.

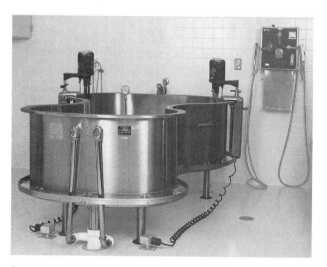

Figure 6–12. **A "Hubbard Tank" Full-Body Whirlpool.** These whirlpools are designed to allow the patient to lay supine and abduct the arms and legs. (Courtesy of Ferno Performance Pools, Wilmington, OH.)

Turf burn: A deep abrasion caused by friction between the skin and artificial playing surfaces.

At a Glance: Hot and Cold Whirlpools

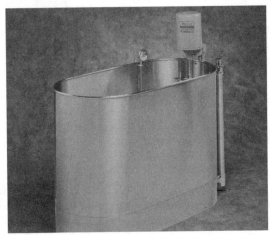

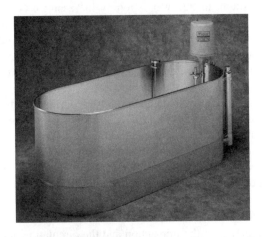

Description

A tub filled with warm or cold water. An attached turbine provides motion and aeration to the water. (A) "High Boy" whirlpool bath. The patient can immerse the extremity and perform ROM exercises. (B) "Lo Boy" whirlpool bath. The patient can sit in this tub with the legs extended. Whirlpools are used for:

- Delivering heat or cold treatment
- ROM exercises
- Promoting muscular relaxation
- Decreasing pain and muscle spasm

Primary Effects

- Provides a supportive medium for range of motion exercises
- The water provides resistance to rapid motions
- Agitation and aeration of the water causes sedation, analgesia, and increased blood flow
- Also includes the effects of hot and cold treatments
- Cold whirlpool treatments result in longer lasting cooling of intramuscular tissues

Temperature Range

COLD WHIRLPOOL
50°F to 65°F (10°C to 16°C). Temperature is increased as the proportion of the body area treated increases.

HOT WHIRLPOOL
90°F to 110°F (32°C to 49°C). Temperature is decreased as the proportion of the body area treated increases.

Treatment Duration

- Initial whirlpool treatments are given for 5 to 10 minutes.
- The duration of treatments may be increased to 20 to 30 minutes as the program progresses. When treating deep structures, the treatment duration should be increased as the amount of adipose tissue increases.
- Treatments may be given once or twice a day.

Indications

- Decreased range of motion
- Subacute or chronic inflammatory conditions
- Peripheral vascular disease (use a neutral temperature)
- Peripheral nerve injuries (avoid the extremes of hot and cold)

Contraindications

- Acute conditions in which water turbulence would further irritate the injured areas or in which the limb is placed in a gravity-dependent position.
- Fever (in hot whirlpool).
- Patients requiring postural support during treatment.
- Skin conditions in spa-type tubs. Otherwise, follow the cleaning instructions noted on page 143.
- General contraindications listed for heat and cold treatments.

Precautions

- The whirlpool must be connected to a ground-fault circuit interrupter (see Box 4–5).
- Instruct the patient not to turn the whirlpool motor on or off while in the water. Ideally, the switch to the motor should be out of the patient's reach.
- Patients who are receiving whirlpool treaments should be in view of a staff member at all times.
- Because of the discomfort associated with cold immersions, the treatment may be started at a comfortable, yet cool, temperature. Decrease the temperature gradually during the treatment by adding cold water.
- The combination of increased circulation and placement of the extremity in a gravity-dependent position tends to increase edema.
- Do not run the whirlpool turbine dry.
- The flowing water may nauseate some patients, especially those prone to motion sickness.[108, 111]
- Patients who are under the influence of drugs (including alcohol) or those who have seizure disorders or heart disease are at risk of losing consciousness during treatment, especially when hot whirlpools are used.[107]
- The pressure associated with full-body immersion may impair breathing in individuals suffering from advanced respiratory disease.

(Lo Boy and High Boy, courtesy of Whitehall Manufacturing, City of Industry, CA.)

4. Add a whirlpool disinfectant according to the manufacturer's directions.
5. If wounds are present on the body part being treated, add a disinfectant such as povidone, povidone-iodine, or sodium hypochlorite to the water.
6. Adjust the temperature for the type of effect desired and for the proportion of the body being treated.
7. The temperature of full-body warm whirlpool immersions should be further reduced if the patient will be performing moderate to strenuous exercise. Exercise increases the body's core temperature and would be magnified by higher water temperatures.
8. If an extremity is being treated, place the patient in a comfortable position using either a high chair or a whirlpool bench. Use rubber padding or a folded terry cloth towel to pad the limb where it contacts the tank.
9. If the entire body is being immersed, use a whirlpool stool or sling seat.
10. Turn the turbine on and adjust the turbulence. With subacute injuries, do not focus the turbulence directly on the affected area.
11. Patients receiving full-body treatments, whether hot or cold, must be monitored continuously.

Maintenance

The presence of electricity, water, and patients in the same room creates unique safety concerns. Refer to Electrical Systems and Hydrotherapy Area, p 85, in Chapter 4 regarding the safe operation of the hydrotherapy area.

Follow the manufacturer's guidelines for quarterly, 6-month, and annual maintenance requirements, including thermometer calibration by qualified personnel as a part of the annual inspection. Unplug the turbine from its power source prior to cleaning or moving the whirlpool tub.

Cleaning the Whirlpool

The whirlpool must be cleaned before and after treating a patient who has open wounds that will be exposed to the water. If no open wounds are permitted in the tub, the whirlpool should then be cleaned at the end of the work day.

1. Drain the whirlpool after treatment.
2. Don appropriate attire such as rubber gloves and a smock.
3. Refill the tub with hot (approximately 120°F [48.9°C]) water to a level sufficient to safely operate the turbine.
4. Add a commercial disinfectant, antibacterial agent, or chlorine bleach to the water, using the concentration indicated on the packaging.
5. Run the turbine for at least 1 minute to allow the cleaning agent to cycle through the internal components.

6. Drain the whirlpool and scrub the interior using a brush with a cleaner, paying close attention to the external turbine, thermometer stem, drains, welds, and other areas that could retain germs.
7. Thoroughly rinse the tub.
8. Clean the exterior surface with a stainless steel (or appropriate) cleaner. Stainless steel tubs should not be cleaned with bleach.
9. Culture kits are available to determine if bacteria are present in the tub.

Monthly or at Regular Intervals

Check the proper functioning of the ground fault circuit interrupter.

Annually

1. Have the whirlpool turbine inspected by a qualified service technician.
2. Calibrate the thermometer or thermometers within the tub or located in the mixing valve.

▮ MOIST HEAT PACKS

The moist heat pack is a canvas pouch filled with silica gel or a similar substance capable of absorbing a large number of water molecules. This pack is kept in a water-filled heating unit that is maintained at a constant temperature ranging between 160°F and 166°F (71.1°C to 74.4°C), although the packs can be heated on a stove top or in a microwave oven for home use (refer to the manufacturer's instructions for at-home heating procedures). This temperature range also assists in killing any bacteria that may collect in the heating unit. Moist heat packs are a superficial heat modality, transferring energy to the patient's skin by way of conduction, with the moisture assisting the transfer of energy. Each subsequent underlying tissue layer is heated through conduction from the overlying tissue. These packs are capable of maintaining a workable therapeutic temperature for 30 to 45 minutes after removal from the heating unit.

The layering around the hot pack (see Set-up and Application) serves as insulation between the pack and the skin (Fig. 6–13). When the pack is placed on the skin, there is little compression of the protective covering, allowing air pockets to form within the layering, providing additional insulation. If the hot pack is compressed, such as when the patient is lying on it, the layering is moved together and the air is forced out. This decreases the available insulation and increases the amount of energy being transferred, increasing the possibility of the patient suffering burns. Lying on the hot pack also decreases capillary flow and energy lost to the environment, further increasing the possibility of burns occurring.

Moist hot packs are suitable for use over localized areas or on areas that normally cannot be treated by immersion in water, such as the cervical spine (Fig. 6–14). The wide array of sizes and styles of moist heat packs make them acceptable for use over the lumbar spine (medium or large size), the cervical spine (cervical pack),

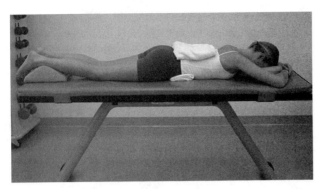

Figure 6–13. **Patient Positioning for Moist Heat Treatments of the Lumbar Spine.** Note the bolsters under the feet, abdomen, and face. This position relieves tension on the lumbar muscles.

the shoulder (medium size), and the knee (medium size). The effectiveness of the moist heat pack is diminished when used over irregular areas such as the ankle or fingers, in which case hot whirlpool or other immersion techniques should be considered.

Some types of dry heat packs are also capable of being frozen and used as cold packs. This style of heat pack delivers dry heat. This style of pack is heated in a moist heating unit or microwave oven. To administer moist heat, wrap the heated pack in a warm, damp towel.

● EFFECTS ON
The Injury Response Process

The specific effects of moist heat packs are the same as described for heat in general. When compared with dry heat, moist heat is considered a more comfortable method of application and may have greater benefit in reducing pain. Dry heating agents, such as an electrical heating pad, do not increase the skin temperature as rapidly as moist agents, allowing fresh blood to keep the tissue temperatures relatively low during normal therapeutic treatment durations. However, because electrical heating maintains a

constant temperature during the treatment, over time the chance of burns increases.

The application of moist heat causes a rapid increase in the surface temperature of the skin. Vasodilation of the vessels produces an influx of blood to the area in an attempt to cool the tissues. Superficial muscle layers can be directly heated by the heat packs, resulting in relaxation of the affected tissues. In areas with low amounts of overlying adipose tissue, blood flow can be affected up to 3 cm deep but not in therapeutic dosages if the overlying adipose tissue layer is thick.[112]

Vasodilation, increased blood flow, and increased pulse rate associated with thermotherapy occur only while the hot packs are in contact with the body.[38] Using the triceps surae muscle group as a model, temperatures at 1 cm deep within the tissues are elevated by 38.5°F (±30.7°F) compared to only 17.6°F (±21.2°F) at a depth of 3 cm.[112]

Relaxation of muscles or muscle layers that are more deeply situated results from soothing of the superficial motor and sensory nerves. When treating obese individuals, the clinician may find that hot packs are less effective in raising subcutaneous tissue temperature because the adipose tissue layer serves as insulation.

■ Set-up and Application

1. Ensure that the patient is free of contraindications for this treatment technique.
2. Cover the pack with a commercial terry cloth covering, or fold a terry cloth towel so that there are five or six layers of towel between the pack and the skin (Fig. 6–15). The treatment temperature can be increased by removing towel layers or decreased by adding layers.
3. Place the pack on the patient in a comfortable manner. If having the patient lie on the pack is unavoidable, additional toweling should be placed between the patient and the hot pack.
4. When treating an infected area, completely cover the skin with sterile gauze. After the treatment, dispose of the gauze in a biowaste container and wash the hot pack's covering according to the universal precautions.
5. Check the patient after the first 5 minutes for comfort and mottling. Recheck the patient regularly, and adjust the toweling if needed.
6. Some clinicians replace the hot pack every 8 to 10 minutes to maintain high treatment temperatures,[58] but properly heated packs contain sufficient energy for a 30-minute treatment.[76] If hot packs are replaced during the treatment, extra caution must be taken to check for burns arising from increased temperatures and rebound vasoconstriction.
7. After the treatment, return the moist heat pack to the heating unit and allow it to reheat for a minimum of 30 to 45 minutes before reuse.

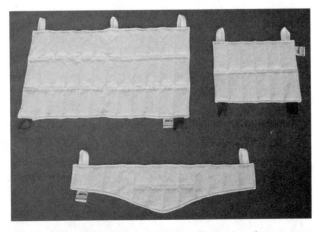

Figure 6–14. **Moist Heat Packs.** Clockwise from upper left: Oversized (15"x24"), standard (10"x12"), and cervical (24" long) packs. Other sizes and shapes are available.

At a Glance: Moist Heat Packs

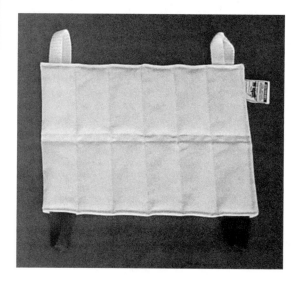

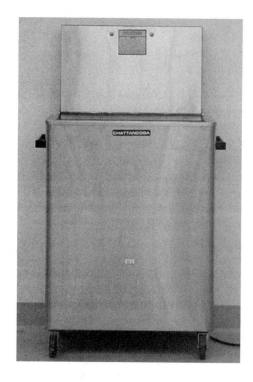

Description

Silica-filled packs are stored in hot water between use. The packs are then removed from the heating unit, wrapped in a terry cloth cover or towel, and used to deliver moist heat to the body. Moist heat packs are used for:

- Localized superficial heating
- Pain
- Muscle spasm
- Chronic inflammatory conditions
- Increasing muscle, tendon, and fascial elasticity

Primary Effects

- Increased blood flow/vasodilation
- Increased cell metabolism
- Muscular relaxation secondary to reducing muscle spindle sensitivity

Temperature Range

- Moist heat packs are stored in 160°F to 166°F (71.1°C to 74.4°C) water between treatments.
- During application, insulation is added to the pack as needed to maintain a comfortable treatment.

Treatment Duration

- Moist heat packs are commonly used in treatment bouts of 20 to 30 minutes. When treating deep structures, the treatment duration should be increased as the amount of adipose tissue increases.
- Treatments may be repeated as needed, but sufficient time should be allowed for the skin to cool before the next treatment is given.

Indications

- Subacute or chronic inflammatory conditions
- Reduction of subacute or chronic pain
- Subacute or chronic muscle spasm
- Decreased ROM
- Hematoma resolution
- Reduction of joint contractures
- Infection (see procedures in Set-up and Application of moist heat packs)

Contraindications

- Acute conditions: This modality will increase the inflammatory response in the area.
- Peripheral vascular disease: The heat cannot be dissipated, thus increasing the chance of burns.
- Impaired circulation.
- Poor thermal regulation.

Precautions

- Do not allow the moist heat pack to come into direct contact with the skin because burns may result.
- If the packs are changed during the course of the treatment, additional care must be taken to prevent burns.
- Infected areas must be covered with sterile gauze or another type of material to collect seepage.
- Do not allow the patient to lay on the heat pack. If this is unavoidable, add extra layers of insulation.

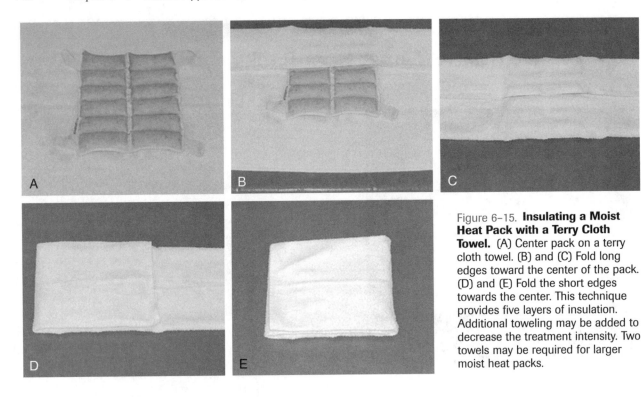

Figure 6–15. **Insulating a Moist Heat Pack with a Terry Cloth Towel.** (A) Center pack on a terry cloth towel. (B) and (C) Fold long edges toward the center of the pack. (D) and (E) Fold the short edges towards the center. This technique provides five layers of insulation. Additional toweling may be added to decrease the treatment intensity. Two towels may be required for larger moist heat packs.

■ Maintenance

Unplug the heating unit before performing any maintenance. Follow the manufacturer's guidelines for quarterly, 6-month, and annual maintenance requirements, including calibration by qualified personnel.

New Moist Heat Packs

Allow new moist heat packs to soak fully immersed in warm water for 2 hours before placing them in the heating unit.

Daily Maintenance

Ensure that the water level covers the top of the moist heating packs.

Biweekly Maintenance

1. Unplug and drain the heating unit.
2. Clean the storage unit, the racks, and the heating element with stainless steal cleanser, a vinegar and water mixture, or a mild abrasive cleanser. If the unit is made from stainless steel, DO NOT use a cleanser that contains chlorine bleach. Chlorine damages stainless steel. If local tap water has high level of chlorine, add a dechlorinator.
3. Remove sediment from the inside metal and heating coil with a firm brush or steel wool. Do not use metal objects to scrape off the sediment as this can damage the metal.

3. Fill the unit with enough water to cover the tops of the moist heat packs.
4. Scented or herbal additives should not be added to the water unless it is specifically approved by the manufacturer.

Care of the Moist Heat Packs

1. Discard any pack that becomes contaminated with germs.
2. Discard any pack that is torn. The contents of the pack will leak out into the storage unit.
3. Do not allow the packs to dry out.
4. To store the packs for long periods, place wet packs in individual sealable plastic bags and store them in a freezer.

▶ PARAFFIN BATH

Paraffin is a superficial agent used for delivering heat to small, irregularly shaped areas, such as the hand, fingers, wrist, and foot. Although its use in sports medicine is limited, it is an effective method for delivering heat, and this form of thermotherapy may increase intra-articular temperature as much as 6.3°F (3.5°C).[23] The application of paraffin is beneficial in chronic conditions in which ROM is not an essential part of the treatment protocol, such as arthritis or chronic inflammatory conditions.

A paraffin bath contains a mixture of wax and mineral oil in a ratio of seven parts wax to one part oil (7:1). Melted paraffin is kept at a constant temperature of 118°F to 126°F (47.8°C to 52.2°C) for upper extremity treatments. Temperatures for treatments given to the lower extremity are decreased to 113°F to 121°F (45.0°C to

At a Glance: Paraffin Bath

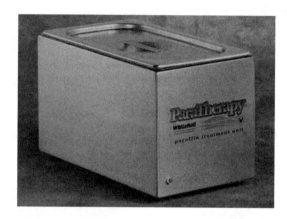

Description

A mixture of wax and mineral oil is melted in the unit. The low specific heat of the mixture allows warm temperatures to be used during treatment. Paraffin is used to deliver heat to small, irregularly shaped areas, especially when ROM exercises are not a part of the treatment, for the treatment of chronic inflammatory conditions, and softening the skin.

Primary Effects

- Increased perspiration
- Increased blood flow/vasodilation
- Increased cell metabolism

Temperature Range

118°F to 126°F (47.8° to 52.2°C)

(ParaTherapy, courtesy of Whitehall Manufacturing, City of Industry, CA.)

Treatment Duration

Paraffin treatments are given for 15 to 20 minutes and may be repeated several times daily.

Indications

- Subacute and chronic inflammatory conditions (e.g., arthritis of the fingers)
- Limitation of motion after immobilization

Contraindications

- Open wounds: Wax and oil would irritate the tissues.
- Skin infections: The warm, dark environment is excellent for breeding bacteria.
- Sensory loss.
- Peripheral vascular disease.

Precautions

- Do not allow the patient to touch the bottom or sides of the paraffin tank. Burns may result.
- The sensation of the paraffin is misleading as to the actual temperature of the treatment. The temperature of the paraffin is sufficient to cause burns, but its specific heat requires more time to transfer the energy (see Box 5–1).
- Avoid using paraffin with athletes who are required to catch or throw a ball (e.g., basketball players) or workers who are required to maintain a good grip (e.g., carpenters) after the treatment. The mineral oil in the paraffin mixture tends to make the hands slippery, making the task of catching a ball or holding onto a hammer difficult.

49.4°C) because the circulation is less efficient.[113] Because of its low specific heat (0.5 to 0.65), paraffin can provide approximately six times the amount of heat as water. Consequently, the paraffin feels cooler and is more tolerable than water at the same temperature (see Box 5–1).

● EFFECTS ON

The Injury Response Process

In addition to the standard effects of heat application, paraffin increases perspiration in the treated area and softens and moisturizes the skin.

■ Set-up and Application

There are several methods of paraffin application, each with its own advantages and disadvantages. The more common methods, immersion and glove, are described here. In addition to providing heat to the area, the paraffin wax may act as an insulator if it is allowed to dry on the skin. With this in mind, the amount of heat delivered can be adjusted by increasing or decreasing the wax layers. During immersion baths, the amount of insulation is increased with the number of layers added.

Preparation for Treatment

To avoid contaminating the paraffin, thoroughly clean and

dry the body part before treatment. Chipped or flaking nail polish should be removed.

Immersion Bath

This is the best method for raising tissue temperature. However, the chance of burns is increased, so the patient must be closely monitored.

1. Ensure that the patient is free of contraindications for this treatment technique.
2. The patient begins by dipping the body part into the paraffin and removing it. If possible, the patient should spread the fingers or toes to allow the paraffin to cover the maximum amount of surface area. Allow this coat to dry (it will turn a dull shade of white).
3. Dip the extremity into the wax 6 to 12 more times to develop the amount of insulation necessary. Allow the wax to dry between dips.
4. The patient then places the body part back into the paraffin for the duration of the treatment.
5. Instruct the patient to avoid touching the sides and bottom of the heating unit because burns may result.
6. Patients who are receiving an immersion treatment must not move the joints that are in the liquid. The cracking of the wax will allow fresh paraffin to touch the skin, increasing the risk of burns.
7. After the treatment, scrape off the hardened paraffin and return it to the unit for reheating, or discard it.

Pack (Glove) Method

The glove method is the safest but least effective method for delivering heat to the body with paraffin wax. This method is recommended for those patients who are in the subacute stage of healing or who have a vascular or nerve condition that would predispose them to burning. The body part may also be elevated during this form of paraffin application (Fig. 6–16).

1. Ensure that the patient is free of contraindications for this treatment technique.
2. Begin the treatment by immersing the extremity in the wax so that it becomes completely covered. Remove the body part and allow the wax to dry.
3. Continue to dip and remove the body part in the wax 7 to 12 times.
4. After the final withdrawal from the wax, cover the extremity with a plastic bag, aluminum foil, or wax paper. Then wrap and secure a terry cloth towel around the area.
5. If indicated, the body part may be elevated.
6. Following the treatment, remove the towel and inner layering. Scrape off the hardened paraffin and return it to the bath for reheating, or discard it.

Maintenance

Refer to the manufacturer's maintenance requirements for the unit being used.

After Each Use

Allow any paraffin that may have dripped onto the outer surface of the heating unit to dry, and then scrape the wax off using a tongue depressor or similar object.

As Needed

The paraffin mixture should be changed when it becomes discolored or debris builds up in the bottom of the tank. Unplug the heating unit prior to performing any maintenance. Follow the manufacturer's guidelines for quarterly, 6-month, and annual maintenance requirements, including calibration by qualified personnel.

1. Unplug the unit and remove the protective grate from the bottom of the unit.
2. Allow the paraffin to harden (this may require several hours).
3. Once the paraffin has hardened, plug the unit back in and allow the paraffin to heat to the point where it dislodges from the unit.
4. Remove and discard the used paraffin.
5. Use paper toweling to remove any residual paraffin.
6. Unplug the unit and cleanse the inner tub with a mild disinfectant.

▌● FLUIDOTHERAPY

Fluidotherapy is a convective modality that delivers dry heat to the extremities. This method of heat application can be used in cases in which paraffin or whirlpool application would be appropriate but results in more heat absorption in the tissues.[114] Air jets circulate heated cellulose particles that have a lower specific heat and thermal capacity than water, allowing higher treatment temperatures to be used. Fluidotherapy applied at 118°F (47.8°C) increases the temperature of the joint capsule by 16.2°F (9°C) and superficial muscle by 9.5°F (5.3°C).[115]

The patient inserts the body part into the fluidotherapy unit through one of the portals located on the machine (Fig. 6–17). The clinician's hands can also be inserted into the unit to assist with ROM exercises or perform joint mobilization techniques. The effect and sensation of fluidotherapy is similar to that of a whirlpool, but without the benefits of buoyancy and hydrostatic pressure. The cellulose medium provides resistance to active exercise. Increasing the amount of airflow decreases resistance and vice versa.

● EFFECTS ON
The Injury Response Process

The effects of fluidotherapy on the injury response cycle are the same as heat treatments in general. An advantage of fluidotherapy is the ability to place the limb in

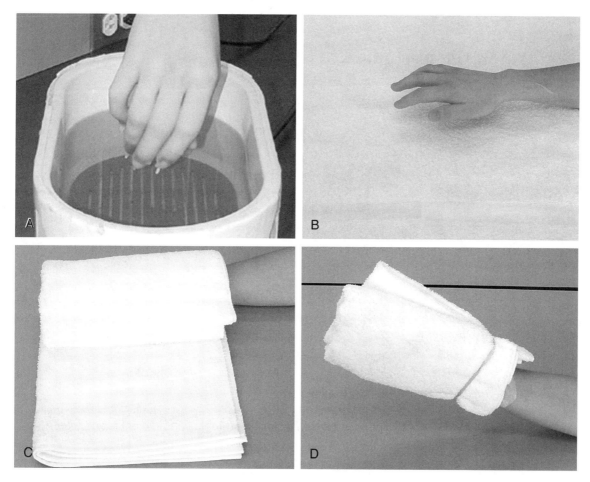

Figure 6–16. **The Glove Method of Paraffin Application.** (A) The body part, usually the hand, is dipped in the paraffin mixture 7 to 12 times. (B) and (C) After the outer layer of the wax dries, the body part is wrapped with a terry cloth towel or aluminum foil. (D) The extremity remains wrapped for the remainder of the treatment. Custom cloth mitts and boots are also sold for this purpose.

the nongravity-dependent position, reducing the formation of edema.

■ Instrumentation

Air Speed: The rate at which the medium is moved through the unit is expressed as a percentage of the total force (0 to 100). The default setting is 50. Lower force increases the viscosity of the mixture, providing more resistance to joint motion.

Preheat Timer: Used for preheating the transmitting medium. Some units are programmable, allowing the unit to automatically preheat at the start of a work day.

Pulse Time: Pulses interrupt the flow of the medium by starting and stopping the air stream. Pulses range from 1 (1 sec on/1 sec off) to 6 (6 on/6 off). Setting the pulse time to OFF provides a constant flow.

Treatment Temperature: Sets the treatment temperature from 88°F to 130°F (31.1° to 54°C).

Treatment Time: Sets the duration of the treatment. The time remaining is displayed on the console, or the timer rotates to display the time remaining.

■ Set-up and Application

Refer to the unit's instruction manual for precise operating instructions.

Patient Preparation

1. Ensure that the patient is free of contraindications for this treatment technique.
2. During the patient preparation period, preheat the fluidotherapy unit. If the unit is so equipped, close the heat flaps to speed preheating. Following the preheating, reopen the flaps.
3. Remove jewelry from the body part being treated.
4. Wash and dry the patient's extremity using an antimicrobial soap and then apply a hospital grade antiseptic skin cleanser.
5. To prevent the medium from entering open wounds, cover skin lesions with a nonpermeable membrane such as a plastic bag, rubber gloves, or surgical skin dressing (e.g., OpSite).

Initiating the Treatment

1. Turn the unit off.
2. Ensure that the unit contains a proper amount of the medium.

At a Glance: Fluidotherapy

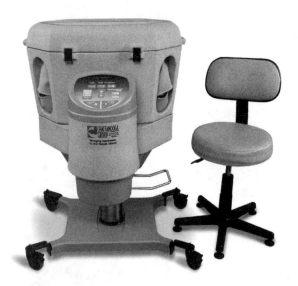

Description

Ground cellulose is heated and circulated by air to deliver dry heat to the extremity. Fluidotherapy is used for superficial heating of the extremities, especially the wrist, hand, and fingers and the ankle and toes.

Primary Effects

- Superficial heating of the skin
- Decreased pain
- Increased ROM

Temperature Range

110°F to 125°F (43.3°C to 51.6°C)

Treatment Duration

Fluidotherapy treatments are given for 20 minutes and can be repeated multiple times per day.

Indications

- Pain reduction
- Prior to or during joint mobilization
- ROM exercises combined with heat therapy
- Non-rheumatoid arthritis

Contraindications

- Uncovered open wounds
- Sensory loss
- Peripheral vascular disease
- Over cancerous lesions
- General medical conditions that reduce the patient's tolerance to heat

Precautions

- Cover open wounds prior to treatment.
- Patients who are sensitive to allergic reactions caused by dust and pollen.

(Fluido CHT, courtesy of the Chattanooga Group, Hixon, TN.)

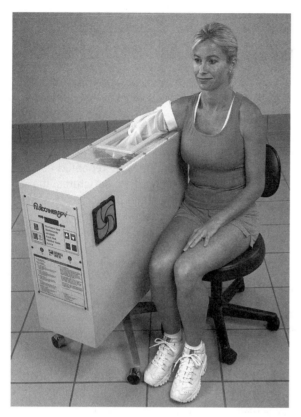

Figure 6–17. **Clinical Application of Fluidotherapy.** Fluidotherapy units are used to deliver dry heat to the extremities. (Fluidotherapy Standard, courtesy of the Chattanooga Group, Hixon, TN.)

3. Secure all nonused entry portals prior to turning the unit on.
4. Select the portal appropriate for the treatment and body part. Have the patient fully insert the body part into the unit.
5. Securely fasten the appliance proximally on the body part.
6. Set thermostat to the desired temperature, usually between 100°F and 123°F (37.8°C to 50.6°C).
7. Set the treatment duration.
8. If indicated, instruct the patient to perform the appropriate ROM exercises.

Terminating the Treatment

1. Turn the unit OFF before removing the patient.
2. Loosen the appliance from the patient's extremity.
3. Before removing the body part from the tank, remove any particles that may have adhered to the patient.
4. Resecure the entry portal used by the patient.

■ Maintenance

Unplug the unit before performing any maintenance. Follow the manufacturer's guidelines for quarterly, 6-month, and annual maintenance requirements, including calibration by qualified personnel.

Daily Maintenance

1. Clean air inlet filters. Remove the filter and wash with antibacterial soap and water. Allow the filter to completely dry before reinstalling it. Older filters are cleaned using a soft-bristle brush.
2. Refill medium. Refill the unit to the indicated level using the manufacturer's recommended medium.
3. Inspect sleeves. Ensure that the portal sleeves are free from rips and weak seams. Porous sleeves will result in the spillage of the medium during treatment.

Weekly Maintenance

Launder all appliance sleeves in a mild antibacterial detergent. Refer to the operator's manual for instructions on removing the sleeves.

▐ CONTRAST THERAPY

Contrast therapy consists of alternating hot and cold treatments. Stationary water immersion, tandem whirlpools, or moist heat packs and ice packs may be used for this application. Alternating heat and cold modalities are thought to produce a kind of vascular exercise, causing a cycle of vasoconstrictions and vasodilations of the superficial blood vessels. This "pumping" action then would stimulate peripheral blood flow and decrease pain and may aid in venous and lymphatic return, although these theories have not been substantiated (see Effects on the Injury Response Cycle).[116]

Contrast therapy is most commonly indicated in subacute or chronic conditions for the removal of edema or ecchymosis, although this result has not been proved. This technique is also used for making the transition from cryotherapy to thermotherapy.

The most effective time ratio between hot and cold has not been determined, but the most commonly used ratios are 3:1 and 4:1 (i.e., 3 and 4 minutes in the hot immersion to 1 minute in the cold). Alternating 6-minute bouts of moist heat pack and cold pack application results in a more pronounced differential in temperatures than immersion techniques used for shorter contact times. This method keeps the temperature gradient high, resulting in a greater exchange of energy.[18]

The treatment may end after either the hot or the cold application, depending on the stage of the injury, the desired effect of the treatment, and the patient's activity plans after the treatment. When a state of vasoconstriction is desired, the treatment is terminated after cold application. If vasodilation is desired, the treatment is terminated after a warm application. In subacute conditions, it is generally beneficial to finish the treatment with following cold exposure. In chronic conditions, the bout is most often ended after the warm exposure.

At a Glance: **Contrast Therapy**

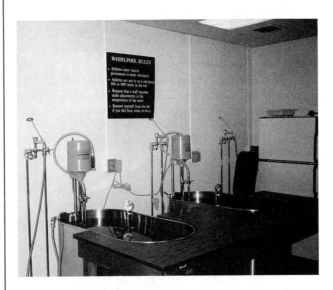

Description

Contrast baths consist of alternating bouts of heat and cold, using a hot and cold whirlpool (shown), hot and cold immersion, or moist heat packs and cold packs. Contrast therapy is used for:
- Removing ecchymosis and reducing edema*
- Transition between cold and heat modalities
- Reducing exercise-induced (delayed onset) muscle soreness

*The efficacy of this treatment has not been fully substantiated.

Primary Effects

Alternating periods of vasoconstriction and vasodilation

Temperature Range

COLD IMMERSION
50°F to 60°F (10°C to 16°C). The temperature is increased as the proportion of the body area immersed increases.

HOT IMMERSION
105°F to 110°F (40.6°C to 43.3°C). Temperature is decreased as the proportion of the body area treated increases.

Treatment Duration

- 20 to 30 minutes and may be repeated as needed. When treating deep structures, the treatment duration should be increased as the amount of adipose tissue increases.
- Hot immersions are typically 3 or 4 minutes in duration.
- Cold immersions are typically 1 or 2 minutes in duration.

Indications

- Ecchymosis removal
- Edema reduction
- Subacute or chronic inflammatory conditions
- Impaired circulation (monitor the patient closely)
- Pain reduction
- Increasing joint ROM

Contraindications

- Acute injuries
- Hypersensitivity to cold
- Contraindications relative to whirlpool use
- Contraindications relative to cold applications
- Contraindications relative to heat applications

Precautions

- If whirlpools are used, see Precautions described in At a Glance: Hot and Cold Whirlpools.
- A Neoprene toe cap may be used to decrease the discomfort associated with cold immersions.
- The combination of increased circulation and placement of the extremity in a gravity-dependent position tends to increase edema.

● E F F E C T S   O N

The Injury Response Process

The exact effects on cellular responses from contrast therapy are not clear. Contrast therapy has long been used under the assumption that the influx of new blood assists in removing edema by unclogging the vasculature. However, arteriole and lymphatic capillaries contain only epithelial cells and are unable to change sizes, that is, they are unable to vasodilate or vasoconstrict. Theoretically, the cellular metabolic rate increases or decreases in response to the temperature of the treatment; however, contrast therapy does not appear to significantly influence subcutaneous tissue temperatures at depths greater than 1 cm.[18, 71]

There is no evidence that supports the efficacy of contrast therapy in reducing edema or removing ecchymosis. If half-leg or half-arm immersion techniques where there is not sufficient hydrostatic pressure placed on the distal extremity is used to deliver contrast therapy, the limb will be placed in the gravity-dependent position, potentially increasing limb volume (see Whirlpools).

■ Set-up and Application

Immersion Technique

1. Ensure that the patient is free of contraindications for this treatment technique.
2. If an immersion technique is being used, position the tubs as close together as possible without touching each other. ("Tubs" refers to either immersion buckets or whirlpool tanks.) The patient should be able to remove the body part from one tub and immediately immerse it in the other.
3. Fill one tub with water in the range from 105°F to 110°F (40.6°C to 43.3°C) and the other with water between 50°F and 60°F (10° to 15.6°C).
4. Position the patient on a chair or bench in a manner requiring a minimal amount of motion from tub to tub.

Hot/Cold Pack Technique

1. Ensure that the patient is free of contraindications for this treatment technique.
2. Position the patient so the hot and cold packs are within reach.
3. Instruct the patient on how and when to remove one pack and apply the other pack.

4. Because of cooling, the original hot pack should be replaced with a fresh, heated pack at approximately 15 minutes into the treatment.

Common Considerations

1. A clock or watch should be available to time the treatment segments.
2. In most cases, heat treatments are given first.
3. Have the patient alternate between the treatments according to the protocol being applied.
4. As with all hot or cold treatments, the patient should be monitored.
5. The treatment ends after the hot immersion if relaxation and vasodilation are desired or after the cold immersion if vasoconstriction is desired.

● Chapter Highlights

- Cold packs are the most common method of applying cryotherapy. With the exception of reusable cold packs or when applied to areas of vascular impairment, the cold pack should be applied directly to the skin.
- Ice massage rapidly reduces intramuscular temperatures and produces relative numbness of the skin; however, these effects are most pronounced when applied to a small area.
- Ice immersion is used to treat irregularly shaped areas such as the foot and ankle, elbow, and wrist and hand.
- Cryostretch uses a vapocoolant spray to desensitize nerve endings while the body part is being stretched. This treatment approach is used for trigger point therapy.
- Whirlpools may be used to deliver hot or cold treatments. Other biophysical effects are based on the turbulence and aeration of the water. Treatment while immersed in water has the effects of buoyancy, resistance, and hydrostatic pressure.
- Moist heat packs are useful for warming local areas of the body and can affect tissues up to 3 cm deep.
- Paraffin baths use a mixture of mineral and wax to treat small, irregularly shaped areas. Paraffin has a low specific heat, allowing the treatment to be administered at higher temperatures than whirlpools or moist heat packs.
- Fluidotherapy uses heated cellulose particles to apply superficial heat to the extremities. The cellulose particles are circulated by a stream of air.
- Contrast therapy involves the alternate application of heat and cold agents.

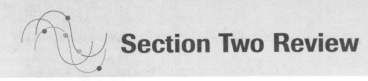

Case Study: Chapter Case Study

Jessica is a 16-year-old basketball player who sustained a left ankle inversion sprain while you are providing medical coverage for this event. You witnessed the incident and noted that her ankle and foot rolled onto the lateral border after landing on another player's foot after a lay-up. After the referee called a time out, you entered the court to assist Jessica. You noted that she was seated on the floor holding her ankle in significant pain. She reports to you that her ankle is in a lot of pain on the lateral aspect of her foot, ankle, and lower leg. After a brief injury assessment, you determine she can be assisted off the court in a non-weightbearing mode to render treatment.

1. What is the best thermal agent to consider in this situation?
2. What are the physiological effects on the injury response cycle from the application of this thermal agent?
3. What are the clinical symptoms that you hope to address with this intervention?
4. At what other phases would this intervention philosophy apply during the injury rehabilitation process?
5. What other thermal modalities may be appropriate over the following 2 weeks for this diagnosis? Why?

Case Study: Continuation of Case Study from Section 1

(The following discussion relates to Case Study 2, found on p 92 of Section One.)

The modalities presented in Chapters 5 and 6 would benefit our patient throughout his rehabilitation program. Various forms of cold modalities can be used throughout the time frame indicated, and moist heat packs can be incorporated in the later stages of the program.

Ice Packs

Either crushed ice packs or reusable cold packs would be used during the early stages of this patient's program, administered in 20-minute treatments throughout the day. The patient would be placed in the supine position, with his head and neck comfortably supported to decrease the amount of electromyographic activity in the trapezius. The cold application will decrease the amount of pain by increasing the pain threshold and by decreasing the rate of the nerve conduction velocity. Muscle spasm will be decreased secondary to reducing the muscle spindle's sensitivity to stretch. Acutely, this method of cold application will also decrease the metabolic activity in the treated area, thereby decreasing the amount of secondary hypoxic injury.

As the patient's treatment progresses, active or passive range of motion exercises (described later) would be performed after the removal of the pack. During the more advanced stages of the rehabilitation program, ice packs would be applied after the rehabilitation session to minimize the postexercise inflammatory response. Lastly, the patient would be instructed to use cold packs as a part of his home treatment program.

Ice Massage

Ice massage could be used in conjunction with stretching exercises. The patient would be in the seated position, with the cervical spine flexed and laterally bent to the left to tolerance. Once the ice massage treatment has begun and the patient reports decreased pain, the trapezius could be further stretched until discomfort is once again reported. This process would be repeated for the 10- to 15-minute duration of the treatment.

This approach relies on ice massage numbing the area and decreasing the sensitivity of the local muscle spindles. This effect, combined with the passive stretching of the muscle, helps to decrease muscle spasm and to increase range of motion.

Moist Heat Packs

When the active inflammatory process subsides, moist heat can safely be applied before therapeutic exercise and other modalities. Similar to the application of cold packs, moist heat decreases the pain and spasm associated with the injury, but other benefits are realized as well. Moist heat promotes relaxation of the cervical musculature and increases tissue extensibility, increasing the effectiveness of the patient's range-of-motion program.

Concurrent Range-of-Motion Exercises

Range-of-motion exercises for side bending and rotation (30-second hold for five repetitions) are first begun with the patient in the supine position to decrease the effects of gravity. As the patient's pain and spasm begin to subside, these exercises can be progressed to being performed in an upright position.

● ● ● Section Two Quiz

1. Which of the following modalities has the greatest likelihood of frostbite?
   A. Ice immersion
   B. Reusable cold packs
   C. Ice massage
   D. Ice bag

2. Which of the following is a contraindication to the use of a paraffin bath?
   A. No range of motion
   B. Chronic conditions
   C. Pain
   D. Skin conditions

3. Which of the following modalities uses convection as the method of heat transfer?
   A. Ice bag
   B. Whirlpool
   C. Hot packs
   D. Infrared lamp

4. Which of the following is not a local effect of cold application?
   A. Decreased rate of cell metabolism
   B. Decreased muscle spindle activity
   C. Decreased nerve conduction velocity
   D. Decreased viscosity of fluids in the area

5. Which of the following modalities has the greatest depth of penetration into the tissues?
   A. Moist heat pack
   B. Hot whirlpool
   C. Infrared lamp
   D. Ice bag

6. Heat application by itself (i.e., without stretching exercises) is sufficient to elongate collagen-rich tissues.
   A. True
   B. False

7. Which of the following is not a local effect of heat application?
   A. Increased rate of cell metabolism
   B. Increased blood flow
   C. Increased muscle tone
   D. Decreased muscle spasm

8. A ____ degree F drop in skin temperature is needed to reduce the sensitivity of muscle spindles.
   A. 5
   B. 9
   C. 13
   D. 17

9. As the size (area) of the body exposed to cold immersion increases, the temperature of the immersion should:
   A. Increase
   B. Decrease

10. The primary reason for the use of cold during the immediate treatment of an injury is:
    A. To decrease swelling
    B. To limit hemorrhage
    C. To reduce pain
    D. To decrease cell metabolism

11. Focal compression serves what purpose?
    A. Prevents swelling from entering the joint capsule
    B. Assisting the lymphatic system in removing solid matter from the area
    C. Providing support to the injured area to assist in ambulating
    D. A and B

12. The "hunting response" has been demonstrated to occur in all body parts during cold application.
    A. True
    B. False

13. Moist heat packs are stored in water having a temperature range between ____ and ____ degrees F.
    A. 140/150
    B. 150/160
    C. 160/170
    D. 170/180

14. The thermal effects obtained from a moist heat pack occur up to ___ cm beneath the skin.
    A. 1
    B. 2
    C. 3
    D. 4

15. Raynaud's phenomenon is a common contraindication to the use of cold and is characterized by:
    A. The skin becoming white and shiny
    B. Alternating bouts of pallor and cyanosis
    C. Welts (wheels) appearing on the skin
    D. Involuntary flexion contraction of the involved muscles

16. Following a 20-minute ice immersion and a short rewarming period, there ___ decreased joint proprioceptive ability.
    A. Is
    B. Is not

17. Which of the follow is not a systemic effect to cold exposure?
    A. Vasoconstriction
    B. Increased heart rate
    C. Decreased respiratory rate
    D. Increased muscle tone

18. If the goal of your treatment is to produce long-lasting cold within the quadriceps muscle prior to exercise (in the subacute or chronic stage of injury), which of the following modalities would be most appropriate?
    A. Ice bag
    B. Ice immersion
    C. Ice massage
    D. Cold whirlpool

19. List the components and effects of intermediate treatment of an acute injury:

Step	Effect
A.	
B.	
C.	
D.	

20. Why does the effect of cold application penetrate deeper and last longer than the effect of heat application?

References

1. Knight, KL: Circulatory effects of therapeutic cold applications. In Knight, KL (ed): Cryotherapy in Sports Injury Management. Human Kinetics, Champaign, IL, 1995, pp 107–125.
2. Halliday, D, et al: Fundamentals of Physics, ed 6. John Wiley & Sons Publishers, Hoboken, NJ, 2000, p 465.
3. Weinberger, A and Lev, A: Temperature elevation of connective tissue by physical modalities. Crit Rev Phys Rehabil Med 3:121, 1991.
4. Low, J and Reed, A: Heat and cold. In Low, J and Reed, A: Electrotherapy Explained: Principles and Practice, ed 2. Butterworth-Heinemann, Oxford, 1994, p. 179.
5. Zemke, JE, et al: Intramuscular temperature responses in the human leg to two forms of cryotherapy: Ice massage and ice bag. J Orthop Sports Phys Ther 27:301, 1998.
6. Lehmann, JF and DeLateur, BJ: Therapeutic heat. In Lehmann, JF (ed): Therapeutic Heat and Cold, ed 4. Williams & Wilkins, Baltimore, 1990, p. 417.
7. Myrer, JW, et al: A comparison of subcutaneous and intramuscular temperature change between ice pack and cold whirlpool cryotherapy (abstract). J Athletic Training 32:S5, 1997.
8. De Coster, D, et al: The value of cryotherapy in the management of trigeminal neuralgia. Acta Stomatol Belg 90:87, 1993.
9. Bolster, MB, et al: Office evaluation and treatment of Raynaud's phenomenon. Cleve Clin J Med 62:51, 1995.
10. Ho, SS, et al: Comparison of various icing times in decreasing bone metabolism and blood flow in the knee. Am J Sports Med 23:74, 1995.
11. Belitsky, RB, et al: Evaluation of the effectiveness of wet ice, dry ice, and cryogen packs in reducing skin temperature. Phys Ther 67:1080, 1987.
12. Merrick, MA, et al: The effects of ice and compression wraps on intramuscular temperatures at various depths. J Athletic Training 28:236, 1993.
13. Myrer, JW, et al: Muscle temperature is affected by overlying adipose when cryotherapy is administered. J Athletic Training 36:32, 2001.
14. Myrer, JW, et al: Temperature changes in the human leg during and after two methods of cryotherapy. J Athletic Training 33:25, 1998.
15. Jameson, AG, et al: Lower-extremity-joint cryotherapy does not affect vertical ground-reaction forces during landing. J Sports Rehabil 10:132, 2001.
16. Myrer, JW, et al: Exercise after cryotherapy greatly enhances intramuscular rewarming. J Athletic Training 35:412, 2000.
17. Ho, SW, et al: The effects of ice on blood flow and bone metabolism in knees. Am J Sports Med 22:537, 1994.
18. Myrer, WJ, et al: Cold- and hot-pack contrast therapy: Subcutaneous and intramuscular temperature change. J Athletic Training 32:238, 1997.
19. Karunakara, RG, et al: Changes in forearm blood flow during single and intermittent cold application. J Orthop Sports Phys Ther 29:177, 1999.
20. Otte, JW, et al: Subcutaneous adipose tissue thickness alters cooling time during cryotherapy. Arch Phys Med Rehabil 83:1501, 2002.
21. Danielson, R, et al: Differences in skin surface temperature and pressure during the application of various cold and compression devices (abstract). J Athletic Training 32:S34, 1997.
22. Dahlstedt, L, et al: Cryotherapy after cruciate knee surgery: Skin, subcutaneous and articular temperatures in 8 patients. Acta Orthop Scand 67:255, 1996.
23. Bocobo, C, et al: The effect of ice on intraarticular temperature in the knee of the dog. Am J Phys Med Rehabil 70:181, 1991.
24. Oosterveld, FG, et al: The effect of local heat and cold therapy on the intraarticular and skin surface temperature of the knee. Arthritis Rheum 35:146, 1992.
25. Jamison, CA, et al: The effects of post cryotherapy exercise on surface and capsular temperature (abstract). J Athletic Training 36:S91, 2001.
26. Allen, JD, et al: Effect of microcurrent stimulation on delayed-onset muscle soreness: A double-blind comparison. J Athletic Training 34:334, 1999.
27. Halar, EM, et al: Nerve conduction velocity: Relationship of skin, subcutaneous, and intramuscular temperatures. Arch Phys Med Rehabil 61:199, 1980.
28. Michalski, WJ and Séguin, JJ: The effects of muscle cooling and stretch on muscle spindle secondary endings in the cat. J Physiol 253:341, 1975.
29. Bugaj, R: The cooling, analgesic, and rewarming effects of ice massage on localized skin. Phys Ther 55:11, 1975.
30. Knight, KL, et al: Circulatory changes in the forearm in 1, 5, 10 and 15°C water. Int J Sports Med 4:281, 1981.
31. Lievens, P and Meevsen, R: The use of cryotherapy in sports injuries. Sports Med 3:398, 1986.
32. Wilkerson, GB: Inflammation in connective tissue: Etiology and management. J Athletic Training 20:299, 1985.
33. Merrick, MA, et al: A preliminary examination of cryotherapy and secondary injury in skeletal muscle. Med Sci Sports Exerc 31:1516, 1999.
34. Menth-Chiari WA, et al: Microcirculation of striated

muscle in closed soft tissue injury: Effect on tissue perfusion, inflammatory cellular response and mechanisms of cryotherapy. A study in rat by means of laser Doppler flow-measurements and intravital microscopy. Unfallchirurg 102:691, 1999.

35. Eston, R and Peters, D: Effects of cold water immersion on the symptoms of exercise-induced muscle damage. J Sports Sciences 17:231, 1999.

36. Taber, C, et al: Measurement of reactive vasodilation during cold gel pack application to nontraumatized ankles. Phys Ther 72:294, 1992.

37. Weston, M, et al: Changes in local blood volume during cold gel pack application to traumatized ankles. J Orthop Sports Phys Ther 19:197, 1994.

38. Baker, RJ and Bell, GW: The effect of therapeutic modalities on blood flow in the human calf. J Orthop Sports Phys Ther 13:23, 1991.

39. Curl, WW, et al: The effect of contusion and cryotherapy on skeletal muscle microcirculation. J Sports Med Phys Fitness 37:279, 1997.

40. Lewis, T: Observations upon the reactions of the vessels of the human skin to cold. Heart 15:177, 1930.

41. Daanen, HA, et al: The effect of body temperature on the hunting response of the middle finger skin temperature. Eur J Appl Physiol Occup Physiol, 76:538, 1997.

42. Hopkins, JT, et al: The effects of cryotherapy and TENS on arthrogenic muscle inhibition of the quadriceps. J Athletic Training 36:S49, 2001.

43. Dolan, MG, et al: Effects of cold water immersion on edema formation after blunt injury to the hind limbs of rats. J Athletic Training 32:233, 1997.

44. Smith, TL, et al: New skeletal muscle model for the longitudinal study of alterations in microcirculation following contusion and cryotherapy. Microsurgery 14:487, 1993.

45. Dervin, GF, et al: Effects of cold and compression dressings on early postoperative outcomes for the arthroscopic anterior cruciate ligament reconstruction patient. J Orthop Sports Phys Ther 27:403, 1998.

46. Allison, SC and Abraham, LD: Sensitivity of qualitative and quantitative spasticity measures to clinical treatment with cryotherapy. Int J Rehabil Res 24:15, 2001.

47. Eldred, E, et al: The effect of cooling on mammalian muscle spindles. Exp Neurol 2:144, 1960.

48. Whitney, SL: Physical agents: Heat and cold modalities. In Scully, RM and Barnes, MR (eds): Physical Therapy. JB Lippincott, Philadelphia, 1989, pp 844–875.

49. Brander, B, et al: Evaluation of the contribution to postoperative analgesia by local cooling of the wound. Anaesthesia 51:1021, 1996.

50. Knight, KL, et al: The effects of cold application on nerve conduction velocity and muscle force (abstract). J Athletic Training 32:S5, 1997.

51. Parker, TJ, et al: Case report: Cold-induced nerve palsy. Athletic Training 18:76, 1983.

52. Green, GA, Zachazewski, JE, and Jordan, SE: A case conference: Peroneal nerve palsy induced by cryotherapy. Physician and Sportsmedicine 17:63, 1989.

53. Ernst, E and Fialka V: Ice freezes pain? A review of the clinical effectiveness of analgesic cold therapy. J Pain Symptom Manage 9:56, 1994.

54. Tremblay, F, et al: Influence of local cooling on proprioceptive acuity in the quadriceps muscle. J Athletic Training 36:119, 2001.

55. Thieme, HA, et al: Cooling does not affect knee proprioception. J Athletic Training 31:8, 1996.

56. Evans, TA, et al: Agility following the application of cold therapy. J Athletic Training 31:232, 1995.

57. Fore, CJ and Smith, BS: The effects of cryotherapy on knee joint position sense in females (abstract). Phys Ther 81:A42, 2001.

58. Halvorson, GA: Therapeutic heat and cold for athletic injuries. Physician and Sportsmedicine 18:87, 1990.

59. Krause, A, et al: The relationship of ankle temperature during cooling and rewarming to the human soleus H reflex. J Sports Rehabil 9:253, 2000.

60. Ruiz, DH, et al: Cryotherapy and sequential exercise bouts following cryotherapy on concentric and eccentric strength in the quadriceps. J Athletic Training 28:320, 1993.

61. Ferretti, G, et al: Effects of temperature on the maximal instantaneous muscle power of humans. Eur J Appl Physiol 64:112, 1992.

62. Thompson, G, et al: Effect of cryotherapy on eccentric peak torque and endurance (abstract). J Athletic Training 29:180, 1994.

63. Mattacola, CG and Perrin, DH: Effects of cold water application on isokinetic strength of the plantar flexors. Isokinetic Exercise Science 3:152, 1993.

64. Kimura, IF, et al: The effect of cryotherapy on eccentric plantar flexion peak torque and endurance. J Athletic Training 32:124, 1997.

65. Verducci, FM: Interval cryotherapy decreases fatigue during repeated weight lifting. J Athletic Training 35:422, 2000.

66. Greenspan, JD, et al: Body site variation of cool perception thresholds, with observations on paradoxical heat. Somatosens Mot Res 10:467, 1993.

67. Ingersoll, CD and Mangus, BC: Sensations of cold reexamined: A study using the McGill Pain Questionnaire. J Athletic Training 26:240, 1991.

68. Streator, S, et al: Sensory information can decrease cold-induced pain perception. J Athletic Training 30:293, 1995.

69. Misasi, S, et al: The effect of a toe cap and bias on perceived pain during cold water immersion. J Athletic Training 30:49, 1995.

70. Ingersoll, CD, et al: Cold induced pain: Habituation to cold immersions (abstract). J Athletic Training 25:126, 1990.

71. Myrer, JW, et al: Contrast therapy and intramuscular temperature in the human leg. J Athletic Training 29:318, 1994.

72. Perlau, R, et al: The effect of elastic bandages on human knee proprioception in the uninjured population. Am J Sports Med 23:251, 1995.

73. Wilkerson, GB: Treatment of the inversion ankle sprain through synchronous application of focal compression and cold. J Athletic Training 26:220, 1991.

74. Lekakis, J, et al: Cold-induced coronary Raynaud's phenomenon in patients with systemic sclerosis. Clin Exp Rheumatol 16:135, 1998.

75. Lehman, JF, et al: Therapeutic heat and cold. Clin Orthop 99:207, 1974.

76. Tomaszewski, D, et al: A comparison of skin interface temperature response between the ProHeaty instant reusable hot pack and the standard hydrocollator steam pack. J Athletic Training 27:355, 1992.

77. Greenberg, RS: The effects of hot packs and exercise on local blood flow. Phys Ther 52:273, 1972.

78. Lehmann, JF, et al: Temperature distributions in the human thigh, produced by infrared, hot pack and microwave applications. Arch Phys Med Rehabil 47:291, 1966.

79. Guyton, AC and Hall, JE: Textbook of Medical Physiology, ed 9. WB Saunders, Philadelphia, 1996, pp 918–919.

80. Draper DO, et al: Temperature change in human muscle

during and after pulsed short-wave diathermy. J Orthop Sports Phys Ther 29:13, 1999.

81. Perkins, SA and Massie, JE: Patient satisfaction after thermal shrinkage of the glenohumeral-joint capsule. J Sport Rehabil 10:157, 2001.

82. Cox, JS, et al: Heat modalities. In Drez, D (ed): Therapeutic Modalities for Sports Injuries. Year Book Medical Publishers, Chicago, 1989, pp 1–23.

83. Knight, KL and Londeree, BR: Comparison of blood flow in the ankle of uninjured subjects during application of heat, cold, and exercise. Med Sci Sports Exerc 12:76, 1980.

84. Abramson, DI, et al: Changes in blood flow, oxygen uptake and tissue temperatures produced by the topical application of wet heat. Arch Phys Med Rehabil 42:305, 1961.

85. Erasala, GN, et al: The effect of topical heat treatment on trapezius muscle blood flow using power Doppler ultrasound (abstract). Phys Ther 81:A5, 2001.

86. McCulloch, J and Boyd, VB: The effects of whirlpool and the dependent position on lower extremity volume. J Orthop Sport Phys Ther 16:169, 1992.

87. Curkovic, B, et al: The influence of heat and cold on the pain threshold in rheumatoid arthritis. Z Rheumatol 52:289, 1993.

88. Fischer, E and Solomon, S: Physiological response to heat and cold. In Licht, S (ed): Therapeutic Heat and Cold, ed 2. Waverly Press, Baltimore, 1965, p. 126.

89. Swenson, C, et al: Cryotherapy in sports medicine. Scand J Med Sci Sports 6:193, 1996.

90. Funk, D, et al: Efficacy of moist heat pack application over static stretching on hamstring flexibility. J Strength Cond Res 15:123, 2001.

91. Benoit, TG, et al: Hot and cold whirlpool treatments and knee joint laxity. J Athletic Training 31:242, 1996.

92. Taylor, BF, et al: The effects of therapeutic application of heat or cold followed by static stretch on hamstring muscle length. J Orthop Sports Phys Ther 21:283, 1995.

93. Wirth, VJ, et al: Temperature changes in deep muscles of humans during upper and lower extremity exercise. J Athletic Training 33:211, 1998.

94. Crumley, ML, et al: Do ultrasound, active warm-up, and passive motion differ on their ability to cause temperature and range of motion changes? J Athletic Training 36(S): S-92, 2001.

95. Merrick, MA. Personal communication.

96. Reed, BV: Wound healing and the use of thermal agents. In Michlovitz, SL (ed): Thermal Agents in Rehabilitation, ed 3. FA Davis, Philadelphia, 1990, pp 5–27.

97. Tsang, KW, et al: The effects of cryotherapy applied through various barriers. J Sports Rehabil 6:345, 1997.

98. Healy, WL, et al: Cold compressive dressing after total knee arthroplasty. Clin Orthop 299:143, 1994.

99. Schroder, D and Passler, HH: Combination of cold and compression after knee surgery. A prospective randomized study. Knee Surg Sports Traumatol Arthrosc 2:158, 1994.

100. Levy, AS and Marmar, E: The role of cold compression dressings in the postoperative treatment of total knee arthroplasty. Clin Orthop 297:174, 1993.

101. Scheffler, NM, et al: Use of Cryo/Cuff for the control of postoperative pain and edema. J Foot Ankle Surg 31:141, 1992.

102. Whitelaw, GP, et al: The use of the Cryo/Cuff versus ice and elastic wrap in the postoperative care of knee arthroscopy patients. Am J Knee Surg 8:28, 1995.

103. Serwa, J, et al: Effect of varying application pressures on skin surface and intramuscular temperatures during cryotherapy (abstract). J Athletic Training 36:S90, 2001.

104. Barr, E, et al: Effect of different types of cold applications on surface and intramuscular temperature (abstract). J Athletic Training 32:S33, 1997.

105. Rogers, JW, et al: Increased pressure of application during ice massage results in an increase in calf skin numbing. J Athletic Training 36:S90, 2001.

106. Nimchick, PSR and Knight, KL: Effects of wearing a toe cap or a sock on temperature and perceived pain during ice immersion. J Athletic Training 18:144, 1983.

107. Newton, RA: Effects of vapocoolants on passive hip flexion in healthy subjects. Phys Ther 65:1034, 1985.

108. Downer, AH: Physical Therapy Procedures: Selected Techniques, ed 3. Charles C Thomas, Springfield, IL, 1981.

109. Cohen, L, et al: Effects of whirlpool bath with and without agitation on the circulation in normal and diseased extremities. Arch Phys Med Rehabil 30:212, 1949.

110. Burke, DT, et al: Effects of hydrotherapy on pressure ulcer healing. Am J Phys Med Rehabil 77:394, 1998.

111. Press, E: The health hazards of saunas and spas and how to minimize them. Am J Public Health 81:1034, 1991.

112. Smith, K, et al: The effect of silicate gel hot packs on human muscle temperature (abstract). J Athletic Training 29:S33, 1994.

113. Griffin, JE and Karselis, TC: Physical Agents for Physical Therapists, ed 3. Charles C Thomas, Springfield, IL, 1988.

114. Borrell, RM, et al: Fluidotherapy: Evaluation of a new heat modality. Arch Phys Med Rehabil 58:69, 1977.

115. Borrell, RM, et al: Comparison of in vivo temperatures produced by hydrotherapy, paraffin wax treatment, and fluidotherapy. Phys Ther 60:1273, 1980.

116. Kuligowski, LA, et al: Effect of whirlpool therapy on the signs and symptoms of delayed-onset muscle soreness. J Athletic Training 33:222, 1998.

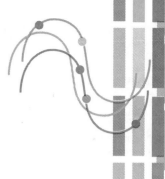

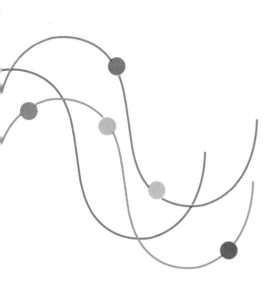

Deep-Heating Agents

This section describes therapeutic ultrasound, a modality that uses acoustical energy, and shortwave diathermy, an electrical modality that produces radio waves, which produce heat deep within the body's tissues. The physics, biophysical effects, and clinical application of each modality are described.

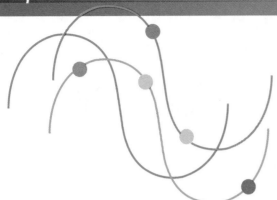

Chapter 7

Therapeutic Ultrasound

Ultrasound is presented in this section rather than in the thermal agents section for two reasons: (1) it is an acoustical modality rather than an electromagnetic or infrared modality and (2) it is a deep-heating agent. In addition, ultrasound is capable of producing mechanical, nonthermal effects in addition to its thermal effects. The reader should also refer to the basic physiological responses to heat described in Chapter 5.

Ultrasound is a deep-penetrating modality capable of producing changes in tissue through both thermal and nonthermal (mechanical) mechanisms. Unlike most other electrically driven modalities, ultrasound is not a part of the **electromagnetic spectrum** ■, but uses acoustical energy (Box 7–1). Depending on the frequency of the waves, ultrasound is used for diagnostic imaging, therapeutic deep tissue heating, or tissue destruction. This chapter focuses on the thermal and nonthermal effects of ultrasound.

Traditionally, therapeutic ultrasound has been used for musculoskeletal conditions primarily for its deep-heating effects. Depending on the output parameters, the effects of ultrasound application include increased rate of tissue repair

and wound healing, increased blood flow, increased tissue extensibility, breakdown of calcium deposits, reduction of pain and muscle spasm by altering nerve conduction velocity, and changes in cell membrane permeability (Table 7–1). Ultrasonic energy is also used to deliver medications to the subcutaneous tissues (phonophoresis) and a specialized form of ultrasound is used to promote fracture healing.

The human ear is capable of detecting sound waves ranging from 16,000 to 20,000 **hertz** ■ (Hz). Any sound wave above this range is considered ultrasound (Box 7–2). Therapeutic ultrasound ranges from 750,000 to 3,300,000 Hz (0.75 to 3.3 **megahertz** ■). In the United States, the most frequently used ultrasound frequencies are 1 and 3 MHz.

Electromagnetic spectrum: A continuum ordered by the wavelength or frequency of the energy produced.

Hertz (Hz): The number of cycles per second.

Megahertz (MHz): One million cycles per second.

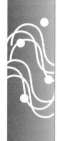

Box 7-1. The Acoustical Spectrum

Acoustical energy is transmitted differently than electromagnetic energy. Electromagnetic radiation involves the transmission of individual particles that prefer not to be hindered by a medium. The sun emits a particle of light that travels unhindered through the vast void of space. This particle stays in motion until it strikes a differing density, such as the earth or the earth's atmosphere.

Acoustical energy requires a dense medium to be transmitted through. In contrast to the emission of individual particles, acoustical energy is transmitted by mechanical waves (vibration) that deform the medium. Therefore, the transmission of acoustical energy is impossible in the vacuum of space. If you yell at a person across the street, your voice causes a deformation in the air. This wave travels through the air and is received by the other person's ear.

In a uniform environment, sound travels at a constant speed based on the frequency and wavelength: Velocity = Frequency × Wavelength. For sounds of different frequencies to travel at the same speed, their wavelengths must be different. Shorter wavelengths must have a higher frequency to match the velocity of longer wavelengths. This concept can be illustrated by picturing two people walking side by side. One of these people is 7 feet tall (the amplitude) and has a stride length of 3 feet. The other is 5 feet tall and has a stride length of 1.5 feet. For the two people to walk together, the taller person must take 30 steps to travel 90 feet; the shorter must take 60 steps.

Ultrasound, and its effects, is differentiated by the frequency and amplitude of the wave. Ultrasound used to produce images of the body's internal structures has a frequency of 2 to 15 MHz, but has a low amplitude. Therapeutic ultrasound has a frequency of 0.75 to 3.3 MHz and has a greater amplitude, meaning that more energy is delivered to the body per pulse.

TABLE 7-1 Ultrasound Output Parameters and Measures

Parameter	Description
Beam nonuniformity ratio (BNR)	The BNR describes the consistency (uniformity) of the ultrasound output as a ratio between the spatial peak intensity and the spatial average intensity. The lower the ratio, the more uniform the beam. A BNR greater than 8:1 is considered unsafe.
Duty cycle (DC)	The percentage of time that ultrasonic energy is being emitted from the sound head. A 100% duty cycle indicates a constant ultrasound output and produces primarily thermal effects within the body. A low duty cycle produces nonthermal effects.
Effective radiating area (ERA)	The area of the sound head that produces ultrasonic waves. Measured in square centimeters (cm²). The actual ERA is usually significantly smaller than the contact area of the sound head. Frequently the frequency determines the effective depth of penetration. A 1-MHz output targets tissues up to 5 cm deep; 3 MHz has a penetrating depth of at least 2 cm.
Intensity	The intensity describes the amount of power generated by unit.
Half layer (depth) value	Tissue depth where half of the initial output intensity has been lost.
Spatial average intensity (SAI)	Measured in watts per square centimeter, the SAI describes the amount of power per unit area of the sound head's ERA.
Spatial peak intensity (SPI)	The maximum output across the ERA.
Spatial average temporal peak (SATP)	The SAI during the "On" time of a pulse and is displayed as intensity on the ultrasound output meter. Meaningful only with pulsed output.
Spatial average temporal average (SATA)	Describes the SATP as calculated across the duty cycle: 1.0 W/cm² * 50% DC = 0.5 W/cm² SATA. The SATA is meaningful only when delivering pulsed ultrasound.
Treatment duration	The treatment duration is determined by the output intensity and the specific goals of the treatment.

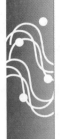

Box 7–2. **Contrast and Comparison of Ultrasound and Audible Sound**

The way in which piezoelectric crystals produce ultrasound bears some striking similarities to the way in which a CD player produces audible sound. When a CD plays music, it detects the patterns of recorded sound impulses. These patterns are converted to electrical energy that is transferred to a speaker. Once the electrical impulses reach the speaker, it activates a magnet, causing a cone to expand and contract. The vibration of the cone produces mechanical waves that are transmitted through the air and subsequently strike our eardrums.

Ultrasound generators operate on basically the same principle. An alternating current is passed through a crystal, causing it to expand and contract. The vibration of this crystal produces mechanical waves that are passed along to the body.

The difference between the production of these two sound waves lies in the frequency at which the "speaker" vibrates. Stereos use a much lower acoustical frequency than ultrasound, so the waves can be transmitted through air and detected by the human ear. Ultrasound units use such a high frequency that the waves cannot be transmitted without the use of a dense medium and cannot be detected by the human ear.

■ Production of Ultrasound

Ultrasound is produced by an **alternating current** ■ flowing through a piezoelectric crystal housed in a **transducer** ■ (Fig. 7–1). Quartz crystals were once used to produce ultrasound, but synthetic crystals such as zirconate titanate have replaced natural crystals, yielding a more consistent field of energy. Experimental work has begun on the development of a laser-driven ultrasound generator, potentially providing a more precise and more flexible ultrasonic output.[1]

Piezoelectric crystals produce positive and negative electrical charges when they contract or expand (Fig. 7–2). A reverse (indirect) piezoelectric effect occurs when an alternating current is passed through a piezoelectric crystal, resulting in contraction and expansion of the crystal. This mechanism, referred to as the **electropiezo effect**, is

used to produce therapeutic ultrasound. The vibration of the crystals results in the mechanical production of high-frequency sound waves.

■ Transmission of Ultrasound Waves

Ultrasound has a sinusoidal waveform and displays the properties of wavelength, frequency, **amplitude** ■, and velocity (see Box 7–1). Acoustical energy is transferred by one molecule jostling against its neighbor and exchanging kinetic energy without actually displacing the molecules. Consider a leaf floating in a pond. If a pebble is dropped near it, the leaf bobs up and down as the ripples pass beneath it but does not change its position.

Because of the high frequencies involved, ultrasound is unable to pass through the air and requires a dense transmission medium. A coupling medium must be used for the ultrasonic energy to pass from the transducer to the tissues. Coupling media are discussed in Chapter 8.

Longitudinal Waves

Particle displacement in longitudinal waves occurs parallel to the direction of the sound. A person dangling from the end of a bungee cord is an example of longitudinal waves. Longitudinal waves result in the elongation and contraction of the cord, causing the jumper to bob up and down. In this case, the energy, as represented by the jumper, is transmitted parallel to the direction of the wave.

The alternation of high and low pressure exerted by the ultrasound beam results in regions of high particle

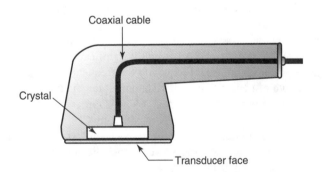

Figure 7–1. Cross-section of an Ultrasound Transducer. Note that the surface area of the crystal (the effective radiating area) is smaller than the face of the transducer.

Alternating current: The uninterrupted flow of electrons marked by a change in the direction and magnitude of the movement.

Amplitude: The maximum departure of a wave from the baseline.

Transducer: A device that converts one form of energy to another.

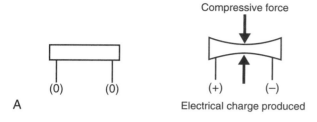

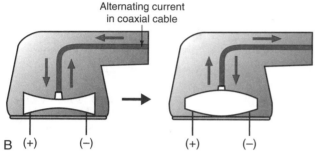

Figure 7–2. **Piezoelectric Crystals.** (A) The direct piezoelectric effect. Crystals possessing piezoelectric properties produce positive and negative electrical charges when they are compressed or expanded. (B) The reverse piezoelectric effect or electropiezo effect. These same crystals expand and contract when an electrical current is passed through them.

density (compression) and low particle density (rarefaction) along the path of the wave (Fig. 7–3). These pressure fluctuations transmit the energy within the tissues and, as discussed in subsequent sections, produce physiological effects. Longitudinal waves are capable of traveling through both solid and liquid media. Ultrasound passes through soft tissue as a longitudinal wave.

Transverse (Shear) Waves

Particles in transverse waves are displaced perpendicular to the direction of the sound wave. Plucking a guitar string, making it vibrate parallel to its length, is an example of a transverse wave. When the longitudinal waves of the ultrasonic beam strike bone, they become transverse waves. Transverse waves cannot pass through fluids and are found in the body only when ultrasound strikes bone.

■ ULTRASONIC ENERGY

Low-frequency sound waves, such as those produced by human speech, diverge in all directions, making it possible to hear a person talking behind you. The greater the frequency of the sound wave, the less the sound beam diverges.[2] The frequencies used in therapeutic ultrasound produce relatively cylindrical beams that have a width somewhat smaller than the diameter of the sound head. Like all sound waves, ultrasound waves are capable of reflection, refraction, penetration, and absorption (Box 7–3).

There is some degree of divergence (spreading) as the ultrasound waves travel through a medium, but it is not as pronounced as sound waves within the range of human

Resonating: Vibrating.

hearing. Consider the difference between a beam of light produced by a spotlight and the light produced by an ordinary light bulb. If the spotlight and lamp were held 1 foot from a wall, the spotlight would concentrate the light within an area approximately the same diameter as the lens. The light produced from the bare bulb would illuminate an area significantly larger than the bulb itself. As the distance between the lights and the wall is increased, the beams' diameters will increase, but much more so with the bare bulb than with the spotlight. Likewise, the treatment area effectively exposed to the ultrasonic energy is limited to the diameter of the sound head.

Close to the transducer head, the pressure of the sound field is nonuniform, forming peaks of high intensity and valleys of low intensity (Fig. 7–4). This area, the **near field** or **Fresnel zone**, is the portion of the ultrasound beam used for therapeutic purposes. The pressure variations occur because the transducer head acts as if it were made up of many smaller heads, each producing its own sound wave. Close to the transducer, these areas are individually distinguishable. As the distance from the head is increased, the waves begin to interact to produce a more unified beam. An example of this can be found in a television set. If you look very closely at the screen, individual colored elements are seen. As the distance between your eye and the screen is increased, the dots lose their individuality, and a complete picture is formed.

Effective Radiating Area

Ultrasound heads are available in different sizes and with different crystal **resonating** ■ frequencies (Fig. 7–5). The effective radiating area (ERA) of the ultrasound head

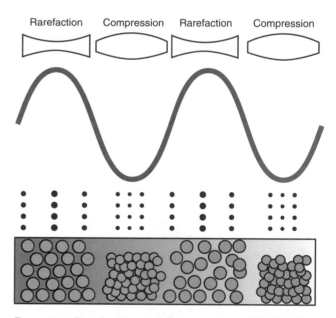

Figure 7–3. **Rarefaction and Compression of Molecules.** An ultrasound wave passing through the tissues creates alternating periods of low and high pressure. Molecules in the low-pressure areas expand (rarefaction), and molecules in the high-pressure area compress.

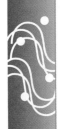

Box 7–3. Influences on the Transmission of Energy

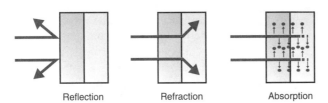

Reflection   Refraction   Absorption

Most energy prefers to travel in a straight line. However, when traveling through a medium, its course is influenced by changes in density. Energy striking the interface between two different densities may be reflected, refracted, or absorbed by the material, or continue through—penetrate— the material unaffected by the change.

Reflection occurs when the wave cannot pass through the next density. The wave strikes the object (tissues) and reverses its direction away from the material. Reflection may be complete, as when all energy is precluded from entering the next density layer, or it may be partial. An echo is an example of reflection that involves acoustical energy.

Refraction is the bending of waves as a result of a change in the speed of a wave as it enters a medium of different density. When the energy leaves a dense layer and enters a less dense layer, its speed increases. When moving from a low-density to a high-density layer, the energy decreases. A prism refracts light rays. As the light is bent within the prism each of the seven color bands becomes visible.

Absorption occurs by the tissue collecting the wave's energy and changing it into kinetic energy within the cell and then possibly into heat. The tissues may absorb part or all of the energy being delivered to the tissue. Any energy not reflected or absorbed by one tissue layer continues to pass through the tissue until it strikes another density layer. At this point, it may again be reflected, refracted, absorbed, or passed on to the next tissue layer. Each time the wave is partially reflected, refracted, or absorbed, the remaining energy available to deeper tissue is reduced.

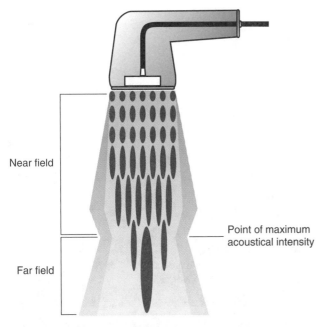

Near field

Point of maximum
acoustical intensity

Far field

Figure 7–4. **A Schematic Representation of an Ultrasound Beam.** Note the irregular intensity of the near field and the spatial peak intensity.

represents the portion of the transducer's surface area that actually produces ultrasound waves and is described in terms of square centimeters (cm^2). Measured 5 mm from the face of the sound head, the ERA represents all areas producing more than 5 percent of the maximum power output of the transducer. Based on this calculation, the ERA is always of lesser area than the actual size of the transducer's face (see Fig. 7–1).[3] Most energy is concentrated at the center of the head, with less energy being emitted away from this point and no energy is produced in the outermost part of the sound head. Large ERAs produce a beam that is more **collimated** ■. Smaller ERAs yield a more divergent beam.

Frequency

The output frequency of an ultrasound generator is measured in megahertz and describes the number of waves occurring in 1 second. Most commercial therapeutic ultrasound units offer 1-, 2-, and/or 3-MHz outputs, although "longwave" ultrasound is now being produced (Box 7–4). Low-frequency (1-MHz) ultrasound has a beam that diverges more than high-frequency (3-MHz) ultrasound.

Collimated: Possessing a beam of parallel rays or waves that form a column of energy.

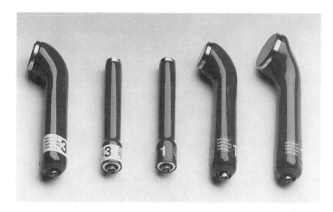

Figure 7–5. **Variety of Ultrasound Heads.** Ultrasonic transducers are available in a range of sizes and frequencies. Note the labels indicating the effective radiating area (ERA), beam nonuniformity ratio (BNR), and frequency (1 or 3 MHz). (Courtesy of Mettler Electronics Corporation, Inc., Anaheim, CA.)

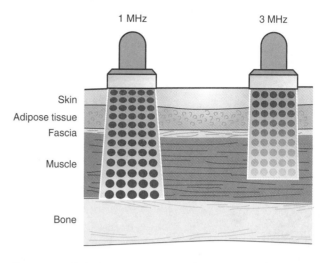

Figure 7–6. **Relative Depth of Penetration of 1-MHz and 3-MHz Ultrasound.** The effects of 1-MHz ultrasound occur more deeply within the tissues than 3-MHz ultrasound, which attenuates in the superficial tissues. Note that the 1-MHz beam diverges more than the 3-MHz beam. The actual depth of penetration is based on the half-layer value of the ultrasonic energy.

The depth of penetration is inversely related to the output frequency.[5] The rate of absorption, and therefore **attenuation** ■, increases as the frequency of the ultrasound is increased because of the molecular friction that the sound waves must overcome in order to pass through the tissues.[6] Because of this, less energy is available to pass deeper into the tissues.[2] Traditionally, 3-MHz ultrasound is thought to affect tissues 2 cm deep, but it may have an affect on tissues 2.5 to 3 cm deep.[7, 8]

High-frequency (3-MHz) ultrasound generators provide treatment to superficial tissues because the energy is rapidly absorbed and heats 3 times faster than 1-MHz ultrasound (Fig. 7–6). The 1-MHz output offers a compromise between deep penetration, adequate heating, and preventing **unstable cavitation** ■ from occurring.[2] Because of the depth of heating, the heat produced by 1-MHz ultrasound is longer lasting than heat produced by 3-MHz ultrasound.[9]

Changing the output frequency sometimes requires that the sound head be changed, but most contemporary units have transducers that are capable of delivering output of varying frequencies through the same crystal. Each crystal is calibrated to its generator.

Power and Intensity

The power produced by an ultrasound generator is measured in watts (W) and represents the amount of energy being produced by the transducer. Intensity describes the strength of the sound waves at a given location within the tissues being treated. There are several methods for describing the output and intensity (see Table 7–1).

Spatial Average Intensity

Spatial average intensity (SAI) describes the amount of energy passing through a unit of area, in this case, the sound head's effective radiating area. Expressed in watts per square centimeter (W/cm^2), the SAI is a measure of the power per unit area of the sound head. This value is calculated by dividing the power of the output (watts) by the ERA of the transducer head (square centimeters):

$$SAI = \frac{\text{Total Watts (W)}}{\text{Effective Radiating Area (cm}^2\text{)}} = \text{W/cm}^2$$

For example, if 10 W were being delivered through a transducer head with an ERA of 5 cm^2, the SAI would be 2 W/cm^2.

Ultrasound units can display their output as either total watts or watts per square centimeter. Standard treatment doses range from 0.3 to 5 watts. If the radiating area of the sound head is smaller than specified, or if a portion of the sound head is obstructed from transmitting sound (such as not being in full contact with the skin), a higher SAI is produced than that indicated on the meter.

As seen with electrical current density, altering the size of the sound head affects the power density. Passing 10 W of energy through a transducer of 10 cm^2 results in a lower density than if a head of 5 cm^2 is used (Table 7–2). Therapeutic ultrasound generators are limited to a maximum output of 3.0 W/cm^2.

Attenuation: The decrease in a wave's intensity resulting from the absorption, reflection, and refraction of energy.

Unstable cavitation: The violent oscillation and subsequent rupture of bubbles during ultrasound application at too high an intensity.

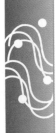

Box 7–4. Longwave Ultrasound

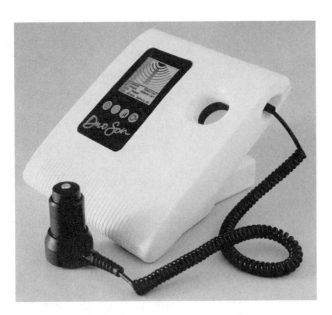

Therapeutic ultrasound traditionally has been used with an output frequency that ranges between 1.0 and 3.3 MHz. Longwave ultrasound employs a wavelength ranging between 20 and 45 **kilohertz** ■ (kHz) and is used for both deep heating and for phonophoresis application. The longer wavelength is capable of effectively penetrating the body's tissues and can produce bone-depth heating in even the largest muscle mass.

The longer wavelength results in greater particle displacement within the tissues and produces a more uniform beam. The increased overall power and homogeneity of the ultrasonic wave requires lower output intensities to reach therapeutic levels than traditional ultrasound units. Heating can be obtained with an output intensity of 0.3 to 0.8 W/cm² and nonthermal effects occur at levels below 0.3 W/cm². Application above 0.8 W/cm² can result in tissue damage.[4]

Unlike shortwave ultrasound, longwave generators do not require the use of a transmission medium. However, a lubricant is used to assist in moving the sound head over the skin. The indications and contraindications for the use of longwave ultrasound are similar to those of traditional ultrasound.

Duoson, courtesy of Orthosonics, Devon, England.

Spatial Average Temporal Peak Intensity

Spatial average temporal peak (SATP) intensity describes the average intensity during the "on" time of the pulse. The output meter on an ultrasound unit displays the SATP intensity.

Spatial Average Temporal Average Intensity

Spatial average temporal average (SATA) intensity measures the power of ultrasonic energy delivered to the tissues over a given period and is meaningful only for the application of pulsed ultrasound. The energy delivered to the tissues per unit time with ultrasound operating at a 50-percent duty cycle is half of that delivered in a continuous mode. If we take a SAI of 2 W/cm² and pulse it with a 50-percent duty cycle, the temporal average density of

the treatment would be 1 W/cm² (2 W/cm² × 0.5 = 1 W/cm²). It is important to distinguish between the SATP intensity, the average amount of power delivered during a single cycle, and the temporal peak intensity, the maximum amount of energy delivered by a single pulse (Fig. 7–7).

Half-Layer Value

The **half-layer** value indicates the depth at which 50 percent of the ultrasonic energy has been absorbed by the tissues. If ultrasound is applied at 1 W/cm² and loses 50 percent of its energy at a depth of 2.3 cm, the beam intensity is now 0.5 W/cm². At twice this depth (4.6 cm), the ultrasound intensity is reduced to 0.25 W/cm².[10] The effect of the half-layer value and the penetrating effects of 1- and

---

Kilohertz (kHz): One thousand cycles per second.

TABLE 7–2 Relationship of Ultrasound Radiating Area and the Total Amount of Energy Produced

Intensity (W/cm^2)	Effective Radiating Area (ERA) of the Sound Head (cm^2)	Total Power Produced (W)
1.5	5	7.5
1.5	6	9.0
1.5	10	15.0

3-MHz (which has a half-layer depth of 0.8 cm) output frequencies are used to target the tissues during treatment (e.g., use 1-MHz ultrasound for deep structures).

Duty Cycle

As we learned in the first few paragraphs of this chapter, therapeutic ultrasound is capable of producing thermal or nonthermal physiological changes within the body, depending on the duty cycle. A continuous (100-percent duty cycle) output causes primarily thermal effects. A pulsed (e.g., 25-percent duty cycle) output produces primarily nonthermal effects.[11] The decision to use thermal or nonthermal ultrasound depends on the stage of healing and the treatment goals. Nonthermal ultrasound can be used during acute inflammation and thermal ultrasound is used later in the healing process (see the Biophysical Effects of Ultrasound Application section on p 165).

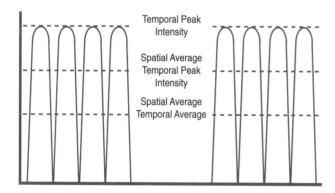

Figure 7–7. **Measures of Pulsed Ultrasound Output.** The temporal peak intensity represents the amplitude of a single wave. The spatial average temporal peak intensity is the average amount of energy delivered by a single pulse. The spatial average temporal average intensity is the average amount of energy delivered to the tissues during the application of pulsed ultrasound.

Continuous Output

Continuous ultrasound application can effectively heat tissues located 5 (or more) cm deep, depending on the frequency used. Because the output is being delivered 100 percent of the time, the ultrasonic energy is measured in terms of the SATP intensity. The spatial peak intensity, as determined using the beam nonuniformity ratio (BNR), should not be allowed to exceed 8 W per square centimeter (metered output × BNR).

Pulsed Output

Pulsing the ultrasound beam decreases the temporal average intensity of the output, reducing the thermal effects while still allowing for the nonthermal effects of ultrasound. The duty cycle describes the percentage of time that ultrasound is actually being emitted from the sound head (Fig. 7–8). The ratio between the **pulse length** ■ and the **pulse interval** ■ is expressed as a percentage duty cycle:

$$\text{Duty cycle} = \frac{\text{Pulse length}}{(\text{Pulse length} + \text{Pulse interval}) \times 100}$$

Pulsing the output reduces the temperature rise proportionally to the duty cycle, but it does not entirely eliminate tissue heating.[5] The closer the duty cycle is to 100 percent, the greater the net thermal effects of the treatment; lower duty cycles produce greater proportions of nonthermal effects, although a proportion of thermal and nonthermal effects occur at all duty cycles. The output of pulsed ultrasound is measured by the SATA intensity, but the actual amount of energy delivered to the tissue is dependent on the duty cycle.

Ultrasound Beam Nonuniformity

The degree to which the intensity within the ultrasound beam varies is measured by the BNR. This is the ratio of the highest intensity within the beam, the spatial peak intensity (Fig. 7–9), to the average intensity reported on the output meter:

$$\text{BNR} = \text{spatial peak intensity/SAI}$$

A perfectly uniform ultrasound beam, one that has no "peaks and valleys" would have a BNR of 1:1, but the mass manufacturing process makes this impractical. A BNR greater than 8:1 is unacceptable because the energy delivered to the body would be harmful. The Food and Drug Administration (FDA) Center for Devices and Radiological Health requires that the BNR must be indicated on the ultrasound unit.[12, 13] Companies do not have to report the BNR of individual crystals, so the BNR of the sound head being used may be different from that indi-

---

Pulse interval: The amount of time between ultrasonic pulses.

Pulse length: The amount of time from the initial nonzero charge to the return to a zero charge, forming one complete cycle.

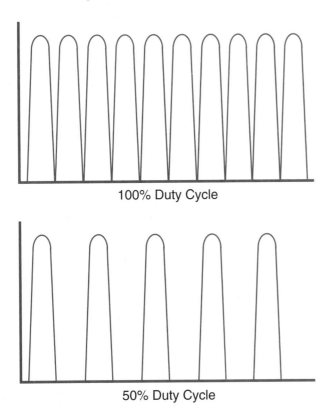

100% Duty Cycle

50% Duty Cycle

Figure 7–8. **Ultrasound Duty Cycle.** The amount of time that the ultrasonic energy is being produced. The top figure shows a 100% duty cycle. The bottom figure shows the ultrasound that would be emitted during the same time period if a 50% duty cycle were selected.

cated on the label. The FDA allows companies to randomly sample their transducers and report the maximum BNR found. The BNR is then labeled as "BNR <5:1" or "6:1 Max."

If the BNR is indicated as 3:1 and the meter displays an output of 2 W/cm², then at some point in the beam the actual intensity is equivalent to 6 W/cm² (3 x 2 W = 6 W). The existence of high-intensity areas in the beam, "hot spots," is the primary reason for keeping the sound head moving during the treatment.

■ Transfer of Ultrasound Through the Tissues

Air is not dense enough to transmit ultrasonic energy. A coupling agent must be used to allow the energy to pass out of the transducer into the tissues (see Chapter 8). Longitudinal waves of ultrasound pass through soft tissue until it strikes bone, where some of the energy is reflected and the rest is converted into transverse waves. The propa-

gation of ultrasonic energy depends on the frequency of the sound waves and the density of the tissues. Passage of ultrasound through the body and the subsequent penetration of cell membranes cause the tissues to acquire kinetic energy, resulting in cellular vibration.

When the ultrasound beam strikes an **acoustical interface** ■ (such as different tissue layers), some of the energy is reflected or refracted. The amount of reflection depends on the degree of change in density at the junction between the two tissues (Table 7–3). Ultrasound meeting with air reflects the energy, preventing it from being transferred. The interface between soft tissue and bone is also highly reflective. Other highly reflective interfaces include the musculotendinous junction and intermuscular interfaces. Unlike infrared energy, ultrasound is not greatly affected by adipose tissue and easily passes through it.[14]

If a reflected wave meets the incoming incident wave, a **standing wave** ■ is created, increasing the intensity of the energy by creating areas of high and low pressure. Free-floating gas bubbles move toward the low-pressure areas. Free-moving cells collect at the high-pressure centers.[15] Because of this condition, a high level of energy is formed in a limited amount of space, increasing the risk of tissue damage. Standing waves can be avoided by keeping the sound head moving.

Reflecting intense ultrasonic energy off bone can pro-

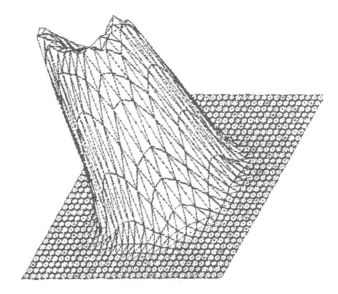

Figure 7–9. **Ultrasound Beam Profile.** This topographical map of an ultrasound beam was plotted from the intensities produced from various points on the transducer. The peak on the left side represents the beam's peak intensity. (Courtesy of IAPT. Used with permission.)

Acoustical interface: A surface where two materials of different densities meet.

Standing wave: A single-frequency wave formed by the collision of two waves of equal frequency and speed traveling in opposite directions. The energy with a standing wave cannot be transmitted from one area to another and is focused in a confined area

TABLE 7–3	Percent Reflection of Ultrasonic Energy at Various Interfaces
Interface	*Energy Reflected (%)*
Water–Soft tissue	0.2
Soft tissue–Fat	1
Soft tissue–Bone	15–40
Soft tissue–Air	99.9

duce **periosteal pain** ■, an unwanted effect. Caution is needed when applying ultrasound over bony protuberances, such as the patella or acromion process. The intensity used to treat the muscle or tendon can produce periosteal pain if applied over relatively subcutaneous bone.

Any energy not reflected or absorbed is passed on to the underlying tissues (see Law of Grotthus-Draper, Appendix B). The intensity of ultrasonic energy decreases as the distance it travels through the tissues increases. This process, called attenuation, occurs through the scattering and absorption of the waves within the tissues.

Absorption of the sound waves transfers energy from the beam into the surrounding tissues through conversion of mechanical energy into thermal energy. The amount of absorption that occurs depends on the protein content of the tissues (especially collagen). Tissues such as bone, cartilage, and tendon absorb much more ultrasonic energy than muscle, fat, or blood.[2] Ultrasound tends to reflect as it strikes bone and refract as it passes through joint spaces.[14]

■ Biophysical Effects of Ultrasound Application

The physiological changes within the tissues associated with ultrasound application can be grouped into two classifications, although they do not occur exclusively from one another[16]:

- Nonthermal effects: changes within the tissues resulting from the mechanical effect of ultrasonic energy
- Thermal effects: changes within the tissues as a direct result of ultrasound's elevation of the tissue temperature

Nonthermal treatment is accompanied by some degree of heating, and thermal treatments is accompanied by nonthermal effects (Table 7–4).

These effects are limited to the treatment area, which should be no more than two to three times the ERA of the sound head, but the smaller the area treated, the greater the

temperature increase.[17] The proportion and magnitude of each are based on the duty cycle and the output intensity. The higher the duty cycle, the greater are the thermal effects; the higher the output intensity, the greater is the magnitude of the effects.

Nonthermal Effects

Ultrasound is applied in a nonthermal mode when acute injuries are being treated or in other cases when increasing the tissue temperature is undesirable. Nonthermal ultrasound is administered by either (1) using a pulsed output (20- to 25-percent duty cycle) and normal treatment intensities or (2) using a continuous (100-percent duty cycle) and a low-output intensity (below 0.3 W/cm^2). The individual pulses of ultrasonic waves cause acoustical streaming and cavitation, two interrelated events that are thought to cause the nonthermal effects during ultrasound treatment.

The amount of cavitation is in direct proportion to the intensity of the sound wave. Low-intensity output with a continuous output leads to more stable, prolonged cavitation than pulsed ultrasound applied at higher intensities. Low-intensity treatments are becoming the method of choice for delivering nonthermal ultrasound.

Acoustical streaming (microstreaming) is the one-directional motion of fluid caused by the sound wave. When the acoustical stream strikes cell membranes, **eddies** ■ of fluid flow around the cell membranes and its **organelles** ■. Free-floating ions and small molecules can be displaced by the acoustical stream.[17] The flow of bubbles in the acoustical streams causes changes in cell membrane permeability that alters the diffusion rate across the cell membrane. This energy can also result in the displacement of ions and small molecules.[17]

Cavitation occurs as a result of the pressure changes created by the ultrasonic wave. The individual sound waves cause gas bubbles to oscillate in a cyclical manner. **Stable cavitation** occurs when the bubbles compress during the high-pressure peaks as ultrasonic energy followed by expansion of the bubbles during the low-pressure troughs (see Fig. 7–3).

Unstable cavitation (transient cavitation) involves the compression of the bubbles during the high-pressure peak, but is followed by a total collapse ("bursting of the bubble") during the trough.[17] Transient cavitation is an unwanted, deleterious effect of ultrasound being applied at too great an intensity and can damage immobile tissue, free-floating blood cells, or other biological structures in the area.[5] When they are in proper working order, therapeutic ultrasound units do not have the output power or frequency required to produce transient cavitation.

Eddy (eddies): A circular current of fluid, often moving against the main flow.

Organelle: A specialized portion of a cell that performs a specific function, such as the mitochondria and the Golgi apparatus.

Periosteal pain: A deep-seated ache resulting from overly intense application of ultrasonic energy that irritates the bone's periosteum.

TABLE 7–4	Local Physiological Effects of Ultrasound Application

Nonthermal Effects	*Thermal Effects*
Increased cell membrane permeability	Increased sensory nerve conduction velocity
Altered rates of diffusion across the cell membrane	Increased motor nerve conduction velocity
Increased vascular permeability	Increased extensibility of collagen-rich structures
Secretion of **cytokines** ■	Increased collagen deposition
Increased blood flow	Increased blood flow
Increased fibroblastic activity	Reduction of muscle spasm
Stimulation of phagocytosis	Increased macrophage activity
Production of healthy granulation tissue	Enhanced adhesion of leukocytes to damaged
Synthesis of protein	endothelial cells
Synthesis of collagen	
Reduction of edema	
Diffusion of ions	
Tissue regeneration	
Formation of stronger, more deformable connective tissue	

A current theory to explain the nonthermal effects of ultrasound is based on the **frequency resonance** of the cellular and molecular structures. The mechanical energy of the ultrasound wave is absorbed by proteins, which alters the structure and function of individual proteins or molecules.[17]

Pulsed ultrasound, often delivered with a 20- or 25-percent duty cycle and an output intensity of 0.5 W/cm², or continuous output at an intensity of less than 0.3 W/cm² may trigger a series of physiological events that stimulate the healing process.[17] Application in this mode stimulates phagocytosis (assisting in the removal of inflammatory debris),[18] increases the quantity of **free radicals** ■ in the area (increasing ionic conductance and acting on the cell membrane),[19] alters cell membrane permeability and cellular proliferation,[17] and accelerates **fibrinolysis** ■.[17, 20, 21]

Increased permeability allows calcium to enter the cell, which, in turn, encourages the release of protein. Potassium and other ions and metabolites also move into and out of the cell. Glycosaminoglycan, the primary component needed for the proper remodeling of collagen, and hydroxyproline, one of the essential amino acids of collagen, are increased following low-dose pulsed ultrasound.[17, 22] These events lead to the healing connective tissue being stronger and more deformable, and thus able to withstand greater loads.

Collagen synthesis, secretion of cytokines, increased uptake of calcium in fibroblasts, increased fibroblastic activity (essential for the production of functional, healthy granulation tissue and scar tissue), mast cell degranulation, and increased macrophage activity are also promoted (see Table 7–4).[15] This mild acceleration of the inflammatory stage helps the body reach the proliferation stage sooner.

Thermal Effects

The amount of temperature increase during an ultrasound treatment depends on the mode of application (100% duty cycle), the intensity and frequency of the output, the vascularity and type of tissues, the size of the treatment area, and the speed with which the sound head is moved over the tissues. The amount of temperature increase may also be generator dependent, with some brands potentially producing more heating than other brands.[23] A treatment area 2 times the ERA can raise the subcutaneous tissues 6.3°F (3.5°C) using 1-MHz ultrasound and 14.9°F (8.3°C) using 3-MHz ultrasound.[24] Using the same output parameters, but increasing the treatment area to 6 times the ERA (much larger than the recommended treatment area) results in only a 2.3°F (1.3°C) temperature increase.[9]

The thermal effects of ultrasound are the same as those described in Chapter 5. The primary differences are ultrasound heats deeper tissues and affects a smaller area. The physiological changes within the tissues are based on the amount of temperature increase and are the greatest when ultrasound is applied in the continuous mode (Table 7–5). Ultrasound applied with a 1-MHz output frequency can affect tissues located up to 5 cm deep; 3-MHz ultrasound is effective on tissues located up to 2 to 3 cm deep. Tissues heated with 1-MHz ultrasound retains heat approx-

---

Cytokine: A protein produced by white blood cells.

Fibrinolysis: Pathological breaking up of fibrin.

Free radical: A highly reactive molecule having an odd number of electrons. Free radical production plays an important role in the progression of an ischemic injury.

imately twice as long as heat generated by 3-MHz ultrasound.[9] Preheating the treatment area for 15 minutes using a moist heat pack will decrease the treatment time required to reach vigorous heating levels by 2 to 3 minutes in deep (3-cm) tissues using a 1-MHz output.[25]

To achieve a therapeutic effect through ultrasound heating, the tissue temperatures must be elevated for a minimum of 3 to 5 minutes.[15, 26] Three-MHz ultrasound heats 3 to 4 times faster than 1-MHz ultrasound, although the thermal effects of 1-MHz ultrasound last longer (see Table 9–1).[10, 27] The relationship between the output intensity and treatment duration cannot be understated. Lower treatment output intensities require a longer duration to elevate the tissue temperature to the desired level.

Heat production is related to the amount of attenuation of the sound waves in the tissues.[28] The process involved in attenuation, absorption, and scattering creates friction between the molecules and results in a temperature increase. Collagen-rich tissues—such as tendon, joint menisci, superficial bone, large nerve roots, intermuscular fascia, and scar tissue—are preferentially heated.[15] Tissues that are largely fluid filled, such as the fat layer and articular fluid, are relatively transparent to ultrasonic energy.[14] Because of their size and relative fluid content, muscle bellies are not well heated by ultrasound, but scar tissue within the belly is.

Temperatures in poorly vascularized tissues increase by 1.4°F to 2.5°F (0.8°C to 1.4°C) per minute during the application of continuous ultrasound with a frequency of 3 MHz.[5, 10] In highly vascularized areas like muscle, the temperature increase is not as great because incoming, cooler blood continually washes out the local warmer blood. Temperature increases of up to 8.8°F (4.9°C) have been documented 2.5 cm deep within the muscle after the application of ultrasound at 1.5 W/cm^2 for 10 minutes.[14]

Reflected waves also increase the amount of heating. When ultrasound waves are reflected, the energy passes through the tissues more than once, increasing the thermal effects. Standing waves greatly exaggerate the rise in temperature.

The Injury Response Process

The effects of ultrasound application depend on the mode of application (continuous or pulsed), the frequency of the sound, the size of the area treated, and the tissues being treated (vascularity and density). The deep thermal effects are similar to those described in the thermotherapy section. The nonthermal effects are discussed, where relevant, in each of the following sections. A specialized form of ultrasound is used to promote fracture healing.

The effects of therapeutic ultrasound are not universally accepted and a great deal of discrepancy is found in the research. Refer to the Controversies in Treatment section at the end of this chapter.

Cellular Response

Microstreaming increases cell membrane permeability, and changes the diffusion rate across the cell membrane. Thermal effects increase cell metabolism and accelerate the rate of inflammation. Nonthermal cellular responses to ultrasound include increased histamine release, increased intracellular calcium, mast cell degranulation, and increased rate of protein synthesis.[4, 17, 41]

Inflammation

In the acute stage of injury, the use of continuous ultrasound output is contraindicated because of the increased tissue temperature and the associated increased need for oxygen. For this reason, ultrasound application during the acute and subacute inflammatory stages should be delivered with a low duty cycle and at a low intensity.

The acceleration of the inflammatory process results in an earlier onset of the proliferation stage.[42] Changes in cell membrane permeability result in degranulation and the release of growth factors and platelets that stimulate fibroblast proliferation.[4] The application of continuous ultrasound has been shown to positively influence macrophage activity [41] and to increase the adhesion of leukocytes to the damaged endothelial cells.[43] When applied during the proliferation phase, ultrasound stimulates cell division.[44]

One-MHz, continuous output ultrasound enhances the release of preformed fibroblasts. Three-MHz ultrasound increases the cells' ability to synthesize and secrete

TABLE 7–5	Temperature Increases Required to Achieve Specific Therapeutic Effects During Ultrasound Application	
Classification of Ultrasound	Temperature Increase	Used for Thermal Effects
Mild	1°C	Mild inflammation Accelerating metabolic rate
Moderate	2°–3°C	Decreasing muscle spasm Decreasing pain Increasing blood flow Reducing chronic inflammation
Vigorous*	3°–4°C	Tissue elongation, scar tissue reduction Inhibition of sympathetic activity

*Tissue temperatures must be increased to 39° to 45°C for vigorous heating to occur. See the comments for Table 5–10.

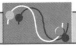

CLINICAL TECHNIQUES: ULTRASONIC BONE GROWTH GENERATORS

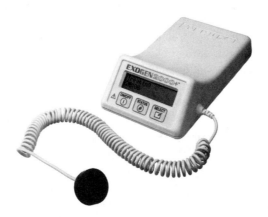

Application over unhealed fracture sites is an absolute contraindication for therapeutic ultrasound. How then can ultrasonic treatment be a promising treatment for accelerating the rate of fracture healing?

The type of ultrasound used for treating fracture sites is different from therapeutic ultrasound. Low-intensity pulsed ultrasound (LIPUS) uses output characteristics that are not available on standard therapeutic ultrasound units to produce low-level mechanical force that stimulates or accelerates bone growth.

Output Characteristics of Ultrasonic Bone Growth Generators

Parameter	Value
Output frequency	1.5 MHz
Burst width	200 microseconds
Repetition rate	1 kilohertz
Effective radiating area	3.88 cm²
Temporal average power	117 milliwatts
Temporal maximum power	625 milliwatts
Spatial average-temporal intensity	30 mW/cm²
Beam nonuniformity ratio	2.16:1

Low-intensity pulsed ultrasound applied in one 20-minute session per day has demonstrated an improved healing rate for acute and nonunion fractures,[29-34] stress fractures,[35] and spinal fusion.[36] This technique is not approved for **nonunion fractures** of the skull or with individuals who are skeletally immature.

Each phase of the bone healing process, inflammation, angiogenesis, chondrogenesis, intramembranous ossification, endochondral ossification, and bone remodeling, appears to be positively affected by LIPUS.[31] The production of the angiogenic factors **interleukin-8**, **basic fibroblast growth factor**, **vascular endothelial growth factor**,[37] bone-forming cell **cyclooxygenase-2**, **and messenger RNA**[34] are also stimulated by LIPUS. The use of medications containing calcium channel blockers, nonsteroidal anti-inflammatory medications, steroids; and smoking decrease the probability of success of LIPUS.[38]

In acute tibial fractures, LIPUS has been demonstrated to reduce the clinical healing time (86 days compared with 144 days for the control group) and radiographic healing time (96 days; control group equals 154 days), an outcome which was found to be both statistically significant and, perhaps most important, clinically significant.[29, 30]

LIPUS has not been demonstrated to be effective in accelerating the healing of tibial fractures that have been surgically reinforced using an **intramedullary rod**.[39] One study found no statistical difference in fracture healing time between direct current electrical stimulation using implanted electrodes and ultrasonic stimulation applied at 0.1 W/cm² at an output frequency of 1 MHz (parameters that do not coincide with LIPUS). However, both groups did demonstrate accelerated healing relative to the control group.[40]
Photograph of Exogen 2000 courtesy of Smith & Nephew, Memphis, TN.

the building blocks of fibroblasts.[41, 42, 44] This response appears to be localized to areas with a high collagen content, especially tendons. Animal studies have shown that the application of continuous ultrasound increased the rate of collagen synthesis in tendon fibroblasts[44] and tendon healing,[45] and increased the tensile strength of tendons.[4, 46]

Blood and Fluid Dynamics

Continuous ultrasound has been reported to increase local blood flow for up to 45 minutes after treatment,[47] although these findings are not universally accepted.[48, 49] It is reasonable to expect increased blood flow during and immediately after the application of continuous ultrasound simply due to its thermal effects. Increased temperature results in increased cell metabolism that thereby increases the need for blood in the area. Other physiological factors may also promote increased blood flow.[50] Alteration of cell membrane permeability could result in decreased vascular tone, leading to a dilation of the vessels, and histamine released in the treated area could also cause vasodilation, further increasing blood flow.

Moist heat,[25] ice massage,[47] and cold packs[26] have been applied before ultrasound to alter blood flow during and after the treatment. The use of moist heat before ultrasound application significantly reduced the relative increase in blood flow.[25] The application of ice massage before ultrasound maintains the increased blood flow at the level found with ultrasound application alone. Cold pack application, long thought to increase the thermal effects of ultrasound, greatly decreases intramuscular temperature increase at a depth of 5 cm below the skin after ultrasound, 3.2°F (1.8°C) compared with a 7.2°F (4°C) rise in the temperature of tissues that were not cooled before treatment.[26]

Nerve Conduction and Pain Control

Ultrasound may control pain through the direct effect that the energy has on the peripheral nervous system, or pain control may be the result of the other tissue changes with ultrasound application. Ultrasound directly influences the transmission of nerve impulses by eliciting changes within the nerve fibers themselves. Cell membrane permeability to sodium ions is affected, altering the electrical activity of the nerve fiber[15] and elevating the pain threshold.[51] Nerve conduction velocity is increased as a result of the thermal effects of ultrasound application and may also produce a counterirritant effect.[2]

Indirect pain reduction results from the other effects of ultrasound application. Increased blood flow and increased capillary permeability augment the delivery of oxygen to hypoxic areas, reducing the activity of **chemosensitive pain receptors ▪**. Input from mechanical pain receptors is reduced because of a reduction in the amount of muscle spasm and increased muscular relaxation.[51]

Muscle Spasm

As described in Chapter 5, the thermal effects of ultrasound can decrease muscle spasm by reducing the mechanical and chemical triggers that perpetuate the pain-spasm-pain cycle. Alteration of nerve conduction velocity, the counterirritant effect of increased temperature, and increased blood flow can decrease noxious stimulus. Relaxation of muscle tension by increasing blood flow, increased delivery of oxygen, and encouraging the elongation of muscle fibers can decrease the mechanical stimulus.

Tissue Elasticity

Ultrasound preferentially heats collagen-rich tissues, especially tendon, ligament, fascia, and scar tissue. To promote tissue elongation, the temperature of the target tissues must be elevated 7.2°F (4°C). After ultrasound application, the stretching window is short-lived.[27] The thermal effects associated with vigorous heating (see Table 7–5), when applied at 3 MHz, have an effective stretching time of just over 3 minutes after the end of the treatment, although the window may be slightly longer when 1-MHz ultrasound is used.[27]

Heating or stretching alone is not sufficient to elongate noncontractile tissue. Repeated exposure to heat and stretch is required to stretch these tissues.[52] When the goal of the ultrasound treatment is to elongate tissue, place the tissues on stretch during the treatment. Any subsequent stretching should be performed immediately after the treatment ends. Repeated application across a number of days may be necessary to obtain the desired lengthening.[24, 53]

Therapeutic ultrasound is effective only in heating a relatively small area of tissue. For this reason, it is not an effective device to heat a large area of muscle. Shortwave diathermy (see Chapter 9) or exercise should be used instead of ultrasound in these cases.

Wound Healing

Some superficial wounds have responded favorably to ultrasound application. The use of continuous ultrasound delivered at 1.5 W/cm² for a 5-minute treatment over a 1-week period has been demonstrated to increase the breaking strength of incisional wounds. The same protocol, except applied at 0.5 W/cm² for a 2-week duration, produced the same results of increased breaking strength after 1 week, and facilitation of collagen deposition was demonstrated during the second week.[54] (Note: The preceding studies were performed with a 1-MHz output

---

Chemosensitive pain receptors: Nerves that are excited by the presence of certain chemical substances.

frequency; the results of the same protocol using a 3-MHz output have not been established.)

Pressure ulcers treated with 3-MHz, 5 cm² ERA, 20-percent duty cycle, at an output intensity of 0.1 to 0.5 W/cm² applied around the open wound and also treated with standard wound care techniques demonstrated accelerated healing compared with the use of standard wound care techniques (Fig. 7–10).[55] Ultrasound applied at 1 W/cm² or applied using a continuous output may have an inhibitory effect on wound healing, possibly because the necrotic tissues are unable to dissipate heat.[55]

■ Phonophoresis

Phonophoresis describes the application of therapeutic ultrasound to assist in the diffusion of medication through the skin.[56] Although it is easy to visualize the ultrasound waves physically driving the medication through the skin, phonophoresis does not work this way. Rather, ultrasound opens pathways that allow the medication to diffuse through the skin and pass deeper into the tissues.

The advantage of introducing medications into the body through phonophoresis rather than by injection is that the medication is spread over a larger area, and phonophoresis is noninvasive.[57] Medication that has entered the tissues by phonophoresis bypasses the liver, thus lessening the metabolic elimination of the substances.

Medications that are applied transdermally must first pass through the enzymatic barrier of the epidermis and the stratum corneum, the rate-limiting barrier to diffusion, before being absorbed by the viable subcutaneous tissues. The stratum corneum determines the rate and amount of medication that is transmitted to the deeper tissues. Medications that are absorbed through the skin may be stored in the subcutaneous tissues for some time and require a longer time to be diffused into the deeper tissues.

With this in mind, the type and consistency of the skin overlying the treatment area are important elements in determining the success of the treatment. Factors such as skin composition, hydration, vascularity, and thickness combine to encourage or prohibit medication diffusion through the skin and, therefore, into the deeper tissues (Table 7–6).

Many substances such as medicated lotions or creams can be moved past the skin's barriers simply by massaging them into the skin. However, some medications have been shown to be delivered to depths of 6 cm into the tissues with the assistance of ultrasound.[58, 59] The thermal and nonthermal effects associated with standard ultrasound application may increase the rate and amount of medication absorbed. The thermal effects of ultrasound increase the kinetic energy of both the local cells and the medication, dilating the points of entry (hair follicles, sweat glands, etc.), increasing circulation, increasing capillary permeability, and disordering the structured lipids in the stratum corneum.[60–62] Nonthermal effects enhancing diffusion across the membranes include altering the cell's resting potential, affecting the permeability of ionized and un-ionized molecules, and increasing cell membrane permeability.[61, 63, 64]

Preheating the treatment area with a moist hot pack to increase local blood flow and kinetic energy can further enhance delivery of the medication into the tissues. After the treatment, leave the remaining mixture on the skin and cover the area with an occlusive dressing to encourage further diffusion of the remaining medication. Systemic effects may be promoted by again heating the area after treatment to encourage vascular absorption and distribution of the medication.[61]

Phonophoresis is applied using a prescription or nonprescription medication that has molecules of relatively small size and of low molecular weight (Table 7–7).[65] The small size and weight of the molecules is needed for the medication to diffuse through the skin. The medication is often mixed with an inert base such as ultrasound gel to help transmit the energy to the tissues. If the medication is mixed with a base, the base must be capable of transmitting ultrasonic energy (see Direct Coupling in Chapter 8).

Do not use medication mixtures that are not specifically intended for phonophoresis. Many commonly used phonophoresis mixtures reflect most of the ultrasonic energy; some of the most popular bases that have been used for years result in 100-percent reflection. In this case, the ultrasound had no effect on the treatment.[56, 64]

The majority of thick, white, corticosteroid creams are poor conductors of ultrasound. Topical gel-mixed media, such as commercially available transmission gels, are good conductors.[66] Another approach to administration of phonophoresis is the "invisible method," in which the medication is first directly massaged into the skin and then followed by a traditional ultrasound application.

The efficacy of phonophoresis has not been fully substantiated.[57, 59, 64, 67] Many of the contradictions in the results of studies can be related to the type of coupling agent used and the concentration of the medication. For

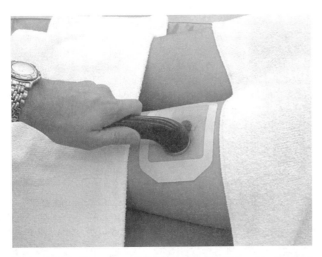

Figure 7–10. Ultrasound Application to Promote Wound Healing. The wound may be covered with an occlusive dressing and MHz low-intensity, pulsed output is applied to the periphery of the wound.

TABLE … …ffecting the Rate of Medication Diffusion During Phonophoresis

Facto…

Hydr… …igher the water content, the more permeable the skin to the passage of medications.
Age… …dration occurs as skin ages; circulation and **lipid ■** content are also decreased.
Con… …easiest passage of medication through the skin is near hair follicles, sebaceous glands,
… d sweat ducts.
… …ough hair follicles encourage the passage of medication through the skin, excessive hair
… hould be shaved off the area being treated.
V… …ghly vascular areas are more apt to allow for the transfer of the medication into the deep
… tissues. Constricted vessels localize the effects, whereas dilated vessels enhance the
… systemic delivery of the medication.
… hick skin presents a much more cumbersome barrier to medication than does thinner skin.
… When applying phonophoresis to an area, attempt to administer it over areas of low skin
… density (e.g., when treating an individual suffering from plantar fasciitis, apply the medica-
… tion to the medioinferior aspect of the calcaneus rather than on its plantar surface).

example, one study examined the subcutaneous absorption of a commercially available **salicylate ■**, Myoflex, and found no difference in the level of salicylates in the bloodstream with or without the use of ultrasound.[64] A later study revealed that Myoflex transmitted no ultrasonic energy compared with water (see Table 8–1).[66]

Still, the actual amount of medication that penetrates to the viable tissues and the effect that ultrasonic energy has on the absorption is unknown. **Hydrocortisone ■** is thought to be delivered into the subcutaneous tissues, where it slowly diffuses into the deeper tissues, but increased serum cortisol levels have not been substantiated after treatment.[68] Hydrocortisone itself is a poor transmitter of acoustical energy.[66] Dexamethasone transmits 95 to 98 percent of ultrasonic energy and is becoming more prevalently used for phonophoresis.[69] Likewise, dexa-

methasone has not been proved to produce a measurable effect in the submuscular or subtendinous tissue[69] or in any amount sufficient to impair adrenal function.[70, 71]

Many of the limitations found in traditional phonophoresis techniques may be circumvented through the use of low-frequency sound generators. These devices use a 20-kHz frequency (at the upper range of human hearing), 125 mW/cm^2, pulsed output to enhance the introduction of medication into the deep tissues. The lower frequency allows medications of a larger molecular size and weight, including insulin and **interferon gamma ■**, to penetrate deeper into the tissues. Initial reports on this technique indicate that low-frequency sonophoresis is capable of delivering a wide range of medications up to 1000 times more effectively than those produced with the traditional ultrasound method (see Box 7–4).[65, 70, 72] The

TABLE 7–7 | **Medications Commonly Administered via Phonophoresis**

Classification	*Indications*	*Target Tissues*	*Examples*
Corticosteroids	Inflammatory conditions	Subcutaneous tissues Nerves Muscle	Hydrocortisone Dexamethasone
Salicylates	Inflammatory conditions Pain	Subdermal tissues	Myoflex*
Anesthetics	Pain Trigger points	Nerves Circulatory system	Lidocaine

Note: Does not transmit ultrasonic energy.

Hydrocortisone: An anti-inflammatory drug that closely resembles cortisol.
Interferon gamma: A group of proteins released by white blood cells and fibroblasts when devouring the unwanted tissues. The gamma classification is also referred to as "angry macrophages" because of their heightened phagocytic activity.
Lipid: A broad category of fatlike substances.
Salicylates: A family of analgesic compounds that includes aspirin.

effect of the treatment may be enhanced by covering the treated area with a dressing following treatment to keep the area hydrated.[61]

Phonophoresis using prescription medication is regulated by most state pharmacy practice acts. Although there is variation from state to state, the law may require that the medication be specifically prescribed to the individual patient.

■ Contraindications to Therapeutic Ultrasound

In cases in which the use of ultrasound is questionable because of underlying medical conditions, consult with the patient's physician to determine if this modality should be used. Thermal ultrasound should not be applied in the presence of the general contraindications to heat application (see Table 5–9). Refer to At a Glance: Therapeutic Ultrasound in Chapter 8 for a complete list of contraindications and precautions in the use of therapeutic ultrasound.

Therapeutic ultrasound must not be applied over areas of impaired circulation, ischemic areas, or areas having sensory deficit. The lack of normal circulation reduces the body's ability to dissipate the heat and may result in burns, a risk that is increased in the absence of normal sensory function. Application over areas of deep vein thrombosis may cause the clot to dislodge and move elsewhere in the circulatory system. Use over sites of active infection may result in the infection spreading. Application of ultrasound over cancerous tumors can increase the tumor's mass and weight.[73]

Specific body regions are potentially hazardous targets of ultrasound, especially fluid-filled cavities. Avoid application over the eyes, heart, skull, and genitals. Application over an implanted pacemaker and its leads is contraindicated because of the risk of damage to the pacemaker or causing it to malfunction. Increased bleeding may occur if ultrasound is applied over the pelvic, lower abdominal region, or lumbar area of menstruating women. Because of the risk to the fetus, do not apply therapeutic ultrasound to the abdominal, pelvic, or lumbar areas during pregnancy.

The use of therapeutic ultrasound over active fracture sites or stress fractures may cause pain and may possibly delay healing (the exception to this is ultrasonic bone growth stimulators). Application of therapeutic ultrasound over unfused epiphyses is commonly listed as a contraindication to therapeutic ultrasound, but no definitive evidence supports this claim. Metal implants are also sometimes listed as a contraindication to ultrasound application. However, metal rapidly conducts heat away from the area and this procedure should be appropriate if the sound head is kept moving.

Although not an outright contraindication, use caution when applying ultrasound over the vertebral column, nerve roots, or large nerve plexus. The tissue densities in these regions may result in a rapid rate of heating. Following a **laminectomy** ■, portions of the muscle and bone covering the spinal cord may retract, potentially directly exposing the spinal cord to the ultrasonic energy.

■ Controversies in Treatment

Despite the relative wealth of published research examining the effects of therapeutic ultrasound, the efficacy of this device is still being questioned. There is sufficient evidence to indicate that continuous ultrasound can significantly increase the temperature of subcutaneous tissues.[9, 10, 14, 25–27, 74] However, another study suggests that the temperature increases seen in these studies are dependent on the ultrasound generator being used. Using the same output parameters, other manufacturers' ultrasound units were unable to reach these temperatures.[23]

In 2001, the *Journal of Physical Therapy* published a two-part review and analysis that questioned the efficacy of therapeutic ultrasound. The authors concluded that most of the published research examining the effectiveness of ultrasound in patient care was methodologically flawed, suffered from a lack of randomized controlled trials, and was limited by an insufficient range of patient problems.[75]

In examining the biophysical effects of ultrasound, the authors concluded that there is no evidence that cavitation actually occurs during therapeutic ultrasound application and initial studies may have been misled by instrumentation errors.[16] If this is the case, then bulk streaming rather than microstreaming may occur in the human body. Bulk streaming has less of a biophysical effect than microstreaming. And if microstreaming does not occur, then the nonthermal effects attributed to ultrasound may not occur.[16] Subsequent research has both supported[17] and refuted[11] the potential of therapeutic ultrasound's nonthermal effects.

Despite all of the recent questions regarding the efficacy of ultrasound, sufficient evidence exists to conclude definitively that when it is applied at the proper intensity for the proper duration and the treatment area is limited to two to three times the transducer's ERA, ultrasound is capable of vigorously heating a small volume of tissue. This may be the inherent limitation to its use. Therapeutic ultrasound is probably incapable of heating a large muscle mass and improving range of motion. This deficit has, in part, given renewed interest in shortwave diathermy as a deep heating agent (see Chapters 9 and 10).

For ultrasound to be effective, it must be used properly, an issue that has plagued this modality since entering the mainstream of health care. Common clinical errors in application include selecting the wrong output frequency, using an output intensity that is too low when attempting to produce thermal effects, treating too large an area, using

---

Laminectomy: Surgical removal of the lamina from a vertebra.

inappropriate coupling media, and moving the sound head too rapidly. Therapeutic ultrasound has its place in the care of musculoskeletal injuries. However, the tool (modality) must fit the job (the treatment goals).

● Chapter Highlights

- Therapeutic ultrasound has a frequency of 1.0 to 3.3 MHz. Because of this high frequency, ultrasound cannot be transmitted through the air and, therefore, requires a transmission medium.
- The electropiezo effect, an alternating current passing through a crystal, produces ultrasound.
- The ERA describes the area of the crystal that produces the majority of the ultrasonic output. The ERA is always less than the size of the sound head.
- The depth of penetration is based on the output frequency. Lower frequencies penetrate into the tissues more deeply than higher frequencies.
- The output intensity can be measured in total watts. Most commonly the spatial average intensity, the total output in watts divided by the effective radiating area of the sound head, is used and is expressed as W/cm^2.
- The beam nonuniformity ratio describes the homo-geneity of the ultrasound beam and is determined by the average output in the near field (Fresnel zone) and the spatial peak intensity.
- Ultrasound can produce thermal and nonthermal effects within the tissues. Temperature increases are obtained by using a 100-percent duty cycle and high output. Nonthermal treatments are applied by using a low number of pulses or a low-output intensity.
- The transmission of ultrasound is not significantly affected by adipose tissue and is selectively absorbed by collagen-rich tissues.
- Ultrasound is capable of producing heat up to 5 cm deep in the tissue. The thermal effects of ultrasound are similar to those described in Chapter 5. However, ultrasound is able to heat only a relatively small volume of tissue.
- Nonthermal effects produce changes in cellular function without a significant increase in tissue temperatures. Nonthermal changes are thought to occur secondary to acoustical streaming and cavitation or by the frequency resonance of the cellular structures.
- Phonophoresis is the use of ultrasound to assist in the diffusion of medications through the skin.

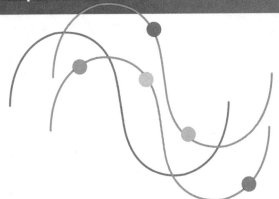

Chapter 8

Clinical Application of Therapeutic Ultrasound

Ultrasound application has evolved from what was once a rote "cookbook" approach to a clinical science. Determining the proper output parameters (indeed, determining if ultrasound is even the proper modality) requires knowledge of the type of tissues involved, the depth of the trauma, the nature and inflammatory state of the injury, and consideration of the skin and tissues overlying the treatment area.

Although finite parameters have been established, much of the application of ultrasound is as much an art (and a learning process) as it is a science. Patient feedback and reevaluation of the patient's physical response to prior treatments should be the basis for adjusting the treatment parameters. Communicate the expectations and sensations that are to be expected during the treatment and inform the patient to report any uncomfortable, unusual, or unexpected sensations.

To ensure safe application of this modality, ultrasound units must be calibrated at least once a year (many manufacturers recommend that this be done twice a year). The U.S. Food and Drug Administration (FDA) requires

that the output frequency, effective radiating area (ERA), and date of last calibration be indicated on the generator or the transducer[13] (Fig. 8–1). The ERA represents the average for that make and model. The size of the transducer face may also be included if it is significantly different than the size of the ERA.

■ Treatment Area

Ultrasound is only effective in increasing tissue temperatures when the treatment area is approximately two, but no more than three, times the size of the sound head's ERA.[9] Attempting to heat a larger area will significantly reduce

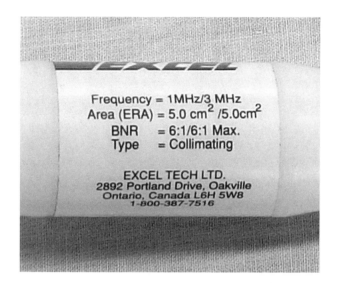

Figure 8–1. FDA Labeling Requirements for Therapeutic Ultrasound. The sound head pictured here is capable of producing an output of 1 or 3 MHz and has an effective radiating area of 5.0 cm². Note that the BNR is listed as 6:1 for the 1 MHz output and 6:1 for 3 MHz. The "Max." indicates that this was the maximum BNR found in a sample of sound heads. (Courtesy of Excel Tech LTD., Ontario, Canada.)

tive medium can damage the crystal. For this reason, only approved conducting agents should be used, and the intensity of the unit should not be increased without the sound head in contact with the body. Most ultrasound generators automatically shut down if application is attempted without a medium, if an unacceptable medium is used, or if sufficient contact is not made with the skin. Operating an improperly coupled ultrasound head causes the temperature of the sound head to increase and may damage the crystal.

Direct Coupling

In this method of ultrasound application, the transducer is applied directly to the skin, with a gel or cream used to transfer the energy between the ultrasound head and the skin. Coupling agents are made of distilled water and an inert, nonreflective material that increases the viscosity of the mixture. Not all substances efficiently transfer the ultrasonic energy from the transducer to the tissues, and many block the energy altogether (Table 8–1). For this reason, only approved transmission media should be used.

the temperature increase. If the size of the target tissues is larger than three times the ERA, break the area down into two or more treatment zones (Fig. 8–2).

When treating two treatment zones, allow time for the first zone to cool before treating the second zone. Consecutive treatments can result in a potentially hazardous increase in temperatures at the borders of the two zones. If more than two zones are being treated, stagger the treatment order to prevent contiguous zones from being heated consecutively. However, this does not increase the collagen elasticity of large body areas sufficiently enough to promote their elongation. The effectiveness of thermal ultrasound treatment decreases as the area treated increases.

The size of the treatment area for nonthermal treatments may be slightly larger. However, no definitive guidelines have been established for this mode of application.

■ Coupling Methods

Ultrasonic waves cannot pass through the air; a transmission medium must be used to allow the waves to pass out of the transducer and into the tissues. A good medium is characterized by the ability to transmit a significant percentage of the ultrasound; therefore, it should be nonreflective. The optimal medium for transmission is distilled water, which reflects only 0.2 percent of the energy.[76]

When large, regularly shaped body areas (such as the quadriceps muscle group) are being treated, good coupling is relatively easy. However, irregularly shaped areas decrease the contact area between the transducer and the skin, causing uneven amounts of energy to be delivered to the tissues, requiring modified coupling methods.

Attempting to pass ultrasound through a nonconduc-

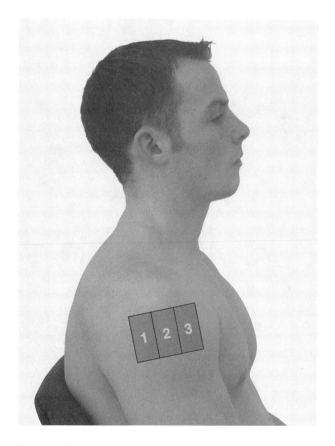

Figure 8–2. Treatment Zones. When treating an area more than twice the size of the sound head's ERA, divide the area into two or more "treatment zones." Use caution when treating overlapping areas. In this example treat the two outer zones and then the center zone. As one treatment zone is being heated, the prior treatment areas will cool, thus limiting the ability to effectively heat the muscle mass as a whole.

TABLE 8–1	Coupling Ability of Potential Ultrasound Media

Substance	Transmission Relative to Distilled Water (%)
Saran Wrap	98
Lidex gel, fluocinonide 0.05%	97
Thera-Gesic cream, methyl salicylate	97
Mineral oil	97
Ultrasound transmission gel	96
Ultrasound transmission lotion	90
Chempad-L	68
Hydrocortisone powder (1%) in US gel	29
Hydrocortisone powder (10%) in US gel	7
Eucerin cream	0
Myoflex cream, trolamine salicylate 10%	0
White petrolatum gel	0

US = ultrasound.

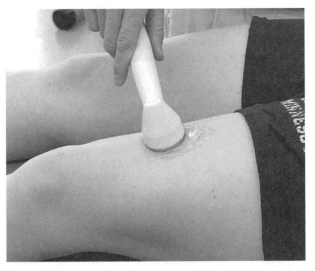

Figure 8–3. **Direct Coupling Method Using an Ultrasound Gel.** Note that the treatment area is only twice as large as the sound head.

Topical counterirritants and analgesics are sometimes used as coupling agents, but these products can decrease the effectiveness of the treatment or altogether render the treatment ineffective. Although some analgesic creams are good conductors of ultrasonic energy (e.g., Thera-Gesic), others do not transmit ultrasonic energy (e.g., trolamine salicylate [Myoflex]) (see Table 8–1). The use of counterirritants as an ultrasound transmission agent increases the patient's perception of heat, but the actual amount of intramuscular heating may be less than that obtained from ultrasound gel.[77, 78]

Apply the gel liberally to the area and ensure a consistent thickness and that no large air bubbles are present (Fig. 8–3). The effectiveness of ultrasound transmission gel or cream is decreased if the body part is hairy or irregularly shaped. Each of these conditions can increase the spatial average intensity by decreasing the contact area between the transducer and the tissues. The application of gel causes air bubbles to cling to hair. The greater amount of hair on the body part, the greater the reduction of ultrasound delivered to the tissues. If the body hair is excessive, consider shaving the treatment area.

Firm, constant pressure should be used to hold the sound head in contact with the skin.[79] Too little pressure creates an insufficient couple. Too much pressure decreases the amount of energy transferred to the tissues, and the pressure may cause the patient discomfort. Move the sound head slowly, using approximately 0.44 to 1.32 pounds of pressure.[79]

A warmer can be used to preheat the transmission gel, but this is primarily for patient comfort. Heating the skin with a moist heat pack results in a more rapid increase in intramuscular temperature; the use of warm transmission gel does not. Overwarming the gel can reduce its density and decrease the efficiency of ultrasonic energy transmission.[80]

Immersion Technique

When treating irregularly shaped areas such as the distal extremities, a more uniform dose of ultrasound can be given using water as the transmission medium. The body part is immersed in a tub of water (**degassed water** ■ is the ideal). Water can be degassed by first boiling it for 30 to 45 minutes and then storing it in an air-tight container (sterile or distilled water may be used as well).

The transducer is then placed in the water with the sound head facing the body part approximately 1 inch away (Fig. 8–4). The face of the transducer should be parallel with the surface of the skin so that the energy strikes the tissues at a 90-degree angle. Angles of less than 80 degrees significantly reduce the effectiveness of the treatment (see the Cosine Law in Appendix B).[81]

A ceramic tub is recommended for underwater ultrasound application.[76] The ceramic sides make an excellent reflective surface, creating an "echo chamber" that allows the sound waves to strike the body part from all angles. The operator's hand should not be continually immersed in the water. Although this is not necessarily dangerous in a single treatment, immersion could unnecessarily expose the hand to ultrasonic energy over repeated exposures.

If nondistilled water is being used, the intensity of the

Degassed water: Water that has been allowed to sit undisturbed for 4 to 24 hours, allowing the gaseous bubbles to escape.

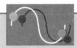

CLINICAL TECHNIQUES: SPEED LIMIT... SLOW DOWN WHEN MOVING THE SOUND HEAD

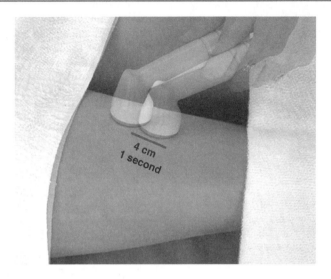

4 cm
1 second

There is a tendency to move the sound head too rapidly during treatment. When thermal ultrasound is being applied, moving the sound head too quickly can decrease the amount of temperature increase to the point of ineffectiveness. An analogy can be made between the speed that the sound head is moved and ironing a pair of pants. If the iron is moved too quickly across the pant leg, it will not be heated to the point required to remove the wrinkles. Moving the iron too slowly can scorch the cloth.

The same holds true for ultrasound. Slow precise strokes are needed to allow the tissues to warm, but moving the sound head too slowly can overheat the tissues. The speed limit for moving the sound head is approximately 4 cm per second, but the slower the better.[79]

If the patient experiences discomfort from the treatment, move the head slightly faster and/or decrease the output intensity. This is probably related to a high BNR creating "hot spots" in the ultrasound output. However, the patient should feel warmth if a thermal treatment is being applied.

The **stationary head technique** is when the sound head is held over the target tissue (e.g., a trigger point or area of muscle spasm). This technique is no longer advocated because of standing waves overheating the tissue and hot spots associated with the beam.

ultrasound can be increased by approximately 0.5 W per square centimeter to account for attenuation caused by minerals in the water. Tap water immersion, using ultrasound delivered at 3 MHz, is less effective in increasing subcutaneous tissue temperatures than the direct coupling method.[74, 82]

During the treatment, air bubbles tend to form along the patient's skin, potentially interfering with the transmission of ultrasound and the energy striking the tissues. Wisp away any bubbles that form on the patient's skin or on the transducer face during treatment.

Pad (Bladder) Method

This technique originally used a balloon, condom, or plastic bag filled with water or ultrasound transmission gel that was coated with a coupling agent.[82] The advantage of the bladder is its ability to conform to irregularly shaped areas such as the acromioclavicular or talocrural joints. The disadvantage is the formation of air pockets within the

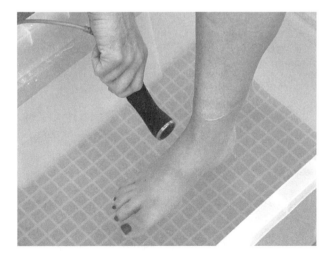

Figure 8–4. **Underwater Application of Ultrasound.** Water is used as a coupling medium to distribute the energy evenly over irregularly shaped areas. The sound head does not come into contact with the body part.

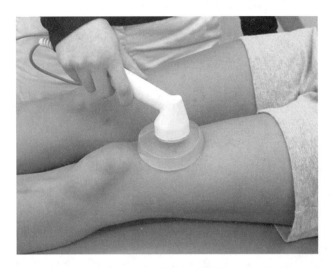

Figure 8–5. **Ultrasound Application Using an Ultrasound Gel Pad.** This method is used to deliver ultrasound to irregularly shaped areas when the underwater area is not practical. These pads also limit the treatment area to an appropriate size.

bladder that prohibit the transmission of sound waves and the difficulty holding the gel-coated bladder in place. The bladder should be made from thin plastic, such as Saran Wrap. Rubber products may absorb more energy as the ultrasound wave passes through the bladder on one side and then again on the other, resulting in less energy being available to be delivered to the tissues.[82]

The bladder is first filled with degassed water (see the Immersion Technique) or ultrasound gel. To prevent blockage of the ultrasonic energy, all air pockets must be eliminated. A transmission medium is applied to the skin and the outer surface of the bladder. The bladder is then held against the body part while the sound applicator is moved over its surface.

Commercially produced gel pads have become a popular and effective alternative to the bladder method.[82] Gel pads are formed from ultrasound gel in a tight matrix that allows them to hold their shape while also conforming to the contours of the body (Fig. 8–5). Another advantage of gel pads is that they limit the treatment area to the size selected, thus focusing the energy on an area approximately twice the size of the sound head.

■ Selecting the Output Parameters

The following sections describe the methodology used to select the various output parameters. This information is described in more detail in Chapter 7.

Output Frequency

The effective depth of the ultrasonic energy and the rate of heating is based on the output frequency (Table 8–2). An output frequency of 1 MHz targets tissues up to at least 5 cm deep. Three megahertz output has traditionally been thought to target tissues up to 2 cm deep, although there is evidence that indicates that heating may occur up to 2.5 to

3 cm deep.[7, 8] Table 8–3 details the differences in 1- and 3-MHz-ultrasound application.

Superficial structures such as the patellar tendon, medial collateral ligament, and brachialis would require a 3-MHz output. Deep structures such as the rotator cuff, vastus intermedius, and the gastrocnemius call for a 1-MHz output. Keep in mind that subcutaneous adipose tissue is relatively transparent to ultrasonic energy.

Treatment Duration

The length of the treatment depends on the size of the area being treated, the output intensity, and the therapeutic goals of the treatment. In all circumstances, the area for any particular treatment should be no larger than two to three times the surface area of the sound head's ERA.[3, 9]

When vigorous heating effects are desired, the treatment duration should be in the range of 10 to 12 minutes for 1-MHz output and 3 to 4 minutes for 3-MHz ultrasound.[3] Table 8–3 should be used as a guide for determining the actual treatment duration based on the frequency of the ultrasound being applied and the goals of the treatment. Ultrasound treatments are generally delivered for a 10- to 14-day period, at which time the efficacy of the treatment approach is reevaluated.

Duty Cycle

The duty cycle determines if the thermal or nonthermal effects of ultrasound will be predominant, although the two are never truly separate. Nonthermal effects are always accompanied by thermal effects and vice versa. However, the rate and magnitude of temperature increase is markedly reduced when a low duty cycle is used. Based on the relative magnitude of the thermal effects, a low duty cycle is used for acute injuries and a continuous output is used when thermal effects are desired.

The duty cycles available on most units range from 20 to 100 percent (continuous output) with gradations ranging

TABLE 8–2	**Comparison of 1-MHz and 3-MHz Thermal Ultrasound Application**	
	1-MHz	*3-MHz*
Beam profile	Relatively divergent	Relatively collimating
Depth of penetration	5 or more cm	0.8 to 3 cm
Maximum rate of heating[3]	0.36F° (0.2°C) per min per W/cm²	1.1°F (0.6°C) per min per W/cm²
Heat latency	Retains heat twice as long as 3-MHz ultrasound	Retains heat half as long as 1-MHz ultrasound

TABLE 8–3 Rate of Ultrasound Heating

	Temperature Increase per Minute	
Intensity (W/cm²) *Tissue Depth*	*1 MHz* *5 cm*	*3 MHz* *1.2 cm*
0.5	0.04°C	0.3°C
1.0	0.2°C	0.6°C
1.5	0.3°C	0.9°C
2.0	0.4°C	1.4°C

Applied at two to three times the effective radiating area.

from 5 to 25 percent. Although it is clear that a 100 percent duty cycle should be used for thermal effects and the lowest duty cycle for the treatment of acute injuries (or when nonthermal effects are desired), it is less clear when, or even if, to use the intermediate duty cycles.

Output Intensity

The effects of the ultrasound treatment depend on the output intensity, the treatment duration, and the duty cycle. The overall amount of energy delivered to the body also depends the BNR and the ERA. When a continuous output is used, the output meter displays the spatial average temporal peak intensity in watts per square centimeter (W/cm²) or the total output in watts. When the output is pulsed, the overall intensity must be thought of in terms of the spatial average temporal average (SATA) intensity, the amount of energy per unit of time. Remember that the metered output displays

only the average intensity in the near field and does not reflect the peak intensity as represented by the BNR.

For thermal treatments, 1-MHz ultrasound applied at 1.5 W/cm² heats at the approximate rate of 0.2°C per W/cm²; 3 MHz heats at approximately 0.2°C per W/cm² (Fig. 8–6).[10] Approximately 10 minutes of treatment time is required to heat tissues to 0.72°F (4°C) using 1-MHz output and a treatment area twice the size of the ERA and an output of 2 W/cm². For 3-MHz ultrasound, just under 4 minutes at an output intensity of 1.75 W/cm² is required.[3]

The values presented in Figure 8–6 are estimates of the treatment duration required to reach the target temperature. The body area being treated and the depth of the target tissue, the ultrasound unit's BNR, application techniques, individual generator variations, and even the coupling medium used influence the rate and degree of temperature increase.

The patient should describe "warmth" or heat during thermal treatments but not pain or burning. Discomfort could indicate that the sound head is not being moved fast enough, approximately 4 cm/sec. Adjust the output intensity to the patient's tolerance and comfort. Erring on the side of caution, use shorter treatment durations and lower treatment intensities, and make subsequent adjustments based on the patient's response to the treatment. Note that the patient's report of heat may not reflect the actual temperature increase within the muscle.[78]

The treatment intensity and duration for nonthermal treatments is largely based on experience and anecdotal evidence. In general, shorter treatment durations and lower intensities—as well as the lowest possible duty cycle—are used for this method of ultrasound application. An intensity of 0.5 W/cm² is recommended for treatment of

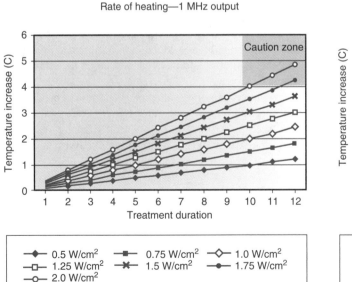

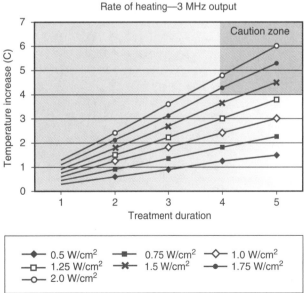

Figure 8–6. **Approximate Treatment Time Based on Target Temperature Increase.** Assuming a continuous output (100% duty cycle), the approximate treatment times required to obtain specific tissue temperatures at different output intensities. The patient should report warmth, but not pain or discomfort, during the treatment.

acute injuries.[18, 54] Superficial skin lesions, such as pressure sores, respond well to 3-MHz ultrasound applied using a 20-percent duty cycle and an output intensity of 0.1 to 0.5 W/cm^2.[55]

Dose-Oriented Treatments

Improvements in the quality of ultrasound generators, microprocessors, and research regarding the heating effects of ultrasound have led to the development of dose-oriented treatment parameters. The desired amount of temperature increase is entered and the unit calculates the output intensity and treatment duration. The clinician may still adjust the treatment intensity, but the treatment duration would change inversely. Decreasing the intensity would increase the duration and vice versa.

■ Ultrasound and Electrical Stimulation

Ultrasound and electrical stimulation have long been applied concurrently for treatment of trigger points and other superficial painful areas, although research supporting the benefits of this combined treatment approach is lacking. In this technique, the ultrasound head serves as an electrode for an electrical stimulating current (Fig. 8–7). Theoretically, this application method would provide the same benefits as ultrasound (thermal and nonthermal) and electrical stimulation if they were applied separately, namely, improved circulation, reduction of muscle spasm, and decreased adhesion of scar tissue.

Trigger points and other stimulation points display a decreased resistance to electrical current flow (see Chapter 12). When a moderate pulse duration and moderate pulse frequency are applied at an intensity sufficient to produce a strong muscle contraction, the muscle fibers within the

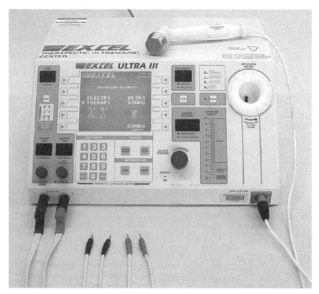

Figure 8–8. **Ultrasound–Electrical Stimulation Combo Unit.** These devices are electrical stimulators and ultrasound generators housed in the same unit. Electrical stimulation and ultrasound can be applied at the same time (see Ultrasound and Electrical Stimulation).

trigger point may fatigue to the point where they no longer have the biochemical ability to spasm. Low-amperage electrical stimulation is capable of increasing adenosine triphosphate activity within the cells, increasing their ability to repair themselves. Increased phagocytosis and increased circulation would assist in the collection and removal of cellular wastes from the treatment area.[83]

A wide range of combined ultrasound and electrical stimulation units are being marketed. The electrical stimulation part of these units delivers a monophasic, biphasic, or alternating current. Each of these parameters would affect the target tissues differently. Likewise, many ultrasound generators in this configuration, especially older ones, deliver only a 1-MHz output. In most instances, a 3-MHz output would be needed to target the stimulation points.

A slowly moving sound head is needed to produce the required amount of subcutaneous tissue temperature increase, approximately 7.2°F (4°C). Placing the target tissues on stretch during treatment could assist the reduction of trigger points and muscle spasm.

■ Set-up and Application of Therapeutic Ultrasound

Ultrasound generators are available in a wide range of makes and models. Although most models have unique features, most are capable of delivering ultrasound at different frequencies (1 and 3.3 MHz being the most common), have adjustable duty cycles, and are capable of using sound heads of different effective radiating areas. Many manufacturers produce "combo units" that are both ultrasound generators and electrical stimulators (Fig. 8–8).

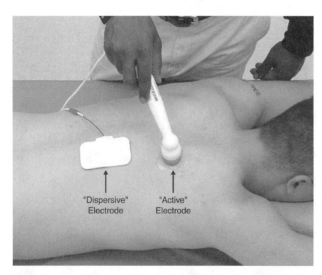

"Dispersive"   "Active"
Electrode   Electrode

Figure. 8–7 **Ultrasound and Electrical Stimulation Combination Therapy.** Using a sound/stimulation combination unit, one electrode is attached to the patient's body while the ultrasound head serves as the active "probe" electrode.

At a Glance: **Therapeutic Ultrasound**

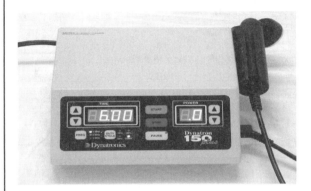

Description

High-frequency (1 to 3.3 MHz) sound waves applied to the body to produce thermal and nonthermal effects that are useful in treating:

- Calcific bursitis
- Inflammatory conditions
- Joint contractures
- Pain
- Acute orthopedic injuries (low pulses, low intensity)

Primary Effects

THERMAL
- Increased nerve conduction velocity
- Increased extensibility of collagen-rich structures
- Increased blood flow
- Increased macrophage activity

NONTHERMAL
- Increased cell membrane permeability
- Tissue regeneration
- Stimulating phagocytosis
- Synthesis of collagen

Treatment Duration

- The treatment time is from 3 to 12 minutes, depending on the size of the area being treated, the intensity of the treatment, and the goal of the treatment.
- Ultrasound is normally given once a day for 10 to 14 days, at which time the efficacy of the treatment protocol should be evaluated.

Indications

- Joint contractures
- Muscle spasm
- Neuroma
- Scar tissue
- Sympathetic nervous system disorders
- Trigger areas
- Warts
- Spasticity
- Postacute reduction of **myositis ossificans**
- Acute inflammatory conditions (pulsed output)
- Chronic inflammatory conditions (pulsed or continuous output)

Contraindications

- Acute conditions (continuous output)
- Ischemic areas
- Areas of impaired circulation including arterial disease
- Over areas of deep vein thrombosis
- Anesthetic areas
- Over cancerous tumors
- Over sites of active infection or sepsis
- Over the spinal cord or large nerve plexus in high doses
- Exposed metal that penetrates the skin (e.g., **external fixation** devices)
- Areas around the eyes, heart, skull, or genitals
- Over the thorax in the presence of an implanted pacemaker
- Pregnancy when used over the pelvic or lumbar areas
- Over a fracture site before healing is complete
- Stress fracture sites or sites of osteoporosis
- Over the pelvic or lumbar area in menstruating female patients

Precautions

- Symptoms may increase after the first two treatments because of an increase in inflammation in the area. If the symptoms do not improve after the third or fourth treatment, discontinue the use of the modality.[84]
- Use caution when applying ultrasound around the spinal cord, especially after laminectomy. Many manufacturers list this as a contraindication to ultrasound application. The various densities provided by the spinal cord and its covering may result in a rapid temperature rise, causing trauma to the spinal cord.
- The use of ultrasound over metal implants is not contraindicated as long as the sound head is kept moving and the treatment area has normal sensory function.
- The use of ultrasound over the **epiphyseal plates** of growing bone should be performed with caution.

Instrumentation

Duty cycle: Adjusts between continuous and pulsed ultrasound application. Most units display the duty cycle as a percentage, with 100 percent representing continuous ultrasound.

Frequency: Selects the output frequency—and therefore the depth of penetration—of the ultrasound. A 3-MHz frequency should be used for tissues 2 cm or less; 1 MHZ is used for greater tissue depth.[7]

Gel warmer: A heating element is used to preheat the transmission gel. This is primarily for patient comfort and has little, if any, additive effect on the treatment. Overwarming (or overcooling) the transmission medium may possibly decrease the thermal effects of ultrasound treatments.[80]

Intensity: Adjusts the intensity of the ultrasound beam. The WATT METER displays the output in either total watts or watts per square centimeter.

Maximum head temperature: Sets the maximum heat tolerance in the sound head in case the head is not properly coupled.

Pause: Interrupts the treatment but retains the remaining amount of treatment time when the treatment is reinstated.

Power: Allows the source current to flow into the internal components of the generator. On many units, a POWER light goes on, or the WATT METER illuminates.

Start-Stop: Initiates or terminates the production of ultrasound from the transducer.

Timer: Sets the duration of the treatment. The time remaining is displayed on the console, or the timer rotates to display the time remaining.

Watt meter: Displays the output of ultrasound in total watts or watts per square centimeter. Digital meters may require that the user manually switch between the two displays. Most **analog ■** meters display the total watts on an upper scale while simultaneously displaying output in watts per square centimeter on the lower scale. These typically have a sound head with a fixed ERA.

Patient Preparation

1. Establish that no contraindications are present.
2. Determine the method and mode of ultrasound application to be used during this treatment.
3. Clean the area to be treated to remove any body oils, dirt, or grime.
4. Determine the type of coupling method to be used.

5. For thermal treatments, identify a treatment area that is no larger than two to three times the size of the ERA.
6. If the direct coupling method is used, spread the gel over the area to be treated. Use the sound head to evenly distribute the gel.
7. Explain the sensations to be expected during the treatment. During the application of continuous ultrasound, a sensation of mild to moderate warmth (but not pain or burning) should be expected.[3] No subcutaneous sensations should be felt during the application of pulsed ultrasound. Advise the patient to inform you of any unexpected sensations.
8. For thermal treatments applied using a 1 MHz output, preheating with a moist heat pack will decrease the treatment time required to reach vigorous heating levels.[25]
9. Advise the patient to report any adverse, unusual, or painful sensations during the treatment. Improper application of therapeutic ultrasound can result in skin burns.

Initiation of the Treatment

1. Reduce the INTENSITY to zero before turning on the POWER.
2. Select the appropriate mode for the output. Use CONTINUOUS to increase the thermal effects of ultrasound application or PULSED output for nonthermal effects. The more acute the injury or the more active the inflammation process, the lower the duty cycle that is used.
3. Ensure that the WATT METER displays the appropriate output for the type of treatment.
4. Set the TIMER to the appropriate treatment length, but treat an area no larger than two to three times the size of the unit's ERA. The actual duration of the treatment depends on the desired effects of the treatment, the output intensity, and the body area being treated. Nonthermal effects require a shorter treatment duration than thermal effects. Refer to Figure 8–6 for the approximate times required to reach various therapeutic heating levels.
5. Begin slowly moving the sound head over the medium and depress the START button to begin the treatment session. Units having low BNR may be moved at a slower rate than those with a higher BNR.
6. Slowly increase the INTENSITY to the appropriate level while keeping the sound head moving and in contact with the patient's body, immersion bath, or coupling bladder.
7. Move the sound head at a moderate pace (4 cm

Analog: A readout on a continuously variable scale. A clock with hands is a type of analog display.

per second or slower) using firm, yet not strong, overlapping strokes.[79]

8. If periosteal pain is experienced, move the sound head at a faster rate, use a reduced duty cycle, or lower the intensity. If the pain continues, discontinue the treatment.

9. If the gel begins to wear away or if the sound head begins sticking on the skin, depress the PAUSE button and apply more gel.

Phonophoresis Application

1. For phonophoresis, preheating of the area to be treated is recommended to decrease skin resistance and increase the absorption of the medication.[58]

2. Use only approved ultrasound transmission media. The direct coupling method is recommended because the efficacy of phonophoresis for the bladder method has not been established.

3. Ensure that the skin is well moistened; areas of dry skin should be avoided.

4. Apply ultrasound or moist heat or shave the area before treatment to improve the medication's ability to diffuse through the skin and into the tissues.

5. Position the extremity to encourage circulation.

6. Use a continuous output to maximize the effect of phonophoresis (unless the thermal effects of ultrasound are contraindicated).

7. Follow the procedures described in Initiation of the Treatment.

8. After treatment, cover the remaining medication with an occlusive dressing.[61]

Termination of the Treatment

1. Most units automatically terminate the production of ultrasound when the time expires. If this is not the case, or if the treatment is being terminated prematurely, the intensity must be reduced before removing the transducer from the medium.

2. Remove the remaining gel or water from the patient's skin.

3. To ensure continuity of treatment sessions, record the parameters used for this treatment in the individual's file; specifically, record the output frequency, intensity, duration, and duty cycle. A

running count of ultrasound treatments given for this condition should also be made.

4. Immediately initiate any post-treatment stretching.

■ Maintenance

Federal regulations require that therapeutic ultrasound units be recalibrated annually by an authorized service technician.

Daily Maintenance

Clean ultrasound head and transducer face as recommended by the manufacturer.

Monthly Maintenance

1. Check all electrical cords for tears, fraying, or kinks.

2. Check the sound head cable for tears, fraying, or kinks.

3. Clean the transmitter face as recommended by the manufacturer.

● Chapter Highlights

- The treatment area should be no larger than two to three times the size of the ultrasound unit's effective radiating area.

- A coupling medium is needed to apply ultrasound. Gels and lotions are used for regularly shaped areas. Irregularly shaped areas can be treated using the immersion or bladder method.

- Only approved ultrasound transmission media or degassed water should be used as a coupling agent.

- The sound head should be moved at approximately 5 cm/sec.

- A 1-MHz output is used for deep tissues. A 3-MHz output is used for superficial tissues.

- The rate of heating is greater for a 3-MHz output than that for a 1-MHz output.

- The duty cycle controls the proportion of thermal and nonthermal effects produced during the treatment.

- The higher the duty cycle, the greater the proportion of thermal effects.

- The amount of heating depends on the output intensity, treatment duration, and the duty cycle.

Chapter 9

Shortwave Diathermy

Shortwave diathermy is a high-frequency electrical current that produces deep heating within the body's tissues. Similar to therapeutic ultrasound, shortwave diathermy can be delivered in pulsed or continuous output modes to produce thermal and nonthermal effects within the tissues. Another type of diathermy, microwave diathermy, is not approved for clinical use in the United States and is not covered in detail in this chapter. Also refer to the basic physiological responses to heat described in Chapter 5.

Shortwave diathermy uses high-frequency electromagnetic energy (similar to broadcast radio waves) to produce deep heat within the tissues. The Federal Communications Commission has reserved the frequencies of 13.56, 27.12, and 40.68 MHz for medical use, with the 27.12 MHz (wavelength of 11 m) frequency being the most commonly used.[85] The energy delivered to the body is a high-frequency alternating electrical current, but the wavelength lacks the duration needed to depolarize motor or sensory nerves. One of two electromagnetic diathermies, shortwave is more prevalent in the treatment of musculoskeletal injuries than its counterpart, microwave diathermy (MWD) (Box 9–1).

The thermal effects of shortwave diathermy are similar to those described in Chapter 5 , but occur deeper in the tissues. Shortwave diathermy can also be applied in a nonthermal mode. The thermal and nonthermal effects are similar to therapeutic ultrasound, but shortwave diathermy does not reflect from bone and is less likely to create hotspots.[85] Shortwave diathermy also affects a significantly greater volume of tissue

than does ultrasound, roughly the size of a cereal bowl for shortwave diathermy compared with approximately the size of a ketchup packet for therapeutic ultrasound.[85]

Different forms of diathermy, a Greek word meaning "through heat," have been used since the late 1800s to treat a wide range of musculoskeletal conditions, diseases, and general medical conditions. The prevalence and popularity of shortwave diathermy and microwave diathermy (which was developed in the mid-1900s) has been cyclical. Leakage of the energy away from the intended target ("scatter") created concerns about patient and clinician safety that negatively impacted the use of these devices. Diathermy also has caused interference with electronic devices such as cell phones and computers.[86] Improved shielding, the ability to better focus the energy, and a more uniform control of the dosage have led to a renewed interest in shortwave diathermy as a clinical treatment. Shortwave diathermy is becoming a more frequently used alternative to therapeutic ultrasound because of its ability to heat a greater volume of tissue.

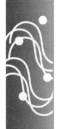

Box 9-1. Microwave Diathermy

Microwave diathermy (MWD) is a deep-heating modality that uses a magnetron to produce high-frequency electromagnetic energy that is converted into heat within the body. The Federal Communications Commission has reserved 915 Hz and 2450 Hz for the medical use of microwave diathermy. Although microwave diathermy is similar to shortwave diathermy, there are differences between the two.

Electrical fields are predominant with microwave diathermy, in contrast to the magnetic fields that predominate in shortwave diathermy. Heating occurs through a dipole response created within the cell membrane. The rotation of these molecules causes friction, resulting in heat production. Because of the spreading of the radio waves and absorption of the energy, superficial tissues tend to be heated more than deeper tissues. Although microwave diathermy produces biophysical effects similar to those of shortwave diathermy, the treatment is more superficial because the microwave radiation cannot penetrate the fat layer to the same extent as shortwave radiation. Because the energy is collected by the adipose tissue, the effects occur at about one third the depth of shortwave diathermy effects, but the energy is reflected at tissue interfaces, creating standing waves that can result in unsafe increases in tissue temperatures.

The indications and contraindications for the use of microwave diathermy are similar to those for shortwave diathermy. However, there can be no metal within the treatment field (4 feet from the pads, drums, or coils). This includes not only metal on the patient but implanted metal (e.g., plates, screws, **intrauterine devices ■**) as well.

Microwave diathermy is not commercially available in the United States, partially because the energy tends to be reflected and scattered into the surrounding environment and has been associated with an unacceptably high incidence of miscarriages among female therapists who regularly operate these units.[87]

■ Types of Shortwave Diathermy Application

There are two types of shortwave diathermy generators: (1) induction field generators and (2) capacitive field generators. The type of shortwave diathermy application is generator specific. The induction field method places the patient in the **electromagnetic field ■** (EMF) produced by the equipment. A capacitive field (also referred to as a "condenser field") shortwave diathermy unit uses the patient's tissues in the actual electrical circuit. The tissues' resistance to the flow of energy produces heating.

The type and depth of tissues affected and the subsequent increase in temperature varies between the two types of shortwave diathermy units. Induction generators produce the greatest amount of heat within the muscular layer directly beneath the coil. Capacitive generators affect tissues under each plate and selectively heat adipose tissue and bone (Fig. 9–1). Heating with capacitive shortwave diathermy is highly dependent on the tissue's constitution

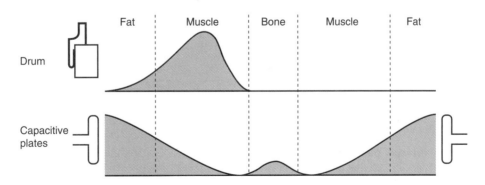

Figure 9–1. Heat distribution for shortwave diathermy, inductive drum and capacitive plate methods.

Electromagnetic field: The lines of force created by positive and negative poles.

Intrauterine device (IUD): A plastic or metal coil inserted within the uterus to prevent pregnancy.

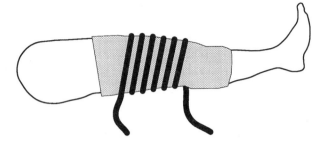

Figure 9-2. Shortwave Diathermy Application Through an Induction Cable. The cable is wrapped around the body part with equal spacing between the coils and an equal length leading to and from the generator. Cables that are too close together will concentrate the heat and may result in burns. Because of these risks cables are seldom used for treatment.

and is not recommended for patients who have a thick layer of adipose tissue. Inductive shortwave diathermy is not tissue-type specific and is considered to be safer.

Induction Field Diathermy

A high-frequency alternating current (see Chapter 11) flowing through a coiled cable creates an EMF that radiates away from the cable. The patient's tissues are placed in the EMF but are not an actual part of the circuit. Induction field shortwave diathermy, sometimes referred to as **magnetic field diathermy,** is delivered to the patient using either the cable method or the induction drum method.

The cable method involves wrapping a conducting cable around an extremity or coiling it and placing the cable on the patient, with terry cloth toweling buffering the cable from the patient's skin (Fig. 9–2). Because of the complexities of set-up and the potential of burns if done improperly, the cable method is infrequently used.

The more common drum applicators have the cable coiled within a plastic drum, which is then positioned over the target tissues (Fig. 9–3). Inductive drums, approximately 200 cm^2 in size, have built-in space plates to keep the source of the energy away from the patient's skin, decreasing the risk of burns.

Electromagnetic fields arise perpendicular from the cable, causing ions to oscillate and create eddy currents (Fig. 9–4). Friction caused by the movement of ions produces heat. The amount of heat produced depends on the strength of the EMF and the distance between the tissues and the source. As the distance between the source of the EMF and the tissues increases, the strength of the field decreases by the square of the distance (see **inverse square law** ■ in Appendix B).

The number and magnitude of eddy currents are based on the strength of the EMF and the electrical conductivity of the tissues. Most of the heat is produced near the source and just below the adipose tissue/muscle interface (see Fig. 9–1). Increased adipose tissue thickness will diminish the rate and magnitude of intramuscular heating.[88]

Capacitive Field Diathermy

In the capacitive field method of diathermy, the patient's tissues are placed between two electrodes and actually conduct the shortwave diathermy's electrical energy. Two insulated plates, electrodes, are placed on either side of the

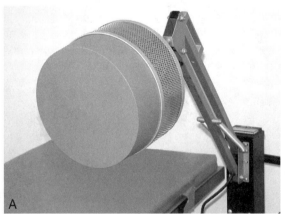
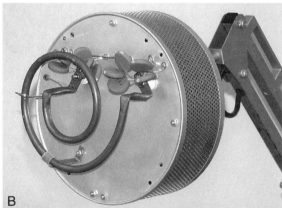

Figure 9-3. Shortwave Diathermy Induction Drum. (A) Plastic housing of the drum. (B) Drum removed to expose the coil that produces the electromagnetic field. The resulting electromagnetic field will produce a circular flow of energy similar to that of the coil. (Note: Do not remove the plastic housing.)

Inverse square law: A law stating that the intensity of the energy striking the tissues is proportional to the square of the distance between the source of the energy and the tissues: Energy received = Energy at the source ÷ Distance from the source squared.

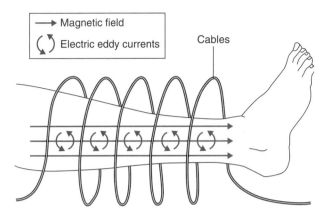

Figure 9-4. Circular electrical fields—eddy currents—form in the presence of an electromagnetic field. The subsequent molecular oscillation produces tissue heating.

site being treated. When an alternating current is applied to the circuit, the plates will always have opposite electrical charges, creating a strong electrical force between them. The flow of electrical energy passes through the tissues as a series circuit, which acts as an electrical resistor and produces frictional heating. Those tissues that present the most electrical resistance produce the most heat. Unlike the inductive technique, capacitive shortwave diathermy heats the body on each side.

The current flows along the path of least resistance, concentrating the heat in the superficial tissues and less in the deep tissues. Adipose tissue is a poor **conductor** ■ of electrical energy, so this layer will insulate the underlying tissues, yielding more heating in the skin than in the muscle. The capacitive method is not recommended for patients who have a large layer of adipose tissue.

The strength of the EMF is closest to the plates and weakest in the middle. The intensity near the plates causes more intense superficial heating than the magnetic field method, occurring at depths of 2.5 to 5 cm but is uneven because of differences in the electrical resistance posed by various tissue types. Altering the distance between the plates and the skin helps maintain superficial temperature within a safe range.

Heat is produced by the **dipole** ■ effect. Dipole molecules, molecules having no net electrical charge but having oppositely charged ends, are randomly arranged within the tissues. When they are exposed to the intense electrical field produced by the diathermy unit, the molecules rotate in the opposite direction of their charge. Positively charged molecules move toward the negative pole, and negatively charged molecules move toward the positive pole (Fig 9–5). The number of times the molecules rotate each second is based on the frequency of the current. High-

frequency currents such as those used in shortwave diathermy cause a great deal of rotation that produces kinetic energy, which is then released as heat within the tissues.

Capacitive shortwave diathermy is administered using air space plate electrodes or pad electrodes. Most contemporary capacitive units use air space plates. To provide uniform heating, pad electrodes require even contact pressure and be a uniform distance from the skin, otherwise burns may occur. To prevent the density of energy from becoming too great, these electrodes must be spaced at least their diameter apart.

Air space electrodes are similar to induction drums in that metallic coils or plates are shielded by a nonconductive material such as plastic (see Fig. 9–3). An electrical charge builds on each plate until it discharges to the opposite one. The number of times this occurs in each second is based on the unit's output frequency. A unit of 27.12 MHz would repeat this cycle 27,120,000 times per second.

To ensure even heating, the electrodes must be placed an equal distance from the skin on opposite sides of the body part, with the conducting plate typically about 3 cm from the skin (Fig. 9–6). A method of spacing the electrodes, usually an adjustment between the insulating cover and the electrode, helps to ensure precise placement. Uneven spacing can cause uneven heating, with more heat accumulation on the side where the electrode is closer.

(A) Tissue Ions Before Application of Electromagnetic Energy

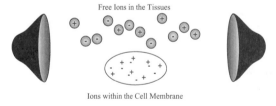

Free Ions in the Tissues

Ions within the Cell Membrane

(B) Ionic Reaction to Electromagnetic Energy

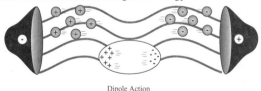

Dipole Action

Figure 9-5. **Dipole Response to an Electromagnetic Field.** *(A)* Tissue ions before the application of electromagnetic energy. (B) Ionic reaction to electromagnetic energy. The ions move toward the pole having the opposite electrical charge.

Conductor (electrical): A material having the ability to transmit electricity. Conductors have many free electrons and provide relatively little resistance to electrical flow. Within the body, tissues having a high water content are considered conductors.

Dipole: A pair of equal and opposite charges separated by a distance.

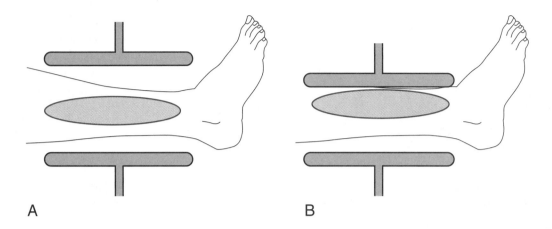

Figure 9–6. **Heating Using Capacitive Pads.** (A) Plates are spaced evenly from the tissue, resulting in even heating. (B) If the plates are unequally spaced (note the top electrode is closer to the skin than the bottom electrode), more heating will occur under the electrode that is closer to the skin.

■ Modes of Application

Shortwave diathermy can be delivered in either continuous or pulsed forms. Continuous shortwave diathermy increases subcutaneous tissue temperature, but its use is generally limited to chronic conditions. The output may also be pulsed, allowing this form of shortwave diathermy to be used on some acute and subacute conditions and preventing tissue temperatures from increasing too fast or too high.

The amount of heating that occurs is based on the total amount of power (measured in watts) and the ratio between the length of the "on" pulse and the duration of the "off" cycle. Pulsed output allows for increased treatment intensities and longer treatment durations than continuous shortwave diathermy application.[89] Unlike therapeutic ultrasound, pulsed output can be used to produce thermal effects, **so the term "pulsed" must not be confused with "nonthermal."**

Pulsed shortwave diathermy (PSWD) is referred to by several other names, including: pulsed electromagnetic fields (PEF), pulsed electromagnetic energy (PEME), and pulsed radiofrequency radiation (PRFR). Nonthermal effects occur when a low average intensity, short pulse duration, and low duty cycle are used. Heat is still generated within the tissues, but the tissues are rapidly cooled by the influx of new, relatively cool blood before heat accumulates.

Regardless of what it is called, PSWD operates by interrupting the continuous output at an interval determined by the pulse frequency creating burst trains similar to those used in electrotherapy (see p 213). Decreasing the pulse frequency decreases the average amount of power delivered to the body during a given period of time. The higher the pulse frequency, the greater the amount of tissue heating that occurs.

Thermal effects are obtained when the total amount of

energy delivered to the patient's body is greater than 38 watts and a high pulse frequency is used.[90] Unlike therapeutic ultrasound, the energy produced by shortwave diathermy generators is not reflected by bone or other tissues and therefore does not create standing waves.

■ Biophysical Effects of Shortwave Diathermy Application

High-frequency electromagnetic energy (greater than 10 MHz) passing through the patient's body is absorbed by the tissues. The rate of energy absorption per unit of area tissue is described as the **specific absorption rate**. The friction caused by the movement of ions produces the heating effect. Free ions within the treatment field are attracted to the pole having the opposite charge and are repelled from the pole having the like charge. Some molecules have ions that are capable of moving only within the cell membrane, causing a dipole action in which the ions within the membrane align themselves along the charges, or creating eddy currents (see Figs. 9–4 and 9–5).[91]

The heating effects occur as a result of friction between the moving ions and the surrounding tissues, and are similar to those associated with therapeutic ultrasound (Table 9–1). Nonthermal effects are obtained when a low-output power or a low-duty cycle, or both, are used.

Nonthermal Effects

Nonthermal effects are obtained by using a low number of pulses, short pulse duration, and a low average output intensity and an output of less than 38 W. Because heat is not produced, nonthermal shortwave diathermy application is advocated for the use of acute trauma and postsurgical treatment.[89, 90, 92]

Nonthermal effects are thought to be caused by

TABLE 9-1   Comparison of Thermal Ultrasound and Shortwave Diathermy

	Ultrasound	*Shortwave Diathermy*
Type of Energy	Acoustical	Electromagnetic
Tissue Heated	Collagen-rich	C: Adipose tissue, skin
		I: Muscle, blood vessels
Volume of tissue heated	Small (20 cm^2)	Large (200 cm^2)
Temperature increase	1 MHz: More than 6.3°F (3.5°C)	C: More than 7°F (3.9°C) (Adipose tissue)
	3 MHz: More than 14.9°F (8.3°C)	I: More than 18°F (10°C) (Intramuscular tissue)
Heat retention	Short (approximately 3 minutes)	Long (approximately 9 minutes)

C: capacitive method
I: inductive method

changes in the way that ions bind to the cell membrane and changes in cellular function caused by the EMF. The nonthermal effects of shortwave diathermy include increased microvascular perfusion, activation of fibroblast growth factors, and increased macrophage activity.[93, 94] Nonthermal shortwave diathermy has been reported to promote edema reduction.

Thermal Effects

The primary advantage of shortwave diathermy is the relatively large volume of tissue it can heat. The heating characteristics of shortwave diathermy are similar to those of ultrasound, but the heat is retained three times longer following the treatment than with ultrasound.[9, 95] However, capacitive shortwave diathermy is less effective on those persons who have a large amount of subcutaneous fat.

Inductive Method

Induction field shortwave diathermy preferentially heats tissues that are good electrical conductors, such as muscle and blood vessels. Adipose tissue is not substantially heated by induction fields because an electrical current is not actually passed through the tissues (see Fig. 9–1). Induction field diathermy is now the most common form of shortwave unit currently being marketed.[85]

An inductive drum heats an area approximately equal to its face, reaching peak temperatures approximately 15 min into the treatment and can increase the temperature of muscle at a depth of 1.2 cm by more than 18°F (10°C).[88] A 10-minute treatment increases subcutaneous tissue temperatures 5.0°F (2.8°C).[9] The most intense heating is at the center of the drum, with slightly lower temperatures (approximately 20 percent less) around the periphery caused by the tissues losing heat via conduction to the surrounding tissues.[9]

Capacitive Method

Capacitive field shortwave diathermy preferentially heats tissues that are not good electrical conductors, such as the skin and adipose tissue. The capacitive method can increase skin temperature approximately 4.3°F (2.4°C) and intra-articular temperatures 2.5°F (1.4°C).[96] Structures with high water content, such as adipose tissue, blood, and muscle, are selectively heated at depths of 2 to 5 cm.

Local tissue temperature may reach 107°F (41.7°C), but the subcutaneous fat layer dissipates a significant portion of the energy. This leads to a secondary heating of the superficial muscle layer by heat conducted from the adipose tissue The amount of intramuscular temperature increase compares favorably with that seen during ultrasound application, producing an increase of more than 7°F (3.9°C).[95, 97]

● EFFECTS ON
The Injury Response Process

The healing properties of shortwave diathermy are similar to those of other forms of heat application but tend to occur deeper within the tissues and are based on the treatment intensity, the number of pulses per second, and the pulse duration. The biophysical effects of shortwave diathermy are also similar to those of therapeutic ultrasound (see Chapter 7). Also refer to the general effects of heat in Chapter 5 (p 119).

Inflammation

The nonthermal effects of shortwave diathermy are believed to alter the rate of diffusion across the cell membrane, whereas the thermal effects increase the rate of cell metabolism. As inductive shortwave diathermy preferentially heats muscle, it is reasonable to expect that the Q10 effect is enhanced deep within the muscle. An 18°F (10°C) increase in intramuscular temperature will approximately double the rate of cell metabolism.

The cellular level effects of shortwave diathermy combined with increased blood flow result in the increased delivery and concentration of white blood cells (WBC). Increased cell membrane permeability assists in the removal of cellular debris and metabolic toxins that may have collected in the area.[92]

Blood and Fluid Dynamics

As with all thermal modalities, the heat produced by shortwave diathermy results in a vasodilation that increases blood flow, increased capillary filtration, increased capillary pressure, and increased oxygen perfusion.[98] Because of its deep-heating characteristics, increased blood flow, increased fibroblastic activity, increased collagen deposition, and new capillary growth are stimulated deeper in the tissues than superficial heating agents.[99] The depth of effective heating and volume of tissue affected also makes shortwave diathermy useful in the resolution of hematoma.[100]

Tissue Elasticity

Shortwave diathermy is capable of reaching vigorous heating levels (5.4°F/3°C) at depths greater than 2 cm. Tissue elongation is obtained by altering the viscoelastic properties of collagen-rich fibrous tissues by increasing the temperature and applying an external force to elongate the tissues.[9] Tissues heated by shortwave diathermy retain heat for longer periods than tissues heated by therapeutic ultrasound, increasing the post-treatment stretching window.

Single treatment sessions of heat and stretch are not sufficient for elongating tissues.[101] Repeated sessions of combined heat and stretching are needed to obtain actual elongation of muscles and tendons.[102] Any increases in range of motion seen following a single treatment are most probably related to decreased muscle tone.

Wound Healing

Pulsed shortwave diathermy increases WBC infiltration and increases the rate of phagocytosis, resulting in more rapid healing time and decreased need for pain medications.[92] The number and quality of mature collagen bundles are increased in the treated area, the result of increased adenosine triphosphatase (ATP) activity, and the proportion of necrosed muscle fibers decreases.[103] Superficial open wounds should not be treated because of the associated moisture.

■ Contraindications to Shortwave Diathermy

Technological advancements have made shortwave diathermy a relatively safe and effective modality, although the electromagnetic radiation creates several contraindications and precautions to its use. This list is also further complicated by individual manufacturing techniques may overcome some contraindications or present unique ones (refer to Chapter 10, At a Glance: Shortwave Diathermy).

The application of thermal shortwave diathermy follows is held to the same contraindications of heat application in general, including acute inflammation, ischemia, and hemorrhage (see Table 5–9). Questions regarding the suitability of shortwave diathermy for the condition being treated should be referred to the patient's physician.

Metal within the output field is often a contraindication to the use of shortwave diathermy, including metal on clothing, jewelry, and so on (see Table 10–3). Circular metal, such as that found with some internal fixation devices and other implants, bedsprings, etc. is always contraindicated because of the potential to create a second EMF within the metal. Metal tends to heat more rapidly than skin and other tissues, thus increasing the risk of burns. Certain forms of pulsed shortwave diathermy may be used over some metal implants. Refer to the manufacturer's operating instructions to determine how to handle metal in the treatment field.

The presence of an implanted cardiac pacemaker is an absolute contraindication to the use of shortwave diathermy. The EMF produced by the diathermy unit can disrupt the pacemaker's rhythm, and the implanted metal will overheat.

The presence of moisture in the EMF will increase the rate of heating and will cause overheating of the skin. Moist dressings, adhesive tape, and skin creams must be removed before the treatment. If moisture collects during the treatment, pause the shortwave diathermy output and dry the skin. Wet towels must not be used to attempt to provide moist heat during the treatment.

Shortwave diathermy applied through the skull using capacitive plates, transcerebral application, should be performed with extreme caution. The energy passing through the skull can result in headaches, dizziness, and vomiting. The eyes, frontal sinuses, and ears are particularly sensitive to shortwave diathermy. Contact lenses must be removed before the application of shortwave diathermy to the face or head, or both.

Application of shortwave diathermy to the female pelvic region (including use of vaginal electrodes), abdomen, and lumbar spine may increase menstrual flow. Likewise, the application of shortwave diathermy to these regions during pregnancy or suspected pregnancy is an absolute contraindication.

Use over unfused epiphyseal plates must be done with caution. Although there are no documented cases, repeated overheating of the growth plate can result in nonunion or malunion of the **physis ■**.

■ Controversies in Treatment

Several recent studies[9, 86, 90, 97, 101] have revalidated the thermal effects of shortwave diathermy, although the

---

Physis: The growth plate of bone.

inductive technique has been the focus of this research. There remains a limited amount of published research that investigates the efficacy of shortwave diathermy in the treatment of musculoskeletal conditions. Similar to the controversies associated with therapeutic ultrasound, other published studies suffer from a lack of randomized control trials and investigated a relatively small number of patient problems.

Several shortwave diathermy units are capable of producing a pulsed output. On some models, the pulses are used to regulate the amount of heat generated. Low-intensity treatments (either by decreasing the output power and/or using a low number of pulses) have been promoted to produce nonthermal (mechanical) effects similar to those associated with nonthermal therapeutic ultrasound. However, a review of the literature produces no studies that investigate the efficacy of nonthermal shortwave diathermy.

Because electromagnetic energy is produced in relatively high quantities by shortwave diathermy units, there are potential hazards associated with repeated exposure to diathermy radiation, especially for the clinician. Harm associated with exposure to microwave diathermy is well documented, and many of these effects have also been attributed to shortwave diathermy. Although care should be taken to avoid repeated exposure to shortwave diathermy energy, this modality does not have the scatter and leakage of radiation found with microwave diathermy. This is especially true with newer models.

● Chapter Highlights

- Shortwave diathermy uses electromagnetic energy that is similar to broadcast radio waves. The most commonly used frequency is 27.12 MHz.
- There are two types of shortwave diathermy: The induction field method places the patient's tissues in a magnetic field. The capacitive field method uses the patient's tissues to form an electrical circuit.
- Shortwave diathermy can be applied in continuous or pulsed mode. Unlike ultrasound, pulsed shortwave diathermy is often used for heating.
- The induction field method most often is performed using an induction drum, but coiled cables may also be used. Induction shortwave diathermy preferentially heats muscle and other structures that are good electrical conductors.
- Capacitive shortwave diathermy is most commonly applied using pairs of electrode plates. This method selectively heats tissues that are poor electrical conductors such as adipose tissue.
- The heating effects are similar to those of therapeutic ultrasound, but affect a larger volume of tissue.
- The presence of metal within the treatment field is often a contraindication to the use of shortwave diathermy.

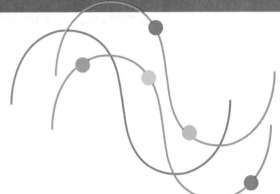

Chapter 10

Clinical Application of Shortwave Diathermy

This chapter describes the general procedures used to set up and apply shortwave diathermy. Because of the variability between units, the instruction manual for your particular brand and model must be the clinical guide for the set-up and application of shortwave diathermy. The information presented here is intended to serve only as a guide.

Shortwave diathermy application involves placing the patient in the unit's electromagnetic field for the induction method or directly in the electrical path for the capacitive method. The body then acts as the radio receiver, converting the energy into heat.

Shortwave diathermy units are capable of producing up to 1000 watts of output energy. However, the output intensity does not reflect the amount of energy that is actually absorbed by the tissues. Unlike superficial heating agents or therapeutic ultrasound, shortwave diathermy is capable of penetrating through all tissue layers. The tissues affected depend on the type of shortwave diathermy being applied (inductive or capacitive field method), the location of the tissues relative to the source of the energy, and the composition of the tissues (see Fig. 9–1).

Medical diathermy, including shortwave diathermy, is regulated under Chapter V, Subchapter C—Electronic Product Radiation Control (Sections 531 to 542) of the Federal Food, Drug, and Cosmetic Act. The Center for Devices and Radiological Health is the U.S. Food and Drug Administration (FDA) center responsible for the oversight of these devices. The exact regulations can be located in Title 21, Code of Federal Regulations, Parts 1000 to 1050.

■ Treatment Dosages

The general output parameters for pulsed shortwave diathermy treatment doses are presented in Table 10–1, but dosage techniques and protocol are generator-specific. The output intensity for thermal treatments is largely based on the patient's report of heat. Parameters for vigorous heating using pulsed shortwave diathermy are presented in Table 10–2.

TABLE 10–1	Dosage Parameters Used with Pulsed Shortwave Diathermy			
Dose	*Temperature Sensation*	*Indications*	*Pulse Width*	*Pulse Rate*
NT	No detectable warmth	Acute trauma Acute inflammation Edema reduction	65 msec	100–200 pps
1	Mild warmth	Subacute inflammation	100 msec	800 pps
2	Moderate warmth	Pain syndromes Muscle spasm Chronic inflammation To increase blood flow	200 msec	800 pps
3	Vigorous heating	Stretching collagen-rich tissues	400 msec	800 pps

NT = Nonthermal

■ Set-up and Application

Only the induction drum and capacitive plate methods of shortwave diathermy set-up and application will be described in this section (Fig. 10–1). Because of their relatively difficult set-up procedure and potential harm, namely burns, associated with their inappropriate use, inductive shortwave cables and capacitive electrode pads are becoming uncommon and are not discussed in this section.

Instrumentation

This section presents a list of controls that are commonly found on shortwave diathermy units (Fig. 10–2). Because of the wide range of generator types and the array of manufacturers, this list serves only as an orientation. Refer to the operator's manual of the specific unit you are using for precise details. Also note that dual head shortwave diathermy units may have dual controls.

Shortwave diathermy units that use cables, either as therapeutic electrodes to be placed on the body or as electrical leads to inductive drums or capacitive plates require particular attention. Therapeutic cables (or their leads) will overheat and rapidly burn the patient if they are allowed to cross over each other or are spaced too closely together. On some drum or capacitive plate units the leads are "hot,"

meaning that they can cause burns if they are placed too close together and may potentially cause an electrical short if they come into contact with each other. Consult the unit's operator's manual for specific details regarding the intricacies of the cables.

Master Power Switch: Initiates current flow to the generator as a whole. Dual head, dual control units may have individual power switches for each.

Output Intensity: Also referred to as "power" on some units. Adjusts the amount of energy delivered to the patient.

Patient Interrupt Switch (Safety Switch): A pushbutton switch held by the patient that allows immediate termination of the treatment in the event of pain, burning, or anxiety. The Interrupt Switch must not be allowed to enter the shortwave diathermy treatment field. If the right extremity is being treated, have the patient hold the switch in the left hand and vice versa.

Pause: Interrupts the treatment (while preserving the remaining treatment time) to allow repositioning of the patient, removing perspiration, or other similar situations.

Pulse Rate (Pulse Frequency): Sets the number of pulses per second (PPS) for the output. Higher PPS produce increased thermal effects.

Start/Stop: Initiates or terminates the treatment. Dual head generators may have separate "start/stop" switches for each head.

Treatment Timer: Sets the duration of the treatment. Some units may use the treatment timer to "start" the treatment: turning the timer past zero initiates the treatment.

Tuning: Adjusts the output resonance to match the patient's tissues. Tuning maximizes the energy exchange between the generator and the patient. Some units will shut off if an out-of-tune state is detected.

TABLE 10–2	Typical Parameters—Pulsed Shortwave Diathermy
Parameter	*Setting*
Output Mode	Pulsed
Bursts per Second	800
Burst Duration	400 microseconds
Interburst Interval	850 microseconds
Output Intensity	RMS amplitude of 150 W RMS output of 48 w per bust

At a Glance: **Shortwave Diathermy**

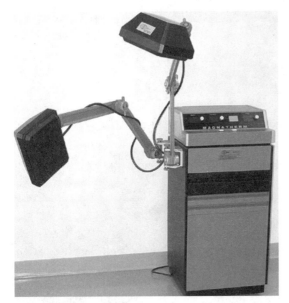

Description

- High-frequency electrical currents produce deep heating to a large volume of tissue. Shortwave diathermy is often indicated in cases where thermal therapeutic ultrasound would be appropriate, but the size of the target tissues is too large. Shortwave diathermy is used for:
- Pain reduction
- Decreasing muscle spasm
- Increasing range of motion
- Treatment of trigger points
- Reducing joint contractures

Primary Effects

THERMAL EFFECTS
- Deep heating
- Increased blood flow
- Increased extensibility of collagen-rich tissues
- Increased cell metabolism
- Muscular relaxation
- Possible changes in some enzyme reactions

NONTHERMAL EFFECTS
- Edema reduction
- **Lymphedema** reduction
- Healing of superficial, open wounds
- **Venous stasis ulcers**

Treatment Duration

At moderate intensities, treatments may be given for 20 to 30 minutes and may be repeated as needed for 2 weeks. When higher treatment temperatures are used, decrease the duration of treatment to 15 minutes and apply on alternate days.

Indications

- Acute and chronic pain
- Subacute and chronic inflammatory conditions in deep-tissue layers
- Chronic inflammatory conditions (bursitis, tendinitis, **myositis**, **osteoarthritis**, etc.)
- Range of motion restrictions
- Muscle spasm
- Edema reduction
- Over fracture sites
- Hematomas and contusions

Contraindications

In addition to the general contraindications to the use of heat (see Table 5-9)
- Metal implants or metals such as jewelry or body piercings: The metal collects and concentrates the energy, potentially causing burns. Pulsed SWD possibly may be used over metal implants that is not a circular wire (consult the unit's user's manual).
- Cardiac pacemakers
- Ischemic areas: The increased metabolic rate increases the need for oxygen, causing further hypoxia.
- Peripheral vascular disease
- Perspiration and moist dressings: The water collects and concentrates the heat.
- Tendency to hemorrhage, including menstruation.
- Pregnancy
- Fever
- Sensory loss
- Cancer
- Areas of particular sensitivity:
  - Epiphyseal plates in children
  - The genitals
  - Sites of infection
  - The abdomen with an implanted intrauterine device (IUD)
  - The eyes and face
  - Application through the skull

Precautions

- The skin exposed to the treatment should be covered by at least 0.5 inch of toweling.
- Do not allow perspiration to collect in the treatment field.
- Excessive amounts of adipose tissue overlying the treatment area can result in overheating the skin.
- It is difficult to heat only localized areas. Water pathways within the tissues dissipate heat formed in the treated area.
- Never allow the skin to come into direct contact with the heating unit or cables. Severe burns may result.
- If the cable method is used, do not allow them to touch each other. This may create a short circuit.
- If electrode pads are used, they must be spaced at least the distance of their width or diameter apart (e.g., if two 20-cm-diameter electrodes are used, they must be placed at least 20 cm apart).
- A deep, aching sensation may be a symptom of overheating the tissues.
- Overheating of the patient's tissues may cause tissue damage without any immediate signs. Deep-tissue burning can cause destruction of muscular tissue or subcutaneous fat necrosis.
- The electromagnetic energy is not localized to the treatment area, radiating 2 to 3 feet from the source of continuous SWD and 2 feet from the source of pulsed diathermy.[105] Clinicians may be placed in the field of this scattering radiation, possibly overexposing them to diathermy. A distance of 3 feet from the source of the energy should be maintained to ensure the operator's safety. Refer to the operator's manual for generator-specific information.
- Remove contact lenses when applying SWD around the head, face, or eyes.

Lymphedema: Swelling of the lymph nodes caused by blockage of the vessels by protein-rich substances.

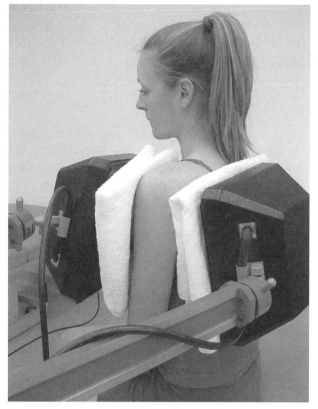

Figure 10–1. Dual Induction Drum Shortwave Diathermy. Twin drums allow for heating on both sides of the body. Note: Dual induction drums should not be confused with capacitive plates.

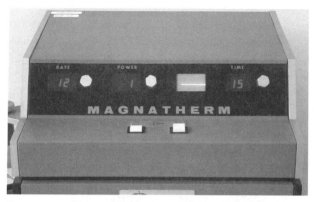

Figure 10–2. Shortwave Diathermy Control Panel. There is a significant amount of difference in the controls between makes and models.

Patient Preparation

1. Ensure that the patient is free of all contraindications to the use of shortwave diathermy.
2. Ensure that any implanted metals (e.g., internal fixation devices, sutures, body jewelry) are not contraindicated by the device (refer to the unit's operator's manual) or by the treatment protocol.
3. Remove all jewelry, clothing, coins, and other metallic items from the patient (Table 10–3).
4. For personal safety, the clinician should remove any rings, watches, bracelets, and so on.
5. There must be no metal within the immediate treatment area, approximately 1 meter for continuous output and 0.5 meters for a pulsed output.[85] The presence of metal will collect and concentrate the energy from the treatment in the same manner that an antenna collects radio waves.[104] Some manufacturers build metal-free tables for use with shortwave diathermy.
6. Keep the patient out of reach of any metal objects that can serve as a ground (e.g., outlets, pipes).
7. Clean and dry the body part. Water, skin oils, or cosmetics can increase superficial heat production.

TABLE 10–3	Precautions Against Metal Within the Field of Shortwave Diathermy	
In the Environment	*Near or on the Patient*	*In the Patient*
Beds	Jewelry	Orthodontic braces
Treatment tables	Body piercings	Dental fillings
Chairs	Earrings	Implanted fixation devices
Wheelchairs	Watches	External fixation devices
Metal stools	Metal in pockets (keys, etc.)	Metal heart valves
CPM units	Belt buckles	Artificial joints
Splints	Zippers	Metal IUDs
Braces	Metal underwire bras	Body piercings
Medical instruments	Hearing aids	Cardiac pacemakers
Electrical modalities		Implanted bone growth generators
		Phrenic pacers

CPM = continuous passive motion; IUDs = intrauterine devices.

8. Position the patient in the most appropriate manner for the body area being treated.
9. The patient must not come into contact with objects that are connected directly to the ground such as whirlpools, pipes, or electrical outlets (see Box 4–5).
10. To encourage venous return, elevate the extremity being treated.
11. Cover the area to be treated with a *dry* terry cloth towel. This provides spacing between the source of the shortwave diathermy and absorbs perspiration, both of which decrease the risk of burns. A portion of the treatment area must remain visible to check for burns during the treatment. Avoid any moisture buildup during the treatment because water tends to collect heat. The intensity must be turned to zero before drying the area.
12. Explain to the patient that mild warmth should be felt. Instruct the patient to inform you if any unusual sensations are experienced. During thermal treatments, only a mild to moderate warmth should be reported.

Patient/Generator Tuning

"Tuning" refers to the resonance between the generator's output and the body's ability to absorb this energy. If more than half of the available power is used to pass the energy through the patient's tissue, the set-up is out of tune and must be calibrated. Older units require that tuning be done manually by the clinician. Newer units are capable of automatically tuning their output to the patient's resonance.

The following section provides an overview for the method used to tune a shortwave diathermy unit manually. Refer to the user's manual and follow the manufacturer's instructions for the specific model being used.

1. Position the electrodes over the patient.
2. Increase the output intensity to approximately 40 percent of the maximum.
3. Adjust (increase or decrease) the TUNING control until the output meter reaches its peak, then decrease the TUNING control to the patient's comfort.
4. A unit is in tune when less than half of the maximum output is used. Some units automatically shut off if more than 50 percent of the maximum output is used. If this occurs, the unit must be tuned again.

Application (General Set-up)

1. Turn the unit on; allow it to warm up if necessary.

2. Some units must be tuned to allow for maximal energy transfer.

Inductive Drum

1. If indicated by the manufacturer's instructions, place a folded layer between the body part and the drum.
2. Position the drum approximately 0.5 to 1 inch above the toweling. There is a direct relationship between the distance of the drum from the patient and the intensity of energy required for the treatment.
3. The surface of the drum must be parallel to the skin surface being treated, otherwise the skin closest to the drum will be overheated, the **cosine law** ■ (see Appendix B) (Fig. 10–3).
4. If appropriate, select the appropriate PULSE RATE.

Capacitive Plate Set-up

1. If indicated by the unit, cover the area to be treated with a towel.
2. Adjust the plates so that they are parallel to the body part, approximately 3 cm from the skin.
3. Both plates must be placed at an equal distance above the tissue. If a spacer is used for this purpose it must be removed before the treatment is started.

Both Methods

1. Instruct the patient not to move until the machine is shut off.
2. Set the TIMER to the desired treatment duration.

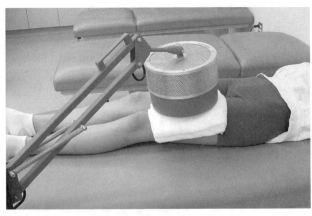

Figure 10–3. **Induction Drum.** Use of shortwave diathermy on the quadriceps muscle group. Note the toweling between the face of the induction drum and the skin.

Cosine law: A law stating that, as an angle deviates away from 90 degrees, the effective energy is reduced by the multiple of the cosine of the angle: Effective energy = Energy × Cosine of the angle. A deviation of ±10 degrees is considered within acceptable limits for therapeutic treatments.

3. Increase the intensity until the patient feels mild warmth.
4. If the electrodes must be moved or if it becomes necessary to dry the area, return the INTENSITY to zero before making any adjustments.
5. The patient must not be left unattended and should be checked regularly. Observe the skin for signs of burns, and inquire as to any unusual sensations. Adjust the INTENSITY, PULSE RATE, or electrode placement as necessary.

Terminating the Treatment

1. After the treatment, return the intensity dial to zero and shut off the unit.
2. Inspect the skin for signs of burns or other abnormal treatment outcomes.
3. Record the treatment parameters in the patient's file.

Maintenance

The production of electromagnetic energy may require additional health and safety precautions because of worker exposure to radiation.

After Each Use
Clean the face of the drum or cables using a cleaning agent recommended by the manufacturer.

At Regular Intervals
Inspect electrical cords for kinks, cuts, and frays.

Annually
The unit must be serviced and calibrated by a qualified service technician.

● Chapter Highlights

- The set-up and application of shortwave diathermy depends on the make, model, and technique being used. Become familiar with the unit's operator's manual before beginning the treatment.
- Inductive shortwave diathermy is applied using an inductive drum or cables.
- Capacitive shortwave diathermy is applied using electrode plates or, less commonly, electrode pads.
- The source of the shortwave diathermy must strike the patient's body at a right angle and be a constant distance from the skin. Otherwise, burning may occur. Avoid metal in the treatment area, including within or on the patient and the clinician.
- Do not allow water (perspiration) to collect on the patient during treatment. The presence of water can result in more rapid heating.
- The report of heat is the primary clinical guide for applying thermal treatments.
- Nonthermal treatments can be applied by using a low number of pulses or an output of less than 38 W.

Case Study: Chapter Case Study

Carlos is a 32-year-old man with marked muscle spasms of his lumbar musculature. He has had progressive symptoms for the past 10 years, but recently he has had significant pain with forward flexion. He also has a lot of difficulty standing up after a prolonged period of a flexed posture, such as with digging or shoveling. He has a 4-×-3-inch gash from getting hit with pipe on the job in the small of his back. Evaluation findings show marked spasm throughout his lumbar paraspinals and 25- to 50-percent limitation in trunk range of motion.

1. What are the best thermal agents to consider for this patient?
2. What are the physiological effects on the injury response cycle from the application of this thermal agent?
3. Why are heat packs, ice, and ultrasound less than optimal choices for this patient?
4. What are the clinical symptoms that you hope to address with this intervention?
5. Name three indications and three precautions for this modality.

Case Study: Continuation of Case Study from Section One

(The following discussion relates to Case Study 2, found on pages 93 to 96 of Section One)

Pulsed ultrasound (20-percent duty cycle) could be incorporated into our patient's program to reduce pain and promote tissue extensibility. Alterations in the cell membrane permeability bring about changes in the nerves' electrical activity, reportedly increasing the pain threshold, and assist in the healing process.

When applied with a continuous output (100-percent duty cycle), ultrasound preferentially heats collagen-rich tissues and assists in reducing muscle spasm. When vigorously heated (3° to 5°C increase), tissue extensibility can be increased. To obtain the maximal benefits of tissue elongation, the trapezius must be placed on stretch during the treatment and any flexibility exercises must be performed within 3 minutes after the conclusion of the treatment.

The treatment area would be limited to an area two to three times the size of the sound head; the output frequency would depend on the depth of our patient's trauma. The intensity and duration of the treatment would be sufficient to produce a vigorous heating effect. Recall that use of ultrasound is a precaution to ultrasound application, so extra care must be taken when applying these treatments.

● ● ● Section Three Quiz

1. When applying ultrasound with metered output of 4 W and an indicated beam nonuniformity ratio (BNR) of 4, the highest intensity in the beam is:
   A. 4 W
   B. 8 W
   C. 16 W
   D. 32 W

2. Which of the following is not an indication for the use of ultrasound?
   A. Scar tissue
   B. Infection
   C. Warts
   D. Trigger points

3. The spreading of an ultrasound beam is a result of the ___ of the waves:
   A. Attenuation
   B. Collimation
   C. Thermal synthesis
   D. Divergence

4. A metered reading of 2 W per square centimeter passing through a sound head having an effective radiating area of 10 cm² produces an output of ___ total watts.
   A. 5 W
   B. 10 W
   C. 15 W
   D. 20 W

5. Reflection of ultrasonic energy occurs least between:
   A. Water and soft tissue
   B. Soft tissue and fat
   C. Soft tissue and bone
   D. Soft tissue and air

6. All of the following are nonthermal (mechanical) effects of ultrasound except:
   A. Increased extensibility of collagen-rich structures
   B. Increased blood flow
   C. Synthesis of protein
   D. Increased cell membrane permeability

7. When treating the patellar tendon with ultrasound, what output frequency should be used?
   A. 1 MHz
   B. 2 MHz
   C. 3 MHz
   D. It does not matter.

8. When cells are exposed to high-pressure ridges, their size
   A. Increases
   B. Decreases

9. Ultrasound that is pulsed so that it flows for 0.5 seconds and does not flow for 1 second is operating at a percent duty cycle.
   A. 33
   B. 50
   C. 66
   D. 133

10. Determining the treatment duration is most closely dependent on what other output characteristic?
    A. Duty cycle
    B. Frequency
    C. Coupling method
    D. Intensity

11. To promote extensibility the tissues must be stretched within how many minutes after the conclusion of the treatment?
    A. 1
    B. 3
    C. 10
    D. 30

12. Standard therapeutic ultrasound generators can be employed to assist in the healing of fractures.
    A. True
    B. False

13. Which of the following substances transmits the highest percentage of ultrasonic energy relative to water?
    A. White petrolatum gel
    B. Eucerin cream
    C. Ultrasound transmission gel
    D. Hydrocortisone powder (1%) in US gel

14. During shortwave diathermy application, high-frequency electromagnetic energy is changed to heat by the process of:
    A. Convection
    B. Conduction
    C. Conversion
    D. Collection

15. Which of the following types of shortwave diathermy application places the athlete's tissues within the generator's physical circuit?
    A. Capacitive method
    B. Inductive method

16. When using a shortwave diathermy induction drum, the drum should be positioned ___ in from the patient's skin.
    A. 1 in
    B. 2 in
    C. 4 in
    D. 8 in

17. The energy from a shortwave diathermy unit may scatter as much as _____ feet from the source.
    A. 1 ft
    B. 3 ft
    C. 6 ft
    D. 9 ft

18. Which form of shortwave diathermy should NOT be used over large areas of adipose tissue?
    A. Capacitive method
    B. Inductive method

19. What four factors determine a medication's ability to diffuse through the tissues?
    A.
    B.
    C.
    D.

20. Complete the following table comparing and contrasting therapeutic ultrasound and shortwave diathermy:

	Ultrasound	Shortwave Diathermy
Type of energy		
Tissue heated		
Volume of tissue heated		
Temperature increase		
Heat retention		

References

1. Chen, QX: A new laser-ultrasound transducer for medical applications. Ultrasonics 32:309, 1994.
2. Ziskin, MC, et al: Therapeutic ultrasound. In Michlovitz, S (ed): Thermal Agents in Rehabilitation, ed 2. FA Davis, Philadelphia, 1990, pp 134–169.
3. Draper, DO: Ten mistakes commonly made with ultrasound use: Current research sheds light on myths. Athletic Training: Sports Health Care Perspect 2:95, 1996.
4. Dyson, M, et al: Longwave ultrasound. Physiotherapy 81:40, 1999.
5. Ter Haar, G: Basic physics of therapeutic ultrasound. Physiotherapy 73:110, 1987.
6. Kitchen, SS and Partridge, CJ: A review of therapeutic ultrasound: I. Background, physiological effects and hazards. Physiotherapy 76:593, 1990.
7. Hayes, BT, et al: The differences between 1 MHz and 3 MHz ultrasound in the heating of subcutaneous tissues (abstract). J Athletic Training 36(S):S-92, 2001.
8. Schneider, NC, et al: 3 MHz continuous ultrasound can elevate tissue temperature at 3-cm depths (abstract). Phys Ther 81:A8, 2001.
9. Garrett, CL, et al: Heat distribution in the lower leg from pulsed short-wave diathermy and ultrasound treatments. J Athletic Training 35:50, 2000.
10. Draper, DO, et al: Rate of temperature increase in human muscle during 1 MHz and 3 MHz continuous ultrasound. J Orthop Sports Phys Ther 22:142, 1995.
11. Tiidus, PM, et al: Ultrasound treatment and recovery from eccentric-exercise-induced muscle damage. J Sport Rehabil 11:305, 2002.
12. Ferguson, BH: A Practitioner's Guide to the Ultrasonic Therapy Equipment Standard. U.S. Department of Health and Human Services, Public Health Service, Food and Drug Administration, Rockville, MD, 1985.
13. U.S. Department of Health and Human Services, Public Health Service: Guide for preparing product reports for ultrasonic therapy products. Food and Drug Administration, Center for Devices and Radiological Health, Rockville, MD, 1996. Available online at: http://www.fda.gov/cdrh/radhlth/pdf/ustrpt0p.pdf.
14. Draper, DO and Sunderland, S: Examination of the law of Grotthus-Draper: Does ultrasound penetrate subcutaneous fat in humans? J Athletic Training 38:246, 1993.
15. Dyson, M: Mechanisms involved in therapeutic ultrasound. Physiotherapy 73:116, 1987.
16. Baker, KG, et al: A review of therapeutic ultrasound: Biophysical effects. Phys Ther 81:1351, 2001.
17. Johns, LD: Nonthermal effects of therapeutic ultrasound: The frequency resonance hypothesis. J Athletic Training 37:293, 2002.
18. De Deyne, P and Kirsch-Volders, M: In vitro effects of therapeutic ultrasound on the nucleus of human fibroblasts. Phys Ther 72:629, 1995.
19. Adinno, MA, et al: Effect of free radical scavengers on changes in ion conductance during exposure to therapeutic ultrasound. Membrane Biochemistry 10:237, 1993.
20. Blinc, A, et al: Characterization of ultrasound-potentiated fibrinolysis in vitro. Blood 81:2636, 1993.
21. Francis, CW, et al: Enhancement of fibrinolysis in vitro by ultrasound. J Clin Invest 90:2063, 1992.
22. Byl, NN, et al: Low-dose ultrasound effects on wound healing: A controlled study with Yucatan pigs. Arch Phys Med Rehabil 73:656, 1992.
23. Holcomb, WR and Joyce, CJ: A comparison of the effectiveness of two commonly used ultrasound units (abstract). J Athletic Training 36(S):S-89, 2001.
24. Chan, AK, et al: Temperature changes in human patellar tendon in response to therapeutic ultrasound. J Athletic Training 33:130, 1998.
25. Draper, DO, et al: Hot-pack and 1-MHz ultrasound treatments have an additive effect on muscle temperature increase. 33:21, 1998.
26. Draper, DO, et al: Temperature changes in deep muscle of humans during ice and ultrasound therapies: An in vivo study. J Orthop Sports Phys Ther 21:153, 1995.
27. Draper, DO and Ricard, MD: Rate of temperature decay in human muscle following 3 MHz ultrasound: The stretching window revealed. J Athletic Training 30:304, 1995.
28. Weinberger, A and Lev, A: Temperature elevation of connective tissue by physical modalities. Crit Rev Phys Rehabil Med 3:121, 1991.
29. Heckman, JD, et al: Acceleration of tibial fracture-healing by non-invasive, low-intensity pulsed ultrasound. J Bone Joint Surg Am 76:26, 1994.
30. Cook, SD, et al: Acceleration of tibia and distal radius fracture healing in patients who smoke. Clin Orthop 337:198, 1997.
31. Azuma, Y, et al: Low-intensity pulsed ultrasound accelerates rat femoral fracture healing by acting on the various cellular reactions in the fracture callus. J Bone Miner Res 16:671, 2001.
32. Hadjiargyrou, M, et al: Enhancement of fracture healing by low intensity ultrasound. Clin Orthop 333(S):S216, 1998.
33. Tsunoda, M, et al: Low-intensity pulsed ultrasound initiates bone healing in rat nonunion fracture model. J Ultrasound Med, 20:197, 2001.
34. Wark, JD, et al: Low-intensity pulsed ultrasound stimulates bone-forming responses in UMR-106 cells. Biochem Biophys Res Commun 288:443, 2001.
35. Jensen, JE: Stress fracture in the world class athlete: A case study. Med Sci Sports Exerc 30:783, 1998.
36. Eck, JC, et al: Techniques for stimulating spinal fusion: Efficacy of electricity, ultrasound, and biologic factors in achieving fusion. Am J Orthop 30:535, 2001.
37. Reher, P, et al: Effect of ultrasound on the production of IL-8, basic FGF, and VEGF. Cytokine 11:416, 1999.
38. Mayr, E, et al: Ultrasound: An alternative healing method for nonunions? Arch Orthop Trauma Surg 120:1, 2000.
39. Emami, A, et al: No effect of low-intensity ultrasound on healing time of intramedullary fixed tibial fractures. J Orthop Trauma 13:252, 1999.
40. Zorlu, U, et al: Comparative study of the effect of ultrasound and electrostimulation on bone healing in rats. Am J Phys Med Rehabil 77:427, 1998.
41. Young, SR and Dyson, M: Macrophage responsiveness to therapeutic ultrasound. Ultrasound Med Biol 16:809, 1990.
42. Kitchen, SS and Partridge, CJ: A review of therapeutic ultrasound: II. The efficacy of ultrasound. Physiotherapy 76:595, 1990.
43. Maxwell, L, et al: The augmentation of leukocyte adhesion to endothelium by therapeutic ultrasound. Ultrasound Med Biol 20:383, 1994.
44. Ramirez, A, et al: The effect of ultrasound on collagen synthesis and fibroblast proliferation in vitro. Med Sci Sports Exerc 29:326, 1997.
45. Jackson, BA, et al: Effect of ultrasound therapy on the repair of Achilles tendon injuries in rats. Med Sci Sports Exerc 23:171, 1991.
46. Enwemeka, CS: The effect of therapeutic ultrasound on tendon healing: A biomechanical study. Am J Phys Med Rehabil 68:283, 1989.

47. Baker, RJ and Bell, GW: The effect of therapeutic modalities on blood flow in the human calf. J Orthop Sports Phys Ther 13:23, 1991.

48. Robinson, SE and Buono, MJ: Effect of continuous-wave ultrasound on blood flow in skeletal muscle. Phys Ther 75:147, 1993.

49. Plaskett C, et al: Ultrasound treatment does not affect postexercise muscle strength recovery or soreness. J Sport Rehabil 8:1, 1999.

50. Fabrizio, PA, et al: Acute effects of therapeutic ultrasound delivered at varying parameters on the blood flow velocity in a muscular distribution artery. J Orthop Sports Phys Ther 24:294, 1996.

51. Downing, DS and Weinstein, A: Ultrasound therapy of subacromial bursitis. A double blind trial. Phys Ther 66:194, 1986.

52. Lehmann, JF, et al: Effect of therapeutic temperatures on tendon extensibility. Arch Phys Med Rehabil 51:481, 1970.

53. Reed, BV, et al: Effects of ultrasound and stretch on knee ligament extensibility. J Orthop Sports Phys Ther 30:341, 2000.

54. Byl, NN, et al: Incisional wound healing: A controlled study of low and high dose ultrasound. J Orthop Sports Phys Ther 18:619, 1993.

55. Nussbaum, EL, et al: Comparison of ultrasound/ultraviolet-c and laser for treatment of pressure ulcers in patients with spinal cord injury. Phys Ther 74:812, 1994.

56. Henley, EJ: Transcutaneous drug delivery: Iontophoresis, phonophoresis. Phys Rehabil Med 2:139, 1991.

57. Davick, JP, et al: Distribution and deposition of tritiated cortisol using phonophoresis. Phys Ther 68:1672, 1988.

58. Quillen, WS: Phonophoresis: A review of the literature and technique. Athletic Training 15:109, 1980.

59. Ciccone, CD, et al: Effects of ultrasound and trolamine salicylate phonophoresis on delayed-onset muscle soreness. Phys Ther 71:666, 1991.

60. Meidan, VM, et al: Phonophoresis of hydrocortisone with enhancers: An acoustically defined model. Int J Pharmacol 170:157, 1998.

61. Byl, NN: The use of ultrasound as an enhancer for transcutaneous drug delivery: Phonophoresis. Phys Ther 75:539, 1995.

62. McElnay, JC, et al: Phonophoresis of methyl nicotinate: A preliminary study to elucidate the mechanism of action. Pharmacol Res 10:1726, 1993.

63. Machluf, M and Kost, J: Ultrasonically enhanced transdermal drug delivery. Experimental approaches to elucidate the mechanism. J Biomater Sci Polym Ed 5:147, 1993.

64. Oziomek, RS, et al: Effect of phonophoresis on serum salicylate levels. Med Sci Sports Exerc 23:397, 1991.

65. Mitragotri, S, et al: Transdermal drug delivery using low-frequency sonophoresis. Pharmacol Res 13:411, 1996.

66. Cameron, MH and Monroe, LG: Relative transmission of ultrasound by media customarily used for phonophoresis. Phys Ther 72:142, 1992.

67. Bensen, HAE, et al: Use of ultrasound to enhance percutaneous absorption of benzydamine. Phys Ther 69:113, 1989.

68. Bare, AC, et al: Phonophoretic delivery of 10% hydrocortisone through the epidermis of humans as determined by serum cortisol concentrations. Phys Ther 76:738, 1996.

69. Byl, NN, et al: The effects of phonophoresis with corticosteroids: A controlled pilot study. J Orthop Sports Phys Ther 18:590, 1993.

70. Franklin, ME, et al: Effect of phonophoresis with dexamethasone on adrenal function. J Orthop Sports Phys Ther 22:103, 1995.

71. Darrow, H, et al: Serum dexamethasone levels after decadron phonophoresis. J Athletic Training 34:338, 1999.

72. Mitragotri, S, et al: Ultrasound-mediated transdermal protein delivery. Science 269:850, 1995.

73. Sicard-Rosenbaum, L, et al: Effects of continuous therapeutic ultrasound on growth and metastasis of subcutaneous murine tumors. Phys Ther 75:3, 1995.

74. Draper, DO, et al: A comparison of temperature rise in human calf muscles following applications of underwater and topical gel ultrasound. J Orthop Sports Phys Ther 17:247, 1993.

75. Robertson, VJ and Baker, KG: A review of therapeutic ultrasound: Effectiveness studies. Phys Ther 81:1339, 2001.

76. Williams, R: Production and transmission of ultrasound. Physiotherapy 73:113, 1987.

77. Ashton, DF, et al: Temperature rise in human muscle during ultrasound treatments using Flex-All as a coupling agent. J Athletic Training 33:136, 1998.

78. Myrer, JW, et al: Intramuscular temperature rises with topical analgesics used as coupling agents during therapeutic ultrasound. J Athletic Training 36:20, 2001.

79. Klucinec, B, et al: The transducer pressure variable: Its influence on acoustic energy transmission. J Sport Rehabil 6:47, 1997.

80. Oshikoya, CA, et al: Effect of coupling medium temperature on rate of intramuscular temperature rise using continuous ultrasound. J Athletic Training 35:417, 2000.

81. Kimura, IF, et al: Effects of two ultrasound devices and angles of application on the temperature of tissue phantom. J Orthop Sports Phys Ther 27:27, 1998.

82. Klucinec, B, et al: Transmissivity of coupling agents used to deliver ultrasound through indirect methods. J Orthop Sports Phys Ther 30:263, 2000.

83. Cheng, N, et al: The effects of electric currents on ATP generation, protein synthesis, and membrane transport in rat skin. Clin Orthop 171:264, 1982.

84. McDiarmid, T and Burns, PN: Clinical application of therapeutic ultrasound. Physiotherapy 73:155, 1987.

85. Merrick, MA: Do You Diathermy? Athletic Ther Today 6:55, 2001.

86. Draper, DO, et al: Temperature change in human muscle during and after pulsed short-wave diathermy. J Orthop Sports Phys Ther 29:13, 1999.

87. Ouellet-Hellstron, R and Stewart, WF: Miscarriages among female physical therapists who report using radio- and microwave-frequency electromagnetic radiation. Am J Epidemiol 138:775, 1993.

88. Lehmann, JF, et al: Selective muscle heating by shortwave diathermy with a helical coil. Arch Phys Med Rehabil 50:117, 1969.

89. Trock, DH, et al: A double-blind trial of the clinical effects of pulsed electromagnetic fields in osteoarthritis. J Rheumatol 20:456, 1993.

90. Murray, CC and Kitchen, S: Effect of pulse repetition rate on the perception of thermal sensation with pulsed shortwave diathermy. Physiother Res Int 5:73, 2000.

91. Kloth, LC and Ziskin, MC: Diathermy and pulsed electromagnetic fields. In Michlovitz, SL (ed): Thermal Agents in Rehabilitation, ed 3. FA Davis, Philadelphia, 1996, pp 213–284.

92. Santiesteban, AJ and Grant, C: Post-surgical effect of pulsed shortwave diathermy. J Am Podiatr Med Assoc 75:306, 1985.

93. Markov, MS: Electric current electromagnetic field effects on soft tissue: Implications for wound healing. Wounds 7:94, 1995.
94. Pilla, AA and Markov, MS: Bioeffects of weak electromagnetic fields. Rev Environ Health 10:155, 1994.
95. Draper, DO, et al: Temperature rise in human muscle during pulsed short wave diathermy: Does this modality parallel ultrasound (abstract)? J Athletic Training 32:S35, 1997.
96. Oosterveld, FG, et al: The effect of local heat and cold therapy on the intraarticular and skin surface temperature of the knee. Arthritis Rheum 35:146, 1992.
97. Castel, JC, et al: Rate of temperature decay in human muscle after treatments of pulsed short wave diathermy. J Athletic Training 32:S34, 1997.
98. McCray, RE and Patton, NJ: Pain relief at trigger points: A comparison of moist heat and shortwave diathermy. J Orthop Sports Phys Ther 5:175, 1984.
99. Brown, M and Baker, RD: Effect of pulsed shortwave diathermy on skeletal muscle injury in rabbits. Phys Ther 67:208, 1987.
100. Schurman DJ, et al: Shortwave diathermy and fracture healing in rabbit fibula model: Preliminary report (abstract). Transactions of the 26th Annual Meeting Orthopedic Research Society, Atlanta, GA, 1980.
101. Draper, DO, et al: The carry-over effects of diathermy and stretching in developing hamstring flexibility. J Athletic Training 37:37, 2002.
102. Peres, SE, et al: Pulsed shortwave diathermy and prolonged long-duration stretching increase dorsiflexion range of motion more than identical stretching without diathermy. J Athletic Training 37:43, 2002.
103. Bansal, PS, et al: Histomorphochemical effects of shortwave diathermy on healing of experimental muscular injury in dogs. Indian J Exp Biol 28:776, 1990.
104. Scott, DG and Wallbank, WA: Electrode burns during local hyperthermia. Br J Anaesth 70:370, 1993.
105. Martin, CJ, McCallum, HM, and Heaton, B: An evaluation of the radiofrequency exposure from therapeutic diathermy equipment in light of current recommendations. Clin Phys Physiol Meas 11:53, 1990.

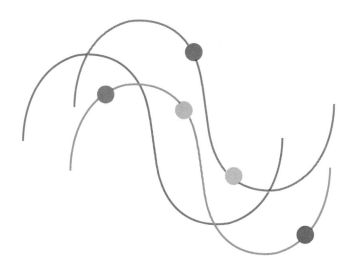

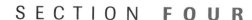

Electrical Stimulation

This section is divided into three chapters concerning the basic electrical principles, concepts, and terms; the effect that an electrical current has on the body and subsequent treatment objectives; and the effects of various electrical stimulation units.

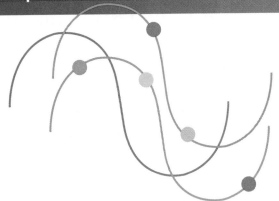

Chapter 11

Principles of Electrical Stimulation

This chapter describes the different types of currents used for therapeutic electrical stimulation. The basic physics and principles of electricity are also presented to build a solid foundation on which to build a good understanding of electrical stimulation goals and techniques.

The effects of electricity on the body can be difficult to comprehend, and the thought of actually sending 500 volts through a person's body can be intimidating. In this chapter, it will become apparent that electrotherapy, when used properly and appropriately, is a safe and effective form of therapy. Just as important, you will also see that electrical stimulation is an adjunct to other therapeutic modalities and rehabilitation exercises. Electrical stimulation is not always an appropriate treatment approach.

Electricity is the force created by an imbalance in the number of **electrons** ■ at two points (these points are referred to as "poles"). This force, known as **electromagnetic force**, **potential difference**, or **voltage**, creates a situation in which electrons flow in an attempt to equalize the difference in charges, creating an electrical current. In its simplest form, an electrical current takes the path of least resistance from the negative pole (**cath-**

ode), an area of high electron concentration, and flows to the positive pole (**anode**), an area of low electron concentration.

In addition to the presence of an imbalance in electrical charge, a complete pathway must be established for flow to occur. A **closed circuit** is formed when a complete path is formed between the two poles, allowing the electrons to flow. An interrupted or incomplete path is an **open circuit** and the electrons are unable to flow. When you walk into a room and flip a switch to turn on the light, you are closing a circuit that allows the electricity to flow from its source, through the light, and back to its source. Likewise, a closed circuit is created between your patient and an electrical stimulator by attaching opposite leads to the body. The electrons flow from the generator, through the patient's body in the form of ions, and back to the generator via electrons.

Electron: A negatively charged atomic particle.

■ Electrical Stimulating Currents

Electrical currents are classified as either being a **direct current** (DC) or an **alternating current** (AC), depending on the course of flow. A third classification, **pulsed current**, represents a type of current that has been modified to produce specific biophysical effects (Box 11–1). The terms "alternating" and "direct" describe the uninterrupted flow of electrons; "pulsed" indicates that the electron flow is interrupted by discrete periods of no electron flow. Pulsed currents may flow in one direction, similarly to a DC, or may have bidirectional movement, as in an AC.[1] **Polyphasic currents** are hybrids that contain multiple current types.[2]

The primary properties of electrical flow are amplitude (intensity) and duration. The **amplitude** is the maximum distance that the pulse rises above or below the baseline. The **isoelectric point** is the baseline at which the electrical potential between the two poles is equal and no current flow occurs. The horizontal distance required to complete the shape represents the **pulse duration**. The term "pulse width" is often incorrectly substituted for pulse duration.[3] The total area within this waveform represents the amount of current the pulse contains, the **pulse charge**.

Direct Currents

DCs are characterized by the uninterrupted, one-directional flow of electrons. The basic pattern of DC is the square wave and is recognized by continuous current flow on only one side of the baseline as the electrons travel from the cathode to the anode (Fig. 11–1). Despite any fluctuations in voltage or amperage, the current flow remains in one direction and stays on one side of the baseline. In medical applications, the term "**galvanic**" is used to describe uninterrupted DC. Iontophoresis is an example of a technique that uses a DC.

Perhaps a flashlight is the simplest example of a DC. The battery possesses a positive pole, which lacks electrons, and a negative pole that has an excess of electrons. Electrons leave the negative pole of the battery and flow through a wire to the bulb. After leaving the bulb, the electrons return to the positive pole of the battery (Fig. 11–2). When the number of electrons at the negative pole equals the number at the positive pole, no further potential for current flow exists. The battery is dead.

Alternating Currents

In an AC, the direction of flow changes from positive to negative in a cyclical manner, although the magnitude of change may not be equal in both directions. Unlike DC, an AC possesses no true positive or negative pole. Rather than constantly moving in one direction, electrons shuffle back and forth between the two electrodes as each take turns being the "positive" and "negative" poles. Household electricity uses AC.

Consider the flashlight example used to describe DC flow (see Fig. 11–2). If a battery were placed on a device that allowed it to rotate between the two wires, we could more or less duplicate an AC. Electrons would flow away from terminal (A) when the cathode is in line with it. When the anode aligns with terminal (A), electrons would flow toward it (Fig. 11–3). The basic pattern of an AC is the sine wave (Fig. 11–4). Interferential stimulators use multiple ACs.

The amplitude, or **peak value**, of an AC wave is the maximum distance that the wave rises above or below the baseline without regard to its duration. In the case of the pure sine wave shown in Figure 11–4, the peak value is the same on both sides of the baseline. The **peak-to-peak** value is the distance from the peak on the positive side of the baseline to the peak on the negative side. In Figure 11–5A, the peak-to-peak value would be the absolute value of the difference between the two peaks. In an **asymmetrical** ■ waveform, such as the faradic wave (Fig. 11–5B), the peak-to-peak amplitude is the absolute value between the two phases.

The cycle duration of an AC is measured from the originating point on the baseline to its terminating point and represents the amount of time required to complete one full cycle. The number of times that the current reverses direction in 1 second is the current's number of cycles per second and is measured in hertz (Hz) (Fig. 11–6). A current of 100 Hz would change its direction of flow 100 times during 1 second. A current of 1 megahertz (MHz) would change its direction 1 million times a second.

Cycle duration and frequency are inversely related. Because ACs are measured in cycles per second, as the duration of the cycles increases, fewer cycles per second can occur. Although amplitude is often used to describe the magnitude of an electrical current, it does not take into account the actual amount of time that the current is flowing. This applies to both alternating and pulsed currents. Box 11–2 presents measures that take into consideration the cycle's duration.

Pulsed Currents

Pulsed currents are the unidirectional (monophasic) or bidirectional (biphasic) flow of electrons that are interrupted by discrete periods of noncurrent flow (see Box 11–1). Using the flashlight analogy from the DC section, turning the switch on and off, causing the light to blink, is an example of a monophasic current. However, the pulses occur in a much more rapid progression and the "switch" is only on for microseconds or milliseconds.

Phases are the building blocks of pulses. A phase is

Asymmetrical: Lacking symmetry (e.g., two halves of unequal size or shape).

Box 11–1. Classification of Electrical Stimulating Currents

Current Classification	Sample Waveform	Uses
Direct Current Uninterrupted, unidirectional flow of electrons.	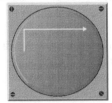	Can produce polarity-based changes in the tissue, resulting in ions being moved to and from the area. Long duration can directly affect muscle fibers and can alter local pH. **Common Generators/Techniques:** Iontophoresis: Medication delivery Low voltage stimulation: Eliciting contractions from **denervated** ■ muscle.
Alternating Current Uninterrupted, bidirectional flow of electrons.	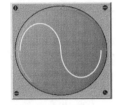	High frequency of the current decreases skin resistance, leading to a more comfortable current. **Common Generators/Techniques:** Interferential Stimulation: Pain control; muscle contractions Premodulated currents; Neuromuscular Stimulation: Muscle contractions

Pulsed Current

Monophasic Unidirectional flow of electrons marked by periods of non-current flow.	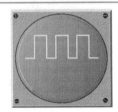	Like a direct current, monophasic currents are applied to the body with a known charge under each electrode. The resulting current can depolarize sensory and motor nerves. **Common Generators/Techniques:** High Voltage Pulsed Stimulation: Muscle contractions, pain control

Biphasic
Bidirectional flow of electrons marked by periods of non-current flow.

Symmetrical Each phase is a mirror image of the other.	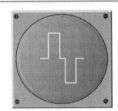	The electrode carries equal positive and negative charges. The effects are equal for both the positive and negative flow and there is no net residual electrical charge. **Common Generators/Techniques:** Neuromuscular electrical stimulation

Asymmetrical
The two phases do not mirror each other.

Balanced The two phases carry equal electrical charges.	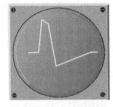	The shape of the pulse allows for greater positive (anodal) or negative (cathodal) effects, but over time the net electrical charge is zero. **Common Generators/Techniques:** Transcutaneous Electrical Nerve Stimulation: Pain control.
Unbalanced The two phases do not carry equal electrical charges.	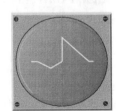	The shape of the pulse allows for greater positive (anodal) or negative (cathodal) effects. Over time there is a net electrical charge. **Common Generators/Techniques:** Neuromuscular Electrical Nerve Stimulation

Denervation (Denervated): Lack of the proper nerve supply or nerve function to, for example, an area or muscle group.

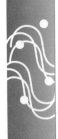

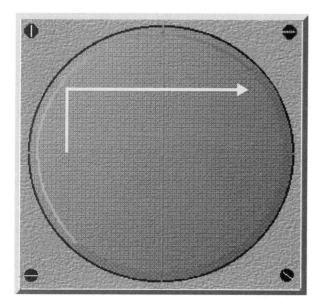

Figure 11-1. **Direct Current.** Characterized by the constant flow of electrons in one direction, a direct current remains uninterrupted (does not return to the baseline) until the path is opened, thus stopping the flow of electrons.

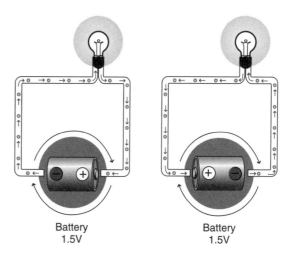

Figure 11-3. **Example of an Alternating Current.** Alternating currents possess no true positive or negative poles. In this type of current, electrons flow back and forth between poles.

the individual section of a pulse that rises above or below the baseline for a measurable period of time. The number and type of phases then classify the pulse as being monophasic or biphasic.

Monophasic Currents

Monophasic pulses have only one phase per pulse, and the current flows in one direction. Notice in Figure 11–7 that each pulse consists of only one component part, the phase. Despite the different shapes involved, there is only one phase, and it remains on one side of the baseline. Monophasic currents are applied to the body with a known polarity under each electrode. With this type of current one electrode is the negative electrode (cathode), and the opposite electrode is the positive electrode (anode). High-

voltage pulsed stimulation is an example of an electrical modality that delivers a monophasic current.

In this type of electrical current, amplitude is the maximum distance that the pulse rises above the baseline. The pulse duration is the horizontal distance required to complete one full waveform (Fig. 11–8). The horizontal baseline is labeled as "time," so the distance a pulse travels represents the duration that the pulse is flowing. With monophasic currents, the terms "pulse," "phase," and "waveform" are synonymous.

Biphasic Currents

Biphasic currents consist of two phases, each occurring on opposite sides of the baseline (Fig. 11–9). The lead phase of the pulse is the first area rising above or below the base-

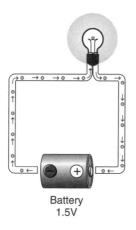

Figure 11-2. **Example of a Direct Current.** Electrons exit the battery through the cathode (negative pole), flow through the wire and bulb, and return to the anode (positive pole).

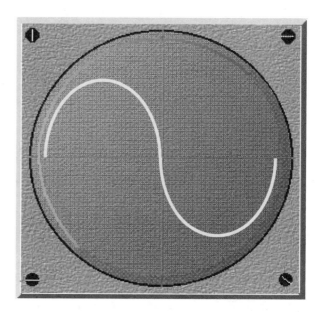

Figure 11-4. **The Sine Wave.** One cycle of an alternating current.

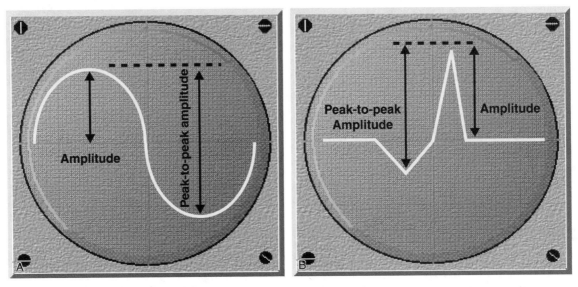

Figure 11–5. **Measures of Amplitude.** Peak amplitude and peak-to-peak values for (A) symmetrical and (B) asymmetrical pulses.

line, and the terminating phase occurs in the opposite direction.

The pulse represented in Figure 11–10A is considered **symmetrical** because the two phases are equal in their magnitude and duration. In this case, each phase has equal, but opposite, electrical balance. Figures 11–10B and C represent **asymmetrical** pulses because each phase in the pulse has a different shape. When asymmetrical pulses are used, the characteristics of each phase should be considered separately. If the charges (area) of both phases are equal, the pulse is electrically **balanced**; otherwise, it is

unbalanced. The phases in a symmetrical pulse or balanced asymmetrical pulse cause the physiological effects of positive and negative current flow to cancel each other out over time. Unbalanced asymmetrical pulses may lead to residual physiological changes based on the remaining net polarity. Symmetrical biphasic waveforms tend to be the most comfortable because they deliver relatively lower charges per phase.[4] Neuromuscular stimulation units often deliver a symmetrical biphasic current; transcutaneous electrical nerve stimulators use a balanced asymmetrical current.

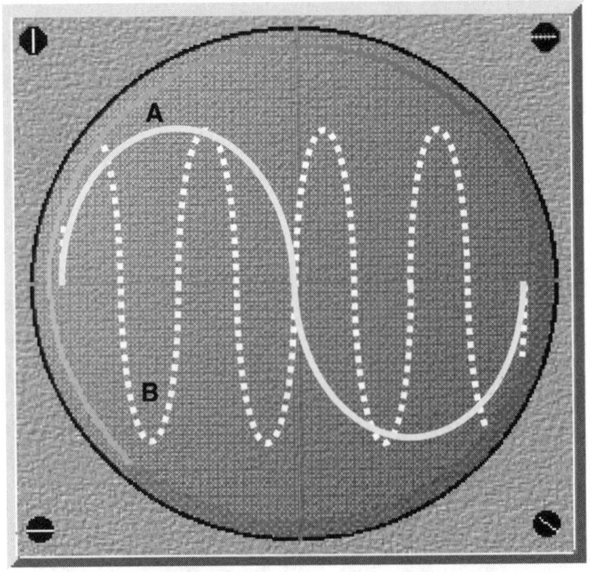

Pulse Attributes

The charge produced by an electrical generator is dependent on the duration and amplitude of the pulse. The relationship between intensity and duration of a single pulse determines the total charge delivered to the body. Increasing the amplitude or duration, or both, increases the total charge of the pulse. Time-dependent pulse characteristics are presented in Table 11–1.

Pulse and Phase Duration

The baseline (horizontal axis) represents time. The distance that a pulse covers on the horizontal axis represents the **pulse duration**: the elapsed time from the beginning of the phase to the conclusion of the final phase, including the intrapulse interval.[1] The duration of biphasic pulses are described by the time required for each phase to complete its shape: the **phase duration** (see Figs. 11–8 and 11–10).

In a monophasic current, the pulse duration and phase duration are equivalent terms. In biphasic currents, the pulse duration is the sum total of the two phase durations plus the intrapulse interval (if present). Note that pulse durations cannot be measured for uninterrupted DCs or ACs.

Figure 11–6. **Frequency of an Alternating Current.** Each complete wave is termed a cycle. The frequency, hertz (Hz), describes the number of cycles per second. If the oscilloscope represents one second, waveform (A–solid line) has a frequency of 1 Hz and waveform (B–dashed line) has a frequency of 4 Hz.

Box 11–2. Measures of a Current's Electrical Power

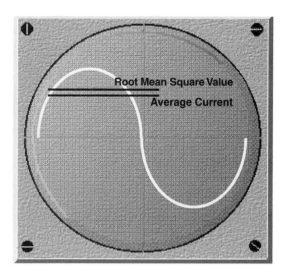

The **average current** of a wave is considered one-half of its complete cycle, taking into account the amount of time the current is flowing. To calculate the average value of a wave, the sine values of all angles up to 180° are added together and divided by the number of measurements. In the case of a perfect sine wave, this value is about 0.637 (63.7% of the peak current). This figure is then multiplied by the peak value to obtain the average value:

Average value = Mean of sines × peak value
Average value = 0.637 × 100 V
Average value = 63.7 V

The **root-mean-square** (RMS) value takes into account the current's amplitude and duration. It describes the total amount of charge delivered by a single cycle and is useful when asymmetrical biphasic currents are used. The RMS is important because it translates the power delivered by a biphasic current into the equivalent amount of power that would be needed by a direct current to produce the same amount of heat. In the case of a pure sine wave, the RMS value is calculated by multiplying the peak value by 0.707.

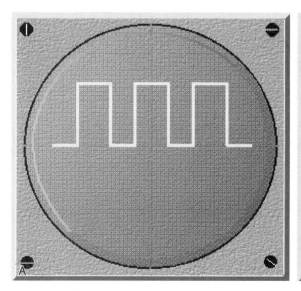
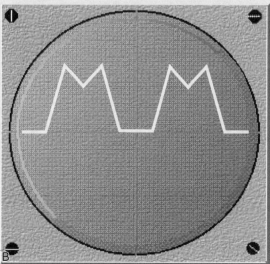

Figure 11–7. **Examples of Monophasic Currents**. Pulsatile current consists of discrete pulses. Like direct current, monophasic currents are characterized by the one-directional flow of electrons. (A) Three square waves. (B) Two twin-peaked monophasic.

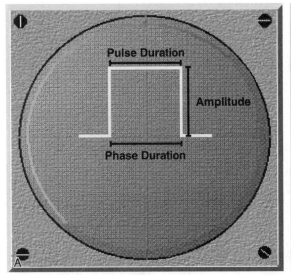

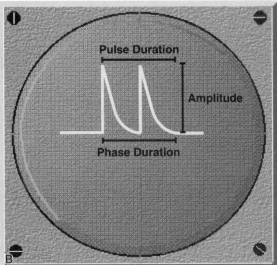

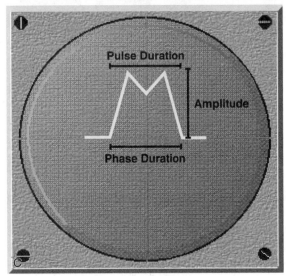

Figure 11-8. **Pulse and Phase Durations for a Monophasic Current.** Monophasic currents have phases and pulses of equal duration. (A) Square wave; (B) sawtooth wave; (C) twin-peaked wave.

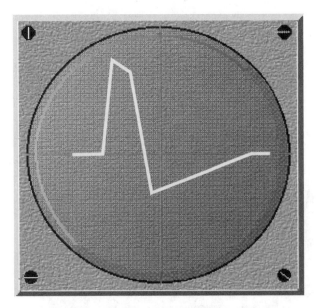

Figure 11-9. **Biphasic Pulse.** An example of biphasic pulsed current commonly used with transcutaneous electrical nerve stimulation (TENS).

The phase duration, and its associated electrical power, is the most important factor in determining what type of tissues will be stimulated. If the phase duration is too short, the current will not be able to overcome the capacitive resistance of the nerve membrane and no action potential will be elicited. As the phase duration is increased, different tissues are depolarized by the electrical current (see Selective Stimulation of Nerves, p 227).

Interpulse Interval, Intrapulse Interval, and Pulse Period

Pulsed currents have periods during which the current is not flowing. The time between the conclusion of one pulse and the start of the next is the **interpulse interval**. A single pulse or phase may be interrupted by an **intrapulse interval**; however, the duration of the intrapulse interval cannot exceed the duration of the interpulse interval (Fig. 11–11).[1] The intrapulse interval allows time for certain metabolic events, such as repolarization of cell membranes to occur. The interpulse interval provides time for mechanical events and chemical recharging to occur. Jointly, the pulse duration and the interpulse interval form the **pulse**

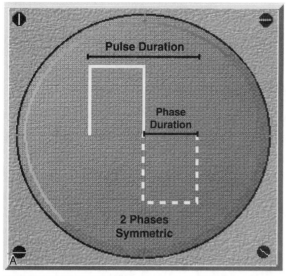

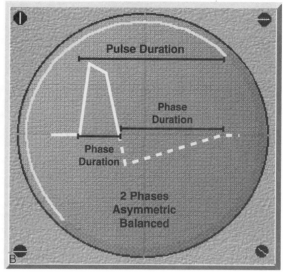

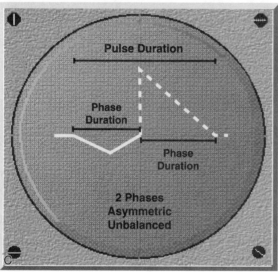

Figure 11–10. **Pulse and Phase Durations for a Biphasic Current.** Pulse and phase durations for (A) symmetrical biphasic, (B) balanced asymmetrical biphasic, and (C) unbalanced asymmetrical pulses. The balanced pulses, A and B, have an equal area on each side of the baseline, yielding an equal net charge during the treatment. Pulse C has unequal areas within each phase. This waveform would yield a net positive charge under this electrode because the charge of the positive (second) phase is larger than the negative (first) phase. (The lead phase is shown using a solid line. The terminating phase uses a dashed line.)

period, the elapsed time between the initiation of one pulse and the start of the subsequent pulse.

By definition, uninterrupted currents (alternating and direct currents) do not possess pulses. Therefore, pulse duration and pulse periods do not exist for these types of currents.

Pulse Charge

A measurement of the number of electrons contained within a pulse, the pulse charge is expressed in **microcoulombs**. A coulomb is too large a unit to use when describing the charge produced by electrical stimulation units. Most electrotherapeutic modalities produce charges measured in microcoulombs (the charge produced by 10^{-6} electrons).

The pulse charge is a function of the amount of area within the waveform. Increasing or decreasing the amplitude or duration alters the charge of the pulse accordingly. The shape of the wave may also be altered to deliver more or less charge to the tissues per pulse (see Electrical Charge, p 213).

Each phase also carries its own charge, the **phase charge**. With biphasic currents, the phase charge is important when trying to evoke a strong muscle contraction. The higher the phase charge, the stronger the contraction.[2]

Pulse Frequency

Any waveform or pulse that repeats at regular intervals may be described in terms of its frequency or the number of events per second.[5] When a pulsed current is being used, the frequency is measured by the number of **pulses per second** (pps). The cycle frequency of an AC is measured by the number of **cycles per second** (cps) or **Hertz** (Hz) (see Fig. 11–6).

TABLE 11–1	Time-Dependent Pulse Characteristics

Phase duration
Pulse duration
  (phase duration + intrapulse interval + phase duration)
Intrapulse interval
Interpulse interval
Pulse period (Pulse duration + interpulse interval)

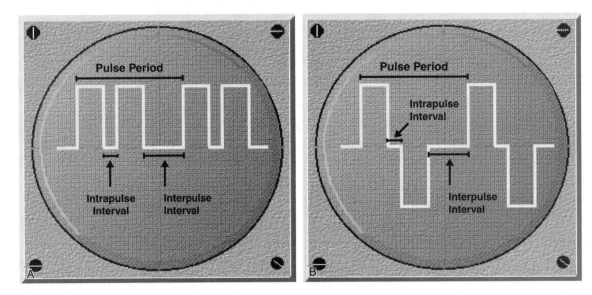

Figure 11–11. **Calculation of Time-Dependent Pulse Characteristics.** (A) Monophasic currents. (B) Biphasic currents. The Pulse Period is the time (horizontal axis) from the start of one pulse to the start of the subsequent pulse. The Interpulse Interval separates two pulses. The Intrapulse Interval interrupts a single pulse.

The use of the term "frequency" can be confusing because it is used to describe base frequency of the electrical stimulator and also to describe the number of electrical pulses (or cycles) delivered to the tissues. Electrical stimulation units are grouped by their carrier frequency. Low-frequency currents, less than 1000 cycles or pulses per second, are used for their biological effects; medium-frequency currents range from 1000 to 100,000 cps; high-frequency currents, greater than 100,000 cps, are used for their heating effects, as seen with diathermy (see Chap. 9). To help alleviate this confusion within this text, the term "pulse frequency" is used to describe an adjustable output parameter. "Stimulation frequency" is used to denote device-specific current frequencies. In each case, the actual numerical value of the frequency is the preferred nomenclature rather than "low," "medium," and "high."

There is an inverse relationship between the pulse frequency of an electrical current and the capacitive resistance offered by the tissues. A current having 10 pps would encounter greater tissue resistance than a current flowing at 1000 pps and would require an increased intensity to overcome the resistance.

Pulse frequencies over 100 pps have little additive effect on nerve depolarization. As the pulse frequency increases beyond 100 pps, the current flow begins to occur during the absolute and relative refractory periods. In most cases, the current intensity is insufficient to cause another depolarization during the relative refractory period. A nerve cannot be depolarized during its absolute refractory period. (Also see Motor-Level Stimulation, p 231.)

Pulse Rise Time and Pulse Decay Time

Pulse rise is the amount of time needed for the pulse to reach its peak value and is usually measured in **nanoseconds** ■ (almost immediate full pulse charge). Rapidly rising pulses cause nerve depolarization. If the rise is slow, the nerve accommodates to the stimulus and an action potential is not elicited. The counterpart of pulse rise time is the pulse decay time, the amount of time required for the pulse to go from its peak back to zero (Fig. 11–12).

Pulse Trains (Bursts)

Pulse trains, or bursts, are individual currents that are regularly interrupted by periods of noncurrent flow. These linked patterns repeat at regular intervals (Fig. 11–13). Bursts can further be described or regulated based on the duration of the bursts, the frequency of the bursts, and the interburst interval, the length of time between bursts.

The gradual rise or fall in amplitude of a pulse train is the **amplitude ramp** (Fig. 11–14). Ramping amplitude causes a gradual increase in the force of muscular contractions by the progressive recruitment of motor units. As the intensity of the ramp continues to rise, more motor units are recruited into the contraction. The patient appreciates a slow rise time because the stimulation is increased gradually and the "shock" of the current is reduced. When muscles are being stimulated, the gradual contraction produced by a slow rise time more closely resembles a voluntary muscle contraction. More and more fibers are recruited as the amplitude of the stimulus, or the phase duration, increases.[6]

Nanosecond: One billionth (10^{-9}) of a second.

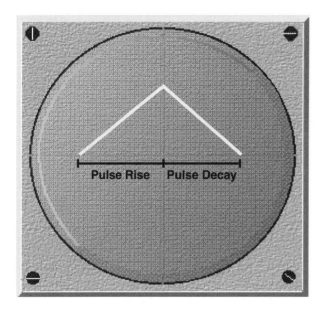

Figure 11–12. Pulse rise and decay time for a monophasic current.

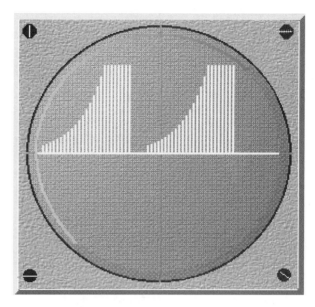

Figure 11–14. **Amplitude Ramp.** The gradual increase in the intensity (amplitude) of a current, allowing for more comfortable muscle contractions.

■ Measures of Electrical Current Flow

The strength of an electrical current is expressed in amperes and is related to the voltage of the current and the resistance it meets. This relationship, Ohm's law, is the fundamental principle governing electrical current flow (Box 11–3). The following sections describe the factors affecting the strength of an electrical current passing through the human body (Table 11–2).

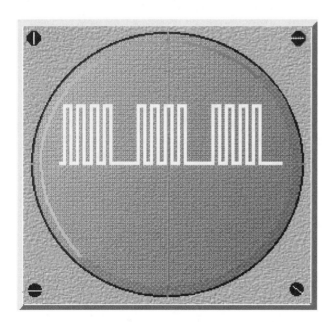

Figure 11–13. **An Example of a Pulse Train (Burst).** A pattern of electrical pulses repeating at regular intervals. In the example presented, each group of four monophasic pulses, the burst, is followed by an interburst interval of noncurrent flow.

Electrical Charge

Electrical current results from the flow of electrons. The number of electrons required for electrical current flow is so great that it is impractical to count each one. Just as we may describe 12 objects as a dozen, or a dozen dozens as a gross, a large number of electrons can be described as a single unit. A **coulomb** ("Q") is used to describe the charge produced by 6.25×10^{-18} electrons (negative charge) or protons (positive charge).

Coulomb's law describes the relationship between like and unlike electrical charges: Opposite charges attract and like charges repel. The strength of the attractive or repulsive forces may be amplified by increasing the magnitude of the charges or by decreasing the distance between the two objects.

Voltage

Voltage, also known as the electromotive force or potential difference between two poles, measures the tendency for current flow to occur. Electrons placed within a field strain themselves to move to the opposite pole, thus creating the potential for work to occur (Work = Force × Distance). The **volt** is the unit of potential difference and represents the amount of work required to move 1 coulomb of charge. The energy required to move this coulomb is termed a **joule**. The symbol used to represent voltage is "E" or "V." The flow of electrons is not the simple movement of particles through a medium. Rather, this flow consists of the passing of electrons between atoms in a manner similar to a bucket brigade. Picture a line of people passing buckets of water. In this analogy, the people represent atoms and the buckets of water are electrons. The first person hands the bucket to the next person. This person then passes the bucket to the next person and the process repeats. The flow

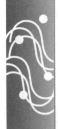

Box 11–3. Ohm's Law

Ohm's law describes the relationship between amperage, voltage, and resistance. Generally stated, current (I) is directly proportional to voltage (V) and inversely proportional to resistance (R):

$$I = V/R$$

By using derivations of Ohm's law, the amperage, voltage, or resistance in a circuit can be calculated if two of the three variables are known. In a circuit where the potential is 120 V with 10 ohms of resistance, the amperage would be calculated as 120 V/10 ohms, or 12 A. Circuits having a very high voltage can still have a very small current flow if the resistance is high. For example, applying 1,000 V to a circuit with a resistance of 1,000,000 ohms would produce only 0.001 A. Likewise, low voltages can give rise to a very high current flow. Consider a 10-V circuit with 0.01 ohms of resistance. The resultant current would be 1,000 A.

To determine the effect that current (I) and resistance (R) have on voltage (V), we may transpose Ohm's law to give:

$$V = IR$$

For current to flow through a resistance, the voltage applied must be equal to or greater than the product of the amperage times the resistance. To produce a current of 12 A flowing through a circuit of 10 ohms, 120 V (12 A × 10 ohms) would be required.

The resistance (R) found in a circuit may be calculated by again transposing the formula so that we divide the voltage (V) by the resistance (I):

$$R = V/I$$

Therefore, if we are using a device that requires 120 V and 12 A, we can calculate the amount of resistance by dividing 120 V by 12 A to give 10 ohms.

You will notice that in all of our equations, current is equal to 10 A, voltage is equal to 120 V, and resistance is equal to 10 ohms. This illustrates the interrelationship between the variables. If we were to reduce the current to 5 A and increase the voltage to 200 V, the resistance would then be 40 ohms. In any case, the voltage applied to the circuit must be greater than the resistance, or no current will flow.

of electrons is similar; rather than a single electron passing through a wire, electrons are passed from atom to atom.

Current

Amperage describes the rate at which the electrical charge (measured in coulombs) flows. More specifically, 1 **ampere** (A) is the current when 1 coulomb passes a single point in 1 second. Conceptually, we may make the analogy to the number of people passing through a turnstile at any given time. If 1 coulomb passes a point in 1 second, the rate of flow is 1 A. If 20 coulombs pass a point in 1 second, the rate of flow is 20 A.

TABLE 11–2   Electrical Terminology

Amperage (I):	The rate at which an electrical current flows. One ampere is equal to the rate of flow of 1 coulomb per second. It is analogous to the rate of flow of water through a pipe. I = V/R.
Charge:	See Coulomb.
Coulomb (Q):	The basic unit of charge is the coulomb, the net positive or negative electrical charge produced by 6.25 × 10^{18} electrons or protons.
Coulomb's law:	Like charges repel and unlike (opposite) charges attract each other.
Joule (J):	Basic unit of work in the International System of Units. Representing the work done by moving 1 coulomb, 1 J equals 0.74 foot-pounds of work. The conversion equation is: J = QV.
Ohm (V):	Unit of electrical resistance (R). R = V/I.
Ohm's law:	Current is directly proportional to voltage and inversely proportional to resistance. I = V/R.
Voltage (V):	The potential for electron flow to occur. Analogous to the height of a waterfall, it indicates how much energy is available in the system. The greater the height of a waterfall, the more energy it can impart to a mill below. V = I/R.
Watt (W):	Unit of electrical power (P). May be calculated from the relation Watts = Volts × Amperage (P = VI). Watts measure the ability to perform work.

The symbol for current flow is "I" or "A." Most electrical modalities have current flow measured in **milliamperes** (mA), 1/1000 of an ampere, or **microamperes** (μA), 1/1,000,000 of an ampere.

Resistance

All materials present some degree of opposition to the flow of electrical current. Those materials allowing current to pass with relative ease are labeled conductors and those that tend to oppose current flow resistors. A material's resistance to the movement of electrons is measured in **ohms**. One ohm is the amount of resistance needed to develop 0.24 calories of heat when 1 A of current is applied for 1 second. The symbol for resistance is "R," and for ohms, Ω (omega). The skin is the primary biological resistor to therapeutic electrical current flow.

Conductance is a measure of the ease with which current is allowed to pass. Conductance is the mathematical reciprocal of resistance and is measured by the unit **mho**—ohm spelled backward.

The type, length, and cross-sectional area of the material and the temperature of the circuit determine electrical resistance (Box 11–4). As we have already discussed, the potential difference at each end of the circuit must be great enough to overcome the resistance, or no current will flow.

Impedance

In an AC, two additional properties, **inductance** and **capacitance**, act to resist the flow of an AC. Collectively known as impedance, this form of resistance is also measured in ohms, but uses the symbol "Z."

Inductance is the ability of a material to store electrical energy by means of an electromagnetic field and is measured by the **henry** ■. Variation in the magnitude and direction of electrical current creates a **flux** ■ that induces voltage. Inductors tend to oppose electrical current flow. A transformer used to convert household current into a lower voltage DC is an example of an inductor. Inductance is negligible in biological systems.[1]

Capacitance is the ability of a material to store energy by means of an **electrostatic field** ■ and provides frequency-dependent opposition to electric current flow. Created by an insulator (dielectric) separating two conductors, charges can be stored even after the applied voltage has been discontinued. Cell membranes act as capacitors that separate positive and negative charges between the inside and outside of the cell. The lipid membrane layer is an electrical insulator between the conducting plates, in this case, the intracellular and extracellular fluids (Fig. 11–15).

Capacitance is a factor in determining the effects of current flow on the body. Higher frequency currents meet less capacitive skin resistance than lower frequency currents. The output of capacitors is measured in farads (F), microfarads, (mF, 10^{-6} F), or picofarads (pF, 10^{-10} F). A farad stores a charge of 1 coulomb when 1 V is applied. As we saw when frequency was discussed, the lower the capacitance of a circuit, the higher the frequency of an AC it allows and vice versa.[7]

Wattage

The relationship between voltage and amperage is expressed in units of wattage (W) and is used to designate the power of a current. Power (P) describes the amount of work being performed in a unit of time. The voltage of the current measures the amount of work being done; amperage defines the time unit. One watt is the power produced by 1 A of current flowing with the force of 1 V. With this in mind, we can then describe wattage as:

$$W = VI$$

Using the variables from Box 11–3, we can calculate the power used by a device requiring 12 A from a 120-V source to be 1440 W.

The change in wattage of an electrical circuit reflects the net change in amperage or voltage, or both. If either amperage or voltage is increased or decreased, the wattage changes accordingly. However, if one variable is increased and the other decreased, the wattage increases or decreases depending on the relative magnitude of the changes in voltage and amperage.

■ Circuit Types

An electrical current introduced into a conductive medium may flow along one set route (**series circuit**), through many different pathways (**parallel circuit**), or through a combination of each. Consider an old-fashioned string of Christmas tree lights. If the string is wired as a series circuit, when one bulb burns out, all the other lights go out as well because the current has no other path to take.

In a string of lights wired in a parallel circuit, a burned-out bulb does not affect the other lights because the current still has other routes by which to reach them. Electricity operates under different constraints when traveling through series and parallel circuits, and each type of circuit has unique properties.

Series Circuit

Electrons in a series circuit have only one pathway available for travel. Connecting a wire between the two poles of

---

Electrostatic field: A field created by static electricity.

Flux: A residual electromagnetic field created by two unlike charges.

Henry: A measure of inductance (H). One henry induces an electromagnetic force of 1 V when the current changes at a rate of 1 A per second.

Box 11–4. Factors Determining the Resistance of an Electrical Circuit

	Material of the Circuit	Length of the Circuit	Cross-Sectional Area of the Circuit	Temperature of the Circuit
Increases resistance/ Decreases resistance	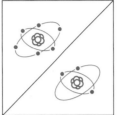	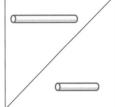	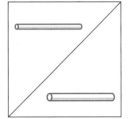	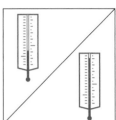
Concept	Materials are classified as resistors or conductors based on the number of free electrons in the **valence shell** ■.	There is proportional relationship between the length of a circuit and the resistance to electron flow.	The resistance of an electrical circuit (path) is inversely proportional to its cross-sectional diameter.	Increased temperature increases the random movement of free electrons.
Relationship	The more free electrons a material has, the better conductor of current it becomes.	The shorter the distance an electron has to travel, the less resistance to electrical current flow.	The greater the cross-sectional area of a path, the less resistance to current flow.	Increasing the temperature of a circuit decreases the resistance to current flow.
Applicability	Not all of the body's tissues conduct an electrical current as well as others.	The distance between an electrical stimulator's two leads affects the output intensity needed to evoke the desired response.	Nerves having a large diameter are depolarized before nerves having smaller diameters.	Preheating the treatment area may increase the comfort of the treatment by decreasing the resistance and the need for higher output intensities.
Example	Blood and nerves have more free electrons than do skin or bone, so the current prefers to travel along this path.	Effects are seen at a lower output intensity if the electrodes are placed closer together rather than farther apart. Superficial tissues are stimulated before deeper tissues.	This, in part, explains how an electrical current selectively stimulates nerves. Sensory nerves tend to be stimulated before motor nerves because sensory nerves have a larger diameter.	The clinical efficacy of body temperature and decreased electrical flow has not been substantiated.

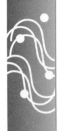

Valence shell: An imaginary shell in which the electrons responsible for chemical reactivity orbit around the nucleus of an atom.

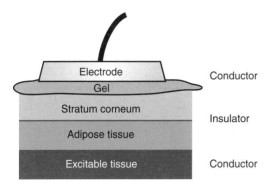

Figure 11–15. **Biological Capacitor.** Charge-carrying conductors, the electrode and excitable tissues, are separated by insulators, the skin and adipose tissue.

a battery forms a simple series circuit (see Fig. 11–2). In more complex series circuits, resistors are aligned "end to end" so that the current leaving one resistor will enter the next. In a series circuit, the current remains the same in all components along the circuit and the total resistance is equal to the sum of the individual resistors. Box 11–5 presents the calculations of Ohm's law within a series and parallel circuit.

Parallel Circuit

Electrons in a parallel circuit are provided with alternative paths to follow, and electrons tend to take the path of least resistance. Paths within the parallel circuit may then branch into other parallel or series circuits, but in either case, each path has its own amperage and the voltage remains constant. The flow in each of these pathways is inversely proportional to the resistance provided. In a parallel circuit, the amperage is varied among the paths, but the voltage remains constant. This is similar to checking out of a grocery store. When we are finished shopping, we tend to get in the line with the fastest clerk rather than the slowest. In any given time frame, more people will check out through the fastest clerk, and fewer through the slowest. Refer to Box 11–5 for the calculations of Ohm's law within a parallel circuit.

■ Characteristics of Electrical Generators

Electrical modalities may be driven by either standard household current (120-V AC) or by batteries (1.5-V to 9-V DC). Before this current is delivered to the body, it must be modified to the desired stimulation parameters.

In a simplified view, the current passes through one or more transformers to change it to the desired type (AC to DC, or DC to AC) and another to control the output current. A device, generically known as a generator, shapes the current (waveform) used by the modality. Other components within the generator control the characteristics of the electrical pulses.

Each element of the waveform has an effect on the

tissues' reaction to the current flow. The following sections discuss each generator characteristic and relate how each affects the treatment.

Current Attributes

The manner in which the stimulating current is applied to the body affects its ability to depolarize excitable tissue. The actual intensity of the current, the amount of current per unit of body area, and the duty cycle influence the effect that the treatment has on human tissues.

Average Current

Average current describes the absolute value of current per unit of time. The physiochemical and thermal changes in the tissues are based on the average current.[8] Average current is meaningful only for monophasic currents and unbalanced biphasic currents. Because the net charge for balanced biphasic currents and ACs is zero, the root-mean-square value should be used for these currents (see Box 11–2).

By increasing the number of pulses per second or by increasing the pulse duration, the average current is increased and so is the perception of the stimulus. There is more current per unit of time in high-frequency generators than with other types. Long pulse durations combined with a high average current result in an increased sensation of pain.

The average current found in most electrical stimulation units is measured in milliamperes. This measure is not meaningful for a balanced symmetrical current because the phase charges for this type of current are equal and for the average current are zero.

Current Density

The physiological effects derived from electrical stimulation are related to the current density and the amount of current per unit area. The current density is inversely proportional to the size of the electrode. For example, if you are passing 300 V through an electrode of 10 square inches, the resulting current density would be 30 V per square inch. If the electrode's surface area is reduced by half, 300 V are then passing through an electrode of 5 square inches, with a current density of 60 V per square inch. If the electrode's surface area is again reduced, to a size of 1 square inch, the result is a current density of 300 V per square inch.

As the current density increases, so does the perception of the stimulus. If the stimulus was comfortable to the patient in our first example, it would be much more uncomfortable in the last example because the same amount of current is being delivered by one-tenth of the initial surface area (see Electrode Size, p 223).

Duty Cycle

The duty cycle describes the amount of time the current is flowing (ON) as opposed to the time the current is not flowing (OFF). Expressed as a percentage, duty cycles are calculated by dividing the time the current is flowing by the total cycle time (the time the current is flowing plus the time it is not). For example, to calculate the duty cycle of a generator producing 10 seconds of stimulation, followed by 10 seconds without current flow, the following equation would be used:

$$\text{Duty cycle (percentage)} =$$

$$\text{Time current is ON/Total cycle time} \times 100$$

$$= 10 \text{ s (ON)}/10 \text{ s (ON)} + 10 \text{ s (OFF)} \times 100$$

$$= 10 \text{ s}/20 \text{ s (Total cycle time)} \times 100 = 0.5 \times 100$$

$$= 50 \text{ percent duty cycle}$$

This relationship may also be expressed as a ratio. Using the parameters from the previous examples:

$$\text{Duty cycle (ratio)} = 10{:}20$$

$$= 1{:}2$$

Muscular stimulation is started with a 25-percent duty cycle and is progressively increased as the condition improves.[9]

● Chapter Highlights

- An electrical current is the flow of electrons through a medium (wires, electrodes, the body).
- Electrons move from the negative pole (cathode) where there is an abundance of electrons and move to the positive pole (anode) where there is a relative absence of electrons.
- Therapeutic currents are classified as being alternating, direct, or pulsed.
- Alternating and DCs are characterized by an uninterrupted flow of electrons.
- All forms of current have the common measures of amplitude, duration, and frequency.

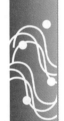

Box 11–5. Calculation of Ohm's Law in Series and Parallel Circuits

In a Series Circuit:

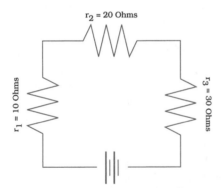

$r_2 = 20$ Ohms

$r_1 = 10$ Ohms

$r_3 = 30$ Ohms

If we know that a potential of 120 V is applied to a circuit with 60 ohms of resistance, the amperage can be calculated by using Ohm's law. Using the values Figure A above, the equation for calculating the current flow through the series of resistors is:

$$I = V/R_t$$
$$I = 120 \text{ V}/60 \text{ ohms}$$
$$I = 2 \text{ A}$$

If each of three resistors has a different resistance (say 10 ohms, 20 ohms, and 30 ohms), the voltage will fluctuate between resistors. By applying a derivation of Ohm's law, $V = IR$, the voltage across each resistor may be calculated as:

$V_1 = Ir_1$	$V_2 = Ir_2$	$V_3 = Ir_3$
$V_1 = 2 \text{ A} \times 10 \text{ ohms}$	$V_2 = 2 \text{ A} \times 20 \text{ ohms}$	$V_3 = 2 \text{ A} \times 30 \text{ ohms}$
$V_1 = 20 \text{ V}$	$V_2 = 40 \text{ V}$	$V_3 = 60 \text{ V}$

By adding V1 + V2 + V3, you can see that the sum of the potential across the individual resistors equals the total power applied to the circuit. The current (amperage) remains the same throughout a series circuit. The voltage and the resistance vary.

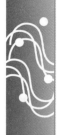

Box 11–5. Calculation of Ohm's Law in Series and Parallel Circuits *(Continued)*

In a Parallel Circuit:

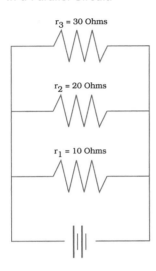

To calculate the total resistance for a parallel circuit, we must keep in mind that the flow in each pathway is inversely proportional to its resistance. Because voltage is constant, this value may be canceled out and the mathematical reciprocal (1/n) of the resistance may be used:

$$I = V/R_t$$
$$I = 120 \text{ V}/5.56 \text{ ohms}$$
$$I = 21.6 \text{ A}$$

The amount of current flowing across each resistor (and path) is calculated by:

$i_1 = v/r_1$	$i_2 = v/r_2$	$i_3 = v/r_3$
$i_1 = 120 \text{ V}/10 \text{ ohms}$	$i_2 = 120 \text{ V}/20 \text{ ohms}$	$i_3 = 120 \text{ V}/30 \text{ ohms}$
$i_1 = 12 \text{ A}$	$i_2 = 6 \text{ A}$	$i_3 = 4 \text{ A}$

where:

i_n = Amperage across resistor n
v = Voltage applied to the circuit
r_n = Resistance in ohms

Unlike series circuits, the parallel circuits have the same voltage across each path. The amperage and resistance differ from path to path. Therefore, if the voltage across one path can be calculated, the voltage for the entire circuit is known.

- In pulsed currents, the flow of electrons is intermittently paused.
- The interpulse interval represents the pause between pulses; the intrapulse interval represents a pause within the pulse itself.
- Pulsed currents are classified as monophasic (one directional electron flow) or biphasic (bidirectional electron flow).
- The shape of the current's pulse or waveform affects the tissue's physiological response to the treatment.
- The current variables are what ultimately differentiate stimulation approaches and the target tissues.
- Ohm's law describes the relationship between amperage, voltage, and resistance. The current is directly proportional to voltage and inversely proportional to resistance: $I = V/R$.
- On entering the body, several different electrical paths develop and form a series or parallel circuit.
- Therapeutic electrical stimulators generate a current that targets different types of tissues (usually nerves) to produce a specific result.

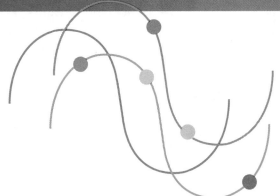

Chapter 12

Electrical Stimulation Techniques

This chapter describes the therapeutic objectives, methods, and effects of passing a therapeutic electrical current through the human body.

The type of current, the current's parameters, and the size and arrangement of the electrodes can produce specific physiological events and target specific tissues. Electrical stimulation has little, if any, direct effect on the cellular level inflammation response, but this is not to imply that it does not have a useful role in injury management.

The primary effects of electrotherapy occur secondary to the depolarization of sensory, motor, or pain nerves. Other effects are caused by electrochemical changes in the tissue. Chapter 11 described the different electrical parameters that can be modified, each type of current producing unique effects within the tissues and causing a wide range of therapeutic responses (Table 12–1).

■ The Body Circuit

The human body is a mass of tissues and fluids, each having varying ability to conduct an electrical current based on its water content. As the percentage of the water in tissue increases, its ability to transmit electricity increases.

Tissues are classified as being either excitable or nonexcitable. Excitable tissues (nerves, muscle fibers, cell membranes, etc) are directly influenced by the current parameters of intensity, pulse or phase duration, and pulse frequency. Nonexcitable tissues such as bone, cartilage, tendons, adipose tissue, and ligaments do not directly respond to current flow but may be influenced by the electrical fields caused by the current (Fig. 12–1).

The outer layer of the skin has a low water content, making it a poor electrical conductor. Bone, tendons, fascia, and adipose tissue are also poor conductors of electrical currents because of their low water content (20 to 30 percent). Muscle, nerve, and blood have a high water content (70 to 75 percent) and are good conductors of electrical currents. Cell membranes produce the greatest resistance to current flow. The internal organs, especially the heart, have a low resistance to electrical current flow (Box 12–1).

The current enters the body through a series circuit. Because the composition and texture of skin are relatively consistent, there is only one path for the flow to take. Once

TABLE 12–1	**Therapeutic Uses of Electrical Currents**

Controlling acute and chronic pain
Reducing edema
Reducing muscle spasm
Reducing joint contractures
Inhibiting muscle spasm
Minimizing disuse atrophy
Facilitating tissue healing
Facilitating muscle reeducation
Facilitating fracture healing
Strengthening muscle
Effecting orthotic substitution (Electrical stimulation can be used to force contractions of specific muscles during gait)

the current enters the tissues, it may take many different paths, forming a parallel circuit, with the current preferring to follow the path of least resistance, such as those formed by muscle, nerves, effusion, and blood. Areas on the skin having decreased electrical resistance form **stimulation points** (see Box 12–3).

The passage of current through living tissues produces varying biophysical effects, including physiochemical effects and physiological reactions. Thermal changes could potentially occur within the tissues using low- and moderate-frequency electrical currents, but at therapeutic doses, the effect is negligible.[8] High-frequency electrical

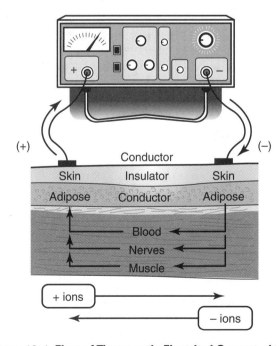

Figure 12–1. **Flow of Therapeutic Electrical Current.** At the skin-electrode interface the flow of electrons is exchanged for the flow of ions within the body. Within the tissues, the current has multiple paths from which to choose. Positively charged ions move toward the cathode and away from the anode. Negatively charged ions move towards the anode and away from the cathode.

currents, such as those used with medical diathermy, do produce thermal effects (see Chapter 9).

Electrode Leads

Electrode leads conduct the current to and from the generator, the electrodes, and the patient. A minimum of two leads are required to complete the electrical path, with each lead representing each side of the circuit. Individual leads can be bifurcated, allowing multiple electrodes to be attached to each leads (Fig. 12–2).

The U.S. Food and Drug Administration (FDA) Performance Standard for Electrode Lead Wires and Patient Cables (Code of Federal Regulations, Chapter 21, Part 898) mandates electrode lead wires to be fitted with jacks that prevent unintended contact between the patient and an unintended electrical power source (Fig. 12–3). Documented instances of electrode leads being plugged directly into alternating current (AC) electrical wall outlets have occurred and the new jack design prevents this from happening. Older units must also be retrofitted with these jacks (Fig. 12–4).

Electrodes

Formed of polymers, metal, or carbon-impregnated silicon rubber, electrodes introduce the current to the body (Fig. 12–5). When the electrons reach the electrode, they will choose the path of least resistance and travel toward the periphery of the electrode.[10] The site where the electrodes touch the skin is the point of conversion between the flow of electrons used by the generator and the flow of ions within the body's tissues (Box 12–2). Ion flow consists of positively charged sodium and potassium ions moving toward the negative pole and negative ions, primarily chlorides, moving toward the positive pole.[5] The interface between the electrode and the skin is also the primary source of resistance to current flow.

To form a closed circuit between the generator and the body's tissues, at least one electrode from each of the generator's output must be in firm contact with the skin. Properly prepared and positioned electrodes increase the efficiency of the electrical current and provide for improved patient comfort (Table 12–2). If the current is not evenly distributed across the electrode, increased current density will cause "hot spots" that may cause discomfort.

The skin creates both capacitive and parallel resistance to current flow. The stratum corneum has dielectric properties and creates a capacitor between the electrode and the underlying excitable tissues (see Fig. 11–15). As the thickness of the stratum corneum decreases, the capacitive resistance decreases. Parallel resistance is formed as the ions pass through portals in the skin, such as glands and pores, to the underlying tissues. As the number of parallel paths increase, the overall parallel resistance decreases. Water, gel, or self-adhesive electrodes more efficiently transmit the current by conforming to the small contours of the skin.

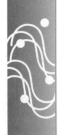

Box 12–1. The Path of Least Resistance

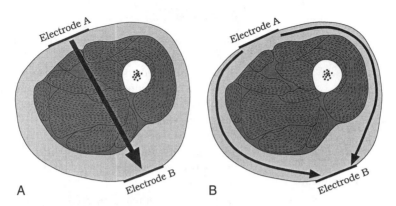

We tend to think of an electrical current flowing in a straight line from one electrode to another, and in some cases this is correct. Recall that electrons follow the path of least resistance and that the amperage and voltage must be sufficient to overcome the total resistance imposed by the circuit.

Consider a situation in which electrodes are placed on the anterior and posterior surfaces of the thigh. We may think that the current will flow directly through the tissues from one electrode to another as presented in A above. Most therapeutic treatment dosages lack the electrical power required to overcome the sum of the resistance formed by the cross-section of the tissues. In most cases, the current travels around the periphery by conducting through superficial blood vessels and nerves (B above). The deeper tissues are affected by stimulation of superficial nerves.

Transthoracic and transcranial stimulation is often contraindicated, but not necessarily out of fear of sending a current through the heart or brain. Appropriately placed electrodes can affect the functions of these organs secondary to stimulation of superficial nerves. Many stimulation techniques, such as those for temporomandibular joint dysfunction and auriculotherapy, involve application of electricity to the head. However, at these intensities the current stays within the tissues that are immediately subcutaneous.

Exercise caution when applying an electrical current anywhere on the upper torso, neck, or head. In these areas the path of least resistance may involves nerves that regulate heart rate, blood pressure, and other involuntary life functions.

The type of electrode and the conductive medium used can affect the efficiency and comfort of electrical stimulation. Of the standard electrode types, carbon-rubber electrodes deliver the most current at the lowest skin impedance, about 200 ohms, allowing for a more comfortable stimulation. Silver electrodes (most commonly used with iontophoresis, microcurrent stimulators, and electrodiagnostic units) provide about 20 ohms of resistance, so less energy is required to pass the current through them.[11, 12] However, silver electrodes are expensive.

Self-adhesive electrodes are commonly used for clinical electrotherapy. With this type of electrode, the conducting gel is a part of the electrode. Although self-adhesive electrodes are convenient and easy to use, they produce the highest resistance to electrical current flow.[10, 12] Self-adhesive electrodes have been shown to produce the most discomfort during the treatment, with an increased burning sensation occurring under the electrode's metal connector.[12] Other types of electrodes require an additional conducting medium to improve the contact between the skin and electrode, improve current distribution, and decrease the resistance formed by the stratum corneum.[10]

Metal electrodes use moistened sponges to make an electrical connection with the skin. Carbon-rubber electrodes may also use moist sponges, gauze, or a conducting gel. Although tap water is commonly used to moisten the sponges, the quality and mineral content of water in many

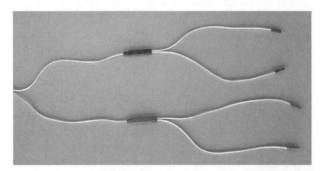

Figure 12-2. **Bifurcated Electrode Lead.** A single lead can be split, or bifurcated, to allow two electrodes to be attached.

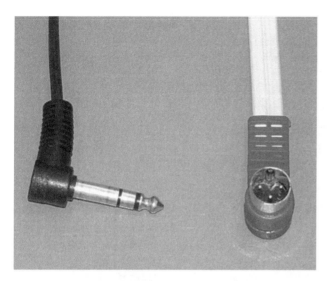

Figure 12–3. **Electrode Leads.** The lead on the left is non-compliant with FDA standards because the current-carrying surfaces are exposed. The lead on the right is compliant because the conductors are shielded.

areas can increase electrical resistance. Usually, this is not a problem, but patients who are sensitive to electrical currents may be more comfortable if the sponge is saturated with a commercially available saline solution.

Conducting gels are salt-free coupling agents designed to minimize skin-electrode resistance and are used with carbon, rubber, or metal electrodes and are a part of adhesive electrodes. The gel contains water with a thickening agent, a bactericide or fungicide, and ionic salts. The salt's ions increase the gel's conductivity, allowing diffusion into the skin, and decreasing the skin's capacitive resistance. The ionic salts can, however, result in skin irritation. Their chemical properties allow long-term use with little breakdown associated with current flow or evaporation, and because of the gel's high water content and low mineral content, skin irritation and allergic reactions are minimized.

Before placing nonadhesive rubberized electrode on the patient's skin, a liberal amount of the gel should be spread over the entire area of the conducting surface. Once the electrode has been positioned on the skin, it should be slightly rotated and slid to ensure even distribution of the medium. Nonadhesive electrodes used during short-term treatments are generally held in place by elastic straps. In the case of long-term treatments, the electrodes are either self-adhesive or they must be secured through the use of adhesive patches. Gel, rather than water, should be used for this type of treatment. Generally, these types of electrodes and their adhesives are very durable and water resistant.

Electrode Size

The size of the electrode inversely affects the current density; as the size of the electrode increases, the current density decreases. Consider, for example, a current passing through two electrodes, one having a surface area of 10 square inches and the other 5 square inches. The smaller electrode (5 square inches) would have twice as much current passing through it per square inch than the larger one (Fig. 12–6).

The electrode's contact with the skin also influences the stimulation parameters, comfort, and muscular tension associated with electrical stimulation.[13] As the electrode surface area increases, there is a greater current flow at any given voltage.[1] **Most electrodes have a maximum current density that must not be exceeded**. This value (e.g., 0.1 watts/cm^2) is included with the electrode's packaging information.

By altering the relative sizes of the electrodes, various physiological responses may be elicited. Smaller electrodes require less current to stimulate tissues than larger electrodes because of the high current density. The size of an electrode to be used is determined by the size of the

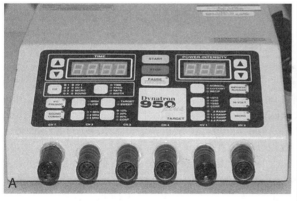

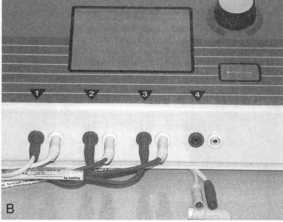

Figure 12–4. **Complying with the FDA Performance Standard for Electrode Lead Wires and Patient Cables.** (A) An older, previously noncompliant generator retrofitted with new jacks to bring the unit into compliance with the standard. (B) A new unit having compliant leads (note the face electrode lead wires in the bottom right).

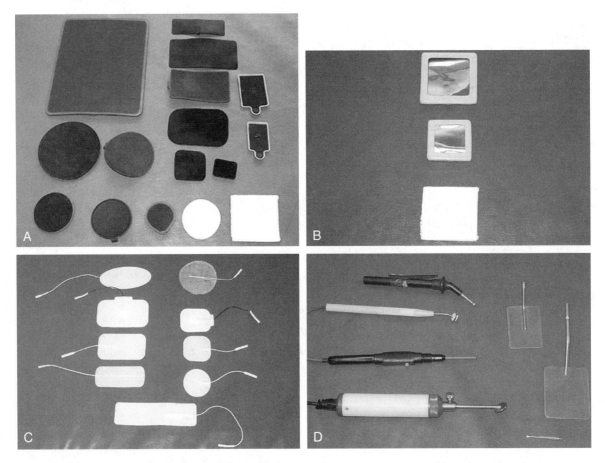

Figure 12–5. **Electrical Stimulation Electrodes.** (A) Carbon-impregnated rubber electrodes. A sponge or other conducting medium is required. (B) Metal electrodes. A moistened sponge (bottom) is needed to conduct the current. (C) Self-adhesive electrodes. (D) Probes (point stimulators) and paddles.

body area being treated or the other electrodes being used. A "small" electrode used on the quadriceps may be a "large" electrode when it is used on the forearm. In addition, as we will see in the next section, the size of an electrode is relative to the other electrode(s) being used.

The strength of isometric contractions increases as the size of the electrode increases.[12] The resistance to current flow (impedance) offered by the skin is reduced as the size of the electrode increases. Larger electrodes produce stronger contractions without causing pain, but

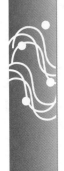

Box 12–2. Ionic Changes

In its normal state, an atom has a number of electrons equal to the number of protons. Because the charges of the electrons (negative) and protons (positive) are equal, the atom has a zero (neutral) charge. Atoms that no longer have a zero net charge are known as ions. When an atom loses one or more electrons, it becomes a positive ion (cation) because the number of protons is greater than the number of electrons. Likewise, atoms that gain electrons become negatively charged ions (anions) because the number of electrons is greater than the number of protons.

Ions behave differently from their neutrally charged relatives. Because they possess an electrical charge, they are subject to electromagnetic and **electro-osmotic** ■ influences. When placed in the path of a direct current, positively charged ions migrate toward the negative pole and vice versa.

Electro-osmotic: Pertaining to the movement of ions as a result of electrical charges. Positive ions move away from the positive pole toward the negative pole; negative ions move away from the negative pole toward the positive pole.

TABLE 12–2 Methods of Reducing Skin-Electrode Resistance

Moisten electrodes with water or conductive gel (sponge or rubber electrodes).

Remove dirt, oil, or flaky skin by washing with soap and water, alcohol, or acetone.

Warm area with a moist heat pack.

Gently scrub area with fine emery paper.

Remove excess hair.

Saturate sponges with commercial saline solution rather than tap water.

Use silver electrodes.

the stimulation of the tissues is less specific because the current is spread over a larger area.[13]

Electrode Placement

The size of the treatment area, current intensity, and type of excitable tissue being stimulated are determined by a combination of electrode size and their relative location on the body. Certain areas of the skin are more conducive to electrical stimulation than other areas. These sites, collectively referred to as stimulation points, represent motor points, trigger points, and acupuncture points (Box 12–3). Anatomically, these points tend to be located close to each other; so one electrode often stimulates multiple points. Likewise, the patient's perceived intensity and the intensity of muscle contractions is dependent on the number of nerve fibers that are stimulated.

The proximity of electrodes to one another deter-

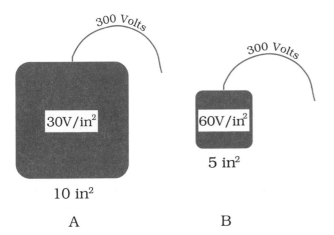

Figure 12-6. **Current Density.** Electrodes must transmit the entire voltage flowing through the circuit. In this case the large electrode, electrode A has 300 volts flowing through it. Electrode B is half the size of A, yet 300 volts must pass through it as well. In this example, electrode A has a current density of 30 volts per square inch (in²); electrode B has 60 volts per square inch. The stimulation would be more intense under electrode B because of the increased current density.

mines which tissues are stimulated, the depth of the stimulation, and the number of parallel circuits that are formed. When electrodes are placed close together, the current flows superficially, forming a relatively small number of parallel paths. As the distance between electrodes is increased, the current is allowed to reach deeper into the tissues. If the distance between the two electrodes is too great, such a large number of parallel circuits is formed that the specificity of the stimulation decreases (Fig. 12–7). Muscle fibers are four times more conductive when the current flows with the direction of the fibers than when it flows across them.[5]

Although each electrical circuit must have two leads from the generator, more than one electrode can be connected to a single lead. Through bifurcation, two or more electrodes can originate from a single lead (see Fig. 12–2). It is common for both leads to possess two electrodes each, or for one lead to have two electrodes and the other lead to have only one. The relationship between the total current density of one electrode (or set of electrodes) to the other electrode determines the electrode configuration, which may be classified as monopolar, bipolar, or quadripolar.

The terms "monopolar" and "bipolar" are often confused with "monophasic" and "biphasic." Remember that electrodes represent electrical poles (mono**polar** technique) and electrical currents are built out of phases (mono**phasic** current).

Bipolar Technique

Bipolar application involves the use of electrodes of equal or near-equal size (Fig. 12–8). Both electrodes are located in the target treatment area. Because the current densities are equal, an equal amount of stimulation should occur under each electrode or set of electrodes. Other factors may affect the quality and equality of stimulation under each electrode. If electrode A is placed over a motor point or other hypersensitive stimulation point (see Box 12–3) and electrode B is not, the effects of the treatment will be weighted toward electrode A. This scenario would be appropriate if a single point, such as a trigger point, were being targeted during the treatment. In this case, a monopolar configuration would be preferable because a single, well-localized area is being targeted. However, if the treatment goal is to elicit a muscle contraction, electrodes A and B both should be placed over motor points within the same muscle or muscle group.

Monopolar Technique

Monopolar application involves the use of two classifications of electrodes: (1) one or more active electrodes placed over the target tissues and (2) a dispersive electrode used to complete the circuit. The active electrode is placed on or near the body part to be treated, and the dispersive electrode is fastened elsewhere on the body (e.g., opposing muscle group, opposite limb, low back) (Fig. 12–9). The high current density focuses the effect of the treatment under the smaller electrodes. As the distance between the

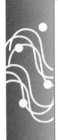

Box 12–3. Stimulation Points

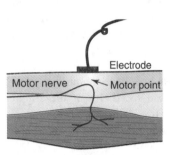

Certain areas of the skin conduct electricity better than other areas. These locations, collectively known as stimulation points, represent areas that require less current to produce muscle contractions, sensation, or pain. Many therapeutic techniques are designed to specifically stimulate one or more of these stimulation points. The proximity of these areas to each other results in a single electrode stimulating all three points.

Motor Points

Each muscle has one or more skin surface areas that are hypersensitive to electrical current flow. These points, known as motor points, are discrete areas above the location where motor nerves and blood vessels enter the muscle mass. Because of their low electrical resistance, stimulation of these points elicits a stronger contraction at lower intensities than the surrounding tissues. Motor points associated with an injured area show an increased sensitivity to current flow and palpation.

Although there is a degree of consistency in the location of motor points, there is some variation between individuals and, depending on the pathology involved, can vary within the same person over time. Appendix C presents commonly accepted motor points and is presented for reference purposes. These points must be located on each athlete by finding the point at which the strongest contraction results from the lowest intensity of stimulation.

Trigger Points

Trigger points are pathological, localized areas of pain that are hypersensitive to stimulation. Stimulation of these areas "triggers" radiating or referred pain. Unlike motor points, trigger points may be found not only in muscle but also in other soft tissues, such as ligament, tendon, and fascia (see Appendix A).

Acupuncture Points

Acupuncture points are specific sites on the skin possessing a decreased electrical skin resistance and increased electrical conductivity. These points are connected by meridians through which blood and energy flow.[14, 15, 16] Superficial **master points** ■, consisting of 12 main channels, 8 secondary channels, and a network of subchannels, connect areas of the skin to deeper channels and allow systemic regulation of many body functions. These master points are often effective in alleviating pain along the entire meridian. Although acupuncture has been successfully used for many centuries, its theoretical basis has never been fully substantiated.

---

active and dispersive electrodes increases, more parallel electrical paths are formed, resulting in less specific stimulation of deep motor nerves.

The surface area of the dispersive electrode is significantly larger, usually more than 2.5 times than that of the total area of the active electrodes. Because of the relatively low current density, little or no stimulation should occur under the dispersive electrode, despite the fact that current is still flowing through it. If sensation is experienced under

this electrode, reapply the dispersive electrode to a different site, re-wet it, or use a larger electrode. Sensation under the dispersive electrode does not negate the effects of the treatment, but it is unnecessary. Motor nerve stimulation under this electrode indicates that the current densities of the electrodes are too similar. In this case, a larger dispersive electrode or a smaller active electrode should be used. Note that the dispersive electrode is often incorrectly referred to as the "ground."

Master points: Points that, according to the theory of acupuncture, connect skin areas to deeper energy channels. Stimulating master points results in systemic changes.

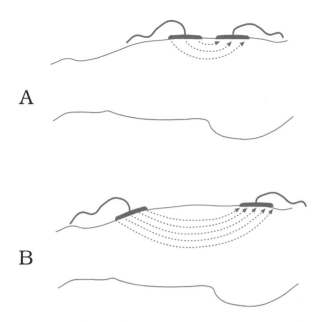

A

B

Figure 12-7. **Electrode Proximity.** (A) When electrodes are placed in close proximity to each other, the current flow forms relatively few parallel paths and does not penetrate as deeply into the tissues. (B) As the distance between the electrodes is increased, the number of parallel paths increases and the current tends to flow more deeply within the tissues. However, along with this the focus of the stimulation becomes less defined because the current meets more resistance and more parallel pathways are formed.

Quadripolar Technique

Quadripolar application involves the use of two sets of electrodes, each originating from its own **channel** ■; it may be considered the concurrent application of two bipolar circuits. The current from each of the two channels may intersect and intensify and localize the treatment effects as is found with interferential stimulation. Other quadripolar configurations include parallel placements, as are found in certain transcutaneous electrical nerve stimulation techniques, or agonist-antagonist placements used in neuromuscular electrical stimulation techniques (Fig. 12–10).

Movement of Electrical Currents Through the Body

Most forms of clinical electrical stimulation are applied transcutaneously. The exceptions are certain bone growth generators that may have electrodes surgically implanted in the muscle or bone. When a current is passed through the skin, it has the potential to upset the resting potential of peripheral axons (Box 12–4).

Once a therapeutic electrical current enters the body, the movement of ions replaces the flow of electrons (see Fig. 12–1). As described by Coulomb's law, ions move away from the pole having the same charge and migrate toward the pole having the opposite charge. When an AC

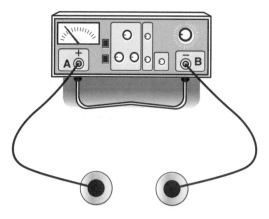

Figure 12-8. **Bipolar Application of Electrical Stimulation.** The surface area of the electrodes originating from each lead is equal. This creates an equal current density, and the effects of the stimulation occur equally under each electrode. Each lead may be split to accommodate two electrodes. As long as the electrodes are of equal size and the resulting current density is equal, the application is classified as bipolar.

or pulsed biphasic current is used, the ions move back and forth between the electrodes based on the number of cycles per second, as shown in Figure 11–6. When a DC or pulsed monophasic current is used, this migration is in one direction only.

Selective Stimulation of Nerves

The different nerve types are depolarized in an orderly, predictable manner. A nerve's response to electrical stimu-

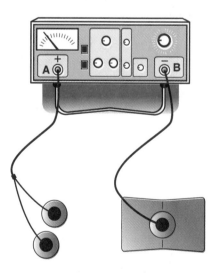

Figure 12-9. **Monopolar Application of Electrical Stimulation.** The total area of the active electrode is significantly less than the area of the dispersive electrode. The imbalance in current density focuses the stimulation to the area under the active electrodes.

Channel (electrical): An electrical circuit consisting of two poles that operate independently of other circuits.

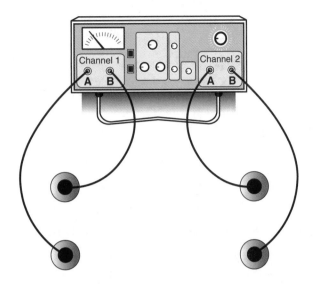

Figure 12–10. Quadripolar Application of Electrical Stimulation. Two sets of electrodes operating with two independent channels.

lation is based on three factors: (1) the relative diameter of the nerve, (2) the depth of the nerve in relation to the electrode, and (3) the duration of the pulse or phase. Sensory nerves are stimulated first, followed by motor nerves, and then pain fibers. Only after these structures have been depolarized (or if these nerves are incapable of depolarizing) can the electrical current directly affect muscle fibers.

Large-diameter nerves are depolarized before smaller diameter nerves. The amplitude necessary to stimulate a nerve is inversely proportional to the nerve's diameter. Because the larger cross-sectional area of the nerve provides less capacitive membrane resistance, less current is required (Box 12–5).

Superficial sensory nerves receive more stimulation than the more deeply placed motor nerves. To activate a deep motor nerve, the current must first pass through the superficial sensory nerves. Pain fibers are more superficial than motor nerves, but they also tend to have a smaller diameter. Their resistance to current flow is so great that motor nerves reach threshold first, allowing muscle contractions to be elicited before pain is felt. Superficial pain fibers may, however, be stimulated before the deeper motor nerves. Surface stimulation of the skin always results in the activation of sensory receptors before motor or pain nerves.[19]

Short pulse durations allow the greatest range in stimulation intensity for excitation of the three nerve types. As the phase duration is increased, two events occur. First, less amplitude is required to stimulate each nerve type. Second, the interval between each nerve level is decreased. Figure 12–11 depicts a typical strength-duration curve between phase duration and the threshold of excitation for the nerve types indicated. Theoretically, if the phase duration were continued out along the baseline, there would be a point at which each type of nerve would be stimulated almost simultaneously and at a very low intensity.

Various electrical stimulation protocols require that the stimulation parameters be sufficient to produce a muscle contraction, edema "milking," muscle re-education, or pain control, for example. Most electrical stimulators produce a muscle contraction by depolarizing motor nerves, not by directly depolarizing muscle fibers. Motor nerves have a larger diameter than muscle fiber; they present decreased electrical resistance relative to muscle fibers, so they are prone to depolarize first. Another reason for this lies in the resting potential of nerves and muscle fibers. On average, nerves have a resting potential of −75 mV and the resting potential of muscle fibers is −90 mV. Therefore a larger charge is needed to cause muscle to depolarize.

Electrical stimulators that have a long phase duration and sufficient amplitude can cause muscle fibers to depolarize and contract. However, referring to the selective stimulation of nerves, these parameters would also cause pain fibers to depolarize. Direct muscle fiber depolarization is used to produce muscle contractions in patients who are suffering from paralysis, enabling them to partially regain use of their limbs.

Stimulation Levels

Stimulation intensities are described with reference to the type of nerve depolarized:

Subsensory-level stimulation occurs between the point at which the output intensity rises from zero to the point where the patient first receives a discrete electrical sensation.

Sensory-level stimulation describes an output that stimulates only sensory nerves. This level is found by increasing the output to the point at which a slight muscle twitch is seen or felt and then decreasing the output intensity by approximately 10 percent.

Motor-level stimulation describes an intensity that produces a visible muscle contraction without causing pain.

Noxious-level stimulation is current applied at an intensity that stimulates pain fibers.

Central and Peripheral Nervous System Interference

When a stimulus sufficient to cause depolarization of a cell membrane remains unchanged, the resting potential of the membrane rises to above its prestimulus level. This process, called **accommodation**, occurs when the rate of discharge of the nerve's action potential decreases while the depolarization stimulus, in this case an electrical current, remains unchanged. Nerves undergoing accommodation require a more intense stimulus to reach the threshold of depolarization (Fig. 12–12).

The threshold for the initiation of an action potential varies according to the stimulation applied. Slowly rising pulses require a greater amount of amplitude to initiate an action potential. Nerves accommodate quickly; thus, an abrupt pulse rise is needed. Muscle fibers accommodate

Box 12–4. Exciting Excitable Tissues

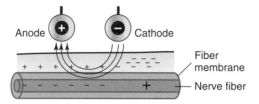

When an excitable tissue (nerves, muscle fibers, cell membranes, etc.) remains undisturbed, its resting potential stays constant. The resulting potential acts as a stored energy source to be used in the transmission of impulses; the energy is stored as separated electrical charges on either side (inside and outside) of the cell membrane. In this sense, the membrane serves as a capacitor.

A decrease (**depolarization**) or increase (**hyperpolarization**) in the cell membrane's electrical charge is required before an action potential can take place. **Rheobase** is the minimum amount of voltage, under the negative pole, required to produce a stimulated response when the phase duration is unlimited (e.g., a direct current is used). Unless specifically noted otherwise, the term "depolarization" will be used to denote the triggering of an action potential by either depolarization or hyperpolarization.

Any stimulus, be it electrical, mechanical, chemical, thermal, or hormonal, at a sufficient magnitude, can cause a depolarization by changing the permeability of the cell, resulting in an action potential. A membrane requires approximately 0.5 mSec to recover its excitability after an action potential. This "down time" after the action potential is the absolute refractory period. If a second impulse at the same intensity occurs within this period, the membrane will not discharge. After the absolute refractory period, there is a relative refractory period, during which another depolarization can occur if the magnitude of the stimulus is increased (see Box 1–2).

Under the cathode, the membrane potential is reduced, resulting in depolarization. Negative charges are repelled from the cathode and migrate to the relatively positively charged outer side of the nerve membrane, increasing the negative charge outside the cell and reducing the electrical potential between the inside and outside of the membrane. The resting potential shifts toward the positive and—given sufficient electrical potential—triggers an action potential.

Excitable tissues under the anode are hyperpolarized. Negative ions migrate from the nerve membrane towards the anode, creating an increased net positive charge outside of the membrane. The relative increase in the negative charge within the membrane triggers an action potential.

To trigger an action potential, the stimulus must be greater than the nerve's threshold potential. Cathodal stimulation, or the negative phase of a biphasic or alternating current tends to more easily trigger an action potential.[10]

Nerve Type	Diameter	Conduction Velocity	Stimulus Level for Depolarization
A-beta	12 to 20 μm	30 to 70 m/s	Low
A-delta	1 to 4 μm	6 to 30 m/s	High
C-fibers	<1 μm	0.5 to 2 m/s	High

more slowly than nerve fibers, so a gradual pulse rise may be used.[8] The pulse rise time is typically preset by the generator and is not changeable by the user.

The central nervous system (CNS) may also play a role in decreasing the long-term sensory stimulation associated with electrical stimulation. Through the process of **habituation**, the CNS filters out a continuous, nonmeaningful stimulus. This can be seen in everyday life: You sit down to study in the kitchen. Your roommates have gone out for the evening, so the apartment is quiet except for the humming of the refrigerator. After you

begin studying, the sound of the refrigerator gets pushed further and further into the background of your consciousness. Eventually, you no longer realize that the sound is there. This stimulus stays in your mental "background" until the refrigerator stops humming. At this point, you are struck by the roaring silence of the room.

The concepts of accommodation and habituation can be demonstrated in applying an electrical modality. Increase the intensity of an electrical modality to the point at which the patient expresses slight displeasure in the comfort of the stimulus. Allow the person to experience the

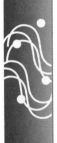

Box 12–5. The Law of Dubois Reymond

Causing a nerve to depolarize is a relatively easy task; simply apply enough voltage with sufficient amperage and depolarization is bound to occur. However, this type of stimulation is rarely therapeutic or selective.

According to the Law of Dubois Reymond, the variation in current density, rather than the absolute current density, causes the depolarization of nerves or muscle tissue.[17] Variations in current density overcome the cell membrane's resistance at a lower intensity than at unchanging densities. To depolarize excitable tissues in an orderly and sequential manner, the following criteria must be met[18]:

- The current must be of sufficient intensity to cause depolarization of the cell membrane.
- The rate of rise of the leading edge of the pulse must be rapid enough to prevent accommodation.
- The duration of the current must be long enough in one direction that the nerve has the time to depolarize and repolarize.

STRENGTH - DURATION CURVE

In neural activation the amplitude and phase duration are usually inversely related.

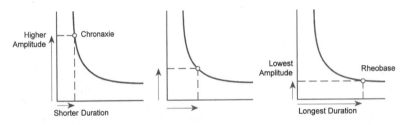

The optimal excitation of the nerve occurs between its rheobase and chronaxie (or simply where the nerve bends) as plotted on the strength - duration curve.

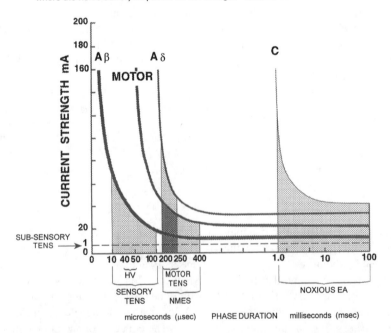

Figure 12–11. **Strength-Duration Curve.** Because of the capacitive resistance formed by the walls of cell membranes, short pulse or phase durations are more selective in the nerve fibers stimulated than pulses having a longer duration. Shorter-duration currents require increasing amounts of current to stimulate the same type of nerve fiber than currents having a longer duration. (Courtesy of IAPT. Used with permission.)

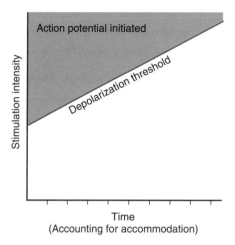

Figure 12–12. Changes in Depolarization Threshold During Accommodation. When excitable tissues are exposed to an unchanging stimulus, the cell membrane adapts to the stimuli, requiring an increased level of stimulation to trigger an action potential. This figure illustrates how the level of stimulation, over time, would have to be increased to cause depolarization of the cell membrane. The onset of accommodation can be combated when using electrical stimulation by adjusting the output parameters such as intensity, frequency, and duration at random intervals. These modulation parameters are built into many electrical stimulators.

current flow for about 5 minutes, and then ask if the intensity can be increased. More times than not, the patient will say "Yes." This ability to increase the intensity represents accommodation of the involved nerves. People become accommodated to an electrical current and are able to tolerate increased intensity as their number of treatment sessions increases.[20]

Many electrotherapeutic modalities have **modulation parameters** to combat the effects of accommodation. The generator randomly alters the intensity, frequency, or duration of the pulses to prevent the body from receiving a constant, unchanging stimulus (Table 12–3).

Medical Galvanism

Galvanic stimulation involves the application of a low-voltage direct current to the body, with a known polarity under each electrode. By controlling the polarity of the electrodes, certain involuntary cellular and biochemical responses may be elicited. True galvanism requires an uninterrupted direct current to achieve a net galvanic change under the electrodes. The **pH ■** of tissues under the cathode becomes basic (the alkalinity of the tissues is increased) and has an increased risk of chemical burns. Acids collect or form under the anode, causing coagulation of proteins and hardening of the tissue. Galvanic stimulation is the only type of current that elicits a muscle contraction from denervated muscle, but the phase duration is so

long that C fibers are also stimulated, making the contraction painful.

Through an electro-osmotic process, ions are attracted to the pole possessing the opposite charge and repelled from the pole having the same charge. Positively charged sodium ions (Na^+) move toward the cathode, where they gain an electron and form an uncharged sodium atom. Through the reaction of sodium with water, proteins are liquefied, causing a general softening of the tissues in the area and a decrease in nerve irritability.[21] Physiological events under the anode are essentially opposite those occurring at the cathode. Here, tissues are thought to harden because chemical mediators force a coagulation of protein.

These effects are not as pronounced when monophasic, biphasic, or alternating currents are used. The short pulse duration and long interpulse interval reduce the chemical effects of pulsed currents.[22] Symmetrical or balanced asymmetrical biphasic currents or ACs result in no galvanic changes because both phases have an equal but opposite charge. An unbalanced asymmetrical current can result in residual chemical changes if the duration of the current is sufficient.

■ Electrical Stimulation Goals

This section presents common goals of electrical stimulation and techniques on how to achieve them. The next chapter relates these goals to the different types of electrical stimulation units commonly used in the treatment of orthopedic and minor neurological conditions.

Motor-Level Stimulation

If it is applied at a sufficient intensity, almost any type of electrical stimulator can elicit a contraction in normal, healthy muscle, but not every electrical stimulator is appropriate for every motor-level treatment (Table 12–4). Through different types of electrical currents, different

TABLE 12–3	Modulation Parameters to Delay Physiological Accommodation to an Electrical Current

Amplitude
Phase/pulse duration
Frequency
Ramp
Surge
Burst
Multiple (the combination of two or more of the above parameters)

---

pH (potential of hydrogen): A measure of acidity or alkalinity (bases). A neutral solution has a pH of 7.

Acids have a pH of less than 7; bases greater than 7.

electrical stimulators allow for more efficient, intense, and comfortable contractions. The rise of the pulse, pulse/phase duration, and the amplitude of the current all factor together to determine the quality and quantity of the contraction.

The amount of torque that can be produced by an electrical stimulator is related to the amount of sensory discomfort associated with the current and the amount of muscular soreness experienced. Generators that are intended for neuromuscular stimulation should produce a strong tetanic contraction with relatively little sensory discomfort.[20]

During voluntary contractions, type I fibers are the first to fire and the strength of the contractions is based on the number of motor units recruited and the firing frequency of the motor units. Electrically induced muscle contractions cause type II fibers to be activated before type I fibers. With electrically induced contractions, all of the involved motor units fire at the same time. Increased tension is based on the firing frequency (pulse frequency) of the motor units.

TABLE 12–4	Common Uses of Motor-Level Stimulation Protocol by Generator Type
Generator/Current Type	*Clinical Usage/Limitations*
High Volt Pulsed Stimulation Monophasic	Neuromuscular reeducation
	Motor-level pain control
	Motor-level edema reduction
	Some units do not have a duty cycle control
	Lacks total current needed for maximum force production
Transcutaneous Electrical Nerve Stimulation Biphasic	Motor-level pain control
	No duty cycle control
	Low total current limits force production
Interferential Stimulation Alternating	Motor-level pain control
	Motor-level edema reduction
	No duty cycle control
	Pre-modulated parameters target current to motor nerves
Neuromuscular Electrical Stimulation Monophasic, biphasic, alternating	Neuromuscular reeducation
	Strength augmentation

Electrical stimulation of **innervated** ■ muscle activates the motor nerve rather than the muscle fibers directly. Because the capacitance of motor nerves is less than that of muscular tissue, the current overcomes the resistance of the nerve first (Table 12–5). When the magnitude of the stimulation is sufficient, an action potential is initiated, sending a signal to the motor unit that results in contraction of the muscle. For this reason, the electrodes should be placed over the muscle's motor points (see Appendix C). These contractions may be used to retard the effects of atrophy, reeducate muscle, reduce edema, or augment the force-generating capacity of healthy muscle.

Motor nerves are recruited into the contraction based on the diameter of their axons and their proximity to the electrodes.[23] Large-diameter motor neurons are recruited before smaller ones, and nerves in proximity to the electrode respond before those more distant. During voluntary muscle contractions, type I motor fibers are recruited before type II fibers. During motor-level electrical stimulation, type II fibers are recruited first.

Pulse Amplitude

The force generated by the muscle contraction is linearly correlated to the amount of current introduced into the tissues. The strength of the contraction increases as the intensity (amplitude) of the current increases.[24, 25] The depth of penetration of the current increases as the peak current increases, thus recruiting more nerve fibers.

The patient's tolerance to the current is often the limiting factor in the strength of the contraction produced. The maximum comfortable intensity tends to be less than 30 percent of the maximum voluntary isometric contraction (MVIC).[26] Prior exposure to electrical stimulation and

TABLE 12–5	Comparison of Physiologically Versus Electrically Induced Muscle Contractions	
Physiologically Induced Contractions		*Electrically Induced Contractions*
• Small-diameter, slow-twitch muscle fibers are recruited first.		• Large-diameter, fast-twitch muscle fibers are recruited first.
• Contractions and recruitment are asynchronous to decrease muscle fatigue.		• Contractions and recruitment are synchronous, based on the number of pulses per second.
• Golgi's tendon organs protect muscles from too much force production.		• Golgi's tendon organs cannot override the developing tension within the musculotendinous unit.

Innervate: Normal and sufficient nerve supply to a muscle, body area, and so on.

an understanding of the treatment and the expected sensations may lead to increased muscular tension.[27]

Cold treatments are often used for their anesthetic effects. Research on the ability of cold application before or during electrical stimulation to improve patient comfort has produced mixed results.[28, 29] The pain experienced during high-amplitude electrical stimulation is caused not only by stimulation of the cutaneous pain receptors but also by the nociceptors located deep within the muscle.[30] This technique could be beneficial for individuals who have increased sensory discomfort during electrical current application.

Phase Duration

The phase charge, the amount of current delivered by each phase, determines the quality and quantity of the muscle contraction. A phase duration of 300 to 500 microseconds (μsec) specifically recruits motor nerves.[8, 31] Short phase durations require greater amplitude to evoke an action potential than phases of longer durations. Phase durations of less than 1 millisecond (msec) will not be able to stimulate denervated muscle, regardless of the current's amplitude.[6, 7]

Pain fibers have a small diameter relative to motor nerves and are normally only stimulated at higher intensities and with longer phase durations, allowing for muscle recruitment without a disproportional amount of discomfort. However, the pain associated with the intensity of the stimulation often prevents maximum contractions from being achieved.

Pulse Frequency

When the stimulation is applied at a pulse rate of less than 15 pps (or in the case of AC, Hz), there are distinguishable muscle contractions for each electrical pulse. At this pulse rate, there is sufficient time for the mechanical process

TABLE 12–6 Pulse Frequency Ranges Commonly Used in Electrotherapy

Descriptor	Pulses per Second (pps)	Neuromuscular Effects
Low	<15	Twitch: Individual muscle contractions
Medium	15–40	Summation: Blending of individual contractions resulting in increased muscle tone
High	>40	Tonic: Steady or constant contraction

Note: The above ranges will differ depending on the individual and muscle group.

required for the muscle fibers to return to their original length before the next pulse begins. Each of these individual contractions is referred to as a **twitch** contraction (Table 12–6).

Because of **summation**, individual contractions become less and less distinguishable between 15 and 25 pulses per second. In this case, the pulses occur in such rapid succession that the muscle fibers do not have the time to return to their original position before the next pulse begins (Fig. 12–13). As the pulse frequency increases, the amount of summation increases as a result of the greater overlap in the mechanical process of muscle contraction.[8]

Summation continues until the muscle reaches the **critical fusion frequency**, the point at which **tetany** ▪ is obtained. At this point, the muscle enters a **tonic contraction** ▪. The critical fusion frequency is slightly different from person to person and between muscle groups, but it usually occurs between 30 to 40 pps.[32] Postural muscles

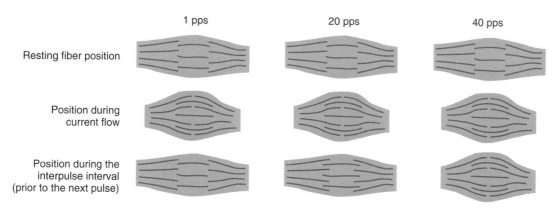

Figure 12–13. **Muscle Fiber's Reaction to Pulse Frequency.** The tone of a muscle undergoing electrically induced contractions varies with the pulse frequency. At less than approximately 15 pps, the muscle fibers have the time to return to their original starting position. As the pulse frequency increases, the duration of the interpulse interval decreases, prohibiting the muscle fibers from returning to their original starting position before the next pulse.

Tetany: Total contraction of a muscle achieved through the recruitment and contraction of all motor units.
Tonic contraction: Prolonged contraction of a muscle.

have been found to reach tetany before nonpostural muscles.[7]

Increasing the frequency of the stimulation will do little to increase the muscle tone further. Pulse frequencies above 60 pps cause an increased rate of muscle fatigue if used for a sufficient duration.

A strong tetanic contraction is required to delay atrophy or enhance strength. Low pulse frequency stimulation (20 pps) reduces fatigue, but the muscle develops 45 percent less force than it could at higher pulse frequencies.[3] Very high pulse frequencies reach tetany more comfortably than lower frequencies. Medium-frequency biphasic currents selectively fatigue type II muscle fibers, resulting in decreased torque production as the treatment progresses.[33] This effect may be counteracted by increasing the amount of rest between treatment cycles or decreasing the pulse frequency during treatment.

Denervated Muscle

Motor nerves that have been denervated for less than 3 weeks are still capable of depolarization and can be selectively recruited through the use of a short pulse duration that has a slowly rising waveform. In this case, motor nerves can continue to produce a muscle contraction via electrical stimulation until **wallerian degeneration** ■ sets in.[8]

When a muscle is denervated, communication with the muscle fibers can no longer occur through the motor nerve, so the fibers must be directly stimulated to evoke a contraction. Denervated muscle reacts to stimulation from a galvanic current or a monophasic current having a long phase duration but not from ACs or pulsed currents having a short duration. This reaction occurs because the current flows for a longer time in one direction when using a DC, allowing depolarization of the muscle fiber membranes to occur. In cases in which the patient has suffered a spinal cord injury but the peripheral nerves are still intact, such as an **upper motor neuron lesion** ■, muscle contractions can still be obtained through the use of a pulsed current.[8]

Neuromuscular Reeducation

Neuromuscular reeducation involves the "teaching" of a muscle how to contract again. Edema, pain, immobilization, disuse, or nerve damage can interfere with the neurological loop between the muscle, peripheral nerve, spinal cord, and brain.[20] Electrical stimulation is used to reestablish the neural pathways that will give way to voluntary contractions. Neuromuscular reeducation differs from strength augmentation, which is electrical stimulation applied to healthy muscle.

Generators that are capable of producing a duty cycle and ramping the current maximize the neuromuscular benefits.[34] A duty cycle, such as 10 seconds on, 50 seconds off, allows the muscle to relax and recover between contractions.[20] Ramping the current allows for a natural increase in tension. The pulse frequency must be sufficient to produce a tetanic contraction, with 60 pps being commonly used. For neuromuscular reeducation programs, the force generated should be at least 10% of the MVIC of the uninvolved leg.[35]

The patient may experience **delayed-onset muscle soreness** ■ following the treatment. As with any exercise program, the intensity should be adjusted to find a proper balance between therapeutic benefits and patient comfort.[27] Neuromuscular reeducation protocols should not be administered when the tendinous attachment is not secure, the muscle cannot tolerate the tension, or joint motion is contraindicated.

Similar to voluntary muscle contractions, electrical stimulation strengthening protocols may affect the contralateral muscle group, increasing strength by as much as 10 percent. These strength gains can be attributed to a neurological crossover effect, motor learning, or subconscious contraction of the nontreated muscle.[20] When the patient is unable to contract a muscle, secondary either to disuse or immobilization (i.e., splint or cast), strengthening the uninvolved limb by voluntary or electrically induced contractions may delay atrophy or assist in the reeducation of the involved limb.

Strength Augmentation

When the goal is to increase the muscle's strength, electrically induced muscle contractions can supplement but should not substitute for voluntary contractions. Electrical stimulation is less effective in increasing quadriceps torque than is biofeedback (see Chap. 18).[36] Strength gains obtained by electrical stimulation follow the same parameters of specificity as any other form of exercise; that is, isometric training improves only isometric strength, and that improvement does not carry over to **isotonic** ■ or **isokinetic** ■ strength.[37]

Delayed-onset muscle soreness: Residual muscle soreness, caused secondary to damage of the muscle cells, which appears within 24 hours after heavy muscular activity, particularly with eccentric muscle actions.

Isokinetic (contraction): A muscle contraction against a variable resistance where limb moves throughout the range of motion at a constant speed.

Isotonic (contractions): Muscle contraction through a range of motion against a constant resistance.

Upper motor neuron lesion: A spinal cord lesion resulting in paralysis, loss of voluntary movement, spasticity, sensory loss, and pathological reflexes.

Wallerian degeneration: Gradual physiological breakdown of a nerve axon that has been severed from its body.

Strength gains realized through the use of electrical stimulation are attributed to two factors[38]:

1. Muscular overload
2. Reversal of type I and type II motor nerves

Strength gains are a response to placement of an increased functional load on the muscle. For strength gains to occur through electrical stimulation, the functional load placed on the muscle must be equal to at least 30 to 60 percent of MVIC.[2, 26] You may recognize this factor as being, in part, the basis of the **overload principle** ■. To produce overload, the muscle must exceed the minimum electrically evoked torque (EET) production threshold, the point at which the contraction produces measurable and meaningful tension on the muscle. As the strength of the muscle increases, the EET also increases.[39]

The increased functional load produced by electrical stimulation is supplemented by the increased recruitment of type II muscle fibers, the second factor in strength augmentation. Because electrical current depolarizes larger diameter nerves first, type II fibers are brought into the contraction sooner and fatigue first.[23, 33, 40] The two elements of type II fiber recruitment and increased functional load work together so that muscle strengthening through electrical stimulation may occur at levels producing 30 percent of the tension found in the MVIC.[3, 38]

Several variables must be considered when attempting to increase muscle strength through electrical stimulation. If the duty cycle is too high, premature fatigue can occur because of increased use of the **phosphocreatine system** ■. Also, the protective function of Golgi's tendon organs is overridden during electrical stimulation. Precautions must be taken to damper the terminal ends of the patient's range of motion. For these reasons, the patient should always be given a safety switch that, when depressed, shuts off the stimulation unit in the event that the stimulation or muscle tension becomes too intense.

Pain Control

Electrical currents are used to reduce the amount of pain experienced by either assisting in the healing process or affecting the transmission and perception of pain. Lessening the mechanical pressure placed on nerve endings or decreasing the degree of muscle spasm or edema eliminates the mechanical and chemical events that stimulate pain transmission. In specific pain control approaches, electrical stimulation simply masks the pain or encourages the body to release its pain-controlling substances, endogenous opiates (Table 12–7).

High-pulse-frequency, short-phase-duration, sensory-level currents are thought to activate the gate mechanism of pain modulation. Stimulating sensory nerves closes the gate to the transmission of pain. Low-pulse-frequency, moderate-pulse duration, high-intensity stimulation and noxious-level stimulation stimulate the release of the body's natural opiates—β-endorphin from the anterior pituitary gland and enkephalins from the spinal cord (Table 12–8). High pulse frequency (more than 80 pps) motor-level stimulation triggers the release of enkephalins.[41]

In the initial phases of pain control, electrical currents stimulate the dorsal horn of the spinal cord. Activation of type I, II, III, and IV neurons may cause the dorsal horn to transmit less noxious information to the supraspinal levels.[42] Decreased nerve conduction of small, pain-carrying nerves reduces the amount and rate of noxious impulses transmitted up the spinal cord. In large motor nerves, decreased nerve conduction decreases the amount of pain-producing muscle spasm in the treated area.[43] Peripheral stimulation could relieve chronic pain if applied to the site of pain or to an area serviced by the involved peripheral nerve.

As mentioned in Chapter 2, the placebo effect of electrotherapeutic modalities cannot be overlooked. Many studies exploring the effects of electrical current flow (and other modalities and medications as well) on pain perception report that patients receiving sham treatments described a decrease in the amount of pain experienced, supporting the theory that cognitive processes are involved in pain modulation.[44–49]

Circulation

Electrically induced contractions increase local blood flow approximately the same amount as voluntary contractions, but heart rate and systemic blood pressure are not affected.[50] The increased blood flow may be caused by the release of endothelial relaxing factors that cause vasodilation.[50] The effect of sensory-level stimulation on local blood flow has not been substantiated.

Wound Healing

The use of a low-intensity DC or HVPS may reduce the time needed for superficial wound healing to 1.5 to 2.5 times that needed for wounds not receiving such treatment.[51–54] The electrical current acts by killing the organism directly, producing antimicrobial factors, and by attracting antimicrobial factors to the wound.[32] Negative polarity has demonstrated the ability to break down and absorb blood clots and other hemorrhagic byproducts. The positive pole may enhance the formation of clots.[52]

Explanations for the effectiveness of tissue repair include increased circulation, antibacterial effects, influ-

Overload principle: For strength gains to occur, the body must be subjected to more stress than it is accustomed to. This is accomplished by increasing the load, frequency, or duration of the exercise.
Phosphocreatine system: A compound that is important in muscle metabolism.

TABLE 12–7   Spinal Levels of Pain Control

Spinal Level	Theory	Activating Stimuli	Physiological Events
I	Presynaptic inhibition	Sensory stimulation of A-beta fibers Phase duration 75 msec	Enkephalin interneurons block the transmission of impulses traveling along small C fibers within the dorsal horn T cell.
II	Descending inhibition	Intense (high-frequency) stimulation of C fibers Phase duration 1000 msec	Central biasing mechanisms in the periaqueductal gray matter and the raphe nucleus activate descending influences along the dorsolateral tract of the spinal cord.
III	β-Endorphin modulation	Noxious, low-frequency, motor stimulation (A-delta) Phase duration 250–300 msec	Activates the tract cell and reticular formation, resulting in the release of b-endorphin from the anterior pituitary gland, causing the degeneration of prostaglandin and dorsal horn inhibition.

ences on migration of cells, and the presence of an **injury potential** ■ in damaged tissues. When tissues are damaged, an electrical potential is created between the healthy and damaged tissues.[55, 56] This injury potential is theorized to electrically control tissue repair. Most of the evidence supporting the use of electrical stimulation in wound healing in humans has involved chronic conditions, with the majority of the cases being **dermal ulcers** ■ or surgical incisions.

Depending on the polarity of the electrode, certain inflammatory mediators, including neutrophils, macrophages, epidermal cells, and fibroblasts, are attracted or repelled from the area.[52, 57] Low-intensity DC encourages hydration, increases the number of growth factor receptors, increases the rate of collagen formation,[58] stimulates the growth of fibroblasts and granulation tissues,[59] reduces the number of mast cells in the injured area,[60] and destroys bacteria and other microbes.[61] Last,

leukocytes migrate toward the anode, resulting in increased blood clotting in the area.[52]

Using animal models, DCs have also shown efficacy in promoting healing of the medial collateral ligament. Traumatized ligaments treated with electrical stimulation demonstrated an increased rupture force, increased amount of energy absorption, and decreased stiffness and laxity compared with nonstimulated ligaments.[62] When applied to healing tendons, DC appeared to suppress the proliferation of adhesion-causing cells compared with untreated tendons.[63]

Control and Reduction of Edema

Electrical stimulation is often used to control or reduce the amount of edema formed following orthopedic trauma, surgery, certain diseases, and burns. Sensory-level stimulation attempts to inhibit edema formation by preventing the fluids, plasma proteins, and other solids from escaping into

TABLE 12–8   Electrical Parameters Used in Pain Control Approaches

Approach	Target Nerves	Phase Duration	Pulse Frequency	Intensity
Sensory level	A-beta	<100 msec	60–100 pps	Submotor
Motor level	Motor nerves	150–250 msec	2–4 pps 80 to 120 pps	Strong contraction Moderate to strong contraction
Noxious level	A-delta C fibers	1 msec	Variable	As painful as can be tolerated

Dermal ulcer: A slow-healing or nonhealing break in the skin.

Injury potential: Disruption of a tissue's normal electrical balance as a result of injury.

surrounding tissues. If edema has already formed, motor-level stimulation assists the venous and lymphatic systems in returning the edema back to the torso, where it can be filtered and removed from the body.

Sensory-Level Stimulation for Edema Control

In acute trauma, sensory-level HVPS applied to, or directly around, the injury site has been found to limit the volume of edema formed in laboratory animals. The central concept of this theory is to limit the formation of edema rather than to remove existing edema. In fact, attempting these techniques when swelling has already formed may inhibit edema reduction.

A possible mechanism for this response is reduced capillary pressure and capillary permeability, which discourages plasma proteins from entering the extracellular tissues.[64] The pulsed monophasic current may cause a vascular spasm that prevents fluids from leaking out of the vessels.[65]

The theoretical and applied approach to sensory-level edema control is described in the section on High-Voltage Pulsed Stimulation of the next chapter.

Motor-Level Stimulation for Edema Reduction

The role of the motor-level response in reducing edema formation is less controversial and has demonstrated more clinical efficacy than the sensory-level approach. Muscular contractions encourage venous and lymphatic return by squeezing the vessels, moving the fluids proximally, and "milking" the fluids out of the area. Many types of electrical stimulation devices can be used to produce an involuntary muscle contraction that forces the fluids out of the area, but the output must be configured so that the current develops a tetanic contraction that forces the fluids proximally along the extremity and then is followed by a relaxation period (e.g. duty cycle). This technique is also referred to as "muscle milking" or the "muscle pump."

Electrodes are arranged on the involved extremity so that they follow the course of the primary vein exiting the swollen area. If the generator does not allow for a duty cycle, a low pulse frequency, usually 1 pps, is used to allow enough time for the contents of the venous and lymphatic system to move between muscle contractions. If a duty cycle is available, increase the number of pulses per second so that a tonic contraction is achieved. A 50-percent duty cycle is then used to obtain the desired off-and-on contractions.

The output intensity is adjusted so that the contraction is within the patient's tolerance, and contraindicated joint movement is avoided. Although electrically induced muscle contractions do increase the rate of venous return, the volume of flow is less than that which occurs with voluntary contractions. If the individual is capable of producing strong contractions, this method should be preferred over electrically induced contractions.

As would be expected from what we know of the venous and lymphatic return mechanisms (see Chap. 1), the efficiency of this technique is improved when the limb is elevated so that gravity may assist in the fluid flow. In addition, the use of an elastic wrap or tubular compressive stockings applied to the extremity assists in edema reduction.

Fracture Healing

Implantation of electrodes into acutely fractured bones and the subsequent introduction of a direct current to the healing structure have shown an increased bending rigidity and bone mineral density in animal models.[66] Normally, fractures heal through the process of **osteogenesis** ■. If the fracture fails to heal properly, further repair must occur through endochondral bone formation, the process by which the soft tissue callus transforms itself into bone.[67] Historically, nonunion fractures required the surgical grafting of bone into the fracture site to assist the healing process.

The use of electrical stimulation to aid in the healing of bone is based on the theory that bone cannot differentiate between the body's innate charges needed for normal bone remodeling (see Wolff's Law in Chap. 1) and those derived from outside sources, such as electrical generators. The natural source of these intrinsic stresses are piezoelectric charges caused by the deformation of the bone's collagen matrix.[68] These piezoelectric charges require an intermittent stress to be delivered to the bone. Static or constant stresses do not produce an electric charge.

Collectively known as bone growth generators, these units attempt to produce electromagnetic fields that mimic the normal electrical signals produced by bone or to activate the bone's piezoelectric properties. Each approach encourages the deposition of calcium through increased osteoblastic activity, regardless of the technique used to introduce the current. Generally, those generators applied transcutaneously use ACs, whereas those having electrodes implanted in the body use DCs.[69] The cathode is placed near the fracture site when the electrodes are implanted into the tissues because new bone callus is electropositive.[70] Implanted electrodes are then surgically removed once successful healing has been obtained.

Generators with external electrodes are similar to diathermy units (see Chap. 9) in that their electrodes produce strong electromagnetic fields. These fields then create electric currents at the fracture site.

The usefulness of bone growth generators is still debatable.[67, 69–71] Evidence exists that electrical bone growth generators may actually delay fracture healing, with stress fractures perhaps being the most negatively impacted.[66] This negative effect may be, at least in part, a result of the fact that many generators use a current "orders of magnitude" more powerful than that required for healing.[68]

Osteogenesis: Healing of fracture sites through the formation of callus, followed by the deposition of collagen and bone salts.

The prescription of bone growth generators is the physician's domain, and it is most likely their use will be prescribed only in extraordinary circumstances. These units appear to be most effective only in certain nonunion fractures and require long-term treatments (6 months or more). Because it appears that the currently proposed protocol for treating acute fractures involves implanting electrodes into the damaged bone, the risks and time delays of the associated surgery may limit use of this device to cases in which the patient is at risk for a nonunion or **malunion fracture** ■. However, clinicians should be familiar with the functions, benefits, and limitations of this device. As this technology grows and the efficacy of this modality is established, its possibilities for use in the treatment of acute fractures increase. A specialized form of ultrasound is also used to improve fracture healing (see Clinical Techniques: Ultrasonic Bone Growth Generators, p 174).

■ Contraindications and Precautions

The general contraindications and precautions in electrical stimulation are presented in Table 12–9. Contraindications particular to specific electrical stimulators are presented in the appropriate sections of the next chapter.

The primary precautions and contraindications to the use of electrical stimulation lie in the placement of the electrodes. Current flow through the heart, **carotid sinus** ■, and pharynx must be avoided because of the potential disruption in normal cardiovascular function. Most therapeutic currents do not directly affect the heart and other deeply-lying tissues (see Box 12–1). However, current flow can affect the heart's superficial stimulation points (e.g., the carotid sinus). Implanted cardiac pacemakers may be affected by stimulation of the thorax, lumbar region, or upper extremity. Because of the unknown and unpredictable effects, electricity is not normally applied over sites of infection.

Electrical stimulation is contraindicated over cancerous sites because of the possibility of accelerating the growth of the tumor or causing the cancer to spread. Electrical stimulation is sometimes used to help control pain in terminal cancer patients. At this point, the treatment approach no longer focuses on controlling the spread of the cancer but rather focuses entirely on patient comfort. The amount of medication needed to control pain in these instances leaves the patient unconscious or incoherent. Sensory-level pain control such as transcutaneous electrical nerve stimulation (TENS) can reduce the reliance on narcotic medications to the point where the patient may remain **lucid** ■ and relatively pain free.

TABLE 12–9	**General Contraindications and Precautions in Electrotherapy**

Cardiac disability: Stimulation of the thorax or neck may result in disruption of normal respiratory or cardiac function.

Demand-type pacemakers: Electrical current flow may interfere with pacemaker's function.

Pregnancy: Stimulation of the abdominal, lumbar, or pelvic region may have an adverse effect on the developing fetus. Specific guidelines, however, have been developed to decrease pain for pregnant women, but these protocols must be closely monitored by a physician. Electrical stimulation has also been used during delivery, although the current may interfere with fetal monitoring machines.

Menstruation: Stimulation of the abdominal, lumbar, or pelvic region may increase hemorrhage.

Cancerous lesions: Electrical current may possibly result in a growth or spread of the tumor.

Sites of infections: Unless the treatment protocol is specifically designed to reduce infection.

Exposed metal implants: An example is a metal rod used for external fixation of fractures. Contact of a metal fixation rod to a grounded object can result in severe electric shock.

Areas of particular nerve sensitivity:

- The carotid sinus
- The esophagus
- The larynx
- The pharynx
- On or around the eyes
- The upper thorax
- The temporal region

Severe obesity: Adipose tissue may provide insulation against effective stimulation. Skin irritation from the gel, adhesive, or current flow in individuals who wear electrodes for extended periods. Altering the position of the electrodes reduces irritation.

Epilepsy: Use adequate precautions and increased monitoring of the patient.

Electronic monitoring equipment: Concurrent use of electrical stimulators may cause the equipment (e.g., ECG monitors, ECG alarms) to not operate properly.

■ Controversies in Treatment

Electrical stimulation is an effective modality for stimulating sensory, motor, and pain nerves and, given the proper phase duration, muscle fiber. Although there is not univer-

---

Carotid sinus: An enlargement of the carotid artery near the branch of the internal carotid artery, located distal to the inferior arch of the mandible. Baroreceptors at this site monitor and assist in the regulation of blood pressure.

Lucid: Of clear and rational mind.

Malunion fracture: The faulty or incorrect healing of bone.

sal agreement in the parameters[19, 25, 72] the use of electrical stimulation to control pain[15, 42, 73] and reeducate muscle has been substantiated,[74, 75] but conflicting results can be found in the literature.[76, 77] Wound healing, stimulation of bone healing, and changes in tissue pH following various forms of electrical stimulation have yet to be conclusively demonstrated.

The theoretical basis for cathodal sensory-level edema control has been substantiated in the laboratory using an animal model.[44, 64, 78] However, there still remains a lack of evidence conclusively demonstrating the clinical effectiveness of this approach.

No evidence exists that suggests that electrical stimulation has an effect on cellular level function. This leads to errors in clinical application of various forms of electrical stimulation. There is no evidence that suggests that subsensory or sensory-level electrical stimulation affects cellular function or affects inflammation. And because the current follows the path of least resistance, the target tissue (e.g., the anterior cruciate ligament) is not affected by the current.

Electrodes are often placed over the edematous area under the guise that the current will "drive" the edema out of this area. This effect has not been demonstrated to occur with any type of current or any type of treatment protocol.[79]

● Chapter Highlights

- Not all of the body's tissues are able to conduct therapeutic currents. Those that can, such as nerves, blood vessels, and cell membranes are called excitable tissues.

- Within the body ions flow instead of electrons.
- Electrodes represent the site where the current enters and exits the body. The size of the electrodes determines the current density.
- Bipolar electrode arrangements are created when the electrodes from lead have equal current densities.
- A monopolar electrode arrangement is created when one electrode has a significantly higher current density than the other electrode.
- Two bipolar electrode arrangements is termed quadripolar.
- Excitable tissues always depolarize in a predictable sequence: sensory nerves, motor nerves, noxious nerves, muscle fiber.
- The pulse duration can selectively stimulate different types of tissues.
- The body can adapt to electrical currents, thus requiring increased intensity to produce the same result. Accommodation occurs in the peripheral nervous system, habituation occurs in the central nervous system.
- Sensory-level stimulation is used for pain control, controlling the formation of edema, iontophoresis, wound healing, and fracture healing.
- Motor-level stimulation is used for muscle re-education, edema reduction, pain control, and increasing circulation.
- Noxious-level stimulation is used for pain control.
- The primary contraindications against the use of electrical stimulation arise from the placement of the electrodes. Electrodes must not be placed over nerves that control involuntary life functions.

Chapter 13

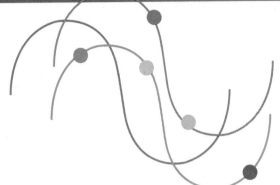

Clinical Application of Electrical Agents

This chapter describes the typical set-up and clinical application of electrical stimulators based on the type of current delivered. Although each stimulation method is presented as a distinct modality, many generators are capable of producing a wide range of electrical characteristics. The information presented in the Biophysical Effects section for each modality should be reinforced with the information presented in Chapter 12. The set-up and application protocol are described in generalized terms. Always familiarize yourself with the operator's manual of the specific equipment being used.

The diverse array of electrical stimulation units, techniques, and theories can make understanding electrical stimulation difficult and can be further complicated by individual manufacturers creating their own terminology. A common question is "When do I use each type of stimulator?" In some cases, there is one obviously correct answer; in other cases, there may be more than one correct option; and in other cases electrical stimulation may not be appropriate.

Some electrical stimulators deliver only one type of current. Multimodalities are capable of generating many different types of currents and may also include therapeutic ultrasound (Box 13–1). Some multimodalities allow for two patients to be treated simultaneously.

State practice acts may require that electrical stimulation devices be applied only under a physician's order. Clinicians must be aware of state practice acts governing their profession's use of these devices as well as the policies and procedures for use at their institution. Likewise, an appropriately credentialed individual should supervise use of these devices.

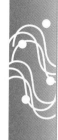

Box 13–1. Multimodalities

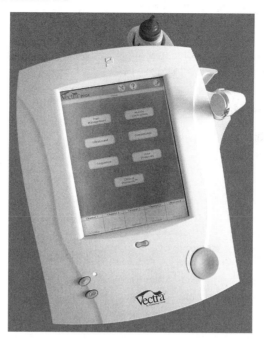

The development of microprocessors, advanced circuitry, and improved battery supplies has led to an evolution in the design and function of electrical stimulators. Until recently, each type of electrical stimulating current described in this chapter required a specific generator. Now a single microprocessor-based multimodality is capable of producing all of the current types described in Chapter 11 and may include other therapeutic agents, such as ultrasound.

The user simply selects the type of output desired, usually described by the type of current, and selects a preprogrammed treatment regimen (e.g., motor-level edema reduction, sensory-level pain control). The instrumentation and output controls are unique to each unit. Because of the differences among multimodalities, their use is not described in this text.

■ BASIC GUIDELINES FOR THE SET-UP AND APPLICATION OF ELECTROTHERAPY

This section describes the general steps used to prepare the generator, the electrodes, and the patient for electrotherapy. The steps involved in using the generator are described in further detail in their individual sections. Electrical stimulation units should not be used in the presence of flammable gases such as anesthetics or oxygen.

Electrical stimulators may operate from either household current or batteries. Clinical units that are driven by household (120 V) current require less output intensity to reach therapeutic goals than do portable, battery-driven stimulators.[2] Portable units may be powered by standard or rechargeable batteries (1.5 V to 9 V). Larger portable units may also have the option of working from a transformer.

■ Preparation of the Generator

1. If a portable or battery-operated unit is being used, make sure the batteries are fully charged. If a clinical model is being used, make sure it is properly plugged into a grounded wall socket. If the treatment involves water immersion, the unit must be plugged into a ground-fault interrupter circuit. Avoid the use of extension cords.
2. Make sure the electrode leads are not tangled. The leads should be inspected regularly for frays, broken insulation, and loose connections. Frayed leads should be repaired or replaced before they are used.
3. Ensure that all controls are in their zero (OFF) position.

■ Preparation of the Electrodes

1. Clean the electrodes to remove any residual gels or skin oils. Rubber electrodes should be cleaned with alcohol, and gel-based, self-adhesive electrodes should be cleaned with soap and water as recommended by the manufacturer.
2. Carbon-impregnated rubber electrodes should be used only with a wet medium, such as a sponge. Gels should not be used unless specifically recommended by the manufacturer.

3. If conductive sponges are used, moisten them with water. If sponges are not required, apply an even coat of conductive gel to the electrodes.

4. Connect the leads to the unit and to the electrodes.

5. In all cases, read and follow the manufacturer's recommendations for the electrodes being used.

■ Preparation of the Patient

1. Ensure that the patient has no contraindications to the treatment about to be performed.

2. Determine the electrode placement technique to be used.

3. Clean the skin with alcohol to remove any body oils, lotions, dirt, and grime. Keep in mind that body hair increases resistance to electrical current flow. When possible, place the electrode over areas of low hair density (see Table 12–2).

4. If a monopolar technique is being used, attach the dispersive electrode to a large body mass, such as the thigh or lower back. If the lower back is selected for the site of the dispersive electrode, place the electrode so that it lies on one side of the spinal column and not across it. The indentation formed by the erector muscles causes incomplete contact with the dispersive electrode and may result in sensation under this electrode. Avoid placing the dispersive electrode over the abdomen or torso.

5. If the electrodes are not self-adhesive, use rubber and Velcro straps, elastic wraps, or sandbags to secure the electrodes in place.

6. If this is the patient's first exposure to electrical stimulation, explain the sensations to be expected (e.g., "tingly sensation" or "muscle twitch"). Be aware that some individuals are apprehensive about electrotherapeutic treatments. The patient should be advised against any unnecessary movements because this may break the circuit between the electrodes.

■ Termination of the Treatment

1. Many units automatically stop the current flow when the treatment time has expired. If this is not the case with your unit, or if the treatment is being terminated prematurely, gradually decrease the INTENSITY and/or depress the STOP button.

2. Remove the electrodes from the body, and wipe away any residual water or gel.

3. Check the treatment area for burns, skin irritation, or discoloration.

4. Interview the patient immediately following the treatment to determine the effectiveness of the parameters used. The results should be noted in the medical or treatment file. Future modifications of the treatment protocol should be indicated.

Maintenance

Adhere to the manufacturer's required maintenance protocol. Failure to follow these recommendations may void the manufacturer's warranty.

Daily Maintenance

1. Clean the exterior housing of the unit using a mild household cleanser.

2. Keep the electrical power cord and electrode leads neatly stored.

Monthly Maintenance

1. Check lead wires for fraying, cut or torn insulation, or loose connections.

2. Check power cord and plug for fraying, kinks, or cuts.

Annual Maintenance

The unit must be recalibrated by an authorized technician.

▶ HIGH-VOLTAGE PULSED STIMULATION

High-voltage pulsed stimulation (HVPS) uses monophasic current, so the polarity of each electrode is known. This type of current is often incorrectly referred to as high-voltage galvanic stimulation (Box 13–2). HVPS is a versatile form of electrical stimulation and has a wide variety of uses,

---

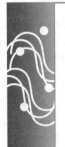

Box 13–2. What's in a Name? (Part I)

The term "high-voltage pulsed galvanic stimulation" is an oxymoron similar to "jumbo shrimp." The contradiction arises from the use of the terms "pulsed" and "galvanic" in describing the flow of the same current. As you will recall from the discussion on direct current flow, galvanic refers to "a continuous, waveless, unidirectional current."[80] Therefore, a galvanic current cannot be pulsed. The confusion stems from the constant use of this term in the literature and in manufacturers' descriptions.

including muscle reeducation, nerve stimulation, reduction of edema, and pain control.[34]

A typical high-voltage generator produces a twin-peaked waveform or a train of two single pulses having a short phase duration and a long interpulse interval. The low pulse charge requires an output voltage of greater than 150 V to stimulate motor and sensory nerves.[3] The short phase duration allows for the activation of sensory and type II motor nerves without stimulating pain fibers.

The interpulse interval is much longer than the pulse duration. Consider a current consisting of pulses having a duration of 140 msec and a frequency of 125 pps. In 1 second, the current is actually flowing for 0.0175 second. Because of the short amount of time the current is flowing, there is time for the ions attracted to each electrode to dissipate. As a result, the amount of physiochemical reaction beneath the electrodes is limited, and no skin significant pH changes occur under the cathode.[81] The fact that galvanic changes do not seem to occur within the tissues indicates that many of the effects attributed to polarity during HVPS may be the result of some other mechanism.

■ Electrode Configuration

HVPS may be applied using either a monopolar or bipolar technique. Monopolar application is used when the focus of the treatment is over a wide area, such as in the control and reduction of edema, sensory-level pain control, and point stimulation. Bipolar techniques are most often used when attempting to evoke a contraction from a specific muscle or in motor-level pain control.

● EFFECTS ON
The Injury Response Process

■ Neuromuscular Stimulation

The short phase duration allows a moderately high-intensity muscle contraction with relatively little patient discomfort. The strength of the contraction produced by high-voltage pulsed stimulators is less than that of neuromuscular electrical nerve stimulators or interferential stimulators.[34] Unlike muscle contractions produced by other electrical modalities, the pulse frequency seems to have little effect on the maximum tension produced in a muscle being stimulated by HVPS. Pulse frequencies above 30 pps appear to have little effect on increasing the strength of the contraction.[20, 74]

Generation of these contractile forces has not been shown to translate into increased muscular strength. The short-term benefits derived from HVPS neuromuscular stimulation are unclear, with study results ranging from significant increases in isometric strength to significant decreases in strength relative to a nonexercising control group.[82]

The most important role for HVPS in neuromuscular stimulation is to "teach," or reeducate, a muscle how to contract after periods of immobilization or transient denervation. Other types of currents, such as biphasic or alternating, that provide for a duty cycle (as found on neuromuscular stimulators) should be used when the treatment goal is strength augmentation.

■ Pain Control

HVPS may be used as an adjunct treatment in controlling acute and chronic pain through both sensory-level (gate control) and motor-level (opiate release) stimulation. The lack of current modulation allows the body to accommodate to the stimulation, decreasing the effectiveness of long-term pain control techniques. The gate control mechanism of pain modulation can be activated through the application of sensory-level currents at 100 to 150 pps. Because of the relative lack of portability of some high-voltage generators, HVPS is not the modality of choice for pain control treatments that require long-term stimulation.

HVPS can also be used to stimulate the release of opiates. Although the phase duration associated with HVPS does not easily activate A-beta fibers, the high output intensity (voltage) can stimulate these fibers. A monopolar electrode configuration should be used, with the active electrodes being only as large as the area being stimulated. A hand-held probe is often used for this method of application (Fig. 13–1). Pain reduction can also be obtained through the brief-intense stimulation protocol.

The polarity of the active electrode (monopolar techniques) or the electrode placed over the target tissue (bipolar) can influence the effectiveness of the treatment.[80] Acute pain is associated with an acid reaction that may be repelled by the positive pole. In the case of chronic pain, the negative pole is used for its reputed liquefying and vasodilative properties.

In practicality, long-term pain relief derived from HVPS application most probably stems from the other

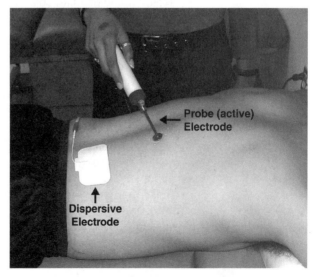

Figure 13–1. **Use of an Electrode Probe with High-Voltage Pulsed Stimulation.** This form of electrical stimulation is used to target stimulation points. Because of the current density under the probe, this type of stimulation is monopolar.

Treatment Strategies
Neuromuscular Stimulation Using High-Voltage Pulsed Stimulation

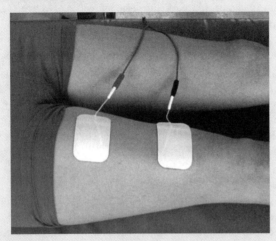

Parameter	Setting
Output intensity	Strong, intense, comfortable contractions.
Pulse frequency	If duty cycle cannot be adjusted: low for individual muscle contractions (<15 pps). If adjustable duty cycle available: moderate for tonic contractions (>50 pps).
Polarity	Negative over primary motor point (if monopolar arrangement is used. Note that bipolar is pictured above).
Duty cycle	Initial treatments should begin with a low (e.g., 20%) duty cycle and be increased as the muscle responds.
Electrode placement	Bipolar: Proximal and distal to the muscle (or muscle group) to be stimulated. This method offers the most direct method of stimulating specific areas. Monopolar: over motor points or muscle belly.

These parameters are modified to meet the goals of the specific treatment regimen being used.

Treatment Strategies
Pain Control Using High-Voltage Pulsed Stimulation via the Gate Control Mechanism

Parameter	Setting
Output intensity	Sensory level
Pulse frequency	60–100 pps
Phase duration	<100 msec*
Mode	Continuous
Electrode arrangement	Monopolar or bipolar
Polarity	Acute: positive Chronic: negative
Electrode placement	Directly over the painful site

* Not adjustable on most HVPS units.

biophysical effects described in the following sections. Reduction of edema, decreased muscle spasm, muscle re-education, and increased blood flow assist in decreasing the mechanical and chemical factors triggering the nociceptors. These factors are usually not sufficient, however, to decrease pain caused by delayed-onset muscle soreness.[83, 84]

■ Control and Reduction of Edema

Sensory-level HVPS has typically been used to limit the formation of acute edema after trauma. Motor-level stimulation is used to reduce the amount of swelling that has formed in the traumatized tissues during the subacute or chronic stages of inflammation.

■ Sensory-Level Edema Control

In acute injuries in which HVPS is intended to prevent or limit the amount of swelling, the polarity, the time of intervention after the onset of the injury, the pulse frequency used, and the sequencing of the treatments are critical in obtaining positive treatment outcomes. The treatment parameters are configured to keep the current flowing as long as possible and to focus the cathodal (negative electrode) over the target tissues.

The output parameters result in decreased permeability of the microvascular structures in the target tissues. Decreased permeability blocks the passage of plasma proteins and helps to maintain the osmotic gradient that is lost during the acute inflammatory response and prevents fluids from escaping into the extracellular tissues.[34]

Treatment Strategies
Pain Control Using High-Voltage Pulsed Stimulation via the Opiate Release Mechanism

Parameter	Setting
Output intensity	Motor level
Pulse rate	2–4 pps
Phase duration	150–250 msec
Mode	Continuous
Electrode arrangement	Monopolar or bipolar
Polarity	Acute: positive
	Chronic: negative
Electrode placement	Directly over painful site, distal to the spinal nerve root origin, trigger points, or acupuncture points

Negatively charged blood cells and plasma proteins are—theoretically—repelled from the cathode, creating a concentration gradient that encourages local reabsorption of fluids.[34]

The permeability of the local microvessels must be decreased before gross edema forms. If the stimulation is applied too late in the injury response process, decreased vascular permeability may inhibit reabsorption of the edematous proteins and fluids back into the venous and lymphatic system, virtually trapping them within the extracellular tissues and preventing edema reduction.[85]

The sensory-level application of HVPS in limiting the formation of edema has been extensively tested in animal models. Cathodal stimulation applied at 10 percent below the motor threshold with a frequency of 120 pps and delivered to the traumatized tissues through immersion may be effective in limiting the formation of post-traumatic edema.[65] When applied immediately after trauma, this protocol, delivered in four 30-minute treatments interspersed with 60-minute rest periods, suppressed edema formation for 17 hours. A single 30-minute treatment curbed edema formation for 4 hours but did not significantly decrease long-term edema formation.[64, 78, 86–88] The pulse frequency also influences the effectiveness of sensory-level edema control. A low pulse frequency (e.g., 1 pps) does not significantly limit edema formation.[86, 89, 90]

For sensory-level edema control to be effective, the treatment must be initiated as soon as possible after injury, preferably within 6 hours.[65] To preserve the benefits associated with the recommended treatment protocol, care must be taken to limit edema formation between treatment sessions and treatment bouts. The injured limb should be elevated or a compression wrap applied to discourage fluids from leaking into the interstitial space while encouraging venous and lymphatic return.

Blood clot formation was once thought to be enhanced under the positive electrode, and the use of anodal stimulation to control acute edema has been suggested. However, this treatment approach has not been substantiated.[65, 80]

High sensory-level stimulation (just below the threshold of visible muscle contractions) of HVPS significantly increases the lymphatic uptake of protein associated with edema but does not reduce limb volume.[91] This technique combined with elevation, sequential compression (see Chapter 14), or muscle contractions may assist in reducing limb volume.

■ Motor-Level Edema Reduction

Chapter 1 of this text described how muscle contractions assist in venous and lymphatic return by manually forcing the contents of these vessels out of the extremity. Motor-level edema reduction attempts to replicate this effect by eliciting the required muscle contractions. This technique is used during the subacute or chronic stage of injury because the force of muscle contraction or the associated joint motion may either limit the effectiveness of this technique or may be contraindicated.

To increase the milking effect, a low pulse frequency (e.g., 1 pps) and a strong, comfortable muscle contraction within the patient's tolerance should be used. The electrodes should be placed over the motor points of the major muscle groups through which the vessels course, following the path from the swollen area proximally to the torso.

Treatment Strategies
Pain Control Using High-Voltage Stimulation via the Brief-Intense Protocol

Parameter	Setting
Output intensity	Noxious
Pulse rate	>120 pps
Phase duration	300–1000 msec
Mode	Probe (15–60 sec at each site)
Electrode arrangement	Monopolar (probe)
Polarity	Acute: positive
	Chronic: negative
Probe placement	Gridding technique, stimulating hypersensitive areas, working distal from the painful area to proximal to it

Treatment Strategies
Sensory-Level Control of Edema Formation Using High-Voltage Pulsed Stimulation

Parameter	Setting
Intensity	Sensory level.
Pulse duration	Maximum duration allowed by the generator.
Pulse frequency	120 pps.
Polarity	Negative electrodes are placed over the injured tissues.
Mode	Continuous.
Electrode placement	The immersion method should be used when possible, or the active electrodes should be grouped over and around the target tissues.
Treatment duration	Four 30-minute treatments, each followed by 60-minute rest periods or Four 30-minute treatments, each followed by 30-minute rest periods
Comments	This treatment approach should be initiated as soon as possible after the onset of the trauma. The treated body part should be wrapped and elevated between sessions. This treatment regimen should not performed if gross swelling is present.

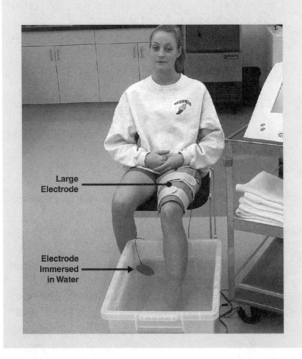

Large Electrode

Electrode Immersed in Water

Elevating the limb, allowing gravity to assist in the venous return process, enhances the effectiveness of this treatment. As with all edema reduction techniques, the patient should be given home-care instruction to keep the limb elevated and wrapped between treatment sessions.

■ Blood Flow

Although it is not clear if HVPS significantly increases local blood flow, any influence would depend on the output intensity and pulse frequency. Motor-level stimulation increases metabolism of the affected tissues, increasing their need for oxygen. This demand is met by increasing the amount of blood delivered to the area. The number of pulses per second may also influence the increase in blood flow, although this relationship is less understood.

Isometric contractions producing muscular tension between 10 and 30 percent of the maximal voluntary contraction produce a slight increase in local blood flow but at a level significantly less than that associated with voluntary contractions.[92] Increasing the output intensity is positively correlated with increased blood flow.[93] However, strong muscle contractions, joint motion, and the associated stresses placed on the involved tissues are often contraindicated.

Pulse frequencies of 10, 20, and 50 pps significantly increased blood flow, although these conclusions have not been obtained by all researchers.[94, 95] Pulse frequencies of 2 and 128 pps have also produced a significant increase in blood flow, but no significant increase has been demonstrated at 32 pps.[93, 95]

If the treatment goal is to increase blood flow, other techniques should probably be considered before HVPS. Ideally, voluntary muscle contractions or therapeutic exercise should be used to meet this goal, providing that the patient is able. If not, the use of moist heat or 3-MHz ultrasound (for superficial blood flow) or 1-MHz ultrasound (deep blood flow) should be considered.

■ Wound Healing

The use of HVPS to facilitate wound healing stems from the results seen with the application of low-intensity direct currents (DCs). The use of HVPS is similar in that each electrode serves as either the positive or negative pole. The possible shortcoming of this technique may be that the pulses are of insufficient duration to cause responses equal to those of a low-intensity DC. HVPS is used to promote healing of decubitus ulcers and surgical incisions.[61]

An antimicrobial effect is obtained during HVPS application that persists after the treatment is discontinued.[61] Depending on the polarity of the treatment electrode, leukocytes, epidermal cells, and fibroblasts are attracted to the area,[57] and the level of collagenase is increased.[96] High-voltage pulsed current has also been shown to inhibit the growth of certain bacteria in infected wounds.[97] No changes in tissue pH or temperature that could affect wound healing occur during a 30-minute HVPS treatment.[61]

Treatment Strategies
Motor-Level Reduction of Edema Using High-Voltage Pulsed Stimulation via the Muscle-Milking Technique

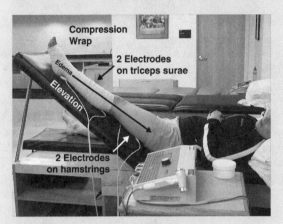

Compression Wrap

2 Electrodes on triceps surae

Edema

Elevation

2 Electrodes on hamstrings

Parameter	Setting
Intensity	Strong, yet comfortable muscle contraction. Avoid joint movement that may be contraindicated.
Pulse frequency	Low.
Polarity	Positive or negative.
Mode	Alternating.
Electrode placement	Bipolar: Proximal and distal ends of the major muscle (or muscle group) proximal to the edematous area. Monopolar: Active electrodes follow the course of the venous return system.
Comment:	Ice may be applied to the injured area, but this could impede venous return by increasing the viscosity of fluids in the area (see Chapter 5).

Negative polarity encourages blood clots to dissolve and increases the inflammatory/hemorrhagic byproducts, promoting the healing of necrotic tissues.[52] Clot formation around the margin of the wound and in granulation tissue is promoted by a positive polarity.[52]

Because most of the biophysical effects of electricity on wound healing are polarity specific, the application protocol should reflect the desired outcomes of the treatment. To account for the effects of polarity during the treatment of cutaneous wounds, the application of 20 minutes of negative polarity followed by 40 minutes of positive polarity stimulation has been recommended.[98]

■ Instrumentation

Power: When this switch is in its ON position, the current is allowed to flow to the internal components of the generator.

Reset: This safety feature ensures that the voltage is reduced to zero before each new treatment is started.

Timer: This control sets the duration of the treatment and subsequently displays the remaining time. On some units, the TIMER serves as the master power switch.

Start-stop: When this button is depressed to start the treatment, the circuit is closed, allowing the current to flow to the patient's tissues. When it is depressed again, the circuit is opened, interrupting the current flow.

Intensity (voltage): This knob adjusts the amplitude of the pulse from zero (OFF) to the maximal value of the unit. The applied output is displayed on the OUTPUT meter.

Pulse (phase) duration: This control selects the duration of each pulse or pair of pulses. Short pulses selectively stimulate sensory nerves, medium-duration pulses stimulate motor nerves, and long pulses activate pain fibers. This parameter may not be available on all units.

Pulse rate: This parameter controls the number of pulses (or pulse trains) per second. Low numbers of pulses per second stimulate endorphin release for pain control, moderate levels produce tetanic contractions, and the upper levels are useful in activating the gate mechanism of pain control.

Pulse multiplier: This switch multiplies the number of pulses per second by a selectable value. For example, if the pulse rate is set at 12 pps and the pulse multiplier is set at 10, the resultant output would be 120 pps.

Polarity: This switch determines the polarity (positive or negative) of the ACTIVE electrode or electrodes. Depending on the manufacturer of the product, the polarity may be changed during the course of the treatment without first decreasing the voltage. Other units require that the voltage be reduced before changing polarity.

Mode: When this switch is set to CONTINUOUS, the current is always flowing to each of the active electrodes. Switching to the ALTERNATING modes causes the current to be routed to only one set of active electrodes at a time. Many units also have a PROBE selection that activates the hand-held electrode.

Alternating rate: This switch sets the amount of time the current is routed to each active electrode. For example, selecting an electrode alternating rate of 2.5 seconds routes the current to one set of electrodes for 2.5 seconds, then the other set for the same amount of time. On many units, this function is meaningful only when the MODE is set to ALTERNATING and two sets of active electrodes are attached to the "ACTIVE" electrode jack.

At a Glance: **High-Voltage Pulsed Stimulation**

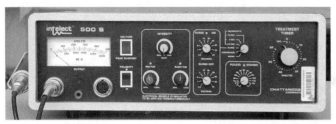

Parameters

CURRENT TYPE: Monophasic
AMPLITUDE: 0 to 500 mA RMS
VOLTAGE: 0 to 500V
PULSE FREQUENCY: 1 to 120 pps
PULSE DURATION: 13 to 100 msec
PHASE DURATION: 20 to 45 msec

Waveforms

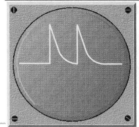 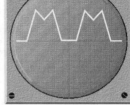 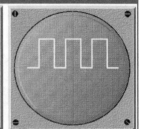

Saw tooth (1 pulse)   M-wave (2 pulses)   Square wave (3 pulses)

Output Modulation

Duty cycle
Electrode alternating rate
Electrode balance
Intensity
Polarity
Probe electrode
Surge/Ramp

Treatment Duration

The typical duration of HVPS treatments is 15 to 30 minutes, and the treatments may be repeated as many times a day as needed.

Indications

- Reeducation of peripheral nerves
- Delay of denervation and disuse atrophy by stimulating muscle contractions
- Reduction of post-traumatic edema
- Increase in local blood circulation (unsubstantiated)
- Restoring range of motion:
  - Reduction of muscle spasm
  - Inhibition of spasticity
  - Reeducation of partially denervated muscle
  - Facilitation of voluntary motor function

Precautions

- Stimulation of muscles can cause unwanted tension to be placed on the muscle fibers, the tendons, or the bony insertion.
- Muscle fatigue can rapidly develop if the duty cycle is too high.
- Improper use can cause electrode burns or irritation.
- Intense or prolonged stimulation may result in muscle spasm and/or muscle soreness.

Note: See Table 12–9 for a list of contraindications to the use of electrical modalities.

Alternating the electrodes is useful for reciprocal stimulation of agonist-antagonist muscle groups. Another use is to stimulate different muscle groups to produce a milking action to reduce edema.

Balance: During the course of a treatment, the greater sensation may be experienced under one set of active electrodes than the other. This situation may be corrected through the BALANCE adjustment dial. When this dial is in its midposition, an equal amount of current is routed to both sets of electrodes. If this dial is moved in one direction, toward the "B" electrodes for example, a greater amount of current flows to the "B" electrodes and less to the "A" electrodes.

The imbalance in stimulation under the electrodes can be the result of many factors. These may include improper preparation of the electrodes, the location of the electrodes, and loose connections between the electrodes and the generator or between the electrodes and the patient's body. If adjusting the BALANCE dial does not equalize the sensation, discontinue the treatment, reapply the electrodes, and start again.

Duty cycle: Not available on all HVPS units. Adjusts the ON/OFF time of current flow.

■ Set-up and Application

Refer to manufacturer's operating instructions for the procedures specific to the unit being used.

Initiation of the Treatment

1. Turn the unit on: Activate the POWER switch.
2. Reset output parameters: Fully reduce the INTENSITY control and depress the RESET button.
3. Select output parameters: Based on the goal of the treatment, adjust the POLARITY, DURATION (width), FREQUENCY, and electrode ALTERNATING rates.
4. Set treatment duration: Indicate the duration of the treatment by adjusting the TIMER.
5. Begin treatment: Press the START button to close the circuit between the generator and the patient's tissues.
6. Increase intensity: Slowly increase the INTENSITY control until the appropriate current level is obtained.
7. Adjust electrode balance: If necessary or applicable, adjust the BALANCE control to maximize comfort.

■ Alternate Methods of Application

Water Immersion

HVPS may be combined with water immersion to treat irregularly shaped areas, such as the hand or foot (see Treatment Strategies: Sensory-Level Control of Edema Formation Using High-Voltage Pulsed Stimulation). The water touching the skin serves as the active electrode. With

this in mind, the dispersive electrode should be as large as possible to keep the focus of the electrical stimulation on the part being treated. Even with the use of a large dispersive electrode, the size of the contact area between the patient's skin and the water creates a current density equal to or less than the dispersive electrode. In many cases, the change in current density causes the treatment configuration to become bipolar.

For safety, place the active electrodes in the tub with the insulated (rubber-coated) side facing toward the body part. Intense stimulation would occur if the patient were to contact one of the electrodes. The dispersive electrode is placed on the closest large body mass. When treating the foot or ankle, the thigh is a logical site. The application of the current is similar to that in all other forms of HVPS. It is important to instruct the person not to remove the treated body part from the water; if the intensity of the treatment is too strong, a greater proportion of the body part should be immersed (see Current Density).

Treatment of acute injuries with water immersion also raises the same concerns about edema management as ice immersion. Because the limb is placed in a gravity-dependent position, the hydrostatic pressure within the capillaries is increased and the formation of edema is encouraged rather than discouraged. After treatment, the treated limb should be wrapped and elevated to encourage venous return.

Probe

A probe electrode can be used to specifically stimulate trigger points or other localized areas. The probe serves as a very small active electrode in a monopolar configuration that results in a very high current density being placed on a limited group of tissues. A dispersive electrode is required to complete the circuit. A typical probe consists of a handle with a metal tip that is designed to hold a conductive medium (see Fig. 13–1).

The handle contains an INTENSITY control knob and an INTERRUPT button. The probe is activated by setting the electrode alternating switch to PROBE or by plugging the probe into a separate jack on the generator. In either case, the INTENSITY adjustment on the probe overrides the adjustment on the generator. This allows the operator to remotely adjust the intensity of the treatment. The INTERRUPT button allows the operator to open and close the circuit. When the button is depressed, the circuit is closed and the patient's tissues are stimulated.

▶ TRANSCUTANEOUS ELECTRICAL NERVE STIMULATION

Although all electrical modalities described in this chapter deliver their current transcutaneously, the term transcutaneous electrical nerve stimulation (TENS) has evolved to describe a specific electrotherapeutic approach to pain control. It describes the process of altering the perception of pain through the use of an electrical current (Box 13–3).

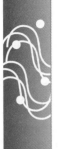

Box 13–3. What's in a Name? (Part II)

Transcutaneous electrical nerve stimulation, or TENS, is the term used to describe an electrotherapeutic modality used in pain control. In reality, each of the electrical modalities described in this chapter could be termed TENS. Transcutaneous means "through the skin," and "nerve stimulation" implies that the current has sufficient intensity to cause the depolarization of sensory, motor, or pain nerves. Therefore, whenever electrodes are attached to the body, an electrical current is passed through them, and the patient first reports a tingling sensation, TENS is being performed.

The names given to electrotherapeutic modalities most probably arise from, and are most certainly reinforced by, marketing of the product. As multimodalities become more prevalent, names such as "TENS" and "HVPS" will most likely be replaced by more accurate descriptors of the current being used (e.g., low-voltage biphasic, high-voltage monophasic). Transcutaneous electrical stimulation is also sometimes used in the literature to describe any electrical stimulation procedure administered through the skin. When conducting a literature review, always check the PROCEDURES section to identify the characteristics of the electrical current being used.

Depending on the parameters used during treatment, electrical stimulation may reduce pain through activation of the gate control mechanism or centrally through the release of **endogenous opiates** ■.

The use of TENS in the treatment of pain is a spin-off of the work conducted by Melzack and Wall during their gate control pain modulation experiments (see Chap. 2).[99] Anecdotal claims of permanent relief from chronic pain after a single, brief TENS treatment—although possibly true—are an exaggeration and oversimplification of the practical effects and application of TENS. This technique is effective in the management of acute or chronic musculoskeletal pain but has little effect on reducing visceral or **psychogenic** ■ pain.

The effectiveness of TENS is as varied as its application techniques. The treatment depends on the nature of the pain, the individual's pain threshold, electrode placement, the intensity of the stimulation, and the electrical characteristics of the stimulus.[76] Traditionally, TENS units incorporate an asymmetrical biphasic pulsed current. However, some manufacturers use variants of this pulsed current including a symmetrical biphasic or monophasic waveform. When this treatment is given for extended periods, the waveform should be designed so that there is no net physiochemical effect on tissues.

● E F F E C T S   O N

The Injury Response Process

■ Pain Control

Despite the fact that a TENS unit can cause muscle contractions, the primary, if not the only, use of TENS is

to control pain. TENS decreases the patient's perception of pain by decreasing the conductivity and transmission of noxious impulses from the small pain fibers to the central nervous system. By affecting the large motor fibers, TENS may interfere with the normal guarding pattern of the muscle (muscle spasm), further reducing painful stimuli.[43, 100] The pulse frequency and pulse duration, combined with the current intensity, activate responses at different pain-modulating levels (Table 13–1).[101] The determination of the exact parameters to use on any given patient is as much of an art as it is a science. The combination of output parameters is more important in obtaining the desired outcome than any single parameter.[100]

The pain reduction associated with TENS application occurs primarily through modulation of the body's nervous system. Neither sensory-level nor moderate motor-level TENS application significantly increases blood flow in the treated area. Indeed, evidence supports the concept that TENS application may activate the preganglionic and postganglionic neurons and produce a mild vasoconstriction.[102] Most prolonged TENS applications can modulate the activity of dorsal horn neurons secondary to stimulation of peripheral nerves and chemical stimulation of visceral organs by the release of endogenous opiates.[42] Last, pain relief obtained through the various forms of TENS application may occur through psychological factors either exclusively from, or in addition to, the neurophysiological effects.[103, 104]

The patient's consumption of moderate levels of caffeine (200 mg, approximately equal to two or three cups of coffee) can decrease the effectiveness of TENS.[105] Caffeine competes with adenosine, a primary mediator of TENS-induced pain reduction, for its receptor sites. Because caffeine binds to these sites, adenosine is prohib-

---

Endogenous opiates: Pain-inhibiting substances produced in the brain. These include endorphins and enkephalins.

Psychogenic: Pain of mental rather than physical origin.

TABLE 13–1 **Protocol for Various Methods of Transcutaneous Electrical Nerve Stimulation Application**

Parameter	High TENS	Low TENS	Brief-Intense TENS
Intensity	Sensory	Motor	Noxious
Pulse frequency	60–100 pps	2–4 pps	Variable
Pulse duration	60–100 msec	150–250 msec	300–1000 msec
Mode	Modulated rate	Modulated burst	Modulated amplitude
Treatment duration	As needed	30 min	15–30 min
Onset of relief	<10 min	20–40 min	<15 min
Duration of relief	Minutes to hours	Hours	<30 min

Source: Adapted from Bechtel and Fan p 41.

ited from filling its receptors, causing a decreased effectiveness in TENS pain reduction.

Note that although the following techniques decrease the individual's perception of pain, the treatment has little effect on the underlying pathology. This modality should be used in conjunction with other therapies that attempt to treat the source of the pain.

■ High-Frequency TENS (Sensory Level)

Conventional TENS treatment, applied with a high pulse frequency (60 to 100 pps), short pulse duration (less than 100 msec), and sensory-level intensity activates the pain-modulating gate at the spinal cord level. Painful impulses are transmitted along slow-transmitting, unmyelinated, small-diameter nerves. Nonpainful sensory information travels at a faster rate along neurons of larger diameter.

The short phase duration and high pulse frequency used with high-frequency TENS selectively targets large-diameter A-beta fiber sensory nerves.[106] Activation of A-beta nerves causes presynaptic inhibition of A-delta and C fibers within the substantia gelatinosa, blocking transmission of painful impulses to the T cells. In other words, the gate is closed to pain transmission and opened to the transmission of sensory information.

High-frequency, low-intensity stimulation decreases the activity of spontaneously firing nerves, decreases the activity in noxiously evoked dorsal horn neurons, and decreases neural activity compared with the low-frequency TENS, high-intensity TENS protocol (described in the following section).[42] In addition, patients who are seeking pain reduction subjectively prefer the high-frequency TENS protocol.[107]

Accommodation and habituation are concerns when high-frequency TENS is used for an extended period. If the stimulation parameters are kept constant, the nervous system will adapt to the unchanging stimulus. Most TENS generators have current modulation parameters designed to diminish these effects. The generator should be adjusted so that the output is modulated to decrease accommodation, with burst and frequency modulation being the most preferred by patients.[108, 109] Even so, the current intensity is normally increased during the course of the treatment.

High-frequency TENS is effective in the treatment of acute soft tissue injury, but care must be taken to avoid unwanted muscle contractions. Other indications for high-frequency TENS include treatment of pain associated with musculoskeletal disorders, postoperative pain, inflammatory conditions, and myofascial pain.

■ Low-Frequency TENS (Motor Level)

Low-frequency TENS (low TENS) is applied with a low pulse frequency (2 to 4 pps), long phase duration (150 to 250 msec), and motor-level intensity in treatment bouts lasting a minimum of 45 minutes. These stimulation parameters activate small-diameter nociceptors and motor fibers. The sensory information travels along the muscle spindle's afferent nerves, which activate descending pain suppression mechanisms. Pain relief obtained through this method is thought to occur by the release of β-endorphin, which results in narcotic-like pain reduction.[103] Low-frequency TENS is sometimes referred to as "acupuncture-like TENS," but this is based on the nerves targeted rather than the stimulation of acupuncture points.[110]

Low-frequency, high-intensity TENS stimulates the pituitary gland to release chemicals that trigger the production of pain-reducing β-endorphins. During the treatment, the pituitary gland releases ACTH and β-lipotropin into the bloodstream. Once present, these two mediators trigger the release of β-endorphin that binds to the receptor sites of A-beta and C fibers, blocking the transmission of pain.

Actual relief of pain may not be experienced for some time after the treatment has been completed, but the effects last much longer than with high-frequency TENS.[14, 22, 111] Suggested uses for low-frequency TENS include the treatment of chronic pain, pain caused by damage to deep tissues, myofascial pain, and pain caused by muscle spasm. Because this method of TENS application involves muscle contractions, care must be taken to avoid any joint movement that may be contraindicated. Studies have indicated little difference between the degree of pain reduction obtained from high- and low-frequency TENS treatments.[15, 76]

■ Brief-Intense TENS (Noxious Level)

This method of TENS application is delivered at a high pulse frequency (greater than 100 pps), long pulse duration (300 to 1000 msec), and motor-level intensity in treatment bouts lasting a few seconds to a few minutes. Pain relief is achieved by activating mechanisms in the brain stem that dampen or amplify pain impulses. Although this application protocol is sometimes referred to as noxious-level TENS, true noxious-level stimulation is not actually obtained because the limited phase duration found on TENS generators is too short to activate C fibers.

Pain relief is obtained in this TENS protocol by the formation of a negative feedback loop within the central nervous system. The intense stimulation activates ascending neural mechanisms that, on reaching the brain, make the person conscious of the pain caused by the stimulation. During the impulse's passage through the midbrain, a "short circuit" occurs, stimulating the release of endogenous opiates in the raphe nuclei. A descending pain suppression system is activated that loops efferent impulses down the spinal cord.[103] Here, the opiates inhibit the release of substance P, a neurotransmitter of noxious impulses, thus blocking the transmission of pain.[112]

A high level of analgesia is achieved through this application protocol, but the effects are more transitory than those derived from high- and low-frequency TENS. Because of the short duration of pain relief, this technique is recommended for pain reduction before rehabilitation exercises.[14]

■ Other Biophysical Effects of TENS

Range of motion and muscle strength may be improved secondary to pain reduction. The use of low-frequency TENS may be more effective at improving range of motion than the high-frequency TENS protocol.[73, 112] During the early stages of rehabilitation, patients using TENS have demonstrated the ability to reduce the need for pain medication and a more rapid return to active exercise relative to patients not using TENS.[46]

■ Electrode Placement

The placement of TENS electrodes for optimal treatment is not an exact science, but the process is made easier if a consistent decision-making process is followed. Placement techniques are described by the electrodes' location relative to the painful area: direct placement, contiguous placement, stimulation points, dermatome placement, and placement at the level of the involved spinal nerve root (Box 13–4).[113]

High-frequency TENS is most commonly employed with direct, contiguous, dermatome, or nerve root–level electrode placement. Low-frequency TENS and brief-intense TENS treatments target the stimulation points. This is not an absolute formula; the parameters can be mixed and matched to obtain the best treatment results.

Most TENS units use four electrodes, two originating from each of two channels used. However, some units may have as few as two electrodes or as many as eight (two electrodes originating from each of four channels). When two or more channels are used, electrode placement is further defined by one channel's electrode placement relative to the other possible placements.

The effects of TENS can be maximized if the nerve or nerves involved in the transmission of pain are targeted. For example, the reduction of pain associated with an injured thumb is facilitated if the radial nerve, or portions of its path, is stimulated, rather than the median or ulnar nerve.

■ Instrumentation

Intensity: On most units there is one intensity dial for each channel. Although the intensity of each channel is controlled individually, the other current parameters (pulse duration and pulse frequency) regulate the activity in all channels.

Pulse duration: Usually labeled "PULSE WIDTH" on the unit, this adjustment should be set according to the treatment method being used.

Pulse frequency: Also labeled "PULSE RATE," this adjustment sets the number of pulses per second used during the treatment.

Mode: Modes are used to alter the current in an attempt to reduce the amount of accommodation that occurs. The various modes that are commonly selectable are:

Constant: Current flow occurs at a constant amplitude, rate, and pulse duration. This mode is best described as unmodulated, to avoid confusion with uninterrupted current. This mode is used when the treatment is not required for an extended length of time and accommodation is not a concern.

Burst: In the burst mode, pulse frequencies are interrupted at regular intervals. Bursts allow "OFF" time from stimulation and assist in reducing muscle fatigue in low-frequency TENS treatments.

Modulated rate: This setting alters, at a preset percentage, the frequency at which the stimulus is delivered. For example, if the pulse rate were adjusted to 100 pps, the unit would alternate the rate between 90 and 110 pps. Modulating the frequency has been found effective in the treatment of chronic musculoskeletal pain.[14]

Modulated amplitude: The pulse amplitude is increased and decreased by a preset percentage. Modulating the amplitude has been shown to provide short-term analgesia in the area.

Multiple modulation: Intensity, frequency, and pulse duration are alternately modulated in such a way that there is delivery of a steady amount of current to the body, but the body has a varying sensory perception of the treatment. This mode decreases the effects of accommodation during prolonged TENS application.

At a Glance: **Transcutaneous Electrical Nerve Stimulation (TENS)**

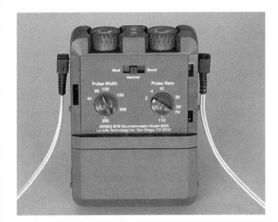

Parameters

CURRENT TYPE: Asymmetrical balanced biphasic
TOTAL CURRENT FLOW: 0 to 100 mA
PULSE FREQUENCY: 1 to 150 pps
PULSE DURATION: 10 to 500 msec
PHASE DURATION: 5 to 250 msec

Waveform

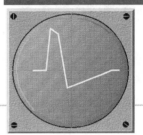

Output Modulation

Intensity   Pulse duration
Mode (output modulation)   Pulse frequency

Treatment Duration

- Conventional high-frequency TENS may be used as needed, but should be used with caution when the patient is sleeping. The use of a TENS device during athletic competition has been attempted; however, because of the potential of TENS to mask pain, its use should be discouraged. An alternate approach would be to keep the electrodes affixed to the athlete and apply stimulation while the athlete is on the sideline.
- Low-frequency TENS may be given as needed in treatment bouts not exceeding 30 minutes.
- Brief-intense–type TENS application should be performed only once a day, in treatment bouts not exceeding 30 minutes.

Indications

- Control of acute or chronic pain
- Management of postsurgical pain
- Reduction of post-traumatic acute pain

Contraindications

In addition to the contraindications presented in Table 12-9
- Pain of central origin
- Pain of unknown origin

Precautions

- Transcutaneous electrical nerve stimulation is a symptomatic treatment that can mask underlying pain and other conditions.
- Improper use can result in electrode burns or skin irritation.
- Intense or prolonged stimulation may result in muscle spasm and/or muscle soreness.
- Intake of 200 mg or more of caffeine may reduce the effectiveness of TENS.[105]
- Narcotic use decreases the effectiveness of TENS.

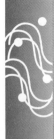

Box 13–4. Tens Electrode Placement

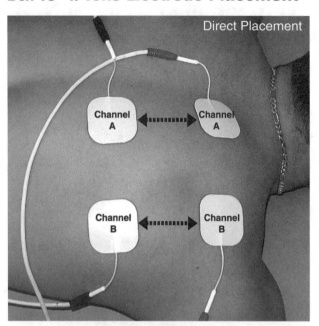

Direct Placement

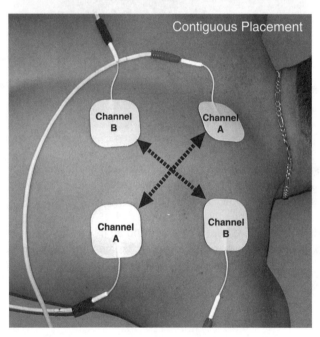

Contiguous Placement

Direct Placement

Electrodes are placed directly on the painful site. The electrical channels run parallel to each other.

Stimulation Point Placement

Motor, trigger, and/or acupuncture points are targeted (see Box 12–3). Because of the close location of these areas, a single TENS electrode may stimulate all three points at once.

Spinal Cord-Level Placement

The spinal cord nerve roots associated with the pain are targeted. The electrodes are placed between the spinous process parallel to the spinal column.

Contiguous Placement

Used when direct placement is contraindicated. Electrodes are placed around the painful tissues. Electrical channels can run parallel to each other or their currents can cross over the target tissue.

Dermatome Placement

One electrode is placed at the corresponding spinal cord nerve root and the other at the distal end of the dermatome. When pain is distributed across one or more dermatomes, place the electrodes within the affected dermatome and the contralateral dermatome.

Contralateral Placement

Based on the concept of bilateral transfer, electrodes are placed on the opposite side of the body, approximating the location from which the pain is arising on the injured side.

■ Set-up and Application

Refer to manufacturer's operating instructions for the procedures specific to the unit being used.

Initiation of the Treatment

1. Adjust output parameters: Depending on the method of TENS application to be used (see Table 13–1), set the pulse duration (WIDTH) and pulse frequency (RATE) dials to the midrange of the parameters to be used.

2. Select the electrodes: High-frequency TENS should be applied with larger electrodes. Low-frequency TENS and brief-intense TENS should use progressively smaller electrodes.
3. Set the output mode: Select the appropriate MODE for the method and duration of the TENS application.
4. Make sure the unit is off: Make sure that the output intensity is reset to zero, and turn the unit on. Note that many TENS units have the power switch built into the intensity knobs. In this case, the intensity level of zero is equal to "OFF."
5. Increase the output intensity (channel 1): Slowly

turn up the INTENSITY of channel 1. If this treatment involves sensory-level stimulation, continue increasing the intensity until a slight muscle contraction is visible, then reduce the intensity by approximately 10 percent. (The patient should be monitored for comfort while the intensity is being increased.)

6. Increase the output intensity (channel 2): If more than one channel is being used, increase the intensity of the remaining channels.

7. Balance the channels: Adjust the intensity of the channels so that an equal amount of stimulation occurs under each set of electrodes.

8. Fine-tune the output: When "fine-tuning" the treatment parameters, most manufacturers recommend first adjusting the intensity, then the pulse duration, and finally the pulse frequency.

9. Provide home-care instructions: If the patient is being sent home or to class while wearing this unit, instruction should be provided on how to adjust the intensity. If indicated, instructions should also be provided on how to disconnect the unit before taking a shower or retiring for the night, and during recharging.

■ Alternate Forms of Application

Point Stimulators

Devices such as the Neuroprobe are modified TENS devices designed to locate and stimulate trigger and acupuncture points by measuring the amount of resistance provided by the skin. Neuroprobes and galvanic stimulators are the only types of current that directly cause activation of C fibers. Point stimulators can decrease the conduction velocity of superficial nerves.[114]

Auriculotherapy

Auriculotherapy describes TENS stimulation of acupuncture points on the ear.[45, 115] This method of application is based on the premise that an injured or diseased body reflects pain or tenderness to specific points on the ear. These points, arranged in the form of an inverted fetus, are said to represent the point at which all the acupuncture channels meet and respond to stimulation by decreasing the perception of pain in the corresponding area of the body (Fig. 13–2). Although not conclusively supported by research, this form of electrostimulation has been found effective in reducing pain caused by musculoskeletal trauma.[115]

▶ INTERFERENTIAL STIMULATION

Interferential stimulation (IFS) units generate two ACs on two separate channels. One channel produces a constant high-frequency sine wave (4000 to 5000 Hz), and the other channel produces a sine wave with a variable frequency. The two currents meet in the body to produce

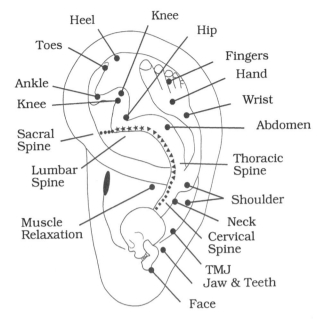

Figure 13–2. Auriculotherapy Points. These acupuncture points are arranged on each ear, roughly in the shape of an inverted fetus. Stimulation of these points reportedly decreases pain in the corresponding body area.

an interference wave having a frequency of 1 to 299 Hz. The medium-frequency carrier currents penetrate the tissues with very little resistance. The resulting interference currents are in a range that allows effective stimulation of biological tissues with relatively little patient discomfort.

Interferential generators combine constructive and destructive interference patterns to form a continuous interference pattern (Box 13–5). These circuits are superimposed in the tissues using a quadripolar technique, two independent electrical currents. **Premodulated currents** are mixed within the generator and use a single channel (bipolar technique).[116]

The rate at which the interference waveform changes is the **beat pattern**, the difference in frequency between the two circuits. One channel has a fixed frequency (for example 5000 Hz), and the second channel has a variable frequency. By selecting a beat frequency of 1 Hz, the second channel produces a current with a frequency of 5001 Hz. Selecting a beat frequency of 100 Hz increases the frequency of the second channel to 5100 Hz. The beat produced by IFS elicits responses similar to the waveforms produced by TENS units but is capable of delivering a greater total current to the tissues (70 to 100 mA).[117]

Capacitive skin resistance is inversely proportional to the frequency of the current. An AC of 50 Hz encounters approximately 3000 ohms of resistance per 100 cm^2 of skin. Increasing the frequency to 4000 Hz reduces capacitive skin resistance to approximately 40 ohms. Consequently, IFS encounters less skin resistance than other low-frequency forms of stimulation. Inside the tissues, the interference between the two waves reduces the frequency to a level that has biological effects on the tissues.

Box 13–5. Electrical Interference

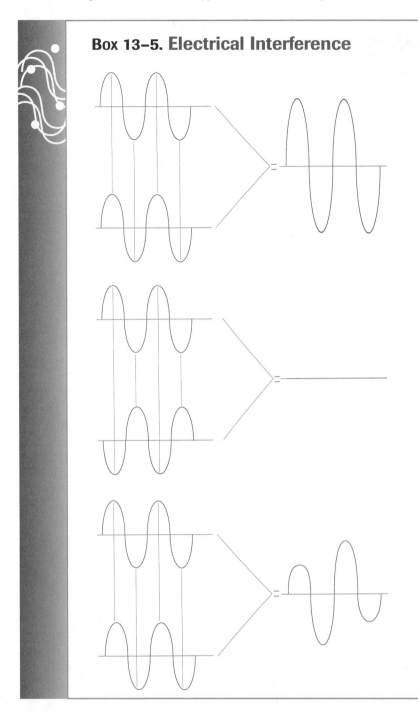

Constructive Interference

When two electrical currents are in perfect phase—that is, the wavelengths are equal and the phases cross the baseline at the same point—the amplitude of the combined wave is equal to the sum of its two parts.

Destructive Interference

Two currents are perfectly out of phase. The positive peak of the first waveform occurs at the same point on the horizontal baseline as the negative peak of the second wave. When these two waves meet, the amplitudes cancel each other out, resulting in a wave intensity of zero.

Continuous Interference

When two currents have slightly different frequencies (e.g., plus or minus 1 Hz), the resulting wave alternates between constructive and destructive interference.

● EFFECTS ON
The Injury Response Process

Interferential stimulation has been used to control pain and elicit muscle contractions to increase venous return. A variation of IFS, with a superimposed duty cycle, is used to reeducate muscle and to increase muscular strength.

■ Pain Control

Mechanisms of pain control are similar to those found with TENS. High beat frequencies, about 100 Hz, when accompanied by sensory-level stimulation, activate the spinal gate, inhibiting the transmission of noxious impulses. Low beat frequencies of 2 to 10 Hz, applied at the motor level, should initiate the release of opiates and result in a narcotic-like pain reduction. Although both high- and low-frequency IFS result in decreased pain perception, the mechanism is probably related to the gate mechanism or occurs secondary to the placebo effect. Serum cortisol levels, an important marker associated with the release of β-endorphin, are not increased following treatment.[41]

Stimulation of acupuncture points with a frequency of 2 Hz or 100 Hz results in pain mediation at specific receptor sites. A 30-Hz frequency affects the widest range of receptors, but the amount of pain reduction is less.[118]

■ Neuromuscular Stimulation

Medium beat frequencies of approximately 15 Hz may be used to reduce edema. Venous and lymphatic return can be increased by motor-level stimulation. The IFS does not appear to significantly increase blood flow in the injured area.[119]

■ Premodulated Currents

A premodulated current is a single AC that is mixed within the generator that produces a sine wave with varying amplitude. The output is interrupted to produce 1 to 100 bursts per second that are capable of producing strong muscle contractions with relatively little discomfort, although it is difficult to balance the parameters required to produce a strong muscle contraction and those that produce pain.[27] Premodulated currents use two electrodes on a single channel and are indicated when the use of four electrodes is impractical because of the size of the treatment area (e.g., the vastus medialis oblique).

Long interburst intervals reduce the root mean square amperage of the applied current but allow for increased treatment intensities per-burst, increasing the intensity of the contraction. The interburst interval is not long enough

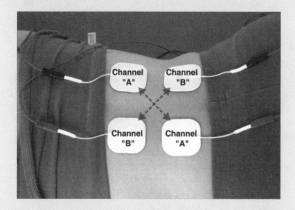

Treatment Strategies
Pain Control via Gate Mechanism Using Interferential Stimulation

Parameter	Setting
Carrier frequency	Based on patient comfort
Burst frequency	80 to 150 Hz
Sweep	Fast
Electrode arrangement	Quadripolar
Electrode placement	Place around the periphery of the target area
Output intensity	Strong sensory level
Treatment duration	20 to 30 minutes

Treatment Strategies
Pain Control via Opiate Release Using Interferential Stimulation

Parameter	Setting
Carrier frequency	Based on patient comfort
Burst frequency	1 to 10 Hz (endorphins) 80 to 120 Hz (enkephalin)
Sweep	Slow
Electrode arrangement	Quadripolar
Electrode placement	Place around the periphery of the target area
Output intensity	Moderate to strong sensory level
Treatment duration	20 to 30 minutes

to allow for muscle relaxation but improves the comfort of the current.[27] "Russian" stimulation is one of the most well known premodulated currents (Box 13–6).

Reduction of Edema

Chronic post-traumatic edema can be reduced by the use of IFS.[121] This effect is attributable to milking of the venous and lymphatic return systems through electrically evoked muscle contractions. Care must be taken to avoid unwanted joint motion that could produce further injury of the involved structures.

■ Electrode Placement

True IFS requires the use of a quadripolar electrode arrangement. Premodulated output may use either bipolar or quadripolar arrangements (see Chapter 12, p 225).

Quadripolar Technique

The four electrodes are positioned around the painful area so that each channel runs perpendicular to the other and the current crosses at the midpoint (Fig. 13–3). The interference effects branch off at 45-degree angles from the center of the treatment, in the shape of a four-leaf clover. Tissues within this area receive the maximal treatment effect. When the electrodes are properly positioned, the stimulation should be felt only between the electrodes, not under the electrodes.

Referring to Figure 13–3, notice that the interference effect covers only about half of the area between the electrodes. If the patient has a very discrete area of pain, the interference pattern should be able to encompass the appropriate tissues. However, in cases in which the pain is

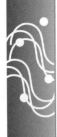

Box 13–6. "Russian" Stimulation

After the 1972 Summer Olympics, much attention was given to an electrical strength training regimen used by Russian athletes. A Soviet physician, Dr. Yakov Kots, reported that athletes training under this technique demonstrated a 30- to 40-percent strength improvement over those training with isometric exercise alone. Other reported benefits of this technique included increased muscular endurance and changes in the velocity of muscular contractions. These results, owing in part to Dr. Kots's failure to specify the parameters used by these athletes, have never been duplicated in the United States.[3, 24, 28, 29, 33, 38, 120, 121] This method of application has gained the name "Russian" stimulation based on its country of origin.

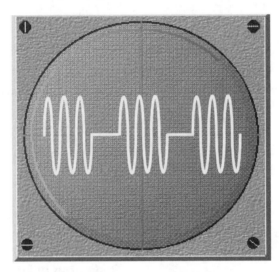

Classic Russian stimulation involves the use of a 2500-Hz carrier sine wave with burst modulation (see At a Glance: Interferential Stimulation, p 260). The theory behind Russian stimulation, as with IFS, is that the higher frequencies would decrease the amount of capacitive skin resistance and allow more current to reach the motor nerve at lower intensities.[3] The 2500-Hz carrier frequency is also thought to "block" superficial sensory nerves while stimulating deeper motor fibers.[27] Although the strength-gain benefits have not been duplicated, this form of electrical stimulation is an excellent method to decrease muscular atrophy.

diffuse, maximal pain reduction may not occur. This problem can be reduced through rotating the interference effect area. By slightly unbalancing the currents, the interference pattern "rotates" or "scans" 45 degrees back and forth between the electrodes, resulting in treatment of a larger area (Fig. 13–4).

Bipolar Electrode Placement

When IFS is applied using a bipolar technique, the mixing of the two channels occurs within the generator rather than in the tissues. Two channels are used within the generator, with a single output channel applied to the tissues. Although bipolar IFS does not penetrate the tissues as deeply as quadripolar application, a more precise mixing occurs.

When muscle contractions are the goal of the treatment session, either through IFS or Russian stimulation, bipolar electrode placements are used. When the effects are targeted for one specific muscle or muscle group, only one channel is used. Four electrodes are incorporated into a dual channel, agonist-antagonist treatment regimen.

■ Instrumentation

Power: When this switch is in its ON position, the current is allowed to flow to the internal components of the generator.

Reset: This safety feature ensures that the intensity is reduced to zero before the treatment is started.

Timer: This control sets the duration of the treatment and subsequently displays the remaining time. On some units, the TIMER serves as the master power switch.

Start-stop: This switch is used to initiate and terminate the treatment.

Intensity: This control adjusts the amplitude of the pulse and is displayed in milliamperes (mA). When quadripolar stimulation is being used, the intensity control regulates both channels simultaneously.

Mode: This switch allows the user to choose between true interferential therapy and bipolar stimulation. The interfer-

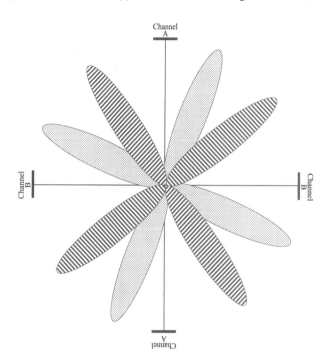

Figure 13-4. **Dynamic Interference Vectoring.** The normal vector pattern is rotated throughout the treatment to stimulate a broader tissue area.

ential mode allows the current to stimulate deep tissue. In the bipolar mode, only one channel is used, and the resultant current flow stimulates relatively subcutaneous nerves.

Premodulated/Russian stimulation: This mode changes the output from amplitude-modulated to burst-modulated

for evoking strong muscle contractions. This technique may use one or both channels. This is an option on many IFS units, and other units provide Russian stimulation as well.

Beat frequency: The "beat" is the result of the fixed rate of the carrier wave and the variable rate of the second channel.

On-off control (duty cycle): When Russian-type stimulation has been selected from the MODE control, this adjusts the duty cycle by determining the amount of time the current is ON versus OFF.

Ramp: Allows the user to determine the amplitude rise time until the peak current is obtained. Often the RAMP represents the percentage of the ON duty cycle time required to reach the maximum intensity.

Balance: This dial allows the user to control the balance of electrical current under each set of electrodes and to equalize the sensory stimulation. It may only be meaningful during quadripolar stimulation.

■ Set-up and Application

Refer to manufacturer's operating instructions for the procedures specific to the unit being used.

Initiation of the Treatment

1. Turn on the unit: Turn on the unit by activating the POWER switch.
2. Reset parameters: Fully reduce the INTENSITY control and depress the RESET button.

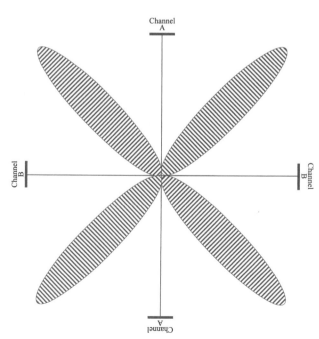

Figure 13-3. **Interference Pattern.** Maximal benefit from interferential stimulation occurs at 45-degree angles from the intersection of the channels.

At a Glance: **Interferential Stimulation**

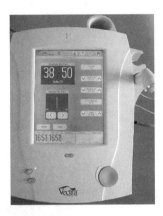

Parameters

CURRENT TYPE:	Two alternating currents forming a single interference current. Premodulated output is based on a single alternating current.
CURRENT FLOW (AMPLITUDE):	1–100 mA
CURRENT FLOW (RMS):	0–50 mA
VOLTAGE:	0 to 200 V
CARRIER FREQUENCY:	Fixed at: 2500 to 5000 Hz
BEAT FREQUENCY:	0–299 Hz
SWEEP FREQUENCY:	10–500 msec

Waveform

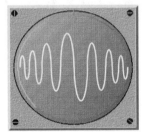

Output Modulation

Beat frequency—Analogous to the number of cycles or pulses per second
Burst duty cycle—Bursts separated by periods of no stimulation (interburst interval)
Intensity
Interburst interval—Duration of time between bursts
Premodulation (e.g., Russian stimulation)
Ramp
Sweep—Variation in the beat frequency; set with a low value and a high value
Vector/Scan—Variation in current intensity

Treatment Duration

- Interferential stimulation may be applied once or twice daily in treatment bouts normally ranging from 15 to 30 minutes.
- Premodulated neuromuscular stimulation bouts are normally applied three times a week in 30-minute bouts (see Neuromuscular electrical stimulation).

Indications

- Acute pain
- Chronic pain
- Muscle spasm

Contraindications

In addition to the contraindications presented in Table 12–9, the use of INF is contraindicated in:
- Pain of central origin
- Pain of unknown origin

Precautions

- Improper use can result in electrode burns or skin irritation.
- Intense or prolonged stimulation may result in muscle spasm and/or muscle soreness.

3. Select application mode: Determine the MODE of application: quadripolar, bipolar, or Russian stimulation.
4. Adjust beat frequency: Select the appropriate BEAT frequencies based on the goals of the treatment.
5. Adjust sweep frequency: Use the appropriate SWEEP frequency for this treatment protocol.
6. Adjust treatment duration: Set the duration of the treatment by adjusting the TIMER.
7. Begin treatment: Press the START button to close the circuit between the generator and the patient's tissues.
8. Increase output intensity: Slowly increase the INTENSITY control until the appropriate current level is obtained.
9. Adjust balance: If necessary, adjust the BALANCE control to obtain maximal treatment comfort.

▶ NEUROMUSCULAR ELECTRICAL STIMULATION

Neuromuscular electrical stimulation (NMES) is used for muscle reeducation, reduction of spasticity, delaying atrophy, and muscle strengthening. The use of electrical stimulation reverses the order in which muscle fibers are recruited into the contraction. During voluntary muscle contractions, small-diameter type I motor nerves are the first to contract. Type I fibers do not generate much force but are able to sustain the contraction for a prolonged period. Electrical stimulation causes large-diameter type II motor nerves to evoke a contraction before type I fibers. Because type II fibers are capable of producing more force, the strength of the contraction is increased.

This reversal in the order of motor nerve recruitment is a result of the relative sizes of the nerves and their depths below the surface of the skin. Electrical stimulation first causes a depolarization of large-diameter type II nerves because their cross-sectional area provides less resistance to current flow. In addition, type II motor nerves, being more superficial, receive greater stimulation than the deeper type I nerves.

The amount of torque produced is directly related to the amount of current introduced into the muscle.[24] The strength of the contraction can be further altered through manipulation of the electrode placement. Generators for NMES use a wide range of waveforms, but the majority of the units currently on the market use a biphasic wave. A review of the literature indicates that no one waveform is universally "comfortable." Perceived comfort is based on individual patient preference. Symmetrical pulses tend to be less painful over a large muscle mass because there is an equal amount of stimulation under both electrodes.[31]

Neuromuscular stimulation is a frequency-dependent modality. The current must be strong enough to overcome the capacitive resistance of the tissues before the motor nerves can be stimulated. The capacitive tissue resistance is inversely proportional to the frequency of the current. Therefore, the relatively low frequencies used by NMES generators must produce a greater current to overcome this resistance.

● EFFECTS ON
The Injury Response Process

■ Neuromuscular Stimulation

Because of the large amplitude and long pulse duration, NMES provides stronger stimulation than other forms of electrical stimulation. The increased pulse duration and amperage, however, tend to result in decreased comfort. Increasing the duration of the pulses results in increased stimulation of pain nerve fibers. When the aim of the treatment session is to increase muscular strength, the output of the treatment should be as high as the patient will allow; if the aim is muscle reeducation, a mild tonic contraction for "cueing" is all that is required.[3]

The efficacy of NMES in improving isometric muscle strength has been substantiated in the literature. The improvement in strength occurs as a result of increasing the functional stress placed on the muscle and as a result of the reversal of motor nerve recruitment.[38] NMES has been shown to elicit a contraction that produces torque equal to 90 percent of the maximal voluntary contraction.[25]

Patients who reeducate muscle with NMES can significantly increase strength as opposed to patients who are not exercising. Patients using NMES applied with a 60 percent duty cycle demonstrated significantly higher strength gains than patients who used only isometric exercise.[122, 123] After ACL reconstruction, high-intensity NMES may increase the strength of the involved quadriceps muscle to 70 percent, compared with 57 percent for voluntary contractions and 51 percent for low-intensity NMES.[124]

Muscular contractions obtained through NMES can increase peripheral blood flow to the extremity being treated. This occurs as a result of the increased metabolic rate associated with the contractions. During treatment, blood flow increases during the first minute, whereas it reaches a steady state for the remainder of the treatment.[125] This response is independent of the stimulation intensity. Sympathetic changes in blood flow may also occur in the opposite side of the body.[126]

Table 13–2 presents several different types of benefits and effects reported to be associated with NMES and various protocols.

■ Edema Reduction

NMES is similar to other forms of electrotherapy for motor-level edema reduction. The protocol described for motor-level reduction of edema using HVPS can be used with this device. Venous and lymphatic return are enhanced through the milking of these vessels by muscle contractions. Because the aim of this method is to produce individual muscle contractions, a low (1 to 10 pps) pulse frequency or a 50-percent duty cycle is used. The intensity of the current should produce a visible contraction but should not cause unwanted movement of the joint. As with other methods of edema reduction, the benefits of this treatment are enhanced if the limb is elevated.

■ Electrode Placement

Bipolar electrode placement is commonly employed in NMES treatments. The electrodes are placed over the proximal and distal ends of the muscle or muscle group. Because large electrodes lie over several muscles or motor points, a more generalized contraction is obtained. The use of small electrodes may elicit a more specific contraction through direct stimulation of the muscle's motor point. As the electrodes are brought closer together, the effect of the stimulation becomes more superficial, and the relative intensity of the contraction decreases.

Quadripolar application requires the use of two separate channels. This method of application is commonly used when stimulating agonist-antagonist muscle groups.

TABLE 13–2	Effects Associated with Neuromuscular Electrical Stimulation

Electrically induced isometric quadriceps contractions can significantly increase strength in certain joint positions:

• Knee joint positions ranged from 30° – 90° of flexion.
• The amount of hip flexion can influence the strength of the contractions, possibly secondary to providing the muscle group with a mechanical advantage.
• Strength gains summarized ranged from 7% – 48%.

Electrical stimulation can increase isokinetic strength at certain speeds.

• No significant strength increases have been reported at speeds greater than 120° per second.
• Speeds of 65° per second showed the most substantial increases.

No statistically significant strength increases have been demonstrated to occur between strength gains obtained via ES, voluntary contractions, and a combination of ES and voluntary contractions.

• Most of the literature reviewed indicated greater strength gains in voluntary contractions than in electrically induced contractions.
• Although the differences in strength gains obtained from voluntary contractions compared with those obtained from ES were not statistically significant, the results may be clinically significant. Strength increases obtained from ES were on average 10% greater than those derived from voluntary contractions.

A monopolar technique may be employed through the use of one small and one large electrode or through the use of a hand-held applicator. This method of electrode placement is useful when a specific muscle, or a small muscle group, is the target of the treatment.

The size of the electrodes should be only as large as is required to stimulate the desired tissues. Electrodes that are too small result in a very high current density, whereas electrodes that are larger than needed may stimulate unwanted nerves.

■ Instrumentation

Power: When this switch is in its ON position, the current is allowed to flow to the internal components of the generator.

Reset: This safety feature ensures that the output is reduced to zero before the treatment is started.

Timer: This control sets the duration of the treatment and subsequently displays the remaining time.

Intensity: This knob adjusts the amplitude of the pulses.

Pulse rate: This parameter determines the type of muscle contraction to be elicited. Depending on the muscle or muscle group being stimulated, a pulse rate of less than 15 pps causes a distinct contraction for each impulse. Between 15 and 25 pps, the muscle begins to contract smoothly, eventually leading to a tonic contraction at approximately 35 to 50 pps.

Mode: This switch allows the user to select the type of waveform used in the treatment.

Duty cycle: This feature allows the user to set the duty cycle for the treatment. Neuromuscular stimulation units have separate dials to adjust the number independently of seconds that the current is flowing and the number of seconds it is not. Other units have preset duty cycles that the user cannot alter. A CONSTANT mode (100% duty cycle) may be provided. This is useful for adjusting the other treatment parameters (intensity, pulse duration, etc.) without waiting for the duty cycle to switch to its ON mode.

External trigger: A hand-held device that allows the user to manually control the ON-OFF time of the stimulation. When the trigger is depressed, current is allowed to flow to the tissues.

Reciprocal rate: When two channels are being used, this feature selects the duration of time that the current is flowing to each channel.

Ramp: The RAMP parameter allows the user to determine the amplitude rise time until the peak current is obtained. Often the RAMP represents the percentage of the ON duty cycle time required to reach the maximum intensity. For example, a 20-percent RAMP with an ON duty cycle time of 5 seconds would require 1 second to reach the maximum intensity.

At a Glance: **Neuromuscular Electrical Stimulation**

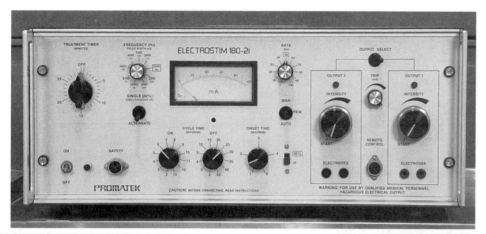

Parameters

CURRENT TYPE: Biphasic or premodulated
TOTAL CURRENT FLOW: 0 to 200 mA
PULSE FREQUENCY: 1 to 200 pps
PHASE DURATION: 20 to 300 msec
INTRAPULSE INTERVAL: Appx. 100 msec

Output Modulation

Intensity   Pulses per second
Duty cycle   Reciprocal rate
Ramp

Waveforms

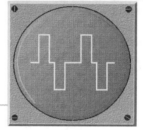

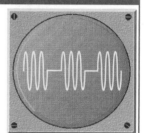

Balanced biphasic   Premodulated

Treatment Duration

Treatments used for muscular reeducation may be given daily, but as with any muscle-building program, the patient should be monitored for undue pain. Treatment to delay atrophy is given throughout the day with the use of a portable stimulator.

Indications

- Maintaining range of motion
- Prevention of joint contractures
- Increasing local blood flow

- Muscle reeducation
- Prevention of disuse atrophy
- Decreasing muscle spasm

Contraindications

In addition to the contraindications presented in Table 12–9, contraindications to the use of NMES include:
- Musculotendinous lesions, in which the tension produced by the contraction will further damage the muscle or tendon fibers
- Cases in which there is not a secure bony attachment of the muscle

Precautions

- Improper use may result in electrode burns or skin irritation.
- Intense or prolonged stimulation may result in muscle spasm and/or muscle soreness.
- An electrically induced contraction can generate too much tension within the muscle (the function of the Golgi tendon organs is overridden).

Interrupt switch: This device is held by the patient and is used to terminate the treatment if the intensity becomes too great or too painful.

■ Set-up and Application

Refer to manufacturer's operating instructions for the procedures specific to the unit being used.

Initiation of the Treatment

1. Prepare the generator: Reduce the output intensity to zero and turn the unit on. If applicable, press the RESET button.
2. Prepare electrodes: Connect the leads to the unit and to the electrodes and secure the electrodes to the patient.
3. Make the interrupt switch available: Give the patient the INTERRUPT SWITCH and provide instruction on its purpose and use.
4. Set pulse variables: Set the phase duration (WIDTH) and pulse frequency (RATE) to the midrange of the parameters to be used.
5. Set current variables: If the RAMP and ON-OFF parameters are manually adjustable on the unit, increase the RAMP to a rapid rise and adjust the ON-OFF controls to a 100-percent duty cycle. This configuration allows the INTENSITY to be increased without waiting for the generator to run through its duty cycle. If these parameters cannot be changed during the course of the treatment, adjust them to the desired settings now. (Certain generators may be designed to allow the intensity to be increased without adjusting these parameters.)
6. Adjust frequency: Adjust the output FREQUENCY to the appropriate level for this treatment (see step 11 below).
7. Set treatment duration: Set the TIMER for this session.
8. Initiate treatment: Press the START button to activate the unit.
9. Increase intensity: Begin the treatment by slowly increasing the INTENSITY until the desired tension is developed in the muscle.
10. Adjust ramp for treatment goals: If applicable, reset the RAMP time to match the treatment goals and patient needs.
11. Adjust the DUTY CYCLE to match the treatment goals: The following protocol may be used as an example: 127.
12. Muscle strengthening: ON = 10 seconds, OFF = 50 seconds.
13. Muscle endurance: ON and OFF have approximately equal durations (4 to 15 seconds). FREQUENCY equals 50 to 200 Hz.

▶ IONTOPHORESIS

Iontophoresis is the introduction of ionized medications into the subcutaneous tissues using a low-voltage DC. The amount of medication entering the tissues is based on the current density and the duration of the treatment. By adapting to fluctuations in tissue resistance, iontophoresis generators (iontophoresors) produce a constant voltage output by adjusting the amperage. The medication types most commonly used for iontophoresis include anesthetics, analgesics, and anti-inflammatory agents. Experimental work has begun that explores the use of iontophoresis as a substitute for certain types of **dialysis** ■ and repeated injections, such as insulin.

Based on the ionic reaction between the positive and negative poles of the generator, ionized medication molecules travel along the lines of force created by the current. At the positive electrode, positive ions are driven through the skin; negative ions are introduced through the skin at the negative pole. This technique has been shown to deliver the medication to depths of 6 to 20 mm below the skin.[128, 129]

Iontophoresis requires the use of custom electrodes that are designed to store medication or a buffer. Electrode sizes are expressed by the amount of medication required to saturate them. For instance, a 3.0 mL electrode will hold 3 mL of medication.

The transdermal introduction of medication has advantages over oral ingestion or injection of medication. An advantage over oral medication includes bypassing the liver, thus reducing the metabolic breakdown of the medication. The medication can also be concentrated in a localized area rather than be absorbed in the gastrointestinal tract, providing local rather than systemic delivery of the drug.[130] Most of these advantages also hold true with injected medication, but iontophoresis is less traumatic and less painful than injected medication. In addition, the injection of medication can result in a high concentration of medication in a localized area, resulting in tissue damage.[128, 131]

Iontophoresis also has its disadvantages. Unreliable results are obtained with certain medications, and the amount of medication that is actually introduced into the tissues is unknown.[21] Areas of thick skin, such as the plantar aspect of the foot, are more difficult to penetrate than thinner skin. Deep structures such as the hip joint are located too deeply to be affected by iontophoresis.

In children, the anxiety caused by iontophoresis was not significantly less than that of an injection. Injections appear to be more tolerable over time. Also, cutaneous anesthesia derived from an injection is more tolerable than that obtained through iontophoresis.[132]

Many of the medications used during iontophoresis are controlled substances requiring a physician's prescription. The use of the iontophoresor may also be regulated by state practice acts.

Dialysis: An external device that is used to assist or replace the kidney's function of filtering blood.

■ Iontophoresis Mechanisms

Traditional iontophoresors deliver a low-voltage, high-amperage DC to the body. The generator's output ranges from 0 to 5 mA at skin impedances ranging from 500 ohms to 100 kilohms.

As we saw in the Phonophoresis section of Chapter 7, the stratum corneum is the primary barrier to the transfer of substances across the skin into the subcutaneous tissues. The electrical charge of the medication helps complete the circuit by carrying the current between the two electrode poles. During iontophoresis, the primary path for current flow, and hence medication transfer, occurs through portals formed by hair follicles and skin pores.[1, 40]

For iontophoresis to occur, the applied current must be sufficient to overcome the skin/electrode resistance and still have enough energy to drive the medication through the skin's portals.[133, 134] As the treatment progresses, the portals' resistance to electrical current flow and medication entry into the body decreases.[135] Once it is within the tissues, the medication is spread locally through passive diffusion and is no longer affected by the current source. The rate of this diffusion is such that the medication tends to remain more highly concentrated within those tissues directly subcutaneous to the introduction site and progressively less concentrated in the deeper tissues and in tissues peripheral to the treatment site.[136]

Iontophoresis uses a monopolar electrode arrangement in which the electrode containing the medication serves as the active electrode. The increased current density under the delivery electrode also decreases the resistance to the iontophoretic current; the higher the current density, the less resistance to electrical flow.[137] Although this trait seems to contradict Ohm's law, the decreased resistance is an artifact of an increase in the size of the skin pores or the creation of new ones.[138, 139]

Local blood flow is increased for 1 hour after the treatment, and the stratum corneum is hydrated for 30 minutes after treatment. Although this assists in the subcutaneous diffusion of the medication, it may result in a wider-than-normal diffusion, spreading the medication systemically and lowering its concentration in the intended treatment area. The increased blood flow may also explain the **hyperemia** ■ after the treatment.[140]

Burns or severe skin irritation are problems inherent to the application of a DC on the human body. Either of these negative reactions is related to the hydrogen and hydroxide ions generated by the current. Experimental work using a low-frequency AC or a combination of ACs and DCs has been shown to be effective in delivering certain forms of medication to the body without the associated skin irritation.[141, 142]

■ Medication Dosage

The medication dosage is measured in terms of milliamperes per minute (mA/min) and is based on the relationship between the amperage of the current and the treatment duration:

$$\text{Current amperage (mA)} \times \text{Treatment duration (min)} = \text{mA} \bullet \text{min}$$

Most iontophoresors use a dose-oriented treatment protocol in which the user indicates the desired treatment dose and the generator calculates the duration and intensity of the treatment. A subsequent change in the output alters the treatment duration; increasing the amperage decreases duration and vice versa. If the treatment duration were shortened, the output intensity would be increased.

For example, if a medication were being used that called for a dose of 50 mA/min, the generator may default to an output of 5 mA and a treatment duration of 10 minutes (5 mA × 10 minutes = 50 mA/min). If this is the patient's first exposure to iontophoresis or if the patient has a history of sensitivity to this treatment, the intensity of the treatment would be decreased. Suppose the intensity was decreased to 3 mA. The generator would then recalculate the treatment duration to approximately 16 minutes and 40 seconds (3 mA × 16.67 minutes = 50 mA/min).

The amperage should be immediately reduced when the patient reports any sensation other than tingling (e.g., reports of burning). The maximum treatment dosage depends on the polarity of the medication delivery electrode. Negative polarity can deliver up to an 80 mA/min dose; positive polarity can deliver up to a 40 mA/min dose.

The dose-oriented approach has led to the development of low-intensity, long-duration treatment in which the patient wears the patch for up to 24 hours (Fig. 13–5). Using a self-contained battery delivering one volt of charge, the patient wears the patch for 12 hours to deliver a dose equivalent to 40 mA/min and 24 hours to deliver a dose equivalent to 80 mA/min.

■ Medications

The type of medication used during iontophoresis depends on the type of pathology and the desired treatment outcome. Table 13–3 presents some common medications used during this treatment, indications for use, and typical treatment dosages. This information should not be viewed as recommended treatment protocols. For this information, refer to the physician's or pharmacist's recommended concentrations and treatment doses.

For the application of iontophoresis, water-soluble

Hyperemia: A red discoloration of the skin caused by increased blood flow. The skin turns white when pressure is applied.

medications are dissolved in a carrier. The amount and rate of medication delivery are based on the total voltage applied, the duration of the treatment, the local pH, and the concentration of the medication in the delivery electrode. As the magnitude of each of these factors increases, the total dosage of the treatment increases. Increased concentrations (percentage) of the medication have the potential to clog the pores and decrease the delivery of the medications to the underlying tissues.[143]

Certain reactions occur that complicate the delivery of medication into the tissues. The medication competes with other ions having the same polarity as the delivery electrodes. There is an equal chance that the medication ions will be driven into the tissues as other ions having the same molecular weight and size. Medications of larger ionic weight and mass require an increased output intensity to drive them through the tissues. Because of the amount of work (energy) required, smaller ions tend to be preferentially moved relative to larger ones.

Passive iontophoresis also alters the amount, rate, and quality of the phoresis. Recall that ions that have unlike charges attract each other. As a charged ion enters the tissues, it tends to "pull" ions having the opposite charge. Consider a negatively charged ion being pushed into the skin by the negative charge of the electrode. A nearby positively charged ion may be within the negative ion's field of attraction. The positively charged ion is pulled behind the negative ion as it enters the tissue.

Different types of medications may be mixed together so long as their ionic charges do cancel each other out or significantly weaken. To achieve equal doses of one medication of a relatively large molecular size and weight

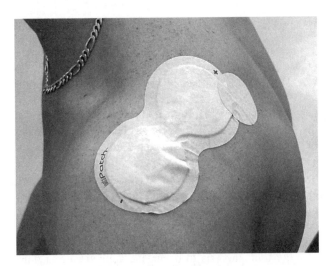

Figure 13–5. **IontoPatch Extended Time-release Iontophoresis System.** This treatment is being applied for inflammation of the acromioclavicular joint. Note the "−" symbol on the lower left of the patch and the "+" symbol in the upper right. In this case, the medication was negatively charged, so it was loaded in the negative electrode. A buffering solution is loaded in the positive electrode to complete the circuit. The small round patch just next to the "+" symbol helps hold the electrode down should it begin to peel away. (IontoPatch courtesy of Birch Point Medical, Oakdale, MN.)

and another one of smaller mass, the concentration of the larger, less mobile medication must be increased.[136]

■ Biophysical Effects

The exact biophysical effects obtained from the treatment depend on the type of medication or medications

---

TABLE 13–3   Sample Medications, Their Indications, and Treatment Dosages Used During Iontophoresis*†

Medication(s)	Pathology	Delivery Concentration	Dosage	Polarity
Acetic acid	Myositis ossificans	2% mixed with distilled water	80 mA/min	Negative
Dexamethasone and lidocaine	Inflammation	4 mg Decadron (1 cm² suspension)	41 mA/min	Negative
	Pain control	4% Xylocaine (2 cm² suspension)	40 mA/min	Positive
Lidocaine and epinephrine	Pain control	4% Lidocaine 0.01 mL 1:50,000 epinephrine	30 mA/min	Positive Positive
Lidocaine and epinephrine	Pain control	4% Lidocaine and 0.25 cc of 1:1000 epinephrine	20 mA/min	Positive
Dexamethasone	Inflammation	2 cc 4 mg/mL dexamethasone	41 mA/min	Negative

Refer to the physician's prescription for exact treatment parameters.
†*Each size electrode has a maximum amperage that should not be exceeded. Consult the packaging information included with the electrodes.*

being used. Medications introduced into the body through iontophoresis can penetrate 6 to 20 mm below the skin and in most instances can reach the depth of tendinous structures and underlying cartilage. However, the exact dose of the medication reaching this depth is undetermined.[21, 128, 129, 144]

When an anti-inflammatory or anesthetic mixture is used (e.g., dexamethasone [Decadron] and lidocaine [Xylocaine]), the onset of relief may take 24 to 48 hours, although immediate relief is sometimes reported. The latent effects may be attributed to a cumulative effect of the treatments.[21] Lidocaine, in concentrations of up to 50 percent, requires a minimum of 10 minutes of electrical current before the skin is anesthetized.[145] Superficial anesthesia can be achieved using iontophoresis, but the lack of depth of penetration prevents a total nerve block from being obtained.

The use of a direct current can potentially alter the pH of skin. However, changes in skin pH do not occur unless the treatment dosage exceeds 80 mA/min (beyond the range of normal dosage).[146]

Electrode Placement

The delivery of iontophoresis involves the use of a delivery electrode ("drug electrode") that serves as the active electrode and a return electrode that serves as the dispersive electrode (Fig. 13–6). Many application procedures use only one delivery electrode, but most units allow two to be used. The delivery electrode is placed over the target tissues. The return electrode is placed 4 to 6 inches away. When placing each electrode on the body, care should be taken to consider the underlying tissues. For example, if iontophoresis is being used to treat plantar fasciitis, the delivery electrode should be placed on the medial aspect of the arch, where the skin is relatively thin, rather than over the thick padding provided under the heel.

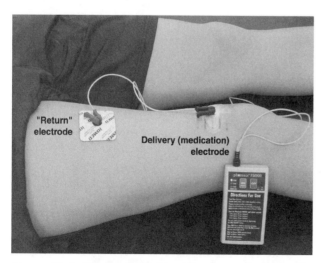

Figure 13–6. **Electrode Set-up for Iontophoresis.** The appropriate medication is introduced to the delivery electrode, and the return electrode is saturated with an electrically neutral buffering solution. The polarity of the delivery electrode must have the same polarity as the medication being used.

Instrumentation

Power: The POWER switch activates or deactivates the generator.

Reset: The RESET switch serves as an "emergency shut-off" in case of patient discomfort or a malfunction within the generator. At the conclusion of the treatment, pressing the RESET button decreases the dosage, output, and duration values to zero.

Dosage: This parameter sets the medication dosage, in milliamperes per minute, for this treatment. Some units allow for the dosage to be keyed in directly (e.g., if a keypad is used, the numerical value is typed in) or set using INCREASE and DECREASE buttons.

Intensity (amperage): By setting the DOSAGE, the amperage increases to a preset level. Increasing the INTENSITY decreases the treatment DURATION; decreasing this value increases the DURATION while keeping the dosage at the level indicated.

Treatment duration: Decreasing the DURATION increases the treatment INTENSITY and vice versa.

Polarity: The polarity of the delivery electrode must be the same as that of the medication currently being applied (i.e., if a medication has a negative polarity, the delivery electrode must have a negative polarity). Units having a POLARITY switch change the polarity of the delivery electrode to either positive or negative. Other units require that the electrode leads be physically plugged into the positive and negative jacks.

Start-stop: Pressing this button the first time begins the current flow to the patient's body. For patient comfort, most generators are programmed so that the current is gradually ramped up from zero to the actual treatment duration. Pressing this button again either creates a pause in the treatment or terminates it, depending on the unit's design.

Set-up and Application

The benefits of preheating or precooling the target tissues have not been substantiated. Preheating the tissues may open skin pathways and ease the passage of the medication through the skin. The increased blood flow, however, may accelerate the removal of the medication from the area. Cold packs decrease blood flow and therefore theoretically maintain the medication concentration in the tissues. However, cold also may decrease the passage of medication into the tissue by tightening the skin portals. Do not apply hot packs or cold packs directly over the iontophoresis electrodes because uneven pressures can result in increased or decreased current densities.

Refer to manufacturer's operating instructions for the procedures specific to the unit being used.

At a Glance: **Iontophoresis**

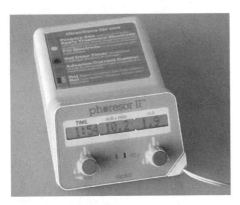

Parameters

CURRENT TYPE: Direct current
TOTAL CURRENT FLOW: Up to 5 mA
VOLTAGE: 80 V
PULSE FREQUENCY: Not applicable
PULSE DURATION: Not applicable
PHASE DURATION: Not applicable
DOSAGE: 0 to 80 mA/min

Waveform

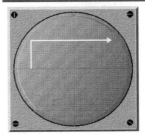

Output Modulation

Amperage
Dosage
Duration
Polarity (medication delivery electrode)

Treatment Duration

The duration of an individual treatment is based on the intensity of the treatment and the desired treatment dose (see Medication Dosage). Treatments are usually given every other day for up to 3 weeks. Consult the patient's prescription for the exact treatment regimen.

Indications

- Acute inflammation
- Chronic inflammation
- Arthritis
- Myositis ossificans
- Myofascial pain syndromes
- As a vehicle for delivering local anesthetics before injection or other minor invasive procedures [130]
- Hyperhidrosis

Contraindications

In addition to the contraindications presented in Table 12-9, iontophoresis should not be used when:
- The patient has a history of adverse reactions or hypersensitivity to electrical stimulation
- The patient has contraindications to the medication(s) being administered
- Pain or other symptoms of unknown origin are present

Precautions

- Controlled medications require a physician's prescription. Pay close attention to any notes or instructions provided by the pharmacist. State practice acts may further regulate the delivery of iontophoresis.
- The exact dosage of the medication delivered to the body is unknown.
- Erythema under the electrodes is common after the treatment.
- A treatment dose that is too intense (in amperage or duration) can result in burns beneath the delivery and/or return electrode.
- Do not reuse an electrode because medications remain in it, contaminating it for future use.

Initiation of the Treatment

1. Clean the treatment site: Using alcohol, cleanse the area where the active and return electrodes are to be affixed to the body.
2. The areas where the electrodes are to be placed should be free of cuts, abrasions, and other open wounds and of excess body hair. Because shaving may cause nicks in the skin, clip excess body hair.
3. Prepare the ACTIVE electrode or electrodes: Fill the delivery electrode with the appropriate medication or medications in the manner applicable to the type of electrode being used. If indicated by the medication being used, add 1 mL of a buffering solution (0.9% saline and 0.5% potassium phosphate) to the active electrode. Buffering may only be required at higher treatment dosages (e.g., 80 mA/min).[146]
4. Wet the RETURN electrode with an appropriate buffering solution.
5. Position electrodes: Place the DELIVERY electrode over the treatment site and the RETURN electrode 4 to 6 inches away.
6. Set electrode polarity: Depending on the type of generator being used, either attach the electrode leads to the generator so that the polarity of the DELIVERY electrode matches the medication's charge or attach the electrode leads as indicated and adjust the POLARITY selector as needed.
7. Provide patient instructions: Inform the patient that tingling and itching may be experienced during the treatment, but the treatment should not be uncomfortable. Advise the patient to inform you of any pain, burning, or other unpleasant sensations.
8. Set treatment dose: Indicate the treatment dose recommended by the physician and pharmacist. Do not exceed the recommended dose or intensity for the electrode being used.
9. Adjust output parameters: Normally, the INTENSITY parameter is adjusted to suit the patient's comfort. If this is the patient's first treatment or if the patient has a history of sensitivity to this treatment or electrical stimulation in general, the output intensity should be decreased. The treatment intensity can be increased if indicated. Remember that decreasing the intensity increases the treatment duration and vice versa.
10. Supplemental treatment: Administer any appropriate follow-up treatments. Pulsed ultrasound (see Chap. 7) may be used after acetic acid iontophoresis for the reduction in the mass of traumatic myositis ossificans.[147]
11. Repeat treatment with the opposite polarity: If medications of different polarities are being used, repeat this procedure with the other medication using the appropriate polarity.
12. Apply a soothing ointment: A mild massage cream, aloe lotion, or skin-soothing ointment may be applied to the electrode sites to aid in reducing the amount of residual skin irritation associated with the treatment.
13. Discard electrodes: Iontophoresis electrodes may be used only for a single treatment.

MICROCURRENT ELECTRICAL STIMULATION

Although there is no universally accepted definition of microcurrent electrical therapy (MET or MENS), some common denominators may be found. The current applied to the body is usually below the depolarization threshold of sensory nerves and has a current of less than 1000 mA. These devices produce an electrical current that has approximately 1/1000 the amperage of TENS but a pulse duration that may be up to 2500 times longer. Microcurrent stimulation is used to restore the body's natural electrical potential to speed healing, reduce edema, and reduce pain. The efficacy of this technique has not been established.

Unlike the other electrical modalities described in this chapter, the distinguishing feature of microcurrent is that it does not attempt to excite peripheral nerves.[148] The subsensory current is thought to regulate cellular activity using a direct, alternating, or pulsed current (in a wide range of waveforms), with each possessing a broad band of pulse durations, frequencies, and treatment durations. Multiple channels may be employed as well. This range of currents makes it difficult to analyze the theoretical and clinical effects of MET.

The efficacy of this form of electrical stimulation has not been substantiated in professional literature. Some controlled studies report decreased pain, increased range of motion, and improved wound healing. However, more often than not, these effects were greater in experimental subjects than those seen in a control group, but less than other modalities, or were conducted in an uncon-trolled manner.[51, 149–152] Likewise, research exists that does not support microcurrent's efficacy as a therapeutic modality.[83, 153–158]

Biophysical Effects

Tissue trauma affects the electrical potential of the involved cells, the previously described injury potential or current of injury.[56] Resistance to electrical current flow increases after trauma, so the body's intrinsic bioelectrical currents take the path of least resistance around, rather than through, the involved tissues. As a result of the diminished bioelectrical activity within the traumatized area, cellular capacitance is decreased, and the cell's homeostasis is further disrupt-ed.[159–161] Theoretically, reestablishing the body's natural electrical balance allows the cell's adenosine triphosphate

(ATP) supply to be replenished, thus providing the metabolic energy for healing to occur.

The theory supporting microcurrent's biophysical effects on the injury response process is based on the effect that a low amperage current has on ATP levels. Currents below 500 mA increase the level of ATP, whereas higher amperages decrease the ATP level. Passing a low-amperage electrical current through mitochondria creates an imbalance in the number of proteins on either side of its cell membrane. As the protons move from the anode to the cathode, they cross the mitochondrial membrane, causing adenosine triphosphatase to produce ATP. The increased ATP production encourages amino acid transport and increased protein synthesis.[162]

Although it seems that a DC would best produce the effects described in this section, many MET protocols use an alternating or pulsed current.[161, 163] It is unlikely that a DC is sufficient to overcome the skin's capacitive resistance because of the low amperage at which MET is applied. As you will recall, capacitive skin resistance decreases as the pulse frequency increases. Therefore, applying MET with an alternating or pulsed current lowers the current threshold required to overcome the skin's resistance. The distances used between the electrodes during treatment also serve to increase the amount of energy needed to complete the circuit.

Research has validated the effects of subthreshold electrical stimulation on cell membrane properties, neurological responses, and ionic responses.[148, 164, 165] These experimental designs most commonly use electrodes that are implanted within the tissues themselves. Other derivations have arisen from the benefits of sensory-level DC application. Unlike MET, the currents used in these studies did not have to overcome the resistance produced by the skin or have the electrical power needed to overcome the resistance posed by the tissues. Any interpolation between these effects and microcurrent may be inappropriate.

MET application has demonstrated increased collagen at the wound site, but this did not correlate to increased tensile strength or increased wound thickness.[151] Transient analgesia[152] and a decrease in postexercise creatine kinase levels[166] have also been attributed to MET therapy.

■ Electrode Placement

The electrodes should be placed so that a line drawn through them transects the target tissues. This, in concept, is similar to the contiguous electrode placement technique described earlier in this chapter. However, proponents of MET view electrode placement in a three-dimensional rather than the traditional two-dimensional manner. This view holds that electrodes should also be placed on opposite sides of the torso or extremity and the current will flow through them. Perhaps if electricity flowed in a perfectly straight line between opposing electrodes, this would be true. However, remember that electricity follows the path of least resistance, which would most likely course the current around the body's circumference rather than

straight through the core. Also remember that the greater the distance between the electrodes, the greater the resistance and the more current required to overcome this resistance.

One technique for treating back pain places an electrode near the spinal cord at the same level as the painful tissues. The opposite electrode is then positioned on the contralateral side of the spinal cord on the anterior side of the body. When the axial skeleton is being treated, MET protocol suggests that treatment occur bilaterally.

The use of MET probes is described in the Set-up and Application section.

■ Instrumentation

Power: When this switch is in its ON position, the current is allowed to flow to the internal components of the generator. Some units have a speaker that emits an audible sound when a certain electrical threshold is met. In this type of generator, the power switch often serves as a VOLUME control as well.

Timer: This control sets the duration of the treatment and subsequently displays the remaining time. On some units, the TIMER serves as the master power switch.

Start-stop: When this button is depressed to start the treatment, the circuit is closed, allowing the current to flow to the patient's tissues. When it is depressed again, the circuit is opened, interrupting the current flow. The START-STOP button may also set the treatment mode on some generators.

Amplitude: This control adjusts the current amperage from zero (OFF) to the maximal value of the unit. The output for each channel has its own AMPLITUDE control. The applied output is displayed on the OUTPUT meter.

Frequency (hertz): When a pulsed current is being applied, the FREQUENCY sets the number of pulses per second; when an AC is being administered, it sets the number of cycles per second. Each channel has its own output control.

Multiplier: A three-position switch that multiplies the output FREQUENCY by the value indicated. The output for each channel has its own multiplier control.

Polarity: This switch selects the output polarity in monophasic mode, or the rate at which the output polarity is alternated in biphasic mode.

Ramp: The ramp selects the rise time of the modulated output in biphasic mode.

Threshold: This button adjusts the level on the power meter at which audible output occurs.

Meter select: This control adjusts which channel is displayed on the power output meter.

Ohm meter: This device is used as a method of identifying stimulation points. When the probe is passed over an

At a Glance: **Microcurrent Electrical Stimulation**

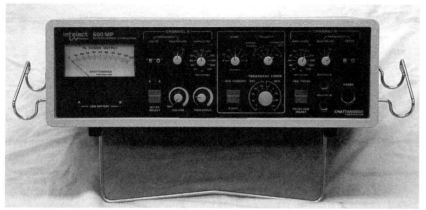

Parameters

CURRENT TYPE	Monophasic, biphasic, direct, or alternating. Monophasic currents may regularly change the electrode polarity.
TOTAL CURRENT FLOW:	1 to 999 μA (Peak current) 25 to 600 μA (RMS)
PULSE FREQUENCY:	0.1 to 1000 Hz
PULSE DURATION:	0.5 to 5000 msec
PHASE DURATION:	0.5 to 5000 msec

Waveform

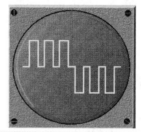

Output Modulation

Intensity
Polarity/alternating polarity
Ramp
Threshold—Ohm meter

Treatment Duration

Most MET treatments range from 30 minutes to 2 hours and may be repeated up to four times per day.

Indications

- Acute and chronic pain
- Acute and chronic inflammation
- Reduction of edema
- Sprains
- Strains
- Contusions
- Temporomandibular joint dysfunction
- Carpal tunnel syndrome
- Superficial wound healing
- Scar tissue
- Neuropathies

Contraindications

In addition to the contraindications presented in Table 12–9, the use of microcurrent electrical stimulation should not be used in:
- Pain or other symptoms of unknown origin
- **Osteomyelitis** ■

Precautions

- The use of MET on dehydrated patients may result in nausea, dizziness, and/or headaches.
- Electrical "shocks" may be reported by the patient when MET is applied to scar tissue. This represents the decreased amount of current required to overcome the scar's electrical resistance.

Osteomyelitis: Inflammation of the bone marrow and adjacent bone.

area of decreased electrical resistance (e.g., stimulation points, traumatized tissues), a tone, light, or numerical readout identifies the point on the skin at which stimulation should occur.

■ Set-up and Application

Refer to manufacturer's operating instructions for the procedures specific to the unit being used.

Initiation of the Treatment

1. Position the electrodes: Most MET stimulators require the use of silver electrodes. Unapproved carbon-rubber electrodes may present too much resistance to current flow and render the treatment ineffective.
2. Wet the electrodes: If felt-tipped electrodes or probes are being used, wet them with saline solution. Tap water should not be used because of its potentially high mineral content. Note that medicinal saline solution requires a physician's prescription. If this type of saline solution is not readily available, a saline-based contact lens cleaner may be used to wet the electrodes.
3. Select the output frequency: Most MET treatment protocols employ a 0.5-Hz frequency. If this frequency proves to be ineffective, a 1.5-Hz output may be attempted. Other protocols suggest using a frequency between 80 to 100 Hz for inflammatory conditions.
4. Increase the output intensity: Increase the intensity to the highest comfortable level, keeping in mind that most treatment applications occur at the subsensory level. Some protocols suggest a series of 5- to 10-minute treatments using a range of output intensities and varying pulse frequencies.
5. Reposition the electrodes: Each treatment bout with the electrode technique lasts from 5 to 10 minutes. At the end of each bout, the electrodes are removed, rewetted, and repositioned around the painful area.
6. Treat the contralateral side: Many MET protocols suggest that the same treatment that was delivered to the injured extremity or injured side of the body be repeated on the noninjured side.

Probe Technique

1. Set the timer: If the MET generator has a PROBE setting, select this. Otherwise, each treatment bout should last approximately 10 seconds.
2. Select output channel: Only one channel is used during the probe technique.
3. Identify target treatment area: Localize the center of pain as accurately as possible. A grease pencil or dry-erase marker may be used to mark the area on the skin.
4. Position probe: The area surrounding the target tissues is treated in an "X" manner. For example, the first treatment bout may have one probe positioned in the upper left-hand quadrant and the opposite probe in the lower right-hand quadrant, relative to the mark identified in step 2. The next treatment bout would have the probes positioned in the upper right-hand and lower left-hand quadrant. The treatment progresses in this manner, with the probes being rotated around the target tissues in varying directions and distances, including anterior-posterior and medial-lateral placements.
5. Determine the number of bout sessions: Each bout in a single session persists for 10 seconds, and each session lasts approximately 2 minutes. Up to four sessions may be used during a single treatment.
6. Reevaluate the patient: The patient should be re-evaluated after each bout session, and treatment parameters adjusted accordingly.

● Chapter Highlights

- HVPS uses a monophasic current that is useful for sensory-level stimulation and producing moderate intensity muscle contractions.
- TENS delivers a balanced, asymmetrical biphasic current that is primarily used for sensory or motor-level pain control.
- IFS uses two ACs that are mixed within the body's tissues to produce a single treatment current. This current is used for pain control and for producing low to moderate intensity muscle contractions.
- Premodulated currents (Premod) are created by modifying an AC within the generator. This type of current is useful for producing strong muscle contractions.
- NMES uses a biphasic or monophasic current to produce high-intensity muscle contractions.
- Iontophoresis uses a direct current to introduce medications into the subcutaneous tissues.
- MET uses monophasic or biphasic currents in an attempt to restore the body's natural electrical balance. The efficacy of this technique has not been substantiated.

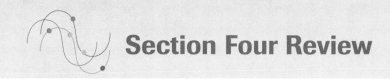

Section Four Review

Case Study: Chapter Case Study

Diana's symptoms began with a sharp, stabbing pain that radiated into her right ear from her mid trapezius/levator scapulae insertion 3 weeks ago. She attributes symptoms to computer use at work, because data entry has dramatically increased in the past 2 months. Her skin temperature is normal, and there is moderate spasm of the levator scapulae with a highly sensitive trigger point at the scapula insertion.

1. What is the best therapeutic modality to consider in this situation?

2. What are the physiological effects on the injury response cycle from the application of this thermal agent?

3. What are the clinical symptoms that you hope to address with this intervention?

Case Study: Continuation of Case Study from Section One

(The following discussion relates to Case Study 2, found on pages 93 through 96 of Section One.)

Based on this patient's condition, the availability of other modalities, and the lack of contraindications to the use of therapeutic modalities and therapeutic exercise, the most probable acute use of electrical stimulation would be that of pain control and trigger point therapy. However, the lack of access to electrotherapeutic modalities probably would not hinder this patient's progress. Other types of modalities could adequately address and resolve the patient's problems.

Pain Control

The problem of acute pain control has been addressed by the use of thermal agents, and the patient has received a prescription for muscle relaxants. If these approaches fail to reduce pain adequately, electrical stimulation could be incorporated into the program.

The acute nature of this injury, the lack of radicular symptoms, and the fact that the patient is taking medication for the pain would make sensory-level pain control an appropriate choice, especially if the patient's symptoms are alleviated during the application of heat and cold. In this case, the use of a portable TENS unit

should be considered and used as a part of the patient's home treatment program.

The electrodes would be positioned so that the current intersects over the primary area of pain. A short pulse duration, a high number of pulses per second, and a sensory-level intensity would be used. Because this unit would be used for long periods, its output must be modulated to help prevent accommodation. The patient would be instructed about how to connect and disconnect the unit, how to adjust the intensity, and if indicated, how to modify the pulse characteristics.

Trigger Point Therapy

If the patient's trigger points do not subside after the other treatment approaches, electrical stimulation could be used to target them. High-voltage pulsed stimulation, delivered with a probe, a Neuroprobe, brief-intense TENS, or noxious-level stimulation can be used to attempt to break down the trigger point. Interrupting the local pain-spasm-pain cycle, decreasing the pain response, or causing the trigger point's fibers to fatigue can bring about long-term relief. The electrodes could safely be worn under the patient's cervical collar.

● ● ● Section Four Quiz

1. Electrons travel from the _____ , which has a _____ of electrons, to the _____ , which has a _____ of electrons.
   A. Anode • high concentration • cathode • low concentration
   B. Anode • low concentration • cathode • high concentration
   C. Cathode • high concentration • anode • low concentration
   D. Cathode • low concentration • anode • high concentration

2. Monopolar stimulation involves the use of active and dispersive electrodes. The parameter that determines which electrode(s) will be active is:
   A. The POLARITY adjustment
   B. The average current
   C. The pulse duration
   D. The current density

3. What is the percent duty cycle for an electrical current that flows for 30 seconds and has no flow for 10 seconds?

A. 33 percent
B. 25 percent
C. 75 percent
D. 3:1

4. All of the following are excitable tissues except:
   A. Muscle fiber
   B. Meniscal cartilage
   C. Sensory nerves
   D. Secretory cells

5. Which of the following would be the modality of choice to cause physiochemical changes within the tissues?
   A. High-voltage pulsed stimulation
   B. Interferential stimulation
   C. Low-voltage alternating current
   D. Low-voltage direct current

6. Under normal circumstances, which of the following nerves would be the first to be stimulated by an electrical current?
   A. A superficial large-diameter nerve
   B. A deep large-diameter nerve
   C. A superficial small-diameter nerve
   D. A deep small-diameter nerve

7. Most tissues provide capacitive resistance to electrical current flow. Which of the following currents would meet the least amount of capacitive resistance?
   A. 1 Hz
   B. 10 Hz
   C. 50 Hz
   D. 100 Hz

8. An electrical stimulation protocol that uses a high pulse frequency (e.g., 120 pps), short pulse duration, and applied at the sensory level is thought to activate which pain control mechanism?
   A. Gate mechanism
   B. Endogenous opiate
   C. Central biasing
   D. Specificity

9. The electrodes from lead (A) have an area of 20 square inches and the electrodes originating from lead (B) have an area of 4 square inches. This type of stimulation would be classified as:
   A. Monopolar
   B. Bipolar
   C. Quadripolar
   D. Polypolar

10. You are setting up an electrical stimulation unit to control pain through the gate-control theory of pain modulation. The correct parameters for this are:
    A. High pulse rate, long pulse duration, short treatment duration, motor level stimulation
    B. Low pulse rate, short pulse duration, short treatment duration, sensory level stimulation
    C. High pulse rate, short pulse duration, long treatment duration, sensory level stimulation
    D. High pulse rate, moderate pulse duration, long treatment duration, noxious level stimulation

11. Iontophoresis is a technique that introduces medication into the tissues through the use of an electric current. For this method to work, the medication must:
    A. Have its outer valence shell filled
    B. Have a net ionic charge
    C. Be electrically neutral
    D. All are correct

12. Interferential stimulation is being applied with a carrier current of 4000 Hz and an interference current of 4130 Hz. The effective frequency of the current within the tissues would be:
    A. 8130 Hz
    B. 130 Hz
    C. 30 Hz
    D. None of these answers are correct

13. Which of the following conditions is a contraindication to the use of electrical stimulation?
    A. Post-traumatic pain
    B. Postsurgical pain
    C. Chronic pain
    D. Pain of unknown origin

14. A high-voltage pulsed stimulator uses what type of current?
    A. Monophasic
    B. Biphasic
    C. Polyphasic
    D. Direct

15. When attempting to reeducate the quadriceps muscle immediately postsurgery, a _____ percent duty cycle should be used.
    A. 20%
    B. 40%
    C. 60%
    D. 80%

16. In general, a tonic contraction occurs when the number of pulses per second exceeds:
    A. 1
    B. 30
    C. 60
    D. 90

17. "The uninterrupted, bidirectional flow of electrons" best describes which of the following types of currents:
    A. Monophasic
    B. Biphasic
    C. Alternating
    D. Direct

18. In an electrical current, electrical flow consists of the movement of electrons; in the body's tissues, therapeutic current flow consists of the flow of:
    A. Protons
    B. Coulombs
    C. Electrons
    D. Ions

19. A POLARITY switch would be found on which of the following modalities?
    A. High-voltage pulsed stimulator
    B. TENS unit
    C. Interferential stimulator
    D. Neuromuscular electrical nerve stimulator

20. Traumatized areas and stimulation points (e.g., motor points, trigger points) display a(n) _____ resistance to current flow.
    A. Increased
    B. Decreased

References

1. Kloth, LC and Cummings, JP: Electrotherapeutic Terminology in Physical Therapy. Section on Clinical Electrophysiology and the American Physical Therapy Association, Alexandria, VA, 1990.
2. Laufer, Y, et al: Quadriceps femoris muscle torques and fatigue generated by neuromuscular electrical stimulation with three different wave forms. Phys Ther 81:1307, 2001.
3. Lake, DA: Neuromuscular electrical stimulation: An overview and its application in the treatment of sports injuries. Sports Med 13:320, 1992.
4. Kantor, G, et al: The effects of selected stimulus waveforms on pulse and phase characteristics at sensory and motor thresholds. Phys Ther 74:951, 1994.
5. Cook, TM: Instrumentation. In Nelson, RM and Currier, DP (eds): Clinical Electrotherapy. Appleton & Lange, Norwalk, CT, 1987, pp 11–28.
6. Baker, LL: Neuromuscular electrical stimulation in the restoration of purposeful limb movements. In Wolf, SL (ed): Electrotherapy. Churchill Livingstone, New York, 1981, pp 25–48.
7. Urbschait, NL: Review of physiology. In Nelson, RM and Currier, DP (eds): Clinical Electrotherapy. Appleton & Lange, Norwalk, CT, 1987, pp 1–9.
8. Binder, SA: Application of low- and high-voltage electrotherapeutic currents. In Wolf, SL (ed): Electrotherapy. Churchill Livingstone, New York, 1981, pp 1–24.
9. DeVahl, J: Neuromuscular electrical stimulation (NMES) in rehabilitation. In Gersh, MR (ed): Electrotherapy in Rehabilitation. FA Davis, Philadelphia, 1992, pp 218–268.
10. Walsh, DM: TENS: Clinical Application and Related Theory. New York, Churchill Livingstone, 1997.
11. Nolan, MF: Conductive differences in electrodes used with transcutaneous electrical nerve stimulation devices. Phys Ther 71:746, 1991.
12. Lieber, RL and Kelly, MJ: Factors influencing quadriceps femoris muscle torque using transcutaneous neuromuscular stimulation. Phys Ther 71:715, 1991.
13. Alon, G, et al: Effects of electrode size on basic excitatory responses on selected stimulus parameters. J Orthop Sports Phys Ther 20:29, 1994.
14. Ottoson, D and Lundeberg, T: Pain Treatment by Transcutaneous Electrical Nerve Stimulation: A Practical Manual. Springer-Verlag, New York, 1988.
15. Denegar, CR and Huff, CB: High and low frequency TENS in the treatment of induced musculoskeletal pain: A comparison study. Athletic Training 23:235, 1988.
16. Berlant, SR: Method of determining optimal stimulation sites for transcutaneous electrical nerve stimulation. Phys Ther 64:924, 1984.
17. Davson, H: A Textbook of General Physiology, vol 2, ed 4. Williams & Wilkins, Baltimore, 1970.
18. Griffin, JE and Karselis, TC: Physical Agents for Physical Therapists, ed 2. Charles C Thomas, Springfield, IL, 1988.
19. Baker, LL, et al: Effects of wave form on comfort during neuromuscular electrical stimulation. Clin Orthop 223:75, 1988.
20. Balogun, JA, et al: High voltage electrical stimulation in the augmentation of muscle strength: Effects of pulse frequency. Arch Phys Med Rehabil 74:910, 1993.
21. Harris, PR: Iontophoresis: Clinical research in musculoskeletal inflammatory conditions. J Orthop Sports Phys Ther 4:109, 1982.
22. De Domenico, G: Interferential Stimulation (monograph). Chattanooga Group, Chattanooga, TN, 1988.
23. Trimble, MH and Enoka, RM: Mechanisms underlying the training effects associated with neuromuscular electrical stimulation. Phys Ther 71:273, 1991.
24. Ferguson, JP, et al: Effects of varying electrode site placements on the torque output of an electrically stimulated involuntary quadriceps femoris muscle contraction. J Orthop Sports Phys Ther 11:24, 1989.
25. Delitto, A and Rose, SJ: Comparative comfort of three wave forms used in electrically eliciting quadriceps femoris muscle contractions. Phys Ther 66:1704, 1986.
26. Holcomb, WR, et al: A comparison of knee-extension torque production with biphasic versus Russian current. J Sports Rehabil 9:229, 2000.
27. McLoda, TA and Carmack, JA: Optimal burst duration during a facilitated quadriceps femoris contraction. J Athletic Training 35:145, 2000.
28. Miller, CR and Webers, RL: The effects of ice massage on an individual's pain tolerance level to electrical stimulation. J Orthop Sports Phys Ther 12:105, 1990.
29. Durst, JW, et al: Effects of ice and recovery time on maximal involuntary isometric torque production using electrical stimulation. J Orthop Sports Phys Ther 13:240, 1991.
30. Belanger, AY, et al: Cutaneous versus muscular perception of electrically evoked tetanic pain. J Orthop Sports Phys Ther 16:162, 1992.
31. Bowman, BR and Baker, LL: Effects of wave form parameters on comfort during transcutaneous neuromuscular electrical stimulation. Ann Biomed Eng 13:59, 1985.

32. Holcomb, WR: A practical guide to electrotherapy. J Sports Rehabil 6:272, 1997.

33. Parker, MG, et al: Fatigue response in human quadriceps femoris muscle during high frequency electrical stimulation. J Orthop Sports Phys Ther 7:145, 1986.

34. Holcomb, WR and Kleiner, DM: Versatile electrotherapy with the high-voltage pulsed stimulator. Athletic Therapy Today, November:37, 1998.

35. Jensen JE: Stress fracture in the world class athlete: A case study. Med Sci Sports Exercise 30:783, 1998.

36. Draper, U and Ballard, L: Electrical stimulation versus electromyographic biofeedback in the recovery of quadriceps femoris muscle function following anterior cruciate ligament surgery. Phys Ther 71:455, 1991.

37. Currier, DP and Mann, R: Muscular strength development by electrical stimulation in healthy individuals. Phys Ther 63:915, 1983.

38. Delitto, A and Snyder-Mackler, L: Two theories of muscle strength augmentation using percutaneous electrical stimulation. Phys Ther 70:158, 1990.

39. Miller, C and Thepaut-Mathieu, C: Strength training by electrostimulation conditions for efficacy. Int J Sports Med 14:20, 1993.

40. Sinacore, DR, et al: Type II fiber activation with electrical stimulation: A preliminary report. Phys Ther 70:416, 1990.

41. Schmitz, RJ, et al: Effect of interferential current on perceived pain and serum cortisol associated with delayed onset muscle soreness. J Sports Rehab 6:30, 1997.

42. Garrison, DW and Foreman, RD: Decreased activity of spontaneous and noxiously evoked dorsal horn cells during transcutaneous electrical nerve stimulation (TENS). Pain 58:309, 1994.

43. Cox, PD, et al: Effect of different TENS stimulus parameters on ulnar motor nerve conduction velocity. Am J Phys Med Rehabil 72:294, 1993.

44. Taylor, K, et al: Effects of interferential current stimulation for treatment of subjects with recurrent jaw pain. Phys Ther 67:346, 1987.

45. Longobardi, AG, et al: Effects of auricular transcutaneous electrical nerve stimulation on distal extremity pain. Phys Ther 69:10, 1989.

46. Jensen, JE, et al: The use of transcutaneous neural stimulation and isokinetic testing in arthroscopic knee surgery. Am J Sports Med 13:27, 1985.

47. Lewers, D, et al: Transcutaneous electrical nerve stimulation in the relief of primary dysmenorrhea. Phys Ther 69:3, 1989.

48. Gersh, MR: Transcutaneous electrical nerve stimulation (TENS) for management of pain and sensory pathology. In Gersh, MR (ed): Electrotherapy in Rehabilitation. FA Davis, Philadelphia, 1992, pp 149–196.

49. French, S: Pain: Some psychological and sociological aspects. Physiotherapy 75:255, 1989.

50. Miller, BF; et al: Circulatory responses to voluntary and electrically induced muscle contractions in humans. Phys Ther 80:53, 2000.

51. Carley, PJ and Wainapel, SF: Electrotherapy for acceleration of wound healing: Low intensity direct current. Arch Phys Med Rehabil 66:443, 1985.

52. Feedar, JA, et al: Chronic dermal ulcer healing enhanced with monophasic pulsed electrical stimulation. Phys Ther 71:639, 1991.

53. Snyder-Mackler, L: Electrical stimulation for tissue repair. In: Snyder-Mackler, L and Robinson, AJ (eds): Clinical Electrophysiology: Electrotherapy and Electrophysiologic Testing. Williams & Wilkins, Baltimore, 1989, pp 229–244.

54. Kloth, LC and Feedar, JA: Electrical stimulation in tissue repair. In Kloth, LC, et al (eds): Wound Healing:

Alternatives in Management. FA Davis, Philadelphia, 1990, pp 221–258.

55. Newton, R: High-voltage pulsed galvanic stimulation: Theoretical bases and clinical application. In Nelson, RM and Currier, DP (eds): Clinical Electrotherapy. Appleton & Lange, Norwalk, CT, 1987, pp 165–182.

56. Hart, FX: Changes in the electric field at an injury site during healing under electrical stimulation. J Bioelectricity 10:33, 1991.

57. Kloth, LC: Physical modalities in wound management: UVC, therapeutic heating and electrical stimulation. Ostomy Wound Management 41:18, 1995.

58. Falanga, V, et al: Electrical stimulation increases the expression of fibroblast receptors for transforming growth factor-beta (abstract). J Invest Dermatol 88:488, 1987.

59. Gentzkow, GD: Electrical stimulation to heal dermal wounds. J Dermatol Surg Oncol 19:753, 1993.

60. Reich, JD, et al: The effect of electrical stimulation on the number of mast cells in healing wounds. J Am Acad Dermatol 25:40, 1991.

61. Szuminsky, NJ, et al: Effect of narrow, pulsed high voltages on bacterial viability. Phys Ther 74:660, 1994.

62. Litke, DS and Dahners, LE: Effects of different levels of direct current on early ligament healing in a rat model. J Orthop Res 12:683, 1994.

63. Fujita, M, et al: The effect of constant direct electrical current on intrinsic healing in the flexor tendon in vitro: An ultrastructural study of differing attitudes in epitendon cells and tenocytes. J Hand Surg [Br]17:94, 1992.

64. Bettany, JA, et al: Influence of high voltage pulsed direct current on edema formation following impact injury. Phys Ther 70:219, 1990.

65. Mendel, FC and Fish, DR: New perspectives in edema control via electrical stimulation. J Athletic Training 28:1, 1993.

66. Chakkalaka, DA, et al: Electrophysiology of direct current stimulation of fracture healing in canine radius. IEEE Trans Biomed Eng 37:1048, 1990.

67. Lilly-Masuda, D and Towne, S: Bioelectricity and bone healing. J Orthop Sports Phys Ther 7:54, 1985.

68. McLeod, KJ and Rubin, CT: The effect of low-frequency electrical fields on osteogenesis. J Bone Joint Surg [Am] 74:920, 1992.

69. Nash, HL and Rogers, CC: Does electricity speed the healing of non-union fractures? Physician and Sportsmedicine 16:156, 1988.

70. Stanish, WD, et al: The use of electricity in ligament and tendon repair. Phys Sports Med 13:110, 1985.

71. Pepper, JR, et al: Effect of capacitive coupled electrical stimulation on regenerate bone. J Orthop Res 14:296, 1996.

72. Robinson, AJ: Transcutaneous electrical nerve stimulation for the control of pain in musculoskeletal disorders. J Orthop Sports Phys Ther 24:208, 1996.

73. Denegar, CR, et al: Influence of transcutaneous electrical nerve stimulation on pain, range of motion, and serum cortisol concentration in females experiencing delayed onset muscle soreness. J Orthop Sports Phys Ther 11:100, 1989.

74. Mohr, T, et al: The effect of high volt galvanic stimulation on quadriceps femoris muscle torque. J Orthop Sports Phys Ther 7:314, 1986.

75. Boutelle, D, et al: A strength study utilizing the Electro-Stim 180. J Orthop Sports Phys Ther 7:50, 1985.

76. Jette, DU: Effect of different forms of transcutaneous electrical nerve stimulation on experimental pain. Phys Ther 66:187, 1986.

77. Angulo, DL and Colwell, CW: Use of postoperative TENS and continuous passive motion following total knee replacement. J Orthop Sports Phys Ther 11:599, 1990.

78. Fish, DR, et al: Effect of anodal high voltage pulsed current on edema formation in frog hind limbs. Phys Ther 71:724, 1991.
79. Cosgrove, KA, et al: The electrical effect of two commonly used clinical stimulators on traumatic edema in rats. Phys Ther 73:227, 1992.
80. Ralston, DJ: High voltage galvanic stimulation: Can there be a "state of the art?" Athletic Training 20:291, 1985.
81. Newton, RA and Karselis, TC: Skin pH following high voltage pulsed galvanic stimulation. Phys Ther 63:1593, 1983.
82. Mohr, T, et al: Comparison of isometric exercise and high volt galvanic stimulation on quadriceps femoris muscle strength. J Orthop Sports Phys Ther 65:606, 1985.
83. Wolcot, C, et al: A comparison of the effects of high volt and microcurrent stimulation on delayed onset muscle soreness. Phys Ther 71:S117, 1991.
84. Butterfield, DL, et al: The effects of high-volt pulsed current electrical stimulation on delayed-onset muscle soreness. Journal of Athletic Training 32:15, 1997.
85. Reed, BV: Effect of high voltage pulsed electrical stimulation on microvascular permeability to plasma proteins: A possible mechanism in minimizing edema. Phys Ther 68:481, 1988.
86. Taylor, K, et al: Effect of electrically induced muscle contractions on posttraumatic edema formation in frog hind limbs. Phys Ther 72:127, 1992.
87. Mohr, TM, et al: Effect of high voltage stimulation on edema reduction in the rat hind limb. Phys Ther 67:1703, 1987.
88. Taylor, K, et al: Effect of a single 30-minute treatment of high voltage pulsed current on edema formation in frog hind limbs. Phys Ther 72:63, 1992.
89. Michlovitz, S, et al: Ice and high voltage pulsed stimulation in treatment of lateral ankle sprains. J Orthop Sports Phys Ther 9:301, 1988.
90. Griffin, JW, et al: Reduction of chronic posttraumatic hand edema: A comparison of high voltage pulsed current, intermittent pneumatic compression, and placebo treatments. Phys Ther 70:279, 1990.
91. Cook, HA, et al: Effects of electrical stimulation on lymphatic flow and limb volume in the rat. Phys Ther, 74:1040, 1994.
92. Walker, DC, et al: Effects of high voltage pulsed electrical stimulation on blood flow. Phys Ther 68:481, 1988.
93. Heath, ME and Gibbs, SB: High-voltage pulsed stimulation: Effects of frequency of current on blood flow in the human calf. Clin Sci (Colch) 82:607, 1992.
95. Tracy, JE, et al: Comparison of selected pulse frequencies from different electrical stimulators on blood flow in healthy subjects. Phys Ther 68:1526, 1988.
96. Agren, MS, et al: Collagenase during burn wound healing: Influence of a hydrogel dressing and pulsed electrical stimulation. Plast Reconstr Surg 94:518, 1994.
97. Kincaid, CB and Lavoie, KH: Inhibition of bacterial growth in vitro following stimulation with high voltage, monophasic, pulsed current. Phys Ther 69:651, 1989.
98. Fitzgerald, GK and Newsome, D: Treatment of a large infected thoracic spine wound using high voltage pulsed monophasic current. Phys Ther 73:355, 1993.
99. Roeser, WM, et al: The use of transcutaneous nerve stimulation for pain control in athletic medicine. A preliminary report. Am J Sports Med 4:210, 1976.
100. Walsh, DM, et al: Transcutaneous electrical nerve stimulation: Relevance of stimulation parameters to neurophysiological and hypoalgesic effects. Am J Phys Med Rehabil 74:199, 1995.
101. Barr, JO, et al: Transcutaneous electrical nerve stimulation characteristics for altering pain perception. Phys Ther 66:1515, 1986.
102. Indergand, HJ and Morgan, BJ: Effects of high-frequency transcutaneous electrical nerve stimulation on limb blood flow in healthy humans. Phys Ther 74:361, 1994.
103. Walsh, DM, et al: A double-blind investigation of the hypoalgesic effects of transcutaneous electrical nerve stimulation upon experimentally induced ischaemic pain. Pain 61:39, 1995.
104. Widerström, EG, et al: Relations between experimentally induced tooth pain threshold changes, psychometrics and clinical pain relief following TENS. A retrospective study in patients with long-lasting pain. Pain 51:281, 1992.
105. Marchand, S, et al: Letter to the Editor: Effects of caffeine on analgesia from transcutaneous electrical nerve stimulation. N Engl J Med 333:325, 1995.
106. Levin, MF and Hui-Chan, CWY: Conventional and acupuncture-like transcutaneous electrical nerve stimulation excite similar afferent nerves. Arch Phys Med Rehabil 74:54, 1993.
107. Buxton, BP, et al: Self selection of transcutaneous electrical nerve stimulation (TENS) parameters for pain relief in injured athletes (Abstract). Journal of Athletic Training 29:178, 1994.
108. Tulgar, M, et al: Comparative effectiveness of different stimulation modes in relieving pain. I. A pilot study. Pain 47:151, 1991.
109. Tulgar, M, et al: Comparative effectiveness of different stimulation modes in relieving pain. II. A double-blind controlled long-term study. Pain 47:157, 1991.
110. Reib, L and Pomeranz, B: Alterations in electrical pain thresholds by use of acupuncture-like transcutaneous electrical nerve stimulation in pain-free subjects. Phys Ther 72:658, 1992.
111. Bechtel, TB and Fan, PT: When is TENS effective and practical for pain relief? Journal of Musculoskeletal Medicine 2:37, 1985.
112. Gersh, MR and Wolf, SL: Applications of transcutaneous electrical nerve stimulation in the management of patients with pain. Phys Ther 65:314, 1985.
113. Somers, DL and Somers, MF: Treatment of neuropathic pain in a patient with diabetic neuropathy using transcutaneous electrical nerve stimulation applied to the skin of the lumbar region. Phys Ther 79:767, 1999.
114. Sung, P: The effect of Genesen® point stimulator the median nerve conduction velocity (abstract). Phys Ther 81:A5, 2001.
115. Paris, DL, et al: Effects of the neuroprobe in the treatment of second-degree ankle sprains. Phys Ther 63:35, 1983.
116. Snyder-Mackler, L: Electrical stimulation for pain modulation. In Snyder-Mackler, L and Robinson, AJ (eds): Clinical Electrophysiology: Electrotherapy and Electrophysiologic Testing. Williams & Wilkins, Baltimore, 1994, pp 205–227.
117. Kloth, LC: Electrotherapeutic alternatives for the treatment of pain. In Gersh, MR (ed): Electrotherapy in Rehabilitation. FA Davis, Philadelphia, 1992, pp 197–217.
118. Chen, XH, et al: Electrical stimulation at traditional acupuncture sites in periphery produces brain opioid-receptor-mediated antinociception in rats. J Pharmacol Exp Ther 227:654, 1996.
119. Nussbaum, E, Rush, P, and Disenhaus, L: The effects of interferential therapy on peripheral blood flow. Physiotherapy 76:803, 1990.
120. Kramer, JF: Effect of electrical stimulation frequencies on isometric knee extension torque. Phys Ther 67:31, 1987.
121. Hobler, CK: Case study: Reduction of chronic posttraumatic knee edema using interferential stimulation. Athletic Training 26:364, 1991.
122. Selkowitz, DM: Improvement in isometric strength of the

quadriceps femoris muscle after training with electrical stimulation. Phys Ther 65:186, 1988.

123. Laughman, RK, et al: Strength changes in the normal quadriceps femoris muscle group as a result of electrical stimulation. Phys Ther 63:494, 1983.

124. Snyder-Mackler, L, et al: Strength of the quadriceps femoris muscle and functional recovery after reconstruction of the anterior cruciate ligament: A prospective, randomized clinical trial of electrical stimulation. J Bone Joint Surg Am 77:1166, 1995.

125. Currier, DP, et al: Effect of graded electrical stimulation on blood flow to healthy muscle. Phys Ther 66:937, 1986.

126. Liu, H, et al: Circulatory response of digital arteries associated with electrical stimulation of calf muscle in healthy subjects. Phys Ther 67:340, 1987.

127. Selkowitz, DM: High frequency electrical stimulation in muscle strengthening: A review and discussion. Am J Sports Med 17:103, 1989.

128. Hasson, SH, et al: Exercise training and dexamethasone iontophoresis in rheumatoid arthritis: A case study. Physiotherapy Canada 43:11, 1991.

129. Glass, JM, et al: The quantity and distribution of radiolabeled dexamethasone delivered to tissue by iontophoresis. Int J Dermatol 19:519, 1980.

130. Henley, EJ: Transcutaneous drug delivery: Iontophoresis, phonophoresis. Physical and Rehabilitation Medicine 2:139, 1991.

131. Gundeman, SD, et al: Treatment of plantar fasciitis by iontophoresis of 0.4% Dexamethasone: A randomized, double blind, placebo controlled study. Am J Sports Med 25:312, 1997.

132. Zeltzer, L, et al: Iontophoresis versus subcutaneous injection: A comparison of two methods of local anesthesia delivery in children. Pain 44:73, 1991.

133. Nimmo, WS: Novel delivery systems: Electrotransport. J Pain Symptom Manage 8:160, 1992.

134. Bertolucci, LE: Introduction of antiinflammatory drugs by iontophoresis: A double blind study. J Orthop Sport Phys Ther 4:103, 1982.

135. Scott, ER, et al: Transport of ionic species in skin: Contribution of pores to the overall skin conductance. Pharmacol Res 10:1699, 1993.

136. Bogner, RB and Ajay, KM: Iontophoresis and phonophoresis. US Pharmacist, August, 1994, p H-10.

137. Kalia, YN and Guy, RH: The electrical characteristics of human skin in vivo. Pharmacol Res 12:1605, 1995.

138. Pikal, MJ and Shah, S: Transport mechanisms in iontophoresis. II. Electroosmotic flow and the transference number measurements for hairless mouse skin. Pharmacol Res 7:213, 1990.

139. Inada, H, et al: Studies on the effects of applied voltage and duration on the human epidural membrane alteration/recovery and the resultant effects upon iontophoresis. Pharmacol Res 11:687, 1994.

140. Grossmann, M, et al: The effect of iontophoresis on the cutaneous vasculature: Evidence for current-induced hyperemia. Microvasc Res 50:444, 1995.

141. Howard, JP, et al: Effects of alternating current iontophoresis on drug delivery. Arch Phys Med Rehabil 76:463, 1995.

142. Reinauer, S, et al: Iontophoresis with alternating current and direct current offset (AC/DC iontophoresis): A new approach for the treatment of hyperhydrosis. Br J Dermatol 129:166, 1993.

143. Evans, TA, et al: The immediate effects of lidocaine iontophoresis on trigger-point pain. J Sports Rehabil 10:287, 2001.

144. Nowicki, KD, et al: Effects of iontophoretic versus injection administration of dexamethasone. Med Sci Sports Exerc 34:1294, 2002.

145. Oshima, T, et al: Cutaneous iontophoresis application of condensed lidocaine. Can J Anaesth 41:667, 1994.

146. Guffey, JS, et al: Skin pH changes associated with iontophoresis. J Orthop Phys Ther 29:656, 1999.

147. Wieder, DL: Treatment of traumatic myositis ossificans with acetic acid iontophoresis. Phys Ther 72:133, 1992.

148. Alon, G: "Microcurrent": Subliminal electric stimulation. Does the research support its clinical use? Sports Med Update 9:8, 1993.

149. Bertolucci, LE and Grey, T: Clinical comparative study of microcurrent electrical stimulation to mid-laser and placebo treatment in degenerative joint disease of the temporomandibular joint. Craniology 13:116, 1995.

150. Lerner, FN and Kirsch, DL: A double-blind comparative study of microstimulation and placebo effect in short-term treatment of chronic back patients. Journal of the American Chiropractic Association 15:S101, 1981.

151. Bach, S, et al: The effect of electrical current on healing skin incision. An experimental study. Eur J Surg 157:171, 1991.

152. Denegar, CR, et al: The effects of low-volt microamperage on delayed onset muscle soreness. J Sport Rehab 1:95, 1992.

153. Byl, NN, et al: Pulsed microamperage stimulation: A controlled study of healing of surgically induced wounds in Yucatan pigs. Phys Ther 74:201, 1994.

154. Leffmann, DL, et al: The effect of subliminal transcutaneous electrical nerve stimulation of the rate of wound healing in rats. Phys Ther 74:195, 1994.

155. Sinnreich, MJ, et al: Microcurrent electrical nerve stimulation (MENS) and coracoacromial arch pain: The effects after one treatment. Phys Ther 72:S68, 1992.

156. Ray, R, et al: Microcurrent therapy versus a placebo for the control of symptoms in mild and moderate acute ankle sprains. Unpublished manuscript, 1996.

157. Weber, MD, et al: The effects of three modalities on delayed onset muscle soreness. J Orthop Sports Phys Ther 20:236, 1994.

158. Allen, JD, et al: Effect of microcurrent stimulation on delayed-onset muscle soreness: A double-blind comparison. Journal of Athletic Training 34:334, 1999.

159. Becker, RO: The Body Electric. William Morrow, New York, 1985.

160. Becker, RO: Electrical control systems and regenerative growth. Journal of Bioelectricity 1:239, 1982.

161. Windsor, RE, et al: Electrical stimulation in clinical practice. Physician and Sportsmedicine 21:85, 1993.

162. Cheng, N, et al: The effects of electric currents on ATP generation, protein synthesis, and membrane transport in rat skin. Clin Orthop 171:264, 1982.

163. Stromberg, BV: Effects of electrical currents on wound contraction. Ann Plast Surg 21:121, 1988.

164. Swadlow, HA: Monitoring the excitability of neocortical efferent neurons to direct activation by extracellular current pulses. J Neurophysiol 68:605, 1992.

165. Pubols, LM: Characteristics of dorsal horn neurons expressing subliminal responses to sural nerve stimulation. Somatosens Mot Res 7:137, 1990.

166. Rapaski, D, et al: Microcurrent electrical stimulation: A comparison of two protocols in reducing delayed onset muscle soreness. Phys Ther 71S:116, 1991.

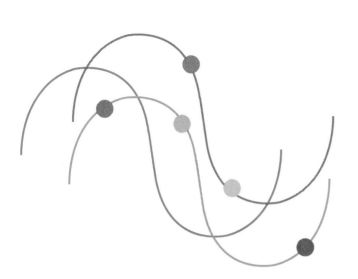

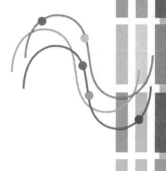

Mechanical and Light Modalities

This section presents the therapeutic agents that rely primarily on mechanical force and on chemical and/or bioelectrical properties to affect the injury response process.

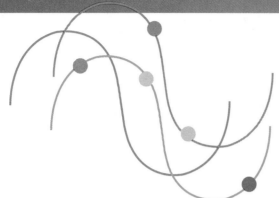

Chapter 14

Intermittent Compression

Intermittent compression units assist in venous and lymphatic drainage by creating a pressure gradient that forces edema out of the extremity through the venous and lymphatic systems. The appliance may be filled with air (pneumatic compression) or chilled water (cryocompression) and may inflate as a single unit or sequentially. The ON/OFF duty cycle assists in milking or pumping edema out of the extremity.

Intermittent compression units use mechanical pressure to encourage venous and lymphatic return from the extremities. Compression units consist of a nylon **appliance** designed to fit the body part (e.g., foot and/or ankle, half leg, full leg) that is connected to the unit through a series of hoses. The compression is then formed by the flow of air or cold water into the appliance.

The compression applied to the extremity is either circumferential or sequential. Circumferential compression applies an equal amount of pressure to all parts of the extremity simultaneously. The pressure is gradually increased to a level determined by the operator and held for a preset time during the ON cycle. The pressure then drops during the OFF cycle. The process then repeats.

Through this cycle, fluids are forced toward the torso through the venous and lymphatic return systems. Sequential compression increases the distal-to-proximal gradient through the sequential filling of pressure chambers within the appliance. The most distal compartment inflates, followed by the next compartment, and so on, until pressure is applied to the length of the appliance (Fig. 14–1).

Compression devices work on two principles. The mechanical pressure forces fluids within the venous system back toward the heart. When the edema is confined to a local area, a limited number of ducts are capable of reabsorbing the solid matter. Lymphatic uptake and return is assisted by spreading the edema over a larger area (usually proximally), allowing more lymphatic ducts to absorb the solid matter within the edema.

Intermittent cold compression units are used to treat acute injuries because of their ease of use and their ability to provide cold and compression while the limb is elevated (ice, compression, and elevation) (Fig. 14–2). Circumferential compression units may also be used immediately between ice bouts to prevent the formation of edema. However, compression units should not be used until the possibility of a fracture or compartment syndrome has been ruled out. In subacute or chronic conditions, intermittent compression is used to reduce edema and decrease ecchymosis from the area.

Controlled cold therapy units, described in Chapter 6, deliver continuous compression and are useful in preventing edema. Intermittent compression units are used to remove edema that has already accumulated.

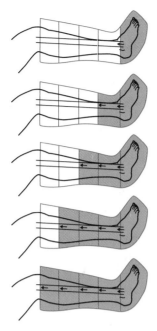

Figure 14-1. Sequential Compression. Compartments within the appliance fill distal to proximal, forcing the fluids toward the torso. Following the cycle, all the compartments deflate and the process repeats.

● EFFECTS ON
The Injury Response Process

The movement of fluids out of the extremity is caused by the formation of a number of pressure gradients. When external compression is applied, the gradient between the tissue hydrostatic pressure and the capillary filtration pressure is reduced, thus encouraging the reabsorption of interstitial fluids. Because the tissues are being compressed, a second pressure gradient is formed between the distal portion of the extremity (high pressure) and the proximal portion (low pressure), forcing the fluids to move from the high-pressure area to a lower pressure area. If the extremity is elevated during this treatment, both of these pressures are enhanced by gravity, speeding venous drainage. Spreading the solid edematous matter over a larger area allows more lymphatic ducts to absorb the wastes.

During the compression sequence, blood flow to the treated area is decreased because of the external pressure on the extremity. The OFF time allows the venous and lymph vessels to re-load, absorbing fluids and proteins from the tissues.

Although deep vein thrombosis (DVT) is a contraindication to intermittent compression, its use can prevent the onset of DVT. The increased venous flow helps prevent the accumulation of the substances that can lead to the formation of a thrombus.

Edema

Both circumferential and sequential compression units can significantly reduce the amount of edema in an injured body part. During the treatment of lower leg edema, low pressure (35 to 55 mm Hg) increases the venous flow velocity 175 percent. When this pressure is increased to the range of 90 to 100 mm Hg, the venous flow accelerates to 336 percent of resting values.[1] Because extracellular debris is removed, the fresh blood flow to the area significantly increases following the treatment.[2]

Intermittent compression may be more effective in reducing fluid-rich post-traumatic edema than lymphedema. Reduced limb volume following intermittent compression may be the result of forcing fluids (water) through the venous system. Movement of protein molecules through the lymphatic system does not appear to be increased by intermittent compression. In this case, intermittent compression may limit the formation of edema by decreasing the blood capillary filtration pressure.[3] A study of post-acute ankle sprains that displayed **pitting edema** ■ found not only that simple elevation was more effective in reducing edema than intermittent compression and elastic wraps but also that the last two techniques actually increased the amount of edema.[4]

Intermittent compression is also sometimes applied concurrently with an electrical stimulation muscle milking protocol (see Treatment Strategies: Motor-Level Reduction of Edema Using High-Voltage Pulsed

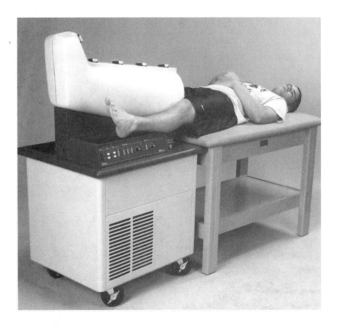

Figure 14-2. Sequential Cold Compression Unit. This device allows for simultaneous sequential cold compression and elevation. (The CRYO*Press*. Courtesy of Grimm Scientific Industries, Inc., Marietta, OH.)

Pitting edema: An exudate-rich form of edema characterized by being easily indented by pressure (hence, "pitting").

Stimulation, p 247). This approach is thought to combine the benefits of both edema reduction techniques into a single treatment session (Fig. 14–3). The effectiveness of this treatment has not been substantiated.

The foot appears to rely on a mechanism other than muscle contractions or range of motion to initiate venous return. The venous foot pump is activated by pressure applied to the plantar aspect of the foot from the calcaneus to the metatarsal heads. This pressure, normally seen during weight bearing, decreases the long and transverse arches of the foot, stretching the veins and causing them to empty.[5] This implies that traditional compression techniques may not be successful for reducing foot edema. In this case, compression would need to be placed on the plantar aspect of the foot through weight bearing or simulated weight bearing by applying pressure to the plantar aspect of the foot.

To reduce the reaccumulation of edema, the extremity should be wrapped with a compression bandage and elevated following treatment. To monitor the effectiveness of intermittent compression on edema reduction, pretreatment and post-treatment limb volume measurements should be taken. Once the edema is sufficiently reduced— and the patient's pathology permits—an active exercise regimen should be implemented.

Range of Motion

Synovial joints such as the knee, interphalangeal joints of the fingers and toes, and the elbow contain synovial fluid that is housed within a relatively dense joint capsule. This fluid must be able to move within the capsule for normal joint motion to occur and moving from extension into flexion increases the amount of pressure within the joint.

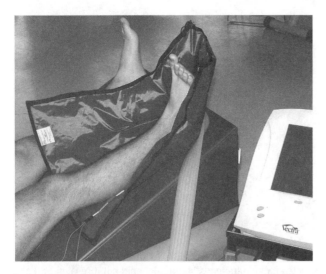

Figure 14-3. **Combination of Electrical Stimulation and Compression.** The electrodes (not visible) are positioned over the calf muscle. The motor-level edema reduction protocol is described on p 247.

Synovitis: Inflammation of the synovial membrane.

When excess fluids form within a joint either as edema or **synovitis ∎**, motion is limited because there is little if any room left within the joint capsule in which to displace the fluid. Excess fluids can trigger arthrogenic muscle inhibition (AMI), an inhibitory reflex that prevents active joint motion (see Chapter 1, p 24).[6, 7] Reducing the joint volume assists in decreasing AMI and restoring normal active range of motion by reducing the hydraulic resistance to motion.[6, 8]

Pain

Pain reduction is achieved by reducing the mechanical pressure caused by the edema and by restoring normal joint range of motion and function. Decreasing vascular clogging helps to restore normal arterial and vascular function. The subsequent increased arterial supply reduces ischemic pain by increasing the rate of delivery of oxygen and nutrients to the tissues.

∎ Contraindications

The primary contraindications to the use of intermittent compression are associated with the pressure applied to the extremity (see At a Glance: Intermittent Compression, p 284). The patient's arterial blood supply, including heart rate, blood pressure, and vessel continuity must be sufficient to deliver oxygenated blood to the extremity. Compression units are also contraindicated in compartment syndromes, such as anterior compartment syndrome, in which the intracompartment pressure hinders normal blood perfusion. Other vascular insufficiencies such as gangrene, peripheral vascular disease, ischemic vascular disease, and arteriosclerosis are generally considered to be contraindications to treatment. On the physician's consent, patients with mild vascular insufficiency may be treated with reduced pressures and/or shortened ON times.

A bit of a paradox exists regarding DVT. Intermittent compression increases venous blood flow, thus helping to remove stagnant debris, thus decreasing the risk of a thrombus forming. However, because of the potential of dislodging a clot that has formed, patients suffering from DVT or thrombophlebitis should not be treated with intermittent compression.

Congestive heart failure is a contraindication to the use of compression devices. The increased pressure on the vasculature may further damage the cardiovascular system or lead to decreased cardiac output. Patients suffering from congestive heart failure may experience increased sodium and water retention following compression therapy, both of which can increase bilateral peripheral edema. Pulmonary edema is aggravated by compression therapy because of the added load on the cardiorespiratory system similar to that described for congestive heart failure.

Insufficiency of valves within the venous network can result in edema being forced distally into the extremity. Because these valves do not adequately close, the pressure from the compression appliance will force fluids both proximally and distally within the extremity (Fig 14–4). In the presence of known venous insufficiency, a full-extremity appliance should be used that maintains a distal to proximal pressure gradient.

The effects of intermittent compression on the reduction of lymphedema have not been conclusively substantiated. However, the treatment of lymphedema can result in edema proximal to the treatment site and the treatment of lower extremity lymphedema with intermittent compression can cause genital edema.[9]

Unhealed fractures, unresolved joint dislocations, or other musculoskeletal instability in the anteroposterior plane are contraindications to the use of compression devices over the involved joint. As the appliance inflates, it will attempt to move the joint into extension and place unwanted stresses on the structures in the area.

■ Controversies in Treatment

The efficacy of intermittent compression for increasing venous flow is widely accepted, but the effect of intermittent compression on lymphedema is not substantiated. Conclusive evidence does not exist that intermittent compression is more effective than a compression wrap and elevation for reducing protein-rich pitting edema[4] but evidence does support that compression units, elevation, and cold reduce edema more than cryotherapy alone.[5]

No published research has conclusively determined the optimal treatment duration and duty cycles for reducing venous flow or lymphedema.

■ Clinical Application of Intermittent Compression

The instrumentation, setup, and application of circumferential and sequential intermittent compression units are similar. Before using an intermittent compression unit, refer to the manufacturer's documentation and protocol for the exact procedures for the model being used.

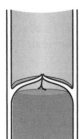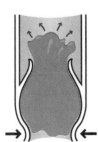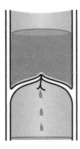

Figure 14-4. **Venous Insufficiency.** The one-way valves do not completely close, allowing venous blood to back fill and collect in the distal extremity, often resulting in swelling of the distal joints.

■ Instrumentation

Refer to the operator's guide for the unit you are using.

Power: Turns the unit on or off.

Temperature: With cold compression units, regulates the temperature of the fluid flowing through a refrigeration device to the appliance. Some portable cold compression units use ice cubes for this purpose. The temperature of the fluid is displayed in the TEMPERATURE GAUGE.

Pressure: Adjusts the amount of compression in millimeters of mercury (mm Hg) applied to the extremity. This value should not exceed the patient's diastolic blood pressure.

On-off time: Controls the proportion of the time that the compression is on and off. This control may be a single switch with selectable duty cycles, or the ON (inflation time) and OFF (deflation time) times may be adjusted separately.

Pump: Turns on the pressure to the appliance.

Drain: Removes the pressure and deflates the appliance.

■ Set-up and Application

Intermittent compression devices should not be used in the presence of flammable gases such as anesthetics or oxygen.

Preparation for the Treatment

1. Establish the absence of contraindications.
2. Remove any jewelry on the patient's extremity being treated.
3. Determine the patient's diastolic blood pressure.
4. To evaluate the effectiveness of the treatment, mark one or more areas on the extremity, measure, and record the girth measurement of the body part being treated.
5. For sanitary purposes, cover the area to be treated with Stockinette or similar material. Care must be taken to ensure that this inner layer is free of wrinkles.
6. Select the appropriate size of appliance for the extremity being treated (Fig. 14–5).
7. Insert the injured limb into the appliance. When full-length appliances are used, avoid bunching the garment in the axilla or groin.
8. For best results, elevate the limb during treatment. (With fluid-filled units it is easier to allow the appliance to initially fill and then to elevate the body part.)
9. Connect the appliance to the compression unit. Note that these units have input and exhaust tubes. The hoses must be properly connected to the appliance and the unit (Fig. 14–6). If a sequential compression unit is being used, the appliance and hoses must be connected so that the appliance fills from distal to proximal.

At a Glance: **Intermittent Compression**

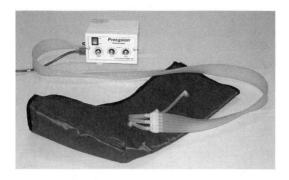

Description

An external pump forces air or water through an appliance fitted to the extremity. The changes in pressure force fluids through the venous system and solids through the lymphatic system to promote edema reduction.

Primary Effects

Increased venous return
May increase lymphatic return. Protein-rich matter is less responsive to intermittent compression than fluids.[3]

Treatment Duration

Intermittent compression can be applied once or twice a day for 20 minutes to several hours per session for post-traumatic edema. Treatment for lymphedema may be given for several hours. If the unit uses cold fluid, increase the temperature as the treatment duration increases.

Indications

- Post-traumatic edema
- Postsurgical edema
- Primary and secondary lymphedema
- Venous stasis ulcers
- *Prevention* of deep vein thrombosis. The presence of deep vein thrombosis is a contraindication to treatment.

Contraindications

- Acute conditions in which the possibility of a fracture has not been eliminated
- Conditions in which the pressure would further damage the structures (e.g., compartment syndromes)
- Peripheral vascular disease
- Arteriosclerosis
- Edema secondary to congestive heart failure
- Ischemic vascular disease
- Gangrene
- Dermatitis
- Deep vein thrombosis
- Thrombophlebitis

Precautions

- Use care when treating the lower leg with a compression device. Even in the absence of a compartment syndrome, inflation devices can elevate intramuscular pressure to a level sufficient to cause ischemia.[10]
- Wrinkling of Stockinette may cause high-pressure areas and subsequent bruising as the pressure in the appliance increases.

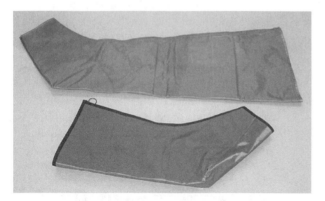

Figure 14-5. **Compression Appliances.** Top: Full-leg; Bottom: Half-leg. Other varieties and sizes are also available.

Initiation of the Treatment

1. If the intermittent compression unit uses a cold fluid, select the TEMPERATURE to be used, generally between 50° and 55°F.
2. Select the maximal PRESSURE for the treatment. Normal pressure ranges are 40 to 60 mm Hg for the upper extremity and 60 to 100 mm Hg for the lower extremity (Table 14–1). This pressure should normally not exceed the diastolic blood pressure. If the treatment pressure must exceed the diastolic pressure, monitor the patient closely and use a lower duty cycle.

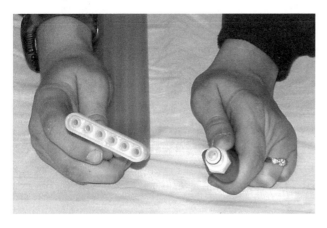

Figure 14-6. Connectors for Intermittent and Sequential Compression Devices. Sequential compression devices have two airways for each chamber in the appliance, one to inflate the chamber and the other to deflate it *(left connector)*. Intermittent or constant compression devices usually only have one airway *(right)*.

3. Select the ON-OFF times. A 3:1 duty cycle (e.g., 45 seconds ON, 15 seconds OFF) is used, although the benefit of this protocol relative to others has not been substantiated. Individual manufacturers may recommend different protocols based on the characteristics of their machine.
4. Select the appropriate TREATMENT TIME. Treatment for post-traumatic edema may be given for 20 to 30 minutes. Treatment of lymphedema may be given for several hours.
5. Inform the individual about the sensations to be expected during the treatment. Instruct the patient to contact you if any unusual sensations, such as pain or a "tingling" feeling, are experienced during the treatment.
6. Encourage the patient to perform gentle range-of-motion exercises or wiggle the fingers (upper extremity treatments) or toes (lower extremity treatments) during the off cycle, if appropriate.
7. If long-term treatments (i.e., more than 60 consecutive minutes) are being administered, regularly interrupt the session and inspect the extremity being treated for proper capillary refill or the presence of unusual markings or unexpected pitting edema.

TABLE 14-1	**Intermittent Compression Treatment Parameters Used for Edema Reduction**	
Extremity	*Inflation Pressure*	*ON:OFF Ratio*
Upper Extremity	40 to 60 mm HG	3:1
Lower Extremity	60 to 100 mm HG	3:1

Termination of the Treatment

1. Reduce ON time or select the DRAIN mode to remove the air or fluid from the appliance.
2. Gently remove the body part from the appliance.
3. Remeasure the circumference of the extremity and determine the amount of edema reduction.
4. Apply a compression wrap and any appropriate supportive devices. Encourage the patient to keep the limb elevated whenever possible between treatments.

Maintenance

Refer to the manufacturer's recommendations for maintenance intervals and procedures. Disconnect the compression unit from the electrical power source before cleaning.

Following Each Treatment

1. Check the appliance for tears or leaks. If a defect is found, repair the defect with an approved patch kit, return the appliance to the manufacturer for repair, or discard the appliance.
2. Clean the appliance using an approved cleanser.
3. If appliances are machine washable, turn them inside out and close them using the zipper.
4. Some appliances can be sterilized using gas systems.

Quarterly or as Indicated

1. Check air/water hoses for defects and replace if necessary.
2. Clean the external unit using an approved cleanser.
3. Check the electrical plug, electrical cord, and control cord (if present) for nicks, frays, or other visible damage.

Annually or as Required

1. A qualified service technician should perform an inspection and perform any needed maintenance.

● Chapter Highlights

- Compression of the extremity forces fluids and solids proximally, thereby reducing edema.
- Intermittent compression can be circumferential where the entire appliance inflates at the same time or sequential where chambers are inflated from distal to proximal.
- The appliance can be inflated using either air or chilled water.
- Intermittent compression is used to reduce edema. Clearing the joint capsule of excess fluids will increase range of motion, decrease muscle inhibition, and reduce pain.

- Unstable fractures or joints in which extension must be avoided and DVT are the primary contraindications to the use of intermittent compression.
- The amount of compression should not exceed the patient's diastolic blood pressure. Lower pressures are often more effective than higher pressure.
- A compression wrap should be applied and the limb elevated following treatment.

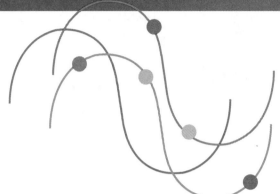

Chapter 15

Continuous Passive Motion

Continuous passive motion units are motorized devices that move one or more joints through a preset range of motion at a controlled speed. The subsequent joint movement allows for improved healing of soft tissue and certain articular pathologies. The method may prevent joint contractures and delay atrophy. Although these devices were originally designed for use on the knee, models have been developed for all of the body's major joints.

Continuous passive motion (CPM) is the antithesis of immobilization, a common postsurgical management technique. To deter the unwanted effects of immobilization, CPM devices are used to deliver gentle stresses to the healing tissues. Still predominantly used for knee injuries, CPM units have been designed for the hand, wrist, hip, shoulder, elbow, and ankle (Fig. 15–1). Although passive motion can be applied through a dedicated CPM unit, it can be delivered manually by the clinician, but for a much shorter time. Some isokinetic units incorporate "robotics" to deliver short-term passive motion treatments.

Robert Salter,[11] a Canadian physician, originally proposed the use of CPM to assist in the healing of synovial joints. On the basis of his clinical observations, Salter hypothesized that the application of CPM would be beneficial in three ways:

- Enhancing the nutrition and metabolic activity of articular cartilage

- Stimulating tissue remodeling and regrowth of articular cartilage
- Accelerating the healing of articular cartilage, tendons, and ligaments

CPM devices are categorized into three types of design: free linkage, anatomic, and nonanatomic.[12, 13] The free linkage design is similar to manually moving the patient's limb through the range of motion (ROM) by grasping it proximal and distal to the joint. Because the joint itself is not supported, free linkage units are not suitable for unstable joints.[13] The CPM devices that incorporate an anatomic design attempt to mimic the natural motion of the involved joints and the proximal joints. Anatomic CPMs are the most suitable for the knee.

Nonanatomically designed CPM units make no attempt to replicate the natural joint motion, with compensatory movement occurring between the patient's extremity and the CPM's carriage. The difference between the

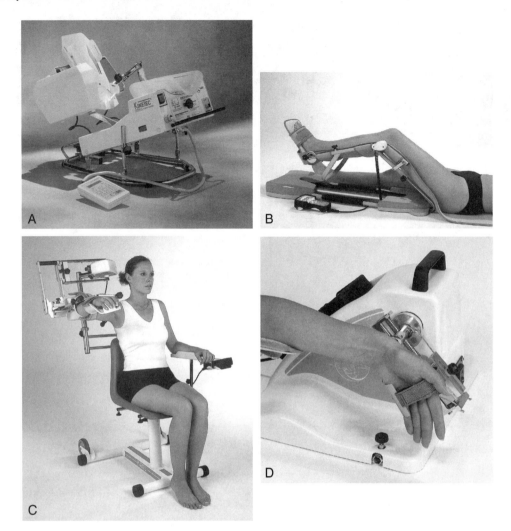

Figure 15–1. **Continuous Passive Motion Devices.** (A) Ankle; (B) Knee; (C) Shoulder; (D) Wrist and hand. (Kinetec courtesy of Sammons Preston Rolyan, an Ability One Company.)

ROM indicated on the CPM and the actual movement of the limb may be in excess of 20 degrees.[13] Table 15–1 summarizes the advantages and disadvantages of each of these styles of CPM units. Regardless of the type of CPM unit being used, care must be taken to avoid placing unwanted stress on the joint's structures.

Incorporating motion early into the patient's rehabilitation routine does not have to include CPM devices. Manual (passive) ROM progressing through active-assisted to fully active motion can decrease hospitalization time (thus decreasing hospital charges) and increase long-term ROM 1 year after total knee **arthroplasty** ■.[14–16]

TABLE 15–1	**Characteristics of Continuous Passive Motion Designs**		
	Continuous Passive Motion Linkage Design		
Parameter	*Free Linkage*	*Anatomic Design*	*Nonanatomic Design*
Joint stability	Very poor	Good	Fair
Control of ROM	Very poor	Excellent	Fair
Total ROM	Poor	Excellent	Good
Multiaxis motion	Good	Poor	Fair
Adjustable to the patient	Excellent	Poor	Fair

ROM = range of motion
Source: Adapted from Saringer[13]

Arthroplasty: Surgical reconstruction or replacement of an articular joint.

● EFFECTS ON
The Injury Response Process

The philosophy regarding the effects of CPM is "Motion that is never lost need never be regained. It is the regaining of movement that is painful."[17] Constant, gentle stresses applied to the injured structure encourage the remodeling of collagen along the lines of force and reduce the negative effects of joint immobilization.[18] When the injured joint is kept in motion, the unwanted effects of immobilization on muscle, tendons, ligaments, articular and hyaline cartilage, blood supply, and nerve supply are reduced (Fig. 15–2).

Under the stress of motion, collagen that would normally be deposited in a random order aligns along the line of applied stress. This realignment reduces functional shortening, cross-linking of collagen, and capsular adhesions, thus maintaining the ROM,[12, 14] enhancing the tensile strength of tendons, **allografts** ■, and skin,[11] and stimulating repair of articular cartilage.[19]

As the joint moves from extension to flexion and back, fluids within the capsule are exposed to low pressure where the joint volume is the greatest (normally extension) and high pressure where the joint volume is least. The greater the amount of joint flexion, the greater the intra-articular pressure. As this cycle is repeated, the change in pressure creates a pumping effect that circulates the synovial fluid. The circulating fluid assists in the removal of joint **hemarthrosis** ■, periarticular edema, and blood from the tissues surrounding the joint.[20] The amount of ROM applied during the CPM sessions must be sufficient to increase intra-articular pressure but not be so great as to damage the surrounding soft tissue or graft.[21]

The effects and benefits associated with CPM are not universally substantiated or accepted. The decision to use CPM should be made on a patient-by-patient basis rather than for specific pathologies. The benefits derived from this treatment and the associated costs versus other treatment techniques should be considered when developing the treatment plan.[22, 23]

Range of Motion

Introducing CPM early into the rehabilitation scheme allows active motion and strength training routines to be incorporated earlier in the patient's program, an important consideration when dealing with an active population.[24–26] In most cases, the benefits of CPM increasing the joint's ROM are seen early in the patient's rehabilitation program, with the differences relative to patients not receiving CPM equalizing over time (assuming that both groups receive proper therapy). When given free rein to control the ROM, patients, using comfort as their guide, increase their ROM by 6 to 7 degrees per day.[27]

CPM is more effective in increasing ROM caused by soft tissue restriction (for example, tightness of the Achilles' tendon during ankle dorsiflexion) than static stretching.[28] When applied immediately following surgery, CPM can be effective in increasing the amount of knee flexion, but this effect has not been substantiated following total knee arthroplasty.[30, 31] The need for manipulation of the knee joint following arthroplasty is significantly reduced or eliminated by the use of CPM.[16, 20, 32]

Increasing ROM may be contingent on the amount of time that the joint spends in the extremes of the ROM, or **total end range time** (TERT). Increasing the TERT delivers a low-load, prolonged stress on the tissues, significantly increasing the ROM compared with a short-duration, high-load stress.[33]

The use of CPM alone does not fully restore ROM and has little effect on muscle strength. Manual or active therapy is required to fully restore strength and ROM. An undocumented benefit of the early application of CPM may be its assistance in helping the patient overcome the apprehension of moving the knee after surgery.

A statistically significant increase in joint ROM has not been documented in all studies. However, the differing protocol, pathologies, and patient base used in these studies make reaching a firm conclusion regarding the efficacy of CPM on ROM impractical, although most studies demonstrate equivalency in the total ROM over the long term.

Lower extremity CPM has also been used to maintain the ROM in patients suffering from advanced cardiovascular pathology that restricts walking. CPM decreases the rate of atrophy and functional shortening of thequad-riceps group with little increase in cardiovascular demands.[34]

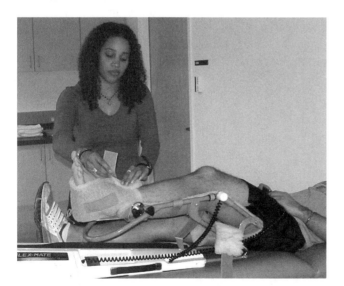

Figure 15–2. **Set-up for Continuous Passive Motion.** The joint axis must be aligned with the hinges on the CPM cradle.

Allograft: A replacement or augmentation of a biological structure with a synthetic one.
Hemarthrosis: Blood in a joint.

Following rotator cuff repair, patients undergoing CPM demonstrated safe improvements in pain, ROM, and other functional measures. However, these outcomes were no better than the results obtained from manual passive ROM exercises.[23]

Joint Nutrition

Both meniscal and articular cartilage are relatively avascular and derive most of their nutrients from synovial fluid. Meniscal and articular cartilage is spongelike and is nourished by expansion and compression; through the natural movement of the joint, the synovial fluid is alternately absorbed by and squeezed out of the cartilage. During immobilization, synovial fluid is not distributed throughout the joint. The application of CPM stimulates the circulation of synovial fluids and causes the meniscal cartilage to increase its uptake of nutrients. The delivery and the subsequent absorption of nutrients assist both types of cartilage in the healing process.[35–37]

The use of early CPM for condylar cartilage defects assists in the healing process, maintains joint ROM, and has a better functional outcome than early active motion.[38–40] Active ROM can place unwanted compressive forces on the joint surfaces, as in the case of osteochondral defects or chondromalacia. By circulating synovial fluid, condylar cartilage healing is accelerated through the deposition of type II collagen.[36, 39, 40] Healing of full-thickness defects may require up to 2 weeks of treatment.[36]

Edema Reduction

The effectiveness of CPM in the reduction of edema is not clearly understood and varies according to the body part and condition being treated.[41] The passive movements of the limb and the elevation of the body part should assist in venous and lymphatic return by milking the muscle (see Treatment Strategies: Edema Reduction, p 23).[42] Significant edema reduction after arthroplasty of the knee and ankle,[20, 26, 43] after anterior cruciate ligament (ACL) surgery, for knee inflammatory conditions,[44] and hand edema[45, 46] has been documented.

Pain Reduction

The movement of the joint activates afferent nerves located in the muscle, joint, and skin, and possibly provides pain control through the gate mechanism. Any associated reduction in edema or muscle spasm, as well as deterrence of functional shortening, would aid in limiting pain. However, CPM is not used as an acute pain-control technique.

Postoperatively, pain control medications may be administered to the patient during the CPM treatment. Narcotic injections or patient-controlled analgesia pumps, local anesthetic injection, or regional nerve blocks are employed to reduce the patient's postoperative pain and the discomfort associated with CPM.[21]

The patient's need for postsurgical analgesic medication does not indicate that CPM reduces pain. Studies show no significant difference in pain (as reported using a visual analog scale) and pain medication between patients receiving CPM and those not receiving CPM,[22, 47] those receiving manual passive ROM treatments,[23] and those patients controlling their own medication dosage.[48]

Ligament Healing

The early use of CPM promotes healing, often more so than surgical correction when a single ligament is involved and there is little rotational instability of the joint.[49] The physiological benefits of CPM application post–ACL surgery are not as promising as its use with other conditions. The ACL does not receive the same nutritional benefits from CPM as meniscal or articular cartilage.[50] The ACL is surrounded by its own synovial lining, which shields the ligament from gaining nutrition from the joint's synovial fluid. Instead, the ligament must rely on its intrinsic blood vessels.

Initial ROM immediately following surgery is increased in patients who receive CPM relative to those patients not receiving CPM. However, as long as proper follow-up therapy is received, there is no long-term difference in the joint's ROM.[51–53] CPM applied immediately following surgery has been demonstrated to be effective in increasing the biomechanical properties of allograft-augmented medial collateral ligament reconstruction.[54]

Many knee CPM units having a proximal posterior tibial bar cause an excessive amount of **translation ■** of the tibia on the femur. In procedures such as ACL surgery, this movement could produce stress sufficient to damage the healing tissue and graft (Fig. 15–3).[55] After surgery, a properly fitted CPM can be used without increasing anterior ACL laxity.[15, 56]

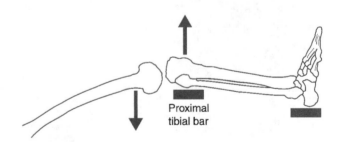

Figure 15–3. **Tibial Translation During Continuous Passive Motion.** A proximal bar supports the tibia while gravity allows the femur to move downward. This effect coupled with the force of motion can place unwanted stresses on the anterior cruciate ligament.

Translation: Sliding or gliding of opposing articular surfaces.

■ Contraindications

Unwanted joint motion and the associated stresses on bones and joint structures are the primary contraindications to CPM (see At a Glance: Continuous Passive Motion). CPM must not be administered in the presence of an unstable fracture. Because of the threat of causing it to spread, CPM should not be used in areas of uncontrolled infection. Likewise, CPM is contraindicated with spastic paralyses because the antagonistic motion may result in muscle damage.

CPM should be used with caution if the patient has a history of deep vein thrombosis. The pressure from the CPM cradle and increased venous return caused by limb motion and elevation may dislodge the clot. Intracompartmental pressures may be increased by the motion and/or supporting cradle straps.

Some CPM designs increase the amount of shear forces crossing the joint and unduly stress the soft tissues and graft. The type of CPM, arc of motion, and speed of motion should be adjusted based on the physician's recommendations for the pathology being treated.

■ Controversies in Treatment

Although the rationale for the use of CPM is sound, many published research articles question the efficacy for most clinical applications. Likewise, CPM has not been demonstrated to be more effective than traditional manual therapies (usually passive ROM).[22] The exception to this are conditions involving the articular cartilage in which compression of the joint surfaces must be avoided.[38, 39]

CPM is often used following total knee arthroplasty and has subsequently been the focus of retrospective and prospective investigation. Some studies have concluded that CPM is beneficial in decreasing the length of hospital stay, decreased need for analgesic medication, earlier implementation of straight leg raises, and improved knee function/satisfaction scores at the time of discharge.[57] Evidence also suggests that the need for knee manipulations following arthroplasty is reduced.[16, 32]

Following total knee arthroplasty, ROM in higher degrees of knee flexion (70 to 110 degrees) required less pain medication than patients receiving CPM within 0 to 50 degrees of flexion or no CPM, but these differences were not statistically significant.[47] Other studies have demonstrated that effects on length of hospital stay [16, 31, 32] and Knee Society Score (a measure of knee function and patient satisfaction) followed similar patterns.[31, 47]

Nearly all studies conclude that there is no significant long-term difference in pain or ROM between patients who received postoperative CPM and those who did not.[16, 20, 23, 31, 32, 47, 57–61] The decision to include CPM in the early treatment protocol must be made by considering the immediate and long-term benefits relative to the associated costs and potential hazards.[22, 30]

■ Clinical Application of Continuous Passive Motion

Instrumentation

Refer to the operator's guide for the unit you are using.

Power: This switch activates the internal circuits of the CPM unit.

Reset: This button clears all previous settings from the CPM unit's memory.

Timer: This control sets the duration of the treatment. A CONTINUOUS setting is provided for long-term treatments

ROM: This control adjusts the ROM from slight hyperextension (approximately + 5 degrees) to full flexion (approximately 130 degrees). Some units have separate controls to adjust the amount of flexion and extension.

Speed: This knob adjusts the rate of motion between 10 and 120 degrees per second. Slow speeds are used immediately postsurgery or postinjury. Increased speed (cycles per second) has been theorized to produce better tensile properties of healing tendons than lower speeds.[62]

TERT: Total end range time. The amount of time the joint is held in the end ROMs. This may be adjustable for both flexion and extension.

Pause (Extension/Flexion Delay): This button stops the motion at the extreme ROM (flexion and/or extension) to allow a passive stretching of the fibers to occur.

Interrupt: This control allows the patient to discontinue the CPM.

Trigger jack: Some units allow synchronization of CPM and electrical stimulation. The TRIGGER JACK allows the neuromuscular electrical stimulation unit to be activated during the PAUSE function.

Program: Microprocessor-controlled CPM devices may have preprogrammed protocols that are selected from a menu. User-defined protocol may also be stored and recalled for later use. Refer to the operator's manual for step-by-step instructions.

Set-up and Application

Often, the CPM unit is applied in the recovery room after surgery by a CPM technician. The following protocol is provided as an example for a post–ACL reconstructive surgery. Refer to the operator's manual for other knee protocol and/or the operation of CPM units designed for other body parts. Advanced units, especially those for the shoulder, may require specialized training to assure proper set-up and protocol selection. CPM devices should not be used in the presence of flammable gases such as anesthetics or oxygen.

At a Glance: Continuous Passive Motion

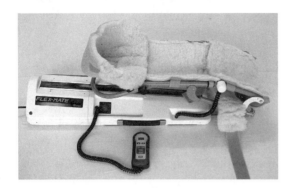

Description

A motorized device that moves one or more joints at a controlled speed through a preset range of motion. Continuous passive motion is used to restore early range of motion, delaying atrophy, improving joint nutrition.

Primary Effects

- Improved nutrition of articular structures
- Increased metabolic activity of articular structures
- Increased remodeling of collagen along the lines of stress
- Increased tensile strength of healing tendons, ligaments, and other soft tissue
- Improved early range of motion
- Potential edema reduction
- Pain reduction via secondary mechanisms (e.g., increased ROM)

Treatment Duration

Continuous passive motion may be applied in long-term bouts where the patient is continuously attached to the unit, or the device may be applied in 1-hour treatment bouts three times a day. After surgery, use is for 6 to 8 hours a day, although the duration preferred by patients is 4 to 8 hours.[27] Patients may also be instructed in the use of CPM for in-home treatments, or a home-care visit by a physical therapist or physical therapist assistant may be required.

Indications

- After surgical repair of stable intra-articular or extra-articular joint fractures
- After joint surgery, including surgery on the ACL [56]
- Following open reduction–internal fixation fracture management
- After joint arthroplasty
- After surgery or chronic pathology to the knee extensor mechanisms
- Joint contractures
- Following meniscectomy
- After knee manipulations
- After joint débridement for **arthrofibrosis** ■
- Tendon lacerations
- After osteochondral repair
- For enhancing the reabsorption of a hemarthrosis
- Thrombophlebitis
- Following surgical correction of chondromalacia patellae

Contraindications

- Cases in which the device causes an unwanted translation of opposing bones, overstressing the healing tissues
- Unstable fractures
- Spastic paralyses
- Uncontrolled infection

Precautions

- The use of continuous passive motion in conjunction with anticoagulation therapy may produce an intracompartmental hematoma [63] or deep vein thrombosis.[21]
- Skin irritation from the straps or carriage cover may develop. Overtightening of the straps and/or dressing can lead to necrosis of the incision sites or other local tissue.[5]

Arthrofibrosis: The repair and replacement of inflamed joint tissue by connective tissues.

Preparation for the Treatment

1. Confirm that the patient is free of contraindications to the use of CPM (see At a Glance: Continuous Passive Motion).
2. Ensure that the unit is clean and fit the CPM unit with a clean carriage cover.
3. Most CPM devices can be adjusted to fit the involved extremity even when the patient is wearing a brace or surgical bandages.
4. The physician may elect to remove circumferential wraps (e.g., cotton batting, elastic wraps) and cover the limb with a single cotton or elastic sleeve.[21]
5. Measure the length of the patient's thigh from the ischial tuberosity to the joint line of the knee. Adjust the proximal carriage so that the proximal end meets the bottom of the buttocks and, if applicable to the unit, aligns with the coxofemoral joint.
6. Determine the length of the lower leg by measuring from the joint line of the knee to approximately 1/4 inch beyond the heel. Adjust the distal portion of the carriage accordingly.
7. Place the lower extremity in the unit with the joint line of the knee aligning to the articular hinge of the CPM unit.
8. Adjust the foot in the footplate so that the tibia is placed in the neutral position. Internally or externally rotating the tibia can result in increased stress on the ACL.

Initiation of the Treatment

1. Give the patient the hand-held control and provide instruction on how and when to use it, including increasing speed and ROM and terminating the treatment.
2. Set the ROM as prescribed by the physician. Generally this protocol is started with a limited ROM (0 to 60 degrees) and progresses to the full ROM as healing occurs and pain decreases.
3. Set the SPEED of the treatment (e.g., cycle time of 4 minutes; 15 cycles per hour). Units may have preprogrammed protocols that are chosen from a menu.
4. The patient may be instructed to increase the ROM at regular intervals as tolerated. Some units do not allow the protocol to be changed once the treatment has been initiated.
5. Instruct the patient and those tending the patient (including family members) to recognize pressure-related problems caused by the CPM carriage. Adjust the carriage accordingly.

6. If this is a home-based treatment, the patient should be provided with written instructions and an emergency contact number.
7. Regularly check the patient for signs of intracompartmental hemorrhage or deep vein thrombosis.

Termination of the Treatment

1. Position the carriage to best suit removing the limb from the unit, usually just short of full extension.
2. Loosen the restraining straps, foot plate, or other supports.
3. Carefully lift the extremity and have an assistant remove the CPM unit.
4. Cut or remove the sleeve from the extremity.
5. Inspect the extremity for pressure sores, distal redness, or swelling that is indicative of increased compartment pressure or deep vein thrombosis, and the surgical sites for proper healing. Notify a physician if any abnormal findings are noted.
6. Clean the extremity according to the physician's protocol.
7. If indicated, redress the surgical wounds and reapply a sterile dressing or compression wrap.

Maintenance

Refer to the manufacturer's recommendations for maintenance intervals and procedures. Disconnect the CPM unit from the electrical power source prior to cleaning.

Following Each Treatment

1. Clean the surfaces with a disinfectant soap. If the unit becomes soiled with blood or other bodily fluids use a 10-percent solution of household chlorine bleach to clean the surfaces.
2. Clean or replace the carriage cover. Some covers can be sterilized by using an **autoclave** ■ at 225°F (125°C). Check the manufacturer's recommendations for additional hygiene concerns. Covers may be reused for the same patient, but patient-to-patient reuse is not recommended.

Quarterly or as Indicated

Some units have an automatic alert that maintenance is needed.

1. Lubricate all moving parts (e.g., joints, ball bearings, threaded rods).
2. Check the electrical plug, electrical cord, and

Autoclave: A device used to sterilize medical instruments using steam heat at 250°F (121°C).

control cord (if present) for nicks, frays, or other visible damage.

● Chapter Highlights

- CPM is used to maintain joint motion and provide nutrition to the articular structures.
- The theory behind the use of CPM is that motion that is never lost does not have to be restored.
- There are two types of CPM units: anatomical design and free linkage design.
- The motion assists in the alignment of collagen and may help remove edema from the joint.
- Increased ROM is dependent on the total end range time (TERT), the time when the joint is held in the end ROM, stretching the soft tissues.
- CPM should not be used when there is an unstable fracture or deep vein thrombosis.

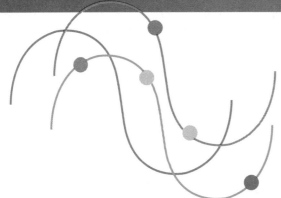

Chapter 16

Therapeutic Massage

Massage is one of the oldest forms of healing techniques. Using therapeutic touch, the body's tissues are manipulated to reduce muscle spasm, promote relaxation, improve blood flow, and increase venous drainage. The scope of massage theories, techniques, and effects is broad. This chapter addresses massage techniques that are most frequently used in the treatment of musculoskeletal conditions.

Massage, the systematic manipulation of the body's tissues, is one of the oldest therapeutic techniques still used in modern medicine. Dating back to the ancient Olympics, massage has been present in most cultures. Regional variations have contributed to the different forms of massage used today. This diverse background leads to differences in application protocol and theory (Table 16–1).

Massage and myofascial release are forms of manual therapy in which the tissues are manipulated to produce the desired effects. Joint mobilizations, another form of manual therapy, are not discussed in this text.

Massage is an effective treatment method for promoting local and systemic relaxation or invigoration, increasing local blood flow, breaking down adhesions, and encouraging venous return. Because it is a time-consuming task that requires the full attention of the clinician, massage is infrequently used in multi-function health care facilities. Still, massage has increased in popularity and massage therapy is a continually growing profession.

Massage is a skill- and knowledge-based technique, and because of the possibility for misuse, many states require licensure for massage therapists. Most other healing professions, including physical therapy and athletic training, incorporate massage techniques into their professional preparation. Massage therapists often work cooperatively with other health-care providers.

■ Massage Strokes

There are several different types of massage strokes, and each may be varied by adding more or less pressure, using different parts of the hand, or changing the direction of the stroke (Table 16–2). These elements are then sequenced to produce different effects. The following sections describe the basic elements of each stroke and discuss how they can be varied.

Effleurage

Effleurage, the stroking of the skin, is performed with the palm of the hand or knuckles to stimulate deep tissues, or with the fingerpads to stimulate sensory nerves. This stroke is categorized as being either superficial or deep. **Superficial stroking** may either follow the contour of the

TABLE 16–1	**Selected Methods of Manual Therapy Techniques**
Technique	*Description*
Acupressure	Pressure is applied along acupuncture meridians, altering the body's energy pattern.
Craniosacral therapy	Alters the flow of cerebrospinal fluid by lightly massaging points along the spinal column, especially the upper cervical spine.
Deep tissue massage	Targets individual deep muscle fibers and attempts to release adhesions.
Lymphatic massage	Targets the lymphatic system and attempts to remove bacteria and toxins from the body using light, rhythmic strokes.
Myofascial release	Breaks adhesions and other restrictions in the body's fascial network to restore normal function.
Myotherapy	Focuses on reducing pain and muscle spasms by breaking up trigger points using focused pressure.
Polarity therapy	Balances positive and negative energies in the body through the use of touch (also referred to as "Polarity Balancing").
Reflexology	Acupressure applied to the feet and hands to affect the body's meridians. Each zone of the feet and hands corresponds to another part of the body. Stimulating the reflexology points stimulates the corresponding area.
Rolfing	A ten-session technique designed to realign the body (also referred to as "Structural Integration").
Shiatsu	The Japanese form of acupressure.
Swedish massage	Traditional massage techniques.

TABLE 16–2	**Summary of Basic Massage Strokes and Their Physiological Effect**	
Stroke	*Technique*	*Effect*
Effleurage	Stroking of the skin	Deep stroking: stimulates deep tissues, forces fluids in the direction of the stroke. Superficial stroking: Slow strokes: promotes relaxation. Fast strokes: stimulates tissues and encourages blood flow
Pétrissage	Lifting and kneading	Stretches and separates muscle fiber, fascia, of the skin and scar tissue
Friction	Deep pressure	Effects muscle mobilization, tissue separation, including the breakup of scar tissue
Tapotement	Tapping or pounding	Promotes relaxation and the desensitization of the skin's nerve endings
Vibration	Rapid shaking	Increases blood flow and provides systemic invigoration of tissues

body itself, or follow the direction of the underlying muscles, but does not attempt to move the underlying muscle. **Deep stroking** requires more pressure to target and elongate the muscle fiber and stretch the fascia.

A slow, light stroke promotes relaxation, introduces the patient to the treatment, and is used to spread the massage lubricant over the area to be treated. Rapid strokes encourage blood flow and stimulate the tissues. Deep stroking should follow the course of veins and lymph vessels to force fluids in these vessels back toward the heart or elongate muscle.

Light effleurage is generally performed at both the beginning and end of the massage and may be used between pétrissage strokes. During the initial stages of the treatment, effleurage relaxes the patient and indicates the areas that will be massaged. At the conclusion of the treatment, this stroke "calms down" any nerves that become irritated during the massage.

Pétrissage

Pétrissage is the lifting, kneading, and rolling of the skin, subcutaneous tissue, and muscle with the fingers or hand. This stroke has some similarity to myofascial skin rolling technique, but pétrissage targets the underlying muscle (see Clinical Techniques: Skin Rolling, p 302). Pétrissage frees adhesions by stretching and separating muscle fiber, fascia, and scar tissue. This technique milks the muscle of waste products, assists in venous return, and can lead to muscular relaxation.

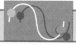

CLINICAL TECHNIQUES: EFFLEURAGE

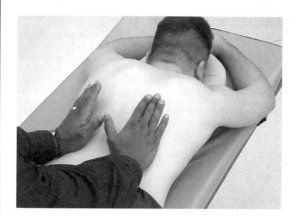

Basic technique

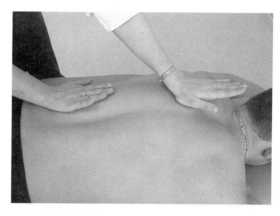

Shingling technique

Technique

- All effleurage strokes are performed in a rhythmic manner.
- Strokes should be directed towards the heart.
- The thumbs can be used to fit into anatomical contours (e.g., between the metatarsals, the posterior portion of the malleoli).
- Ideally, at least one hand should be in contact with the skin at any given point.

Basic effleurage:

1. Place the hands (palms, fingers, or knuckles) parallel to the body part being treated and symmetrical to its long axis.
2. Apply the appropriate amount of pressure for the desired effects.
3. Using a mirrored motion, stroke the body part along its long axis—the strokes may also follow the course of veins and lymph vessels or large muscle masses (e.g., the latissimus dorsi).
4. Still mirroring each other, lightly glide the hands back to the starting point using a light stroke of the fingerpads.

5. Repeat procedures 1 through 4 until the target tissues have been covered and/or the desired effects have been obtained.

"Shingling" technique:

1. Place one palm over the target tissue.
2. Using the palm, make short (e.g., 8 in.) to moderate (e.g., 12 in.) strokes following the path of the underlying muscle or vein, using the amount of pressure appropriate for the desired effects.
3. Just prior to the hand leaving the body, repeat the stroke using the opposite hand, starting approximately one-half the distance between the starting and ending point of the prior stroke, thus overlapping the strokes similar to shingles on a roof and provide the patient with the sensation of unbroken contact.
4. Continue along the length of the treatment area. Keeping the strokes in the original position, progress back towards the starting point.
5. Repeat procedures 1 through 4 until the target tissues have been covered and/or the desired effects have been obtained.

Friction Massage

There are two basic types of friction massage: circular and cross-fiber massage. Circular friction massage is applied with the thumbs working in circular motion and is often effective in the treatment of muscle spasm and trigger points. In transverse friction massage, the thumbs or fingertips stroke the tissue from opposite directions. Friction massage can be painful to receive, especially when it is performed on trigger points. When treating a large muscle mass the elbow or a commercial deep-kneading device can be used in place of the thumbs.

Friction massage mobilizes muscle fibers and separates adhesions in muscle, tendon fibers, or scar tissue that restrict motion and cause pain, and is used to facilitate local blood perfusion.[64] Transverse friction massage is also used for the treatment of trigger points and tendinitis or other forms of joint adhesions.[65]

Tapotement

Tapotement involves the gentle tapping or pounding of the skin. The most common form of tapotement, "hacking," uses the ulnar side of the wrist to contact the skin, in a manner similar to a "karate chop." This stroke is performed with the wrist and fingers limp so that the hand more or less slaps the skin.

In general, tapotement promotes muscular and systemic relaxation. Tapping promotes relaxation and desensitization of irritated nerve endings and is often used following more vigorous techniques (e.g., friction massage or pétrissage) (see Clinical Techniques: Tapotement).

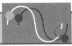

CLINICAL TECHNIQUES: PÉTRISSAGE

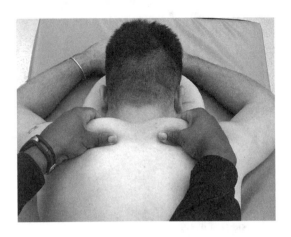

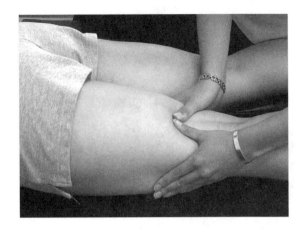

Technique

1. If pétrissage is the only technique being performed, it may be performed without the use of a lubricant.
2. Pétrissage is often administered following effleurage and/or moist heat pack application.

3. Using one or two hands, gently lift the skin and underlying muscle and roll the tissue back and forth.
4. Repeat step three for a few repetitions before progressing to a new location.

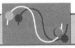

CLINICAL TECHNIQUES: FRICTION MASSAGE

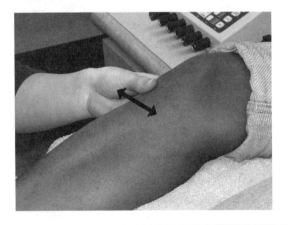

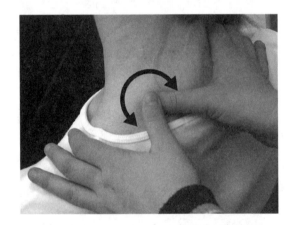

Technique

1. The area may be preheated using a moist heat pack or ultrasound.
2. Position the patient so that the muscle is in a relaxed position.
3. Begin lightly and gradually progress to firmer, deeper circular strokes or strokes that run perpendicular or parallel to the underlying target tissue.
4. The force must be applied so that the pressure will reach deep into the tissues.
5. Friction massage can be followed by a stretching routine to further facilitate range of motion.

Comments

This method of massage is to be avoided in conditions in which the underlying tissues would be further injured by the pressure, such as acute injuries where an unwanted acceleration of the inflammatory response may occur.

Friction massage can be performed by the patient as a part of a home-treatment program.
To reduce soreness this treatment may be followed by ice or ice massage.

CLINICAL TECHNIQUES: TAPOTEMENT

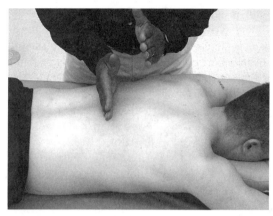

(A) Hacking.

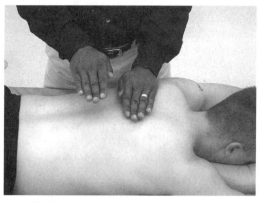

(B) Cupping.

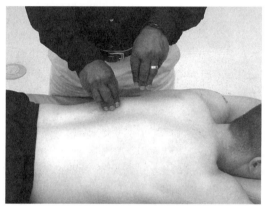

(C) Pincement.

Technique

1. Tapotement is performed with a light, fast tempo.
2. The hands should bounce off the skin as contact is made for each of the following techniques:

   Hacking: Contact is made with the ulnar side of the fifth metacarpal.

   Cupping: The hands are slightly cupped and contact is made with the heel of the hand, palmar aspect of the first metacarpal, and the palmar aspect of the fifth metacarpal.

Pincement: The skin is lightly squeezed (pinched) between the fingers.

Rapping: The hand is made into a loose fist. Contact is made with the distal phalanges.

Tapping: A tapotement variation that promotes relaxation and desensitization of irritated nerve endings is called "raindrops." The fingers lightly touch the skin in an alternating manner, as if you were typing on a keyboard (not shown).

Vibration

This method of massage involves the rapid shaking of the tissue and serves to soothe peripheral nerves and promote muscular relaxation. Although a skilled masseur or masseuse is capable of obtaining therapeutic effects manually, less skilled or untrained individuals often use a mechanical vibration massager.

■ Myofascial Release

Myofascial release involves the traditional effleurage, pétrissage, and friction massage strokes with simultaneous stretching of the muscles and fascia to obtain relaxation of tense or adhered tissues and restore tissue mobility. Fascia forms an interconnected network that connects and surrounds muscle, tendons, and nerves, and separates the skin and adipose tissue from the underlying muscle (Fig. 16–1). Adhesions or restrictions in one area can affect function elsewhere. Abnormalities of the myofascial system are thought to be linked to fibromyalgia, chronic fatigue syndrome, myofascial pain syndrome, postural deviations, and decreased muscular function.[66–68]

Myofascial release attempts to restore normal function by breaking adhesions and restoring normal fascial length. Fascia does not deform when it is exposed to a quick, high-intensity force. Fascia will, however, elongate when a slow, moderate-intensity force is applied to it, an effect referred to as "creep." The pressures used for most myofascial techniques take advantage of this phenomenon to stretch the underlying fascia. These myofascial techniques should then be followed up with traditional muscle stretching techniques.

The actual application of myofascial release techniques tends not to follow a structured pattern. Rather, the clinician receives cues and feedback from the patient's tissues that indicate what strokes and stretches are appropriate. The basic myofascial release techniques involve pulling the tissues in opposite directions, stabilizing the proximal or superior position with one hand while applying a stretch with the opposite hand, or using the patient's body weight to stabilize the extremity while a longitudinal stress is applied.

Areas of myofascial adhesions or shortening are found by gently gliding the skin in multiple directions, seeking to identify areas of restricted motion, or observing the patient's posture and noting areas of possible fascial shortening. Once the restriction is identified, myofascial release can be used to restore mobility. Specialized training in myofascial release techniques is needed to become proficient in these procedures.

The **J-stroke** is one of the most fundamental forms of myofascial release and is used to mobilize superficial fascial restrictions. **Skin rolling** also reduces superficial myofascial adhesions. Depending on the amount and depth of the pressure applied, **focused stretching** can release both superficial and deep fascial restrictions. The **arm pull**, **leg pull**, and **diagonal release** attempt to stretch large areas of fascia in the extremities and torso.

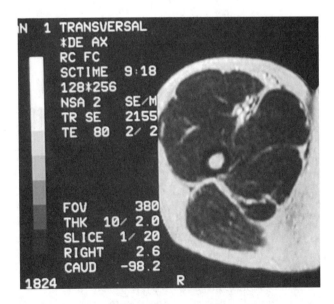

Figure 16–1. **Fascial Network in an Extremity.** An MRI cross-sectional view of the proximal femur. The white bands running through the muscles are the deep fascia. The superficial fascial network lies between the skin and the muscle.

● EFFECTS ON
The Injury Response Process

Massage is promoted to elicit a number of responses within the body. These responses are related to the direct mechanical effects on the tissue (e.g., breaking adhesions), reflexive responses that occur secondary to stimulation of the nerves (e.g, pain reduction), or by psychological means (e.g., systemic relaxation).

In general, massage strokes can produce various responses, depending on the body part, amount of pressure applied, and the speed of the stroke. Light, slow stroking of the skin results in systemic relaxation. Fast, deep strokes cause an increase in blood flow to the area, invigorating the patient.

The lines between the physiological and the psychological effects of massage are often difficult to discern. Athletes who believe that massage will improve their performance, or individuals who believe that massage will assist in the healing process, often will see improvement simply through the power of suggestion.

Cardiovascular Effects

Deep friction or vigorous massage is thought to produce vascular changes similar to those of inflammation, with the treated area being marked by increased blood flow, histamine release, and an increased temperature. Light massage may activate the sympathetic nervous system that causes temporary capillary vasodilation. Deeper, more vigorous massage is used to produce longer lasting vasodilation of the capillaries and arterioles, thus increasing blood flow to the area.

Massage applied for the purpose of inducing systemic relaxation does produce physiological changes in the cardiovascular system. Decreased heart rate, respiratory rate, and blood pressure have been observed in patients after 30 minutes of massage.[69] Massaging acupressure points is reported to decrease systolic and diastolic blood pressure, decrease heart rate, and reduce cutaneous blood flow.[70] Trigger point massage can also reduce systolic and diastolic blood pressure and heart rate and promote systemic relaxation.[71]

Neuromuscular Effects

Pétrissage has been shown to decrease neuromuscular excitability, but only during the duration of the massage, and the effects are confined to the muscles being massaged.[72–74] A massage routine, consisting of deep effleurage, circular friction, and transverse friction applied to the hamstrings, can increase hamstring flexibility.[75] This effect is a result of the combined decrease in neuromuscular excitability (relaxation) and stretching of muscle and scar tissue. Massage or myofascial techniques designed to increase muscular, fascial, or capsular extensibility should be followed by manual stretching of the limb.

CLINICAL TECHNIQUES: MYOFASCIAL TECHNIQUES: J-STROKES

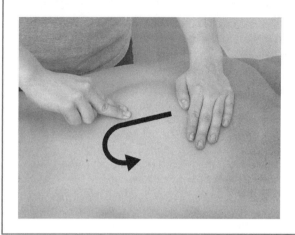

Effects
Release localized superficial fascial restrictions such as scar tissue.

Technique
After locating the adhesion:

1. One hand moves the skin to place the adhesion on stretch.
2. Using the second and third fingers of the other hand, stroke in the opposite direction of the force, terminating in a curl, forming a "J".
3. Repeat until all adhesions have been reduced.

Massage is less effective in decreasing muscular recovery time after exercise but may be effective in reducing the amount of delayed-onset muscle soreness (when applied 2 hours after exercise) by reducing the **emigration** ■ of neutrophils and by increasing serum cortisol levels.[76, 77]

Edema Reduction
When properly performed, massage increases venous and lymphatic flow that assists in the removal of venous and lymphatic edema and increases lymphatic uptake by spreading the extravasated substances, exposing them to more lymphatic absorption points.[78] Manual or mechanical massage (see Chap. 14) forces fluids within the vessels to move toward the heart. Because of the associated pressures, edema reduction massage should not be used on acutely injured tissues.

The key to reducing edema is first to mobilize the proximal area of edema before attempting to move the distal areas. This procedure, known as "uncorking the bottle," can be visualized as removing a traffic jam. Cars at the back of the pack cannot move forward until the car at the front of the line moves. To maintain the level of edema reduction and prevent rebound swelling, apply a compression wrap following treatment and keep the limb elevated whenever possible.[79, 80]

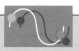

CLINICAL TECHNIQUES: MYOFASCIAL TECHNIQUES: FOCUSED STRETCHING

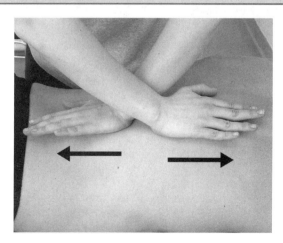

Description
Focused stretching is used to reduce superficial or deep adhesions by moving the skin and fascia in opposite directions. In the case pictured, the force is parallel to the line of the muscles, but this technique can also be performed perpendicular to the muscle fibers.

Technique
After identifying the area of restriction:

1. Place the heel of one hand in the area of the restriction.
2. The opposite arm is crossed in front and the hand is placed below the first hand.
3. Stretch the tissues to take up the slack.
4. Using slow, deep pressure, stretch the tissues.
5. Repeat the above steps in opposite directions until no restrictions are felt.

Emigration: Passage of white blood corpuscles through the walls of capillaries and veins during inflammation.

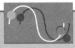

CLINICAL TECHNIQUES: MYOFASCIAL TECHNIQUES: SKIN ROLLING

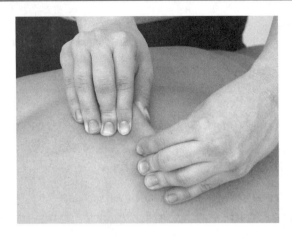

Description

Outwardly, skin rolling in myofascial therapy is similar to petrissage used during traditional massage techniques (see Clinical Techniques: Petrissage). The skin is lifted

and rolled between the fingers, identifying and focusing on areas of superficial myofascial adhesions.

Technique

1. Begin by progressing from the inferior and lateral segment of the body area being treated and progress medially and superiorly.
2. Using the fingers and thumb, lift and separate the skin from the underlying tissues.
3. Roll the skin between the fingers, noting any adhesions, tightness, or other limitations.
4. When an area of adhesion is identified:
   • Lift the skin and move it in the direction of the restriction.
   • Move the skin in the direction of the restriction.
   • If the adhesion is still present, move the skin diagonal to the restriction.
   • Repeat until the restriction has been resolved.
5. Repeat the above steps, this time progressing from the superior and lateral portion of the body segment to the inferior and medial portion.

Pain Control

Pain reduction obtained from massage is the result of several different mechanisms, but the primary effect is derived through the stimulation of cutaneous sensory receptors, activating the spinal gate and the release of endogenous opiates. The benefits of massage-mediated pain reduction can last up to 24 hours after the treatment.[81]

Mechanical pain is reduced through interrupting muscle spasm and reducing edema. Chemical pain is thought to be diminished by increasing blood flow and by encouraging the removal of cellular wastes, but these responses are unsubstantiated. However, simply touching the skin can also reduce the pain by activating cutaneous receptors. Gentle massage activates sensory nerves and, therefore, inhibits pain through the gate mechanism.[82, 83] Massage has also been shown to activate the autonomic nervous system and pacinian receptors, both of which assist in hindering nociceptive impulses[78] and decrease H-reflex amplitude of spinal cord–injured patients, but only

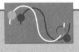

CLINICAL TECHNIQUES: MYOFASCIAL TECHNIQUES: ARM PULL/LEG PULL

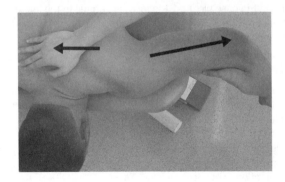

Description

Extremity pulls stretch the fascia first as a single unit and then focus on local areas of adhesion. The theory and technique for the leg pull is similar to the arm pull.

Technique

1. Position the patient supine with the arm relaxed at the side.
2. Grasp the extremity either at the thenar and hypothenar eminence or just proximal to the wrist.
3. Apply a gentle traction force (5 to 10 lb, depending on the size of the patient) that is in line with the anterior deltoid.
4. Hold the stretch until relaxation is felt in the arm.
5. Abduct the shoulder approximately 10 to 15 degrees and repeat the procedure. Continue until full abduction is reached or pain or glenohumeral pathology limits motion.
6. During this process, identify any areas of regional restriction and use the appropriate myofascial techniques to reduce the adhesion.

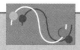

CLINICAL TECHNIQUES: MYOFASCIAL TECHNIQUES: DIAGONAL RELEASE

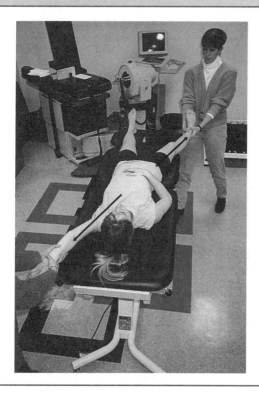

The diagonal release is similar to the arm or leg pull, but affects a larger area of tissue.

Technique

1. Position the patient prone or supine. If the prone position is used, the face should be padded.
2. One clinician grasps the leg just proximal to the talocrural joint.
3. The other clinician grasps the opposite arm proximal to the wrist.
4. Keeping the arm and leg horizontal to each other, one clinician stabilizes the extremity while the other moves the limb until adhesions are felt. A gentle traction force is then applied.
5. Step 4 is repeated until all adhesions have been identified and released (or reduced).
6. Repeat this process with the opposite limb and/or the opposite clinician providing the stabilizing force.

during the actual massage administration.[84, 85] Massage has not been shown to significantly affect serum levels of endogenous opiates, such as β-endorphin, in a treatment group compared with a control group.[86] Further pain reduction may occur secondary to mediation of neural reflexes.[87]

Psychological Benefits

Despite the lack of empirical evidence for many of the physiological benefits that are claimed to be associated with massage, support for the psychological benefits does exist. Much of this benefit extends from the one-on-one interaction required between the clinician and the patient.[82, 88] This interaction reduces patient anxiety, depression, and mental stress.[69, 89] Although pain reduction can be attributed to stimulation of sensory nerves and decreased spasticity within the treated area, administering massage to uninvolved areas also brings about pain relief.[90] Patient compliance in reporting for treatment sessions is greatly enhanced when massage is included as a part of the treatment regimen.[91]

■ Contraindications to Therapeutic Massage

Therapeutic massage is contraindicated in acute injury or inflammation, including sprains, fractures, joint disloca-

tions, and other conditions in which the pressure or motion would worsen the condition. Massage should not be applied directly to open skin wounds or skin conditions (e.g., cellulitis, dermatitis) that should not be touched otherwise or infected areas. Vascular conditions in which direct pressure on the vessels should be avoided or the pressure could loosen a clot are also contraindications to therapeutic massage (see At a Glance: Therapeutic Massage, p 306). Massage is not indicated for the reduction of all forms of edema. Acute edema could cause more inflammation and more swelling. Swelling caused by cardiovascular insufficiency, kidney or liver disease, or pleural effusion is contraindicated.

■ Controversies in Treatment

Massage is often therapeutic because of its "healing touch" effect, spiritual aspects, and other emotional or cognitive effects. As such, the holistic benefits of this treatment approach should not be discounted. However, empirical evidence does call into question many of the effects attributed to therapeutic massage.

The effects of massage on blood flow are unclear. Massaging the forearm and quadriceps muscle groups with effleurage, pétrissage, and tapotement failed to increase the arterial blood flow supplying these groups.[92] Massage before submaximal treadmill testing revealed no significant differences in cardiac output, blood pressure, and lactic acid concentration in a treatment group

Treatment Strategies
Edema Reduction Massage

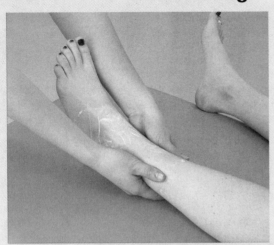

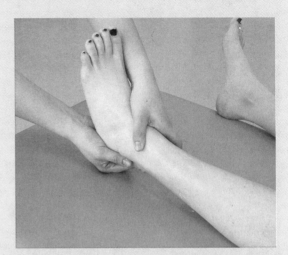

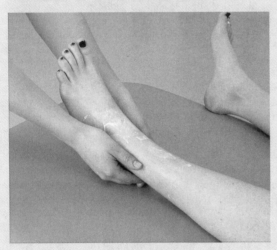

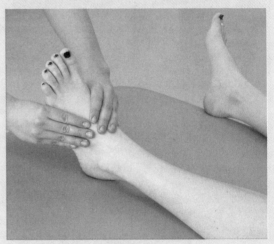

Edema reduction massage is begun proximal to the swollen area, progressing distally to the edema, and then works proximally again, repeating as many times as needed. This effect, "uncorking the bottle," increases lymphatic uptake and venous flow by first mobilizing the proximal fluids, thus allowing the distal edema to flow proximally.

1. Elevate the body part to be treated using an incline board, pillow, or other device.
2. Cover the entire surface to be treated with a lubricating massage lotion.

3. Position yourself distal to the limb. For example, if the ankle is being massaged, stand so that you see the bottom of the foot.
4. Begin by making long, slow strokes toward the heart, starting proximal to the injured area. Every fourth or fifth stroke, move the starting point of the massage slightly distal.
5. Continue stroking longitudinally, with the starting point gradually being moved distally.
6. When the distal portion of the edematous area is reached, begin working back to the original starting point.

compared with a group receiving no massage before testing.[93]

Although massage is often used before athletic competition to improve performance, a study examining the effects of massage before competition concluded that this technique does not significantly increase the stride frequen-

cy of sprinters.[94] Massaging muscles between exercise bouts, be it a sprinter's legs between races or a pitcher's shoulder between innings, does little to reduce muscular fatigue.[75, 95] However, psychological benefits may still be gained from these techniques.

Athletic activity may result in muscle damage,

delayed-onset muscle soreness, and decreased strength, conditions for which massage is often used to treat. However, it appears that "sports massage" techniques fail to address any of these detrimental effects [96] and do not significantly reduce blood lactate concentration.[97]

Recovery from exercise does not appear to be enhanced following massage treatment. Massage has little physiological effect on blood lactate concentrations or other metabolic byproducts [92, 93, 97] and no effect on delayed-onset muscle soreness.[98] Low-intensity active exercises such as stationary bike riding or walking should be used to accelerate the removal of the metabolic byproducts of exercise.[97]

Although anecdotal evidence indicates otherwise, transverse friction massage has not been found to be effective in the treatment of iliotibial band friction syndrome [65] or lateral epicondylitis during controlled studies.[99]

■ Preparation

To be performed properly, the patient must be comfortably positioned and, if applicable, a massage lubricant must be used. Before administering the massage, the patient must be appropriately draped for modesty and the area to be treated must be exposed.

Massage Media

Most massages incorporate some type of lubricant to decrease the friction between the patient's skin and the hand; however, massage can be given without any lubricant being used. Lubricants, including massage lotion, peanut oil, coconut oil, powder, and even counterirritants allow the hands to glide smoothly over the skin and focus the effects on the underlying muscle. If the massage is being given over hairy areas, lubricants are needed to keep from pulling body hair.

The least amount of massage lubricant required to perform the massage should be applied to the patient. Using too much lubricant makes it difficult to adequately manipulate the tissues. Too little lubricant can cause skin irritation or pull the patient's body hair. Patients who have dry skin require that lubricant be added throughout the course of the treatment. Lubricant should not be applied to the face.

Various massage and myofascial release techniques are enhanced when performed without the use of a lubricant. In addition, friction assists in mobilizing the skin over the underlying tissues, making the use of lubricants contraindicated with this style of massage.

Tables and Chairs

Specialized massage tables that have a cutout to comfortably fit the patient's face and upper extremities can be used for treatment. Standard treatment plinths can also be used, but a face bolster or rolled towel should be used when the patient is placed prone. Massage chairs can be used for

thoracic, cervical spine, and upper extremity massage sessions (Fig. 16–2).

■ Clinical Application of Massage

Massage is as much an art as it is a science. There are multiple ways to perform therapeutic massage, but most sessions begin with warming, superficial strokes and conclude with slow, superficial strokes. The proportion of strokes and techniques used in the remainder of the session is based on the patient's pathology and the desired treatment outcomes.

General Considerations

1. Establish the absence of contraindications.
2. Explain the type of massage that will be applied and the expected sensations.
3. If an adjustable-height table is being used, the height should allow the clinician to keep the spine straight during the massages. Any bending or motion should occur at the knees, not at the waist.
4. Cover the table with a sheet.
5. The position of the patient relative to the clinician is important to both parties. When treating small areas the clinician should stand in a place that requires little or no repositioning. Likewise, long strokes, such as those applied to the back or hamstrings, should be performed by taking small steps rather than by bending the back.
6. Position the patient so that the muscles being massaged are relaxed. If an extremity is being massaged to reduce edema, it should be elevated.
7. If a massage lubricant is being used, warm it slightly between the hands so that it is not uncomfortable when applied (i.e., not too hot or too cold). Then spread the lubricant on the skin. Do not pour the lubricant directly on the body.
8. When a painful area is being treated, the massage begins in a nonpainful area, works through the area of pain, and concludes on another pain-free area.
9. Drape the patient to ensure modesty and expose the area to be treated.

Traditional Massage

1. The area may be preheated with moist heat to promote relaxation of the musculature.
2. A bolser may be placed under the ankles and a small pad, such as a folded towel or small pillow, placed under the abdomen to assist in the relaxation of the lumbar musculature.
3. If applicable, apply the massage lubricant on the body parts to be treated.

At a Glance: **Therapeutic Massage**

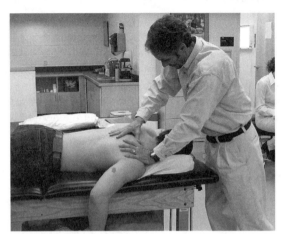

Description

Massage uses touch to produce muscular, nervous, and cardiovascular changes. Targeted techniques are used to break up adhesions and muscle spasm. Therapeutic massage is used for:

Painful conditions of musculoskeletal origin
Muscle strains
Muscle spasm
Muscular/fascial adhesions
Trigger point therapy

Primary Effects

- Increased blood flow
- Increased venous and lymphatic drainage
- Sedation of nerve endings
- Elongation of muscle fibers and other soft tissue
- Decreased muscle tone
- Feeling of wellbeing

Treatment Duration

- The duration of the massage ranges from a few minutes up to an hour.
- Massage for edema reduction is given once a day for an average duration of 5 to 10 minutes.
- Friction massage is performed once a day for 5 minutes or as needed.

Indications

- To relieve fibrosis
- To increase venous return
- Reduction of lymphatic or venous edema
- To break the pain-spasm-pain cycle
- To evoke systemic relaxation
- To improve or stimulate local blood flow
- To increase range of motion

Contraindications

- Acute sprains or strains
- Areas of active inflammation
- Sites where fractures have failed to heal
- Skin conditions in area to be treated
- Open wounds in the area to be treated
- Infection causing **lymphangitis** ■
- Phlebitis or thrombophlebitis
- Varicose veins
- Arteriosclerosis
- Cellulitis
- Abscess or other forms of infection

Precautions

- Massage may increase the inflammatory response when used early in the acute or subacute stage of the injury response cycle.
- Use decreased pressure when applying massage over areas having decreased sensation.
- Do not use massage for swelling caused by cardiovascular insufficiency, kidney or liver disease, or pleural effusion.

Lymphangitis: Inflammation of the lymphatic vessels draining an extremity. This condition is most often associated with inflammation or infection.

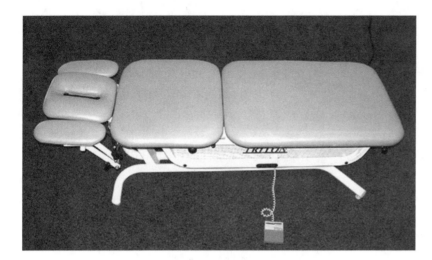

Figure 16–2. **Massage Table and Chair.**

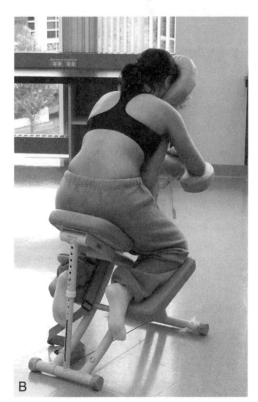

B

4. Follow the application of the lubricant with a light, slow effleurage.
5. Gradually build up to deeper effleurage.
6. Begin pétrissage strokes.
7. Using a towel, wipe the lubricant off the patient's skin before applying deep friction massage where (and if) applicable.
8. Apply tapotement to the back and extremities (if treated).
9. Reapply pétrissage and deep effleurage.
10. End the treatment with light effleurage.

Termination of the Treatment

1. If a lubricant was used, remove it with a towel.
2. If appropriate for the stage of injury, encourage active range-of-motion exercises.
3. Following edema reduction massage, apply a compression wrap and keep the extremity elevated whenever possible.
4. To assist in flushing metabolic waste from the body, the patient should be encouraged to drink water after the treatment.
5. Remove the sheet from the table and launder properly.

● Chapter Highlights

- Massage can be invigorating or relaxing, depending on the type, depth, rate, and intensity of the strokes used.
- Effleurage is the stroking of the skin. Deep stroking encourages venous return. Superficial stroking promotes relaxation.
- Pétrissage is the lifting and kneading of the skin that separates muscle fiber, scar tissue, and fascia.
- Friction massage is used to break up adhesions and to reduce trigger points.
- Tapotement is the shaking or pounding of the skin.
- Vibration is the rapid shaking of the skin to increase blood flow.
- Myofascial release is a targeted technique that breaks fascial adhesions.
- Although the primary benefit of most types of massage carries a large psychological component, it is effective in reducing edema, breaking muscle spasm, and diminishing pain.

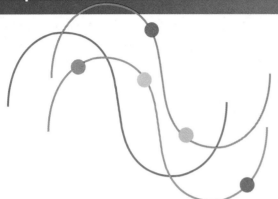

Chapter 17

Cervical and Lumbar Traction

Conceptually, traction devices are best thought of as causing elongation of the soft tissues. Cervical and lumbar traction are applications of a force that separates the vertebrae and opens the intervertebral space in the treated area. The increased space reduces pressure on the intervertebral discs and spinal nerve roots, opens the facet joints, and elongates the soft tissue.

Traction is a technique that applies a longitudinal force to the spine and associated structures, distracting the vertebrae. The distractive force can be administered by gravity (weights or body weight), a machine, the clinician, or by the position of the patient's body. Mechanical force can be applied with continuous or intermittent tension by several different methods. The force of the traction can occur in one plane or multiple planes (polyaxial traction).

Traction is indicated in conditions in which the patient's pain is caused by mechanical pressure on the vertebrae, facet joints, or spinal nerve roots, or other conditions in which removing the mechanical stress results in pain reduction. Unless specifically prescribed by a physician, traction should not be used for acute injuries, hypermobile vertebrae, or other instances when the stability of the vertebral column is in question.

Traction, immobilization, and bed rest were once the common treatments of choice for spinal and back pain. Contemporary practice frequently emphasizes active exercise with traction being used to provide short-term, mechanical relief of pressure placed on nerve roots, articular facets, and other structures.

■ Principles of Traction

The effect and effectiveness of traction is related to the position of the body part, the position of the patient, the force and duration of the traction, and the angle of pull.[100] To distract the vertebrae, the force of the applied traction must be sufficient to overcome the sum of resistance of the weight of the body part being treated, the tension of the surrounding soft tissues, the force of friction between the patient and the table, and the force of gravity. Friction is negligible during cervical traction and lumbar/pelvic traction when a split table is used. Gravity works against traction on the cervical spine when the patient is seated; when the patient is supine, gravity is not a factor.

Traction is an appropriate treatment modality for hypomobile vertebrae. Traction should not be used in the presence of hypermobility of vertebral segments. The tension may lead to subluxation or dislocation of the vertebra or further increase the hypermobility of the segment.

Types of Traction

Traction can either be applied continuously or intermittently. **Sustained traction** maintains the cervical or lumbar spine in an elongated position and is applied with relatively small force for an extended period, usually 45 minutes or less. This method of application stimulates the supporting and stabilizing functions of the structures and, by assisting in support of the spinal segment, allows the musculature to "relax." **Continuous traction** is used to describe tension that does not change over the course of hours.

Sustained traction is applied through a weight-and-pulley system, pneumatic system, motorized device, or patient positioning. **Manual traction** is administered by the clinician. During **auto-traction** the patient controls the amount of traction applied.

Intermittent traction alternates periods of traction force with intervals of relaxation in the tension by way of an **ON/OFF duty cycle**. During the ON cycle, the vertebral segments are distracted and the soft tissues are elongated. The OFF or relaxation phase allows a relative decrease in the amount of neuromuscular activity. Intermittent traction is most commonly applied through the use of a motorized system or manually by the clinician (Fig. 17–1).

The patient may also self-administer **positional traction** techniques (Fig. 17–2). Body position is used to elongate—stretch—the involved tissues or reduce pressure on the vertebral structures.

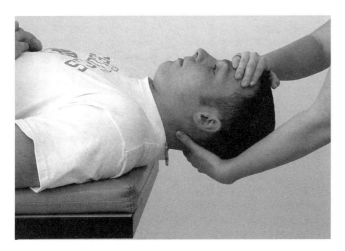

Figure 17–1. **Manual Cervical Traction.** The clinician grasps the patient's occiput to apply traction along the length of the entire cervical spine.

Angle of Pull

The angle of the applied traction is described relative to the long axis of the vertebral column and must be appropriate for the pathology being treated. The resulting angle is then described as neutral (transverse plane), flexion or extension (frontal plane), or unilateral (sagittal plane). Multiaxial (sometimes referred to as polyaxial) traction applies a distractive force in both the frontal and sagittal plane.

Applying an equal amount of tension on the right and left side of the body should result in an approximately equal amount of separation on both sides of the vertebrae. Unilateral muscle spasm and adhesions can cause increased opening on the noninvolved side when traction is applied; unilateral soft tissue laxity can result in increased opening on the involved side. This method of traction is used when lateral bending of the spine reduces the patient's symptoms.

Patient positioning or the use of a polyaxial harness can intentionally increase the unilateral opening of the vertebrae. This method increases the amount of tension applied to the structures on the right or left side of the vertebrae and is useful with unilateral facet joint pathology, nerve root impingement, or muscle spasm. Unilateral traction can often be achieved simply through patient positioning.

The effect of the angle of pull on the facet joints differs between the cervical and lumbar spine. The cervical inferior facet joints are angled anteriorly; in the lumbar spine, they are angled posteriorly. Placing the cervical spine in flexion opens the facet joints and increases the intervertebral space, but too much flexion will result in a decrease in the anterior portion. Because the lumbar facets are angled posteriorly, placing the lumbar spine in extension will open the facet joints. When the traction is applied in the neutral position, the intervertebral disc is allowed to elongate.

Tension

The amount of tension applied to the body can be expressed in terms of pounds (or kilograms) or as a percentage of the patient's body weight. In addition to gravity, friction, and body weight, the force of the traction is absorbed and dissipated by the patient's muscle tone and soft tissue tension. Less force is needed to distract the cervical spine than the lumbar spine. The vertebrae closest to the source of the traction, C1-C2 during cervical traction for example, require less force to separate than those distal to the harness.

There is no clear formula used to determine the amount of tension to apply during the treatment. The general guideline is to use the least amount of tension needed to relieve the symptoms or produce the desired effects. The intensity of the traction should be inversely related to the duration of the treatment. Patients can tolerate more tension if the duration of the traction is reduced.

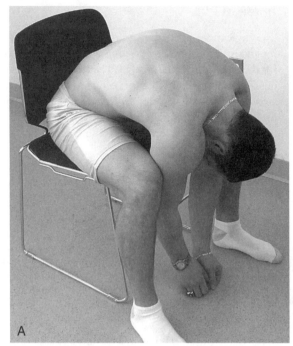
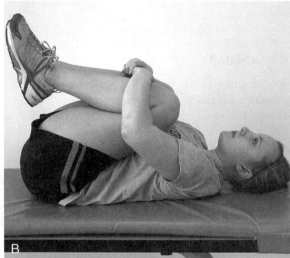

Figure 17–2. **Positional Traction Techniques.** (A) For the thoracic and cervical spine. (B) For the lumbar spine.

As we all know, more is not always better. This is certainly the case with traction, especially in the presence of unstable joints. Too much force can produce muscle guarding or can further injure the soft tissue. As discussed in the following section, too much force or too great a treatment duration can cause an overhydration of the intervertebral discs and increase their chance of rupture.[101]

■ General Uses for Cervical and Lumbar Traction

The fundamental effects of cervical traction and lumbar traction are essentially the same and arise from the distraction of the vertebral segments. Before significant bony separation can occur, the force of the traction must first overcome the resistance exerted by the soft tissues. The benefits of traction tend to be short-lived but may be sufficient to break the pain cycle.

The common effects are presented in this section, and specific effects or influences are described in the appropriate section. Table 17–1 presents general treatment parameters for various spinal pathologies.

Disc Protrusions

Disc protrusions can place pressure on a spinal nerve root, usually the one immediately below the involved disc. Because of their anatomical structure and high water content, discs have the ability to deform (Box 17–1). In the presence of a disc protrusion, body weight (through gravity) and muscle tone compress the disc and force the **nucleus pulposus ■** outward (Fig. 17–3).

Traction affects the discs by decreasing the pressure caused by gravity and the soft tissues. Given sufficient tension, the vertebrae separate and elongate the discs. Negative pressure within the disc removes the forces on the nucleus pulposus, thereby decreasing pressure on the nerve root (Fig. 17–4). Pressure from the posterior longitudinal ligament as it tightens may also force the pulposus inward.[105] Acute disc injuries respond better to traction than chronic lesions.[106] A displaced disc fragment may also be allowed to realign itself on the disc—and subsequently heal—by reducing the pressure and increasing the disc's hydration.

Disc compression is also often reproduced by patient positioning. In Figure 17–4A, if the patient flexes the spine as when bending over, the nucleus pulposus will be forced posteriorly and place pressure on the nerve root. If the symptoms move outwardly (peripheralization), that position should be avoided during treatment. The patient should be taught to always change positions or avoid activities that cause the peripheralization of symptoms.

Traction applied for too long can cause the disc to absorb too much fluid (imbibe). Similarly to an overfilled water balloon, an overly hydrated disc may be predisposed to rupture.[101] Sustained traction can also increase the amount of pressure at the end of the treatment, especially if the tension is not gradually reduced.

Nucleus pulposus: The gelatinous middle of an intervertebral disk.

TABLE 17–1	Guidelines for the Treatment of Various Pathologies with Traction	
Pathology	*Angle*	*Type*
Facet joint	Cervical: Flexion Lumbar: Extension Unilateral (if pathology is unilateral)	Intermittent
Intervertebral space (e.g., degenerative disc disease)	Cervical: Flexion (too much will result in decreased anterior space) Lumbar: Neutral	Sustained
Nerve root impingement	Bilateral: Neutral Unilateral: Neutral with spine laterally flexed to the opposite side	Sustained
Disc protrusion	Extension, neutral, or flexion (based on pain relief obtained)	Intermittent
Muscle spasm	Position the traction to elongate the affected tissues Bilateral—Equal Unilateral—Unilateral	Sustained

Degenerative Disc Disease and Nerve Root Compression

Degenerative disc disease is the gradual, progressive wasting of the intervertebral discs. As the discs lose their mass, the space between the discs decreases (Box 17–2). With time, the vertebrae begin to form spurs and other **osteophytes** ■, causing the vertebral column to straighten, creating a "bamboo pole" appearance (Fig. 17–5).

Increasing the intervertebral space opens the intervertebral foramen and reduces the amount of pressure on the nerve root. Removing the mechanical pressure on the nerve root allows the opportunity for inflammation of the nerve root to decrease. Further nerve root compression can be prevented by reducing adhesions within the dural sleeve by elongating the surrounding structure.[106] In the lumbar nerve roots, traction can also reduce radicular symptoms by restoring the normal slack in the neuromeningeal structures.[107]

Facet Joint Pathology

The inferior facet of the superior vertebrae articulates with the superior facet of the vertebrae below (see Box 17–2). The facet joints significantly contribute to the spine's motion and decrease the stress placed on the vertebral

bodies and discs. In healthy vertebrae, approximately 20 percent of the spine's weight-bearing load is transmitted through the facet joints. When the facet joints are inflamed, up to 47 percent of the load is transmitted by these joints in the lumbar spine.[108]

When the angle of pull places the lumbar spine in extension or the cervical spine in flexion, the resulting tension opens the facet joints. Hypomobility of the facet joints can be reduced by placing the spine in neutral. The resulting traction produces glide between the superior and inferior facets.

In the lumbar spine, approximately twice the tension required to elongate the lumbar spine is required to distract the facet joints.[109] Although less tension would be required in the cervical spine, the proportions of force required to obtain facet distraction would be expected to be reduced. The resulting reduced load can decrease inflammation and other compressive problems.

Muscle Spasm

Traction may be useful in the relief of muscle spasm caused by nerve root impingement or arising from postural disorders. Long, slow stretching can reduce tonic muscle contractions by elongating the involved fibers.[106] Stimulating the muscle's mechanoreceptors can decrease pain and spasm by activating the spinal gate.[107] Intermittent traction promotes relaxation during the OFF phase. Decreased pressure on the spinal nerve roots achieved by increasing the diameter of the intervertebral foramen also results in decreased muscle spasm (see Degenerative Disc Disease and Nerve Root Compression).

Other Effects

Although largely unsubstantiated, traction may also provide other benefits to the paraspinal structures. Improved circulation, increased metabolism, and enhanced nutrition of the structures have all been attributed to the application of cervical or lumbar traction.[105, 106, 110]

▶ CERVICAL TRACTION

The human head accounts for approximately 8.1 percent of the total body weight (approximately 14 lb for the average adult), but more force is needed to produce widening of the vertebral structures because of the cervical musculature and other soft tissues. For most pathologies, separation of the cervical spine begins to occur with an applied force equal to about 20 percent of the body weight with the patient reclined.[111] When the patient is in the seated, gravity-dependent position, a greater proportion of the total body weight is required before separation occurs. The effect of friction during cervical traction is, for the most part, negligible.

Osteophyte: A branching bony outgrowth.

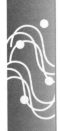

Box 17-1. Intervertebral Discs and Disc Lesions

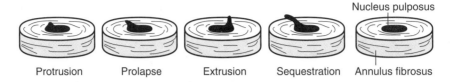

Protrusion   Prolapse   Extrusion   Sequestration   Annulus fibrosus

Nucleus pulposus

Vertebral discs consist of two distinct portions. The outer portion of the disc, the annulus fibrosus, is a relatively inflexible, dense, collagen-rich substance. The middle section, the nucleus pulposus, is a shock-absorbing material having a gelatinous consistency. Each disc is composed of 60 to 70 percent water, allowing it to be deformable, yet not easily compressed.[102]

During the day, the weight of the body slowly compresses the discs, causing them to dehydrate. At night–or when the body is reclined for long periods–the load is taken off the discs, they expand and reabsorb fluids. For this reason, you are slightly taller in the morning than at night.[103] Over time the discs also lose proteoglycan, a molecule that attracts and retains water. The discs become more and more dehydrated between the ages of 40 to 60, resulting in decreased range of motion and a narrowing of the intervertebral **foramen** ■.[104]

Dehydration also weakens the annulus fibrosus, which allows the nucleus pulposus to protrude through and place pressure on the spinal nerve root. Protrusions, as used in this chapter, describe anything from a bulge in the disc to a complete rupture of the disc where the nucleus pulposus exits the disc. A definitive **diagnosis** ■ of these conditions is made using an MRI, CT scan, or other imaging technique.

Traction helps reduce disc protrusions by separating the vertebrae, creating negative pressure within the disc, causing the nucleus pulposus to retreat away from the spinal nerve root and spinal cord.

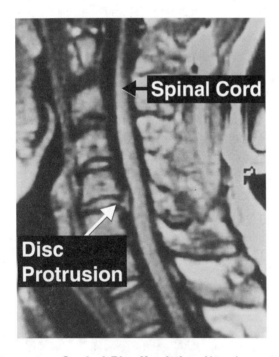

Figure 17-3. **Cervical Disc Herniation.** Note the posterior protrusion of the nucleus pulposus that places pressure on the spinal cord. Cervical traction can decrease the amount of pressure caused by a disc herniation.

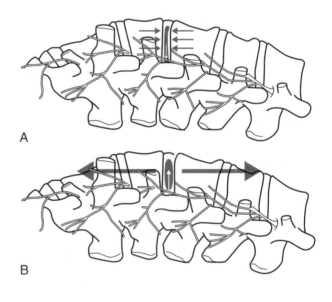

Figure 17-4. **Nerve Root Compression Caused by a Disc Protrusion.** (A) When the vertebrae are load-bearing, the intervertebral disc compresses, forcing the nucleus pulposus posteriorly and laterally outward (similar to squeezing a tube of toothpaste), often placing pressure on a spinal nerve root. (B) Removing the weight-bearing forces causes the pulposus to return into the disc and relieve pressure on the nerve root.

Diagnosis: A physician's determination of the nature and scope of an injury or illness.

Foramen: An opening (e.g., in a bone) to allow the passage of blood vessels or nerves.

Box 17–2. Stenosis of the Intervertebral Foramen

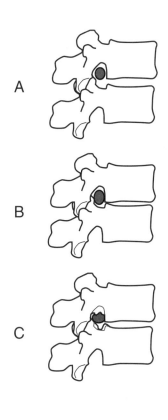

Thirty-one pairs of spinal nerve roots branch off the spinal cord, 8 in the cervical region, 12 in the thoracic region, 5 in the lumbar spine, and 6 in the sacrum. In the mobile spine, these roots exit the vertebral column via the intervertebral foramen, an opening formed by pairs of notches on the inferior surface of one vertebra with a corresponding notch on the superior surface of the vertebrae below. The intervertebral foramen normally allows plenty of room for the nerve root to exit between the vertebrae (Fig. A).

A narrowing of the intervertebral space, the area between the vertebral bodies, such as in the case of disc degeneration (see Box 17–1) can cause a decrease in the diameter of the intervertebral foramen (Fig. B). In some instances, this narrowing is sufficient to produce **radicular** ■ symptoms along the involved nerve root's distribution.

Changes in the weight-bearing load on the vertebral bodies and the facet joints and biomechanical changes can result in the formation of osteophytes (Fig. C). The presence of this bony outgrowth not only decreases the size of the intervertebral foramen, it can cause inflammation of the nerve's sheath. Inflamed nerves occupy more space than healthy nerves, thus increasing the chance of impingement.

Although stenosis of the intervertebral foramen can occur at any level, this condition is most prevalent in the cervical and lumbar regions.

Motorized units can be used to administer intermittent or sustained traction. Intermittent traction may be delivered manually (see Figure 17–1). Sustained traction can also be administered through a weight-and-pulley system or by a pneumatic device (Fig. 17–6).

Mechanical traction is applied to the cervical spine via a harness affixed to the skull. There are two basic types of harnesses: the mandibular-occipital harness and the occipital harness (Fig. 17–7). The mandibular-occipital harness can place too much pressure on the temporomandibular joint (TMJ) and may cause discomfort, especially if there is a preexisting TMJ pathology. Occipital halters place all of the force on the skull's occipital bone and can place the cervical spine in various degrees of flexion, extension, or lateral bending. Other specific styles of halters are designed to allow for specificity of

spinal separation at a lower percentage of the body weight.[112]

■ Treatment Parameters

This section describes the variables in patient positioning and the type and amount of traction to be used during cervical traction. These variables must be consistent with the pathology being treated. Refer to Table 17–1 for general treatment guidelines for common pathologies. Except for where noted, this section refers to mechanical traction techniques.

Patient Position

Cervical traction may be applied with the patient in one of several positions, but the two most common are the seated and supine positions. When the patient is in a seated

---

Radicular: Distally radiating pain caused by spinal nerve root involvement.

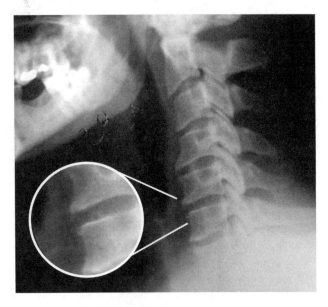

Figure 17-5. **Radiographic View of Degenerative Disc Disease.** Note the absence of the normal spinal curvature and the "beaking" appearance of the anterior and posterior aspects of the vertebral bodies (inset).

position, the traction must first overcome the force of gravity before therapeutic forces are placed on the cervical region. Because of this, more tension is required to separate the vertebrae when the patient is seated than when the patient is horizontal.

The supine position has several advantages. With the patient supine, the cervical musculature is allowed to relax because it is not supporting the weight of the head.

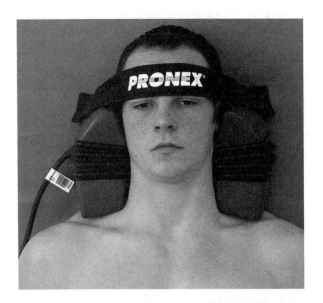

Figure 17-6. **Sustained Traction Using Pneumatic Pressure.** This method has the advantage over door-mounted units because the patient is placed in the horizontal, gravity-eliminated position. (Pronex courtesy of Glacier Cross, Inc., Kalispell, MT.)

Therefore, a lower amount of tension is required to obtain therapeutic effects.

Angle of Pull

To open the intervertebral space, place the cervical spine in approximately 25 to 30 degrees of flexion. This position straightens the normal cervical **lordosis ■** and allows the posterior articulations to open, widening the intervertebral foramen and stretching the posterior soft tissue. The anterior portion of an intervertebral disc is compressed, and the posterior portion elongates when the neck is placed in flexion. When the cervical spine is placed in extension, the opposite effect occurs. To separate the facet joint surfaces, the traction must be administered in at least 15 degrees of flexion (Table 17–2).[113]

Tension

Although treatment bouts with cervical traction can last for hours, the mechanical benefits appear to occur in the first few minutes of treatment.[114] When the patient is placed supine, vertebral separation begins when tension equal to 7 percent of the patient's body weight is applied.[130] Because of the weight of the structures and associated soft tissue, the upper vertebrae, C1-C2, require less force to separate than the lower cervical spine. The least amount of force necessary to produce the desired effects (e.g., decrease in symptoms) should be used.

The force applied to the cervical spine during traction has been suspected of being transmitted to the lumbar area through the dural covering of the spinal cord. This can lead to residual lumbar nerve root impingement and subsequent pain, especially when the patient has a history of lumbar osteoarthritis or other lumbar degenerative changes.[100] During the treatment, question the patient about sensations in the cervical, thoracic, and lumbar spine and the extremities.

● EFFECTS ON
The Injury Response Process

The basic effects of cervical traction are similar to those presented in the biophysical effects section of this chapter. The effects and research specifically related to cervical traction are presented in this section.

Application of cervical traction reduces the amount of pressure on nerve roots as a result of mechanical pressure from bony protuberances or intervertebral discs. Elongating the cervical spine allows separation of the vertebrae and can decompress the structures.

Intermittent cervical traction is incorporated into the treatment plan to reduce the pain and paresthesia associated with cervical nerve root impingement, muscle spasm, or articular dysfunction. The most significant improve-

---

Lordosis: The forward curvature of the cervical and lumbar spine.

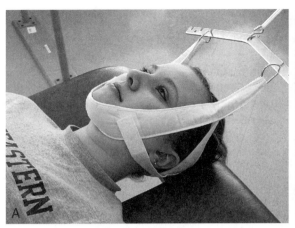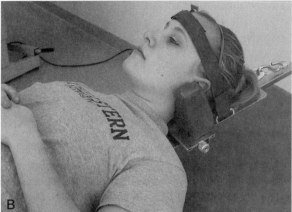

Figure 17–7. **Harnesses Used During the Application of Mechanical Cervical Traction.**
(A) Mandibular-occipital harness. (B) Occipital harness.

ments are seen in patients who had symptoms for less than 12 weeks.[105] This passive treatment can be combined with active exercise to enhance the benefits of the treatment.

■ Muscle Spasm

Traction is often applied in an effort to interrupt the pain-spasm-pain cycle through lengthening of the affected musculature. An analysis of **electromyograms** ■ follow-

ing treatment bouts of intermittent cervical traction showed no decrease in the amount of spasm in the treated tissues when compared with pretreatment activity.[111, 115, 116] However, another study did show reduced excitability of the alpha-motoneuron pool.[117]

The reduction of cervical muscle spasm is contingent on finding the optimal amount of traction force. Too little force will not sufficiently elongate the musculature or open the intervertebral foramen, and little or no benefit will be

		Traction Angle		
Structure	*Spinal Segment*	*Neutral*	*30° Flexion*	*15° Extension*
Anterior intervertebral separation	C2-3	6%	21%	2%
	C3-4	8%	10%	−1%
	C4-5	12%	16%	−1%
	C5-6	5%	15%	−2%
	C6-7	0%	9%	−2%
Posterior intervertebral separation	C2-3	15%	5%	4%
	C3-4	22%	4%	−14%
	C4-5	19%	17%	−26%
	C5-6	19%	19%	−37%
	C6-7	37%	20%	−50%
Facet joint separation	C2-3	2%	−12%	7%
	C3-4	2%	−14%	3%
	C4-5	5%	−19%	15%
	C5-6	3%	−10%	17%
	C6-7	10%	−5%	6%

TABLE 17–2   Amount of Cervical Intervertebral Separation Based on the Angle of Traction

Negative percentages indicate a decrease in the intervertebral space.
Source: Adapted from Wong, AM, et al: Clinical trial of a cervical traction modality with electromyographic biofeedback. Am J Phys Med Rehabil 76:19, 1997.

Electromyogram: A recording of the electrical charges associated with the contraction of a muscle.

gained. If too much force is applied, an unwanted muscle contraction will ensue as the body attempts to protect itself, resulting in the opposite effect of that desired.

■ Pain

In addition to breaking the pain-spasm-pain cycle, as described in the previous section, several other factors have been associated with the reduction of pain. Traction can reduce pain by decreasing the amount of mechanical pressure placed on the cervical nerve roots. Intermittent traction is thought to improve blood flow and to decrease myofascial adhesions. This same rhythm may also stimulate joint and muscular sensory nerves and inhibit the transmission of pain through the gate mechanism.[118]

Cervical traction decreases the radicular symptoms associated with cervical nerve root impingement.[106] If the pain results from a disc lesion, the bulging nucleus pulposus is encouraged to centralize or return to its normal position. Although a disc lesion is not normally responsive to intermittent traction, sustained traction can provide the time necessary for reabsorption of the nucleus pulposus.

■ Contraindications to the Use of Cervical Traction

Clinical cervical traction is absolutely contraindicated in the presence of vertebral fracture or dislocation. The exception to this is the use of traction immobilization such as a halo splint applied by a physician. All acute cervical spine trauma should be evaluated by a physician to rule out fractures, dislocations, or other spinal instability before clinical treatment (see At a Glance: Cervical Traction). Unless specifically ordered by a physician, cervical traction should not be used on patients with diseases, infection, or tumors that affect the cervical vertebrae. Care must also be taken to avoid cervical motions that are contraindicated.

Traction applied to hypermobile joints can elongate the stabilizing tissues and lead to increased instability.[107] Traction should not be used with severe disc herniations because of the possibility of increasing the rate of degeneration. Rheumatoid arthritis and osteoarthritis are contraindications because necrosis can cause ligamentous weakness. The force of the applied traction could result in vertebral subluxation or dislocation and further weaken the soft tissue structures.

Vertebral artery dysfunction is a contraindication to cervical traction, by using unilateral or polyaxial techniques. Cervical traction should not be used on patients who experience dizziness during treatment or when the head is extended or rotated, or who demonstrate a positive vertebral artery test.

Initial treatments should be administered with relatively low tension to determine the patient's response. Discontinue the use of traction if the patient's symptoms increase or if new symptoms develop.

Occiput: The posterior base of the skull.

■ Controversies in Treatment

Although the effects of patient position and angle of pull on the vertebrae have been substantiated, the other treatment parameters are less clear. The exact amount of tension and the duration of the treatment are relatively undefined. Parameters used for individual patients are often derived by trial and error. For this reason, patient interviews to determine the effects of the treatment take on an added level of importance in determining the protocol.

Studies investigating the effects of lumbar and cervical traction indicate that this treatment approach is no better or worse than other modalities in reducing the symptoms of disc compression, but patients receiving treatment showed improvements versus those not receiving treatment.[110] The actual amount of reabsorption of the cervical nucleus pulposus has not been established.

■ Clinical Application of Intermittent Cervical Traction

The following protocol describes the set-up and application of motorized intermittent cervical traction with the patient in a reclined position. Manual traction may be used before mechanized traction to determine the potential benefits of the treatment.

■ Instrumentation

Refer to the operator's manual for the particular unit being used.

Mode: This setting allows the traction to be applied intermittently or continuously.

Type: For multipurpose units that treat both the lumbar and cervical spine. If "Cervical" is selected, the TYPE function presets a maximum amount of tension that can be produced.

Hold time: This control adjusts the duration of the traction phase (in seconds).

Rest time: This control adjusts the duration of the relaxation phase (in seconds). It is applicable only to intermittent traction.

Tension: Controls the amount of tension, in pounds, applied to the halter.

Low tension: Sets the minimum amount of tension to be applied during the OFF cycle.

Duration: Selects the total treatment time.

Harness (halter): The "standard" halter applies force to the mandible and **occiput ■**. Modified halters have been designed that place the force on the occiput and may allow specificity regarding the cervical level where the separation occurs, and decrease the forces placed on the TMJ (see Fig. 17–7).

At a Glance: **Cervical Traction**

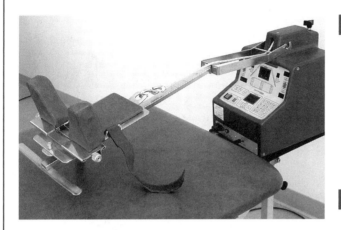

Description

Cervical traction distracts the cervical vertebrae and can be applied continuously or intermittently. This traction can be delivered by way of a motorized unit, weights, gravity, or manually by the clinician. Cervical traction is used for:

- Radicular pain
- Facet joint pathology limiting range of motion including hypomobile facet joints
- Muscle spasm caused by nerve root impingement
- Degenerative disc disease

Primary Effects

- Elongation of the cervical vertebrae, relieving pressure on the intervertebral discs and assisting in the reabsorption of the nucleus pulposus that places pressure on cervical nerve roots.
- Relieves pressure on the spinal nerve roots caused by narrowing of the intervertebral foramen
- Reduces pressure on the facet joints
- Elongates cervical musculature

Treatment Duration

- Facet joint pathology: 25 min
- Degenerative disc disease: 10 min
- Disc protrusion: 8 to 10 min
- Muscle spasm: 20 min

(Approximate treatment durations)

Indications

- Degenerative disc diseases
- Herniated or protruding intervertebral disc
- Nerve root compression
- Osteoarthritis or facet joint inflammation
- Capsulitis of the vertebral joints
- Pathology of the anterior or posterior longitudinal ligaments
- Cervical muscle spasm

Contraindications

- Acute injury
- Unstable spine
- Diseases affecting the vertebrae or spinal cord, including cancer and **meningitis** ■
- Vertebral fractures
- Extruded disc fragmentation
- Spinal cord compression
- Positive vertebral artery test
- Conditions in which vertebral flexion and/or extension is contraindicated
- Osteoporosis
- Rheumatoid arthritis
- Conditions that worsen after traction treatments or motion

Precautions

- Cervical traction should never be attempted in traumatic conditions that have not been evaluated to rule out a fracture or dislocation.
- The patient must be closely monitored throughout the treatment, and the treatment should be immediately discontinued if symptoms increase or if pain or paresthesia is experienced.
- Improper extension traction can result in a rupture of the cervical esophagus.[119]
- Excessive duration and/or traction weight can cause thrombosis of the internal jugular vein.[120]
- Low tension should be used when hypermobility is present (check with a physician prior to treatment).
- Only sustained or continuous traction should be used when motion is contraindicated.
- Mandibular-occipital harnesses should not be used if the patient is suffering from temporomandibular joint pathology.

Meningitis: Inflammation of the membranes of the brain or spinal cord.

Spreader bar: This device connects the older style halter to the traction device through a pulley cable and prevent the cables from rubbing against the patient's face and ears.

Safety switch: This switch allows the patient to interrupt the treatment and decrease tension.

Alarm: Sounds when the patient triggers the safety switch. Will also sound if the amount of tension selected is too great for the cervical spine or a malfunction is detected by the unit.

■ Set-up and Application

Digital units can display force in pounds (lb) or kilograms (kg). Familiarize yourself with the unit of measure that is used by the facility.

Motorized traction devices should not be used in the presence of flammable gas such as oxygen, nitrous oxide, and many anesthetic gases. The unit may interfere with sensitive electrical equipment.

Patient Preparation

1. Determine the presence of any contraindications.
2. Ascertain the patient's body weight.
3. The cervical musculature may be pretreated with moist heat to decrease muscle spasm.
4. Instruct the patient to remove any earrings, glasses, or other clothing that may interfere with the placement of the halter.
5. Lay the patient on the treatment table in the supine position.
6. Place a pillow or other support under the patient's knees.
7. Ensure that the motor unit is firmly attached to its base.
8. For bilateral traction, position the unit so that the line of pull is aligned with the midline of the body (i.e., so that the head is not laterally flexed). For unilateral traction, adjust the halter or position the patient accordingly.
9. Secure the halter to the cervical region according to the manufacturer's instructions. Normally the pressure points are the on occipital processes. Older style halters also place pressure on the chin. To avoid pressure on the mandible or TMJ, use an occipital harness (see Fig. 17–7).
10. Connect the halter to the spreader bar.
11. Align the unit so that the angle of pull corresponds to the pathology being treated (see Table 17–1).
12. Give the patient the SAFETY switch and explain its purpose and use.
13. Explain to the patient the sensations to be expected during the treatment and to report pain, discomfort, or worsening of symptoms.

Initiation of the Treatment

1. Reset all controls to zero and turn unit ON.
2. If applicable, set the TYPE switch to "Cervical."
3. Remove any slack in the pulley cable.
4. Adjust the RATIO to the appropriate on-off sequence, normally a 3:1 or 4:1 ratio.
5. Adjust the TENSION to approximately 10 pounds or 7 percent of the patient's body weight. If this is the patient's first exposure to intermittent cervical traction, or if the person is displaying apprehension about the treatment, use a lower than normal TENSION.
6. If the control is adjustable, set the LOW tension (this value is often set to zero or 10 percent of the maximum tension).
7. Instruct the patient as to what to expect during the treatment and to inform you if any discomfort is experienced. Explain that the force of the pull is felt at the occiput and not at the chin.
8. Set the appropriate treatment DURATION, and initiate the treatment (refer to Table 17–1).
9. Allow the unit to cycle through its first tension cycle. The TENSION may be gradually increased during subsequent cycles. If pain is experienced at any time during the treatment, decrease the amount of force or discontinue the treatment.
10. Instruct the patient to remain relaxed during both the on and off cycles.
11. If the pressure placed on the mandible causes discomfort in the teeth or TMJ, gauze or a mouthpiece may be placed between the teeth to dissipate the force.
12. At regular intervals, question the patient about abnormal sensations in the cervical, thoracic, and lumbar spine and the extremities.

Termination of the Treatment

1. If the traction unit does not automatically do so, gradually reduce the TENSION over a period of three or four cycles.
2. Gain some slack in the cable and turn the unit off.
3. Remove the SPREADER BAR and HALTER.
4. Question the patient regarding any perceived benefit or complications derived from the treatment.
5. Have the patient remain sitting or lying supine for 5 minutes after the conclusion of the treatment. Record the pertinent information (tension, duration, duty cycle) in the patient's medical file.

■ Maintenance

Discontinue the treatment and turn off the unit if unusual noises, or abnormal function are noticed during the treatment. Contact an authorized technician for service.

After Each Use

1. Clean the unit according to the manufacturer's recommendation.
2. Avoid allowing liquids (including cleaning solutions) from entering the unit.

At Regular Intervals

1. Check the electrical power cord for kinks, frays, or cuts.
2. Check the traction cable for knots, twisting, and if applicable, damage to its protective (usually nylon) coating.
3. Recalibrate the unit. Follow the manufacturer's recommended procedures and timetable for recalibrating the traction device.
4. Clean the harness according to the manufacturer's instructions.

Annual

The traction device must be inspected and serviced by an authorized technician.

▐ LUMBAR TRACTION

To be effective, lumbar traction must overcome the weight of the lower extremities (approximately half of the total body weight), pelvis, and the soft tissue tension produced by the paraspinal muscles and ligaments. As with cervical traction, the benefits of lumbar traction are obtained by separating the lumbar vertebrae. Unlike cervical traction, friction is a strong counterforce against the force of the traction and increases the total amount of tension that must be applied during the treatment. A split table (also referred to as a lumbar traction table) in which the lower extremity portion of the table is free to glide on a track reduces the influence of friction between the body and the table (Fig. 17–8).

Lumbar traction is commonly applied using a motorized unit. Manual traction can be applied using a belt that allows the clinician's body weight to help deliver the force. An optional force meter will assist in delivering more precise tension. Each of these methods requires that the patient wear a pelvic traction harness (also referred to as a pelvic corset) and a thoracic stabilization harness that fixates the patient to the table (Fig. 17–9). The effectiveness of the treatment is diminished if there is not good contact between the harness and the patient's skin.

The patient's body weight can be used to deliver traction to the lumbar spine. Inversion traction—in which the patient is suspended upside down by the ankles or legs—

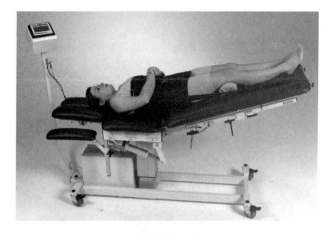

Figure 17–8. **Multiaxial Split Table for Lumbar Traction.** In addition to the lower half of the table gliding on rollers, to eliminate friction and permit vertebral separation to occur at a lower applied force, this unit also flexes, extends, and rotates the lower extremity, allowing for unilateral traction. (Used with permission of The Saunders Group, Inc.)

was a popular method of elongating the lumbar spine. However, this method is hazardous for patients who have hypertension and other cardiovascular disorders and glaucoma.[105]

Gravitational traction can be administered with the patient upright, although some patients find the discomfort caused by the torso harness intolerable.[105] This method does not carry with it the cardiovascular problems associated with inversion traction, only slightly increasing systolic blood pressure and having no effect on diastolic blood pressure. Gravitational traction is capable of increasing the posterior disc space between L1 and S1 (the length of the lumbar spine) by 31 mm.[105]

The patient can also self-administer gravitational traction, called autotraction. Hanging from a bar or supporting the weight of the body on the arms of a chair or between parallel bars while relaxing the spinal muscles can distract the vertebrae (Fig 17–10). This method is, however, limited by the patient's upper body strength.

■ Treatment Parameters

The fundamental parameters for lumbar traction are presented in Table 17–1. The primary difference is the amount of tension required to separate the vertebrae. Except where noted, this section refers to mechanical traction techniques.

Tension

Friction, muscle and soft tissue tension, and the weight of the lower extremity require significantly more tension to separate the lumbar vertebrae than that required for the cervical spine. When lumbar traction is applied using a standard plinth, approximately one half of the force applied is required to overcome the weight of the body

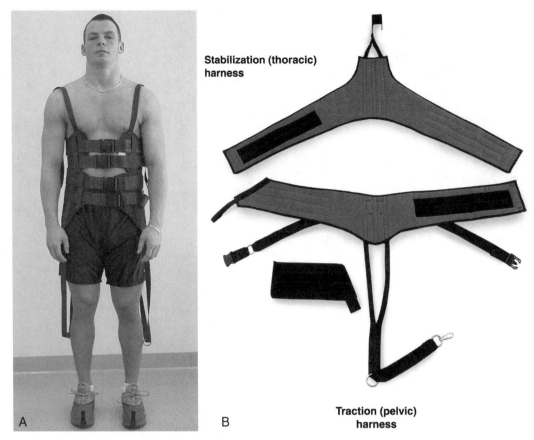

Stabilization (thoracic) harness

Traction (pelvic) harness

A   B

Figure 17–9. **Pelvic and Thoracic Harness Used During Lumbar Traction.** (A) Older style harness using bilateral pulls (note the straps hanging next to each leg). (B) A contemporary harness system that uses a single axis of pull. (B Courtesy of the Chattanooga Group, Hixon, TN.)

part. For example, if a patient's lower extremity and pelvis weighs 100 lb, vertebral separation does not begin until at least 50 lb of tension is applied. Split traction tables remove the effect of friction (see Fig. 17–8).

The range of tension used during lumbar traction is quite variable, and the efficacy of various weights has not been established. Published ranges for the amount of tension used are from 10 to 300 percent of the patient's body weight.[107, 121]

Over 90 percent of the increase in intervertebral separation occurs during the first 15 minutes of static traction.[105, 121] After 25 minutes of static traction, mean torso length increased by an average of 8.9 mm.[121]

Patient Position and Angle of Pull

Patient position has more influence on the angle of pull during lumbar traction than cervical traction. Lumbar traction can be applied with the patient prone or supine (Fig. 17–11). Each of these positions equally decreases the amount of myoelectric activity of the paraspinal muscles.[122] Patient comfort, the pathology being treated, and the spinal segments and structures being treated also help determine the patient position.

Positioning the patient supine tends to increase flexion of the lumbar spine. Flexing the hip and knees further

increases flexion of the lumbar spine and pelvis, flattening the lumbar spine. Flexing the hips from 45 to 60 degrees of flexion increases the laxity in the L5-S1 segment, 60 to 75 degrees in the L4-L5 segment, and 75 to 90 degrees in the L3-L4 segment.[123] Flexing the hips to 90 degrees increases the posterior intervertebral space.[123] In the lumbar spine, extension opens the facet joint and increases distraction in the upper lumbar and, possibly, the lower thoracic segments.

The prone position is used when excessive flexion of the lumbar spine and pelvis or lying supine causes pain or increases peripheral symptoms. This position has the advantage of allowing other modalities to be applied concurrently with the traction.[110] An increased amount of distraction occurs in the lower lumbar segments when the patient is prone, a beneficial effect with lower disc protrusions.

The patient's position and angle of pull should maximize the separation and elongation of the target tissues. An anterior angle of pull increases the amount of lumbar lordosis. A posterior angle of pull increases lumbar kyphosis, but too much flexion can impinge on the posterior spinal ligaments.

The determination of the optimal position and angle of pull is often derived by trial and error and depends on the patient and the pathology (see Table 17–1). For example, a posterior disc protrusion may respond best with

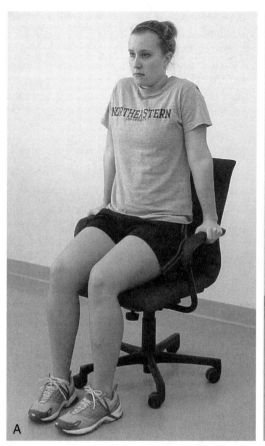
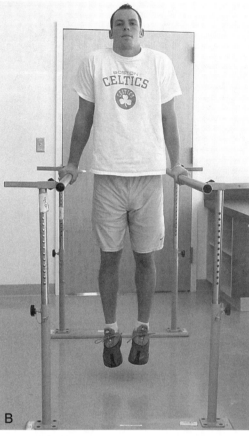

Figure 17–10. **Methods of Self-Administered Autotraction.** (A) Sitting in a chair for the sacroiliac joint. (B) Using parallel bars for the sacroiliac joint and lumbar spine.

the patient prone and the spine placed in extension or neutral. However, if no pain relief is obtained in either of these positions, positioning the patient supine with the lumbar spine placed in flexion may produce beneficial results.

Relief of symptoms caused by nerve root impingement should be obtained with the patient supine and the spine flexed. If the impingement is unilateral, additional pain relief may be obtained by rotating the involved side slightly upward by placing a folded towel or bolster under the involved side.

Unilateral traction is used for the treatment of **functional scoliosis** ■ of the lumbar and thoracic spine (Fig. 17–12). The tension is applied to the convex side of the curvature, straightening the vertebral column and elongating the muscles on the opposite, concave side of the column.[124] Traction is not considered to be effective for the treatment of **structural scoliosis** ■.

● E FFECTS ON

The Injury Response Process

Traction applied to the lumbar area is useful in treating many of the same conditions as cervical traction, resulting in a decrease in lumbar lordosis, distraction of the vertebral bodies, increase in disc height, stretching of lumbar muscles, and widening of the intervertebral foramina.[105] The effects of lumbar traction are similar to those described in the General Uses for Cervical and Lumbar Traction section of this chapter.

Muscle Spasm

Lumbar traction can be effective in reducing muscle spasm caused by nerve root impingement from narrowing of the intervertebral foramen, stenosis, or disc protrusions. To a lesser degree, traumatic muscle spasm can be reduced secondary to stretching of the muscles, although the

---

Functional scoliosis: Lateral curvature of the spinal column in the frontal plane caused as the spinal column attempts to compensate for postural deficits such as leg length discrepancy. Functional scoliosis is also known as protective scoliosis.

Structural scoliosis: Lateral curvature of the spinal column caused by malformed vertebrae and/or inter vertebral discs.

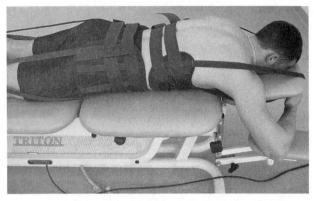

Figure 17-11. Lumbar Traction Applied in the Prone Position. This position permits other modalities to be applied concurrently with the traction.

amount of elongation is less than that obtained by standard stretching routines.

Pain

Increasing the amount of separation between the vertebrae can reduce impingement of the lumbar nerve roots. Nerve entrapment as a result of a disc protrusion can be reduced by allowing the disc to return to its original shape, decompressing the nucleus pulposus to below 100 mm Hg.[125] Radicular pain caused by lumbar disc herniation is reduced with forces of 30 and 60 percent of the body weight.[107] Lumbar traction is not an effective treatment approach for patients with nonspecific low back pain.[126]

■ Contraindications to the Use of Lumbar Traction

The contraindications to the use of lumbar traction are similar to those described for cervical traction. Vertebral body fractures or unstable spinal segments are an absolute contraindication to lumbar traction unless the treatment is specifically approved the patient's physician.

Lumbar traction has been used for **spondylolisthesis** ■ and **spondylolysis** ■, but this should be done with caution and diligence (Fig. 17–13). Spondylolisthesis can lead to hypermobility of the vertebral segment, a contraindication to sustained and intermittent traction. Too much tension can speed the degeneration associated with spondylolysis.

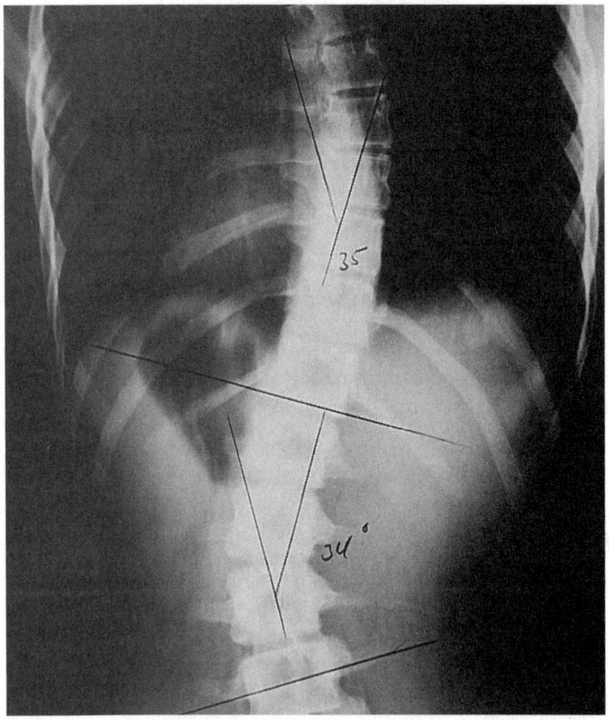

Figure 17-12. Spinal Scoliosis (posterior view). Scoliosis is the lateral curvature of the spinal column in the frontal plane. Focusing on the lumbar segment, this radiograph shows a convex curvature on the left side, elongating the soft tissue on that side. The right lumbar curvature is concave. The muscles on this side are shortened. Note that this radiograph depicts structural scoliosis caused by misshaped vertebrae. Traction is only effective on functional scoliosis.

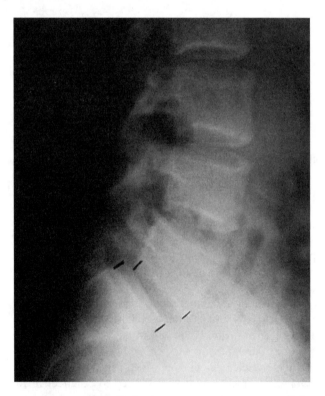

Figure 17-13. Spondylolisthesis of the L5-S1 Vertebrae. Spondylolisthesis is the forward slippage of a vertebra on the one below it. This condition results in pain in the lumbar spine and buttocks that increases when the lumbar spine is placed in extension. Lumbar traction should not be used when the vertebral segment is hypermobile.

Spondylolisthesis: Forward slippage of the lower lumbar vertebra on the vertebra below.
Spondylolysis: The breaking down of a vertebral structure.

Do not use lumbar traction for patients with pain of unknown origin or pain caused by diseases, infections, or tumors (see At a Glance: Lumbar Traction). Traction applied to severely herniated discs may increase the rate of degeneration. Discontinue use if the treatment increases the severity of the patient's symptoms.

Rheumatoid arthritis and osteoarthritis are contraindicated because necrosis can cause ligamentous weakness. The force of the applied traction could result in vertebral subluxation or dislocation and further weaken the soft tissue structures.

■ Controversies in Treatment

The efficacy of lumbar traction has been supported for several types of pathology. Lumbar traction is not considered to be effective in decreasing nonspecific low back pain.[126, 127]

Computed tomographic imaging indicates that lumbar traction increases the reabsorption of the nucleus pulposus. However, the location of the protrusion does affect the efficacy of the treatment. Protrusions closer to the body's midline are more likely to have positive treatment outcomes than lateral protrusions. Factors such as the calcification of the disc also decrease the effectiveness of the treatment.[128] A comparison of lumbar traction and isometric exercise indicated that neither of the interventions was more effective in decreasing pain caused by disc herniations than placebo.[129]

■ Clinical Application of Intermittent Lumbar Traction

The following section describes the use of motorized lumbar traction. The patient position and angle of pull must be appropriate for the condition being treated. Manual traction may be used before mechanized traction to determine the potential benefits of the treatment.

Instrumentation

Refer to the operator's manual for the particular unit being used.

Traction harness: Sometimes referred to as the pelvic "corset." Fits around the patient's pelvis and attaches to the traction unit's pulley cable.

Stabilization harness: Fits around the patient's torso and attaches to the treatment table.

Split table: The lower half of the table glides on rollers, thus eliminating friction and allowing vertebral separation to occur at a lower applied force.

Mode: This setting allows the traction to be applied intermittently or continuously.

Type: For multipurpose units that treat both the lumbar and cervical spine.

Hold time: This control adjusts the duration of the traction phase (in seconds).

Rest time: This control adjusts the duration of the relaxation phase (in seconds). Applicable only to intermittent traction.

Tension: Controls the amount of tension, in pounds, applied to the halter.

Low tension: Sets the minimum amount of tension to be applied during the OFF cycle.

Duration: Selects the total treatment time.

Safety switch: Allows the patient to interrupt the treatment and immediately decrease the tension if pain or other discomfort is experienced.

Alarm: Sounds when the patient triggers the safety switch or a malfunction in the unit is detected.

■ Set-up and Application

The following protocol describes the set-up and application of motorized intermittent lumbar traction with the patient supine and the knees and hip flexed (e.g., for treatment of nerve root impingement) on a split traction table (therefore negating the effect of friction between the patient and the tabletop).

Digital units can display force in pounds (lb) or kilograms (kg). Familiarize yourself with the unit of measure that is used by the facility.

Motorized traction devices should not be used in the presence of flammable gases such as oxygen, nitrous oxide, and many anesthetic gases. The unit may interfere with sensitive electrical equipment.

Patient Preparation

1. Determine the presence of any contraindications.
2. Calculate the patient's body weight.
3. If a split table is being used, unlock the lower section to allow it to slide.
4. The patient's clothing must not interfere with the fit of the halter and not allow the traction or stabilization halter to slide during the treatment.
5. Fit the traction halter on the patient's pelvis. Depending on the type of harness being used, a towel or other type of padding may need to be placed between the harness and the patient's skin.
6. Fit the stabilization harness to the patient's torso, normally fitting over the 8th through 10th ribs. There may be slight overlap between the stabilization and traction harness.
7. If necessary, drape the patient for modesty.
8. If a split table is being used, align the target spinal segment over the opening between the fixed and mobile portion of the table.
9. Position the patient, the patient's hip and knee position, and the angle of pull appropriate for the treatment being treated (refer to Table 17–1).

At a Glance: **Lumbar Traction**

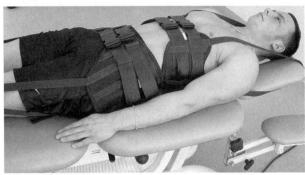

Description

Lumbar traction distracts the lumbar and possibly the lower thoracic vertebrae. Using a motorized unit (shown above), lumbar traction can be applied continuously or intermittently. Lumbar traction can also be applied manually by the clinician, by weights, or by gravity (autotraction). Lumbar traction is used for:

- Degenerative disc disease
- Radicular pain
- Facet joint pathology including hypomobile facet joints
- Muscle spasm caused by nerve root impingement

Primary

- Elongation of the lumbar vertebrae, relieving pressure on the intervertebral discs. Aids in the reabsorption of the nucleus pulposus.
- Relieves pressure on the spinal nerve roots caused by narrowing of the intervertebral foramen.
- Reduces pressure on the facet joints.

Treatment

- Facet joint pathology: 25 min
- Degenerative disc disease: 10 min
- Disc protrusion: 8 to 10 min
- Muscle spasm: 20 min

Indications

- Nerve root compression
- Herniated or protruding intervertebral disc
- Degenerative disc disease
- Lumbar muscle spasm
- Osteoarthritis or facet joint inflammation

Contraindications

- Acute injury
- Unstable spinal segments
- Cancer, meningitis, or other diseases affecting the spinal cord or vertebrae
- Extruded disc fragmentation
- Advanced disc degeneration or advanced herniation
- Spinal cord compression
- Rheumatoid arthritis
- Conditions that worsen after treatment

Precautions

- Monitor the patient closely during the treatment. Discontinue use if symptoms increase.
- Low-tension traction should be used if ligamentous damage is suspected.
- Use only sustained or continuous traction if lumbar motion is contraindicated.

If the patient is supine and lumbar/pelvic flexion is indicated, elevate the lower legs.

10. Align the angle of pull according to the patient's pathology (refer to Table 17–1).
11. If available, give the patient the SAFETY switch and explain its purpose and use.
12. Explain to the patient the sensations to be expected during the treatment and to report pain, discomfort, or worsening of symptoms.

Initiation of the Treatment

1. Reset all controls to zero and turn the unit ON.
2. If applicable, set the TYPE switch to "Lumbar."

3. Remove any slack in the pulley cable.
4. Adjust the RATIO to the appropriate ON-OFF sequence (refer to Table 17–1).
5. Adjust the tension to approximately 25 percent of the patient's body weight. Radicular pain caused by lumbar disc herniation is often reduced with forces of 30 and 60 percent of the body weight.[107, 130]
6. If the setting is adjustable, set the LOW tension (this value is often set to zero or 10 percent of the maximum tension).
7. Instruct the patient as to what to expect during the treatment and to inform you if any discomfort is experienced.

8. Set the appropriate treatment DURATION, and initiate the treatment (refer to Table 17–1).

9. Allow the unit to go through its first tension cycle. The TENSION may be gradually increased during subsequent cycles. Increase the amount of tension as indicated. If pain is experienced at any time during the treatment, decrease the amount of force or discontinue the treatment.

10. Instruct the patient to remain relaxed during both the on and off cycles.

11. At regular intervals question the patient about abnormal sensations in the cervical, thoracic, and lumbar spine and the extremities.

Termination of the Treatment

1. If the traction unit does not automatically do so, gradually reduce the TENSION over a period of three or four cycles.

2. Gain some slack in the cable, and turn the unit off.

3. Remove the traction and stabilization halter.

4. Question the patient regarding any perceived benefit or complications derived from the treatment.

5. Have the patient remain lying for 5 minutes after the conclusion of the treatment.

6. Record the pertinent information (tension, duration, duty cycle) in the patient's medical file.

▤ Maintenance

After Each Use

1. Clean the unit according to the manufacturer's recommendation.

2. Avoid allowing liquids (including cleaning solutions) from entering the unit.

At Regular Intervals

1. Check the electrical power cord for kinks, frays, or cuts.

2. Check the traction cable for knots, twisting, and if applicable, damage to its protective (usually nylon) coating.

3. Recalibrate the unit. Follow the manufacturer's recommended procedures and timetable for recalibrating the traction device.

4. Clean the harness according to the manufacturer's instructions.

Annual

The traction device must be inspected and serviced by an authorized technician.

● Chapter Highlights

- Traction results in the distraction, separation, of the vertebral bodies.

- Sustained traction is constant traction that is applied for less than 45 minutes. Continuous traction is applied for several hours or days. Intermittent traction uses an ON/OFF duty cycle to alternate between periods of traction and relaxation.

- The effects of traction are influenced by the patient position, angle of pull, amount of tension applied, and the duration and type of traction.

- Traction provides short-term mechanical relief of conditions associated with compression of spinal nerve roots, the spinal cord, and associated soft tissue. Common uses include disc protrusions, degenerative disc disease, nerve root compression, facet joint pathology, and muscle spasm.

- Cervical traction requires less force to obtain separation of the vertebral segments when the patient is supine than when seated.

- Lumbar traction is less commonly used than cervical traction and requires more force to obtain separation of the vertebrae than cervical traction.

- Traction should not be used in the presence of unstable vertebral segments.

Chapter 18

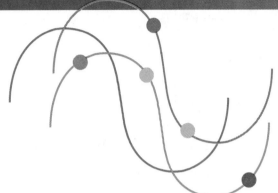

Electromyographic Biofeedback

Unlike other therapeutic modalities presented in this text, electromyographic biofeedback does not deliver energy to the body. Instead, biofeedback measures the amount of a specific type of physiological activity that is occurring. In the case of muscle contractions, the amount of motor nerve activity is being observed. The biofeedback unit then converts this activity into a visual or audible form that can be interpreted by the patient and clinician.

The process of biofeedback involves "tapping into" the body's physiological processes. The body's electrical activity is amplified by the biofeedback unit and converted into auditory or visual signals, or both, that the patient can use to model further activity. Consider for example a patient who is recovering from ACL surgery, but who is unable to voluntarily contract the vastus medialis oblique (VMO) muscle. The patient attempts to get the muscle to contract, but because there is not the normal reinforcement of increased muscle tone, the patient is not sure that the appropriate muscle is being targeted. When a biofeedback unit is placed over the VMO, the feedback indicates that motor nerve impulses are being directed to the muscle (Fig. 18–1).

Biofeedback operates on at least one of four biophysical principles and is used to augment the input lost from these receptors by providing other types of information such as sound or visual feedback (Table 18–1). These

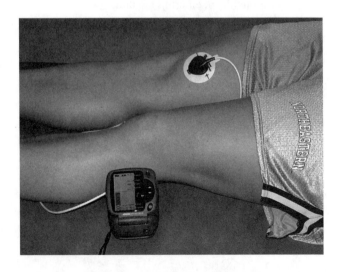

Figure 18–1. **Electromyographic Biofeedback.** Electrode placement for the vastus medialis oblique muscle.

responses can be used to assist in developing the strength of muscular contractions, facilitating muscular relaxation, controlling blood pressure and heart rate, and decreasing the physical manifestation of emotional stress. It also forms the basis of lie detection tests.

Biofeedback does not monitor the actual response itself (e.g., the strength of the contraction), but rather the conditions associated with response (e.g., neurological activity). The normal proprioceptive, and perhaps kinesthetic, input is amplified through the use of sound, light, or meters. This concept applies not only to restoring the function of an injured body part but also to increase the strength of healthy muscle.[131]

With orthopedic patients, biofeedback is most often used as an adjunct to muscle reeducation and training or to encourage the relaxation of a muscle group. Biofeedback is also used for patients suffering central nervous system trauma such as spinal cord injury or stroke. Functional patterns such as gait and grasping and strength training may also be reestablished using biofeedback.

Because the electromyographic (EMG) technique of biofeedback using superficial electrodes is most prevalent in orthopedics, it will be the focus of this chapter (biofeedback is also used to reduce anxiety and improve athletic performance). Conceptually, biofeedback functions by[132]:

• Monitoring the physiological process.
• Objectively measuring the process.

• Converting what is being monitored into feedback that optimizes the desired effects.

The electronic and physiological mechanisms associated with biofeedback are covered in the next section. At this point, a clarification must be made between "monitoring" and "measuring" the electrical activity. **Monitoring** involves determining whether neuromuscular activity is present and, if so, whether it is increasing or decreasing. **Measuring** the activity involves placing an objective scale on the monitored readout.

Consider the two analog meters depicted in Figure 18–2. The meter in Figure 18–2A shows that activity is taking place, and we can tell if it is increasing, decreasing, or holding steady by observing the relative position of the needle. When a scale is placed on the meter in Figure 18–2B, the amount of activity, and therefore the degree of change, can be objectively measured. The scale on a biofeedback unit may use the number of microvolts, a simple 0-to-10 scale, or a bar graph or other visual representation as the measure. Because of the lack of a standard biofeedback scale, measures made on a unit of one brand cannot be compared with measurements on a unit of another brand.[132, 133] Also, placement of skin electrodes from treatment to treatment affects the measurement's reliability.[133]

The meter is only one form of meaningful information that biofeedback units can provide. Most units can

TABLE 18–1	Types of Biofeedback Units
Type	*Principle*
Electromyographic	Measures the electrical activity in skeletal muscle.
Peripheral temperature	Measures temperature changes in the distal extremities (e.g., fingers). Increased temperature indicates a relaxed state (increased superficial blood flow). Decreased temperature indicates stress, fear, or anxiety (decreased superficial blood flow).
Photoplethysmography	Measures the amount of light reflected by subcutaneous tissues based on the amount of blood flow.
Galvanic skin response	Measures the amount of perspiration on the skin by passing a small current through the fingers and/or palm. Sweaty skin contains salt and is a better conductor than dry skin.

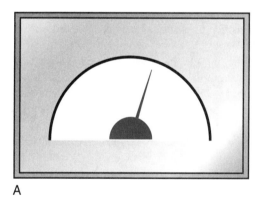

A

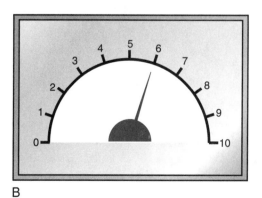

B

Figure 18–2. **Measuring versus Monitoring of Biofeedback.** Meter (A) indicates if activity is occurring, whereas meter (B) places objective measures through the use of a numeric scale.

convert the signals into sound waves, an advantage because they allow the patient to focus on the muscle rather than looking at the biofeedback unit. The pitch of the sound increases and decreases based on the amount of neuromuscular activity. Computer interfaces are also used to create larger renditions of the feedback and may provide increased motivation by creating a game-like, competitive atmosphere.

Biophysical Processes and Electrical Integration

Application of EMG biofeedback involves the use of three electrodes positioned over the muscle or muscle group that is the focus of the session. Basic EMG biofeedback units have one channel composed of three surface electrodes combined on a single self-adhesive electrode. Two of these electrodes are "active electrodes" that actually measure the amount of electrical activity within the muscle. The third electrode, the "reference electrode" is used to filter out non-meaningful electrical activity. The most sensitive EMG surface monitors have electrodes made with silver (Fig. 18–3). Needle electrodes implanted directly in the muscle are used with EMG units for diagnostic and research purposes.

The electrodes monitor the electrical activity within a local area of a muscle, usually the muscle belly (Fig. 18–4). Some EMG units have two or more channels that allow multiple muscles to be monitored or one muscle to be monitored in different areas. Surface electrodes are more sensitive to electrical activity in superficial muscles than in deeper muscles. The amount of electrical activity within the muscle increases as more motor units are recruited into the contraction. These signals are then picked up by the electrodes, amplified, and converted into visual or auditory signals. Although this process seems straightforward, it is complicated by the presence of other electrical activity in our environment. We are always being bombarded by electromagnetic energy. A small portion of this energy is absorbed by the body and is consequently detected by the biofeedback unit. This unwanted energy, referred to as "noise," must be filtered out before the meaningful activity can be determined (Box 18–1).

Although EMG biofeedback requires three electrodes, they are often found on a single self-adhesive patch with the active electrodes spaced approximately 3 cm apart, although some units require that each electrode be applied individually (see Fig. 18–3). Locating the active electrodes close to each other targets the specific muscle, but the raw signal is relatively weak. Spacing the active electrodes farther apart increases the strength of the raw signal and monitors a greater proportion of the muscle. However, as the distance between the electrodes is increased, the reliability of the signal decreases because electrical activity in the surrounding muscles and external electrical interference will be detected by the biofeedback unit.[133]

● EFFECTS ON
The Injury Response Process

EMG biofeedback itself does not affect the injury response process. Unlike other modalities presented in this text, biofeedback units assist voluntary functions to produce the desired results (see At a Glance: Electromyographic Biofeedback, p 332). Other types of biofeedback units monitor functions that are controlled by the autonomic nervous system. Because of this, the effectiveness of biofeedback is judged on a case-by-case basis.[133] However, proper use of biofeedback does facilitate muscle reeducation or promote relaxation and increase range of motion. In turn, these effects can lead to a reduction in pain or an increase in function.[134]

Biofeedback is sometimes combined with electrical stimulation to further restore neuromuscular function. The electrical stimulation unit is programmed to produce a muscle contraction once the patient has reached the threshold established with the biofeedback unit.

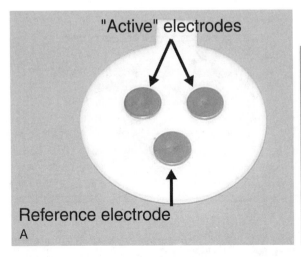

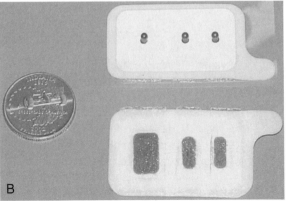

Figure 18–3. **EMG biofeedback surface electrodes.** (A) Standard self-adhesive modeling showing the active and reference electrodes. (B) Silver electrode. A US quarter is used for size reference.

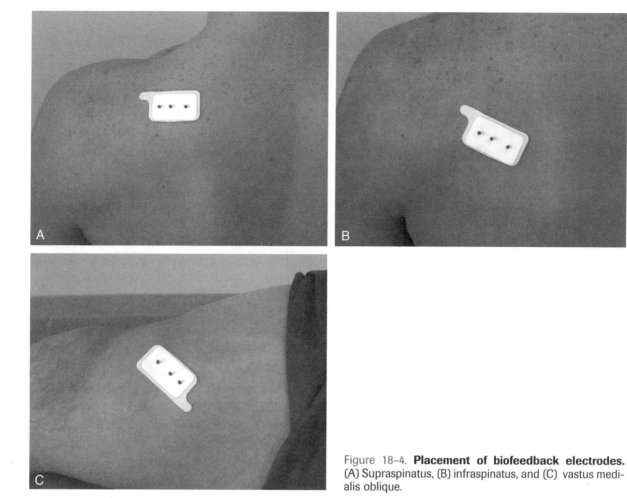

Figure 18–4. **Placement of biofeedback electrodes.** (A) Supraspinatus, (B) infraspinatus, and (C) vastus medialis oblique.

During neuromuscular rehabilitation, EMG biofeedback is most beneficial when it is incorporated early in the patient's program, especially when active motions are involved.[135] Because EMG biofeedback detects the electrical activity associated with muscle contractions, the patient must be able to innervate the muscle. Adjunct strategies can be used to help facilitate a muscle contraction (Table 18–2). The injured tissues must be able to withstand the tension and stresses associated with the motion, and there must be some level of nerve supply to the target muscle or muscle groups.

The benefits of biofeedback are enhanced by educating the patient on the concept of biofeedback, incorporating learning strategies, and setting patient goals.[136, 137] Verbal feedback can reinforce the neuromuscular reeducation and provide positive cognitive reinforcement to the patient. However, this type of feedback while the patient is concentrating on producing a muscle contraction can distract the patient from the task at hand, so refrain from talking to the patient until the exercise has been completed.[138]

Neuromuscular Effects

Biofeedback is most often incorporated into an orthopedic treatment and rehabilitation program after surgery or long-term immobilization. Edema, pain, and decreased input from joint receptors often inhibit voluntary muscle contractions following surgery. The use of biofeedback shapes the response that enables the central nervous system to reestablish sensory-motor loops "forgotten" by the patient.[139, 140] On reaching the brain, afferent stimuli, in this case sound or visual cues, stimulate cerebral areas that normally receive proprioceptive information. These artificial signals, combined with the visual cue of actually watching the muscle contract, assist in reopening a neural loop that sends efferent signals to the appropriate muscles. Facilitative biofeedback can be used to specifically target a specific muscle and modify contraction timing patterns, such as the vastus medialis oblique for patellofemoral conditions.[141]

Dramatic increases in the quality and quantity of a muscle contraction can be seen following a single treatment session. To help the patient retain the newly learned neurological pathways, the patient should perform active muscle contractions without the biofeedback unit immediately following each session. Home exercise programs that target the involved muscles will also facilitate the retention of muscle memory.

The cognitive process of neuromuscular relaxation is similar to that of evoking muscle contractions. However, rather than attempting to reestablish neural loops, these

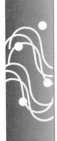

Box 18–1. EMG Biofeedback Signal Processing

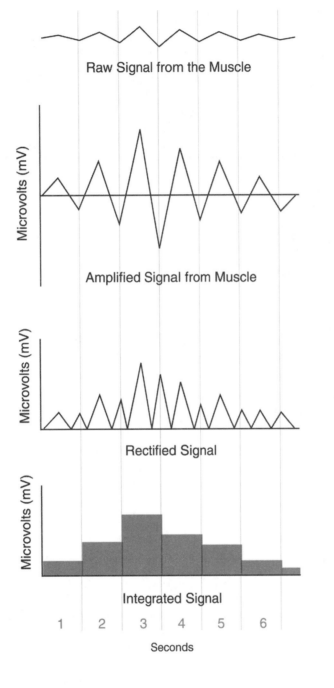

Raw Signal from the Muscle

Amplified Signal from Muscle

Rectified Signal

Integrated Signal

1   2   3   4   5   6

Seconds

Five steps are required to process and provide feedback of the body's neuromuscular electrical activity:

Identify ⇒ Amplify ⇒ Rectify ⇒ Integrate ⇒ Output
Signal   Signal   Signal   Signal   Signal

The EMG unit filters out electrical noise and identifies the raw signal, positive and negative electrical activity associated with the depolarization and repolarization of the involved cells. Referring to Figure 18–3, you will notice that two electrodes are labeled "active" and one as "reference." The reference electrode serves as a measurement point for a very small current passed between the two active electrodes. This results in two sources supplying input to a differential amplifier within the unit. Here, the meaningful information is separated from the meaningless noise. Because the extraneous noise is produced by electromagnetic sources, it occurs at a constant frequency and is detectable anywhere in the body. The differential amplifier compares the input from two sources and eliminates any activity that is common to both. In theory, the remaining activity represents the **raw signal** of the neuromuscular activity. However, the integrity of the final signal depends on the quality of the unit and the number of filters used (more filters lead to a more precise signal). The amplitude of the raw signal is small and must be **amplified** by the unit. **Rectification** involves taking the absolute value of the negative electrical activity and making it a mathematically positive number, causing the plot to move to the positive side of the baseline. The final EMG signal is formed by calculating the root-mean-square average (see At a Glance: Electromyographic Biofeedback, p 332) of the electrical activity per unit of time, **integration.** The integrated signal is then converted into an **output signal** that is normally a visual display or auditory tone.

pathways are inhibited. The goal of relaxation therapy is to decrease the number of motor impulses being relayed to the muscle in spasm. This technique is best used with cases of subconscious muscle guarding. The use of relaxation biofeedback does not significantly increase flexibil-

ity in healthy individuals when compared with standard flexibility exercises. However, athletes combining flexibility with biofeedback displayed a greater retention of improvement than those training without the aid of biofeedback.[142]

TABLE 18–2 Methods to Facilitate a Muscle Contraction

- Have the patient contract the muscle on the opposite limb, then attempt to contract the involved muscle.
- Apply the biofeedback unit to the opposite limb so that the person will "learn" the biofeedback technique.
- Watch and/or touch the contracting muscle.
- Contract surrounding or opposing muscles.
- Contract the proximal portion of the muscle to facilitate neuromuscular activity in the distal motor units.
- Use electrical stimulation to evoke a muscle contraction (note: disconnect the biofeedback device prior to using this technique).

Pain Reduction

The primary benefit of pain reduction stems from restoring normal function of the body part. Reeducating muscle removes the unwanted stress associated with abnormal biomechanics and atrophy. Facilitating reduction of muscle spasm reduces the amount of mechanical pressure placed on nociceptors.

Although its mechanism is beyond the scope of this text, inhibitory biofeedback has also been successfully used in the reduction of myofascial pain, the pain associated with migraine and tension headaches, as well as in general stress reduction.[143] Most inhibitory pain-control approaches also involve cognitive and behavioral aspects that build on the biofeedback sessions.[144, 145]

■ Contraindications

The primary contraindications to the use of biofeedback are conditions in which muscle tension or joint motion would cause further injury (see At a Glance: Electromyographic Biofeedback, p 332). A general rule is that if the patient is prohibited from moving the joint or if isometric contractions are contraindicated, biofeedback should not be used.

Unhealed tendon grafts, avulsed tendons, and third-degree tears of the muscle fibers could potentially be damaged by the tension associated with even moderate muscle contractions. Injury to the joint structure, ligaments, capsule, or articulating surfaces or unstable fractures are also contraindications to biofeedback.

■ Controversies in Treatment

As it relates to musculoskeletal trauma, the efficacy of EMG biofeedback is relatively well accepted for reeducating denervated muscles. The primary concern relates to the unit's accuracy in detecting the muscle's raw signal. Surface electrodes are most sensitive to superficial muscles. Electrode placement, electromagnetic noise, and tissue variability (e.g., hydration) cause significant variability in the signals produced even by the same subject.[133]

■ Clinical Application of Biofeedback

Instrumentation

Biofeedback units range from the very simple to the ultra-complex and may be in the form of clinical models or portable, "take-home" units. The following description is of the typical "midrange" unit. Consult the user's manual of your particular unit for a more detailed description of its operation.

Alarm: Identifies a target range for EMG activity. Provides an alert when the EMG activity is within a specified range of the target value or is significantly above or below preset levels.

Output: This device determines the type of feedback available. Visual feedback appears by way of a meter or bar graph. The audio output is normally adjustable between various frequencies. Many models allow for a computer interface that presents the feedback in a graphical method on the computer's monitor. Computers can also be used to store results of the session.

Sensitivity range: This control provides coarse adjustments on the level needed to obtain feedback. The feedback may be **threshold**, a constant alarm or visual cue that is elicited once the threshold has been reached, or **progressive,** where the level of feedback increases with the intensity once the threshold has been reached.

Statistics: Some biofeedback units calculate statistics of the patient's muscular activity for assessment of the rehabilitation program. Measures such as the mean, maximum, and standard deviation provide quantitative information for evaluating the patient's progress.

Tuner: This knob allows fine adjustments on the threshold required to obtain feedback.

Volume: Adjusts the audible output of the feedback. Audible feedback may come from a built-in speaker or through an earpiece or headphones.

Set-up and Application

Patient Preparation

1. Question the patient to rule out the presence of contraindications.
2. Remove any dirt, oil, or makeup in the area where the electrodes are to be applied by wiping the skin with alcohol. These substances impede the conduction of the bioelectric signals, as may excess body hair where the electrodes are to be placed. Shave the area if applicable.
3. Very sensitive biofeedback units may require that the electrode site be mildly abraded with an emery cloth.
4. Apply a suitable conductive gel to the electrodes.

At a Glance: **Electromyographic Biofeedback**

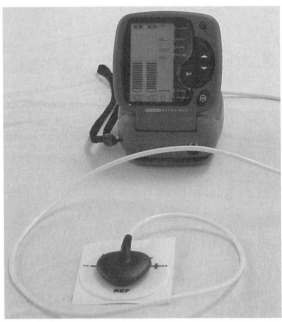

Description

Electromyographic biofeedback detects the amount of electrical activity associated with a muscle contraction and converts it to visual and/or auditory feedback that promotes the strength of the muscular contraction or facilitates relaxation. Common clinical uses include:

- Neuromuscular reeducation
- Gait training
- Relaxation training

Primary

Assists the patient in altering the amount of neuromuscular activity by monitoring the intensity of electrical activity.

Treatment

Biofeedback can be performed daily as needed either in the clinical setting or at home. Be aware of any muscle soreness that may occur after exercise and adjust the treatment protocol accordingly.

Indications

- To facilitate muscular contractions
- To regain neuromuscular control
- To decrease muscle spasm
- To promote systemic relaxation

Contraindications

- Conditions in which muscular contractions would insult the tissues
- Conditions where the contraction will cause joint movement and motion is contraindicated

Precautions

- Do not exceed the prescribed range of motion.
- Avoid undue muscle tension that may affect grafts or other tissue restrictions.

---

5. Secure the electrodes over a motor point near belly of the muscle targeted in this therapy (see Appendix C). If a motor point chart is not available, locate the electrodes over the muscle belly. Note that the active electrodes must be applied over the target muscle. The reference electrode may be secured anywhere on the body, but by convention, it is normally placed between the two active electrodes (see Figure 18–3).

6. Plug the common electrode leads into the INPUT jacks on the unit.

7. Turn the unit ON.

8. Adjust the OUTPUT to the desired mode of feedback (visual, audio, or both).

9. Provide instructions to the individual regarding the proper use of biofeedback, including goal setting.

10. The patient should be free of visual and auditory distractions during the course of the session.

Facilitation of Isometric Muscle Contraction

1. Instruct the patient to relax the body part as much as possible.

3. Place the body part in the desired position.

4. Instruct the patient to maximally contract the muscle.

5. Adjust the SENSITIVITY RANGE to the lowest value that does not provide feedback and note the value.

6. Have the patient relax.

7. Set the SENSITIVITY to approximately 2/3 of the value identified in step 5.

8. Instruct the patient to contract the muscle until maximum feedback is obtained and then hold the contraction for 6 seconds.
9. Have the patient completely relax so that the meter resets to the baseline before the next contraction.
10. If the patient will use an earphone during the treatment, complete two or three contractions using the speaker while the patient is under supervision to familiarize the patient with the treatment prior to its use.
11. Repeat the contractions as indicated. If the muscle group is severely atrophied, the number of contractions is normally limited to 10 to 15 contractions because of fatigue.
12. By decreasing the sensitivity, the patient will have to elicit a stronger contraction to receive feedback.
13. If the individual is unable to evoke a contraction, refer to the strategies presented in Table 18–2.

Termination of the Procedure

1. Remove the electrodes, and wipe away any excess gel.
2. If disposable electrodes are being used, discard after use.
3. To avoid dependency on biofeedback, have the patient perform additional sets of contractions without the aid of the unit to "remember" how to perform the contractions.

Maintenance

Following Each Use

Clean the biofeedback case, lead wire, and earphones following each treatment using a mild cleanser.

At Regular Intervals

Regularly inspect the electrode lead wires and jacks for kinks, frays, and defects.

● Chapter Highlights

* There are four classifications of biofeedback. EMG biofeedback is most commonly used for neuromuscular reeducation or to promote muscular/systemic relaxation.
* Three electrodes are used, two "active" and one "reference." These three electrodes are commonly found on the same adhesive backing.
* The steps involved in EMG signal processing are signal identification, amplification, rectification, integration, and output.
* EMG biofeedback measures the amount of electrical activity within the muscle, not the actual strength of the contraction.
* The strength of muscle contractions is increased by restoring the neurological pathways to the muscle.
* Following biofeedback sessions, the patient should perform active muscle contractions without the aid of the unit to reinforce the muscular reeducation.
* Biofeedback should not be used when muscle tension or joint motion would cause further injury.

Chapter 19

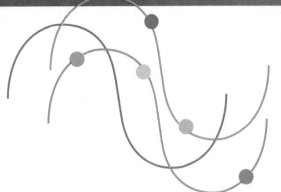

Light Modalities

The light spectrum encompasses ultraviolet, visible, and infrared energy. Although some thermal effects may be obtained from these modalities, the primary benefits are derived from drying the superficial tissues or via superficial photochemical effects.

Electromagnetic energy is the most abundant form of energy in the universe. The energy found in the electromagnetic spectrum, including electricity, radio waves, and x-rays, is categorized by the frequency and length of its wave (Appendix B). Light, another form of electromagnetic energy, is grouped into three general classifications, ultraviolet, visible, and infrared (Fig. 19–1). Energy having a wavelength greater than 780 **nanometers** ■ (nm) (the upper end of visible light) is classified as infrared light. The ultraviolet (UV) spectrum is located in the area below the range of visible light. **Lasers** ■ produce highly refined, **monochromatic** ■ light in the ultraviolet, visible, or infrared range.

Many therapeutic modalities use energy within the light range of the electromagnetic spectrum. UV light is used for the treatment of certain skin conditions. Depending on the relative temperatures involved, transfer of infrared energy is used to heat or cool the body's tissues. Medical lasers produce beams of energy that can cause

either tissue destruction or therapeutic effects within the tissues.

▶ INFRARED LAMP

As with moist heat packs, infrared lamps (also referred to as "heat lamps") are classified as superficial heating agents (see Chapter 5). However, these devices are seldom used for the same purpose as other superficial heating agents. With the range of heating modalities available for use, infrared generators are not common in clinical settings (See At a Glance: Infrared Lamps, p 337). The use of these devices is now primarily limited to drying seeping open wounds or sedating superficial sensory nerves.

Light energy having a wavelength greater than 780 nm is termed infrared light or infrared energy. Because this wavelength is beyond the upper limits of what the human eye is capable of detecting, infrared energy is invisible. Any object possessing a temperature greater than absolute

---

Laser: Acronym for *Light Amplification by Stimulated Emission of Radiation*. A highly organized beam of light.

Monochromatic: Light that consists of only one color.

Nanometer: One-billionth (10^{-9}) of a meter.

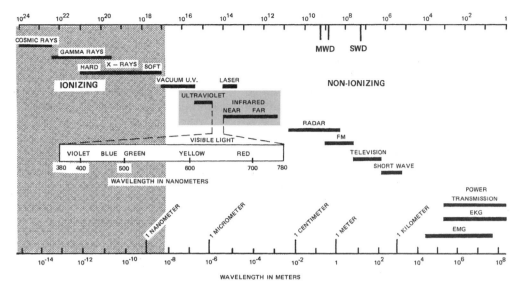

Figure 19–1. **The Light Portion of the Electromagnetic Spectrum.** The visible portion of the light spectrum consists of energy having a wavelength of approximately 380 to 780 nm. Light having a range between 780 and 12,500 nm is infrared light (also referred to as infrared radiation); energy having a wavelength between 180 and 400 nm is in the ultraviolet range. Note that there is a slight amount of overlap between the ultraviolet and visible light and the visible light and infrared ranges.

zero emits infrared energy proportional to its temperature. Hotter sources transmit more infrared energy, because they possess a shorter wavelength than cooler objects.

Infrared lamps are radiant modalities because no medium is required to transmit the energy. The treatment energy is produced by passing an electrical current through a carbon or tungsten filament. The intensity is controlled by adjusting the current flow through the filament or by changing the distance between the lamp and the tissues. The infrared spectrum is divided into two distinct sections: near infrared and far infrared.

Unlike moist heat packs, which lose their energy during treatment, infrared lamps maintain a constant temperature. The constant energy source significantly increases the risk of burns, especially in areas of decreased blood flow or open wounds.

Near-infrared is the portion of the spectrum that is closest to visible light, with wavelengths ranging between 780 and 1500 nm. Because visible light is produced by near-infrared lamps, they are also referred to as luminous infrared lamps. Because visible light is present, some of the treatment energy is reflected by the surface of the skin. Energy in the near-infrared range is capable of producing thermal effects 5 to 10 mm deep in tissue. Luminous infrared radiation is formed by a carbon and tungsten filament similar to a standard household light bulb.

The **far-infrared** portion is located between 1500 and 12,500 nm and results in more superficial heating of the skin (less than 2 mm deep). The energy in the far infrared range is invisible to the human eye. Because they are invisible, these generators are referred to as being nonluminous. Nonluminous infrared radiation penetrates 5 mm beneath the skin, compared with 10 mm for luminous infrared light. Because nonluminous infrared is less penetrating,

the skin being treated will feel warmer than with a luminous generator. Nonluminous infrared radiation is produced by a metal coil similar to an electric stove or space heater (Fig. 19–2).

Heating of the skin depends on the amount of radiation that is absorbed. Pigmented, darker skin will absorb more energy and, therefore, more rapidly heat than lighter skin.

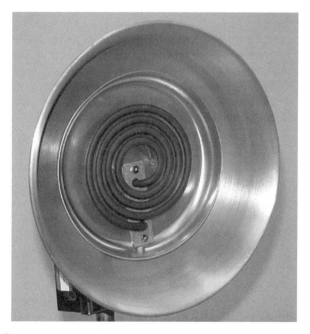

Figure 19–2. **Heating Element for a Nonluminous Infrared Lamp.** These elements are similar to the heating element on an electric stove. Note that the protective screen has been removed.

● EFFECTS ON

The Injury Response Process

Infrared radiation heats the skin almost exclusively and is used when dry heat is indicated, such as dermatological conditions. Deeper tissues are heated by conduction to depths up to 1 cm. The primary physiological effects occur almost entirely in the superficial skin. The increased temperature causes increased cell metabolism, increased superficial blood flow, and other biophysical effects of heat as described in Chapter 5. Hyperemia occurs as a result of increased capillary flow and increased capillary pressure.

If the temperature remains comfortable, superficial muscular relaxation may occur. As the treatment persists, local sweating will begin, an effect that may be unwanted if the goal of the treatment is to dehydrate skin conditions. Note that drying acute open wounds (e.g., abrasions, turf burns) may be counterproductive to the healing process. Infrared application for drying is limited to seeping skin conditions. Treatment of skin conditions must be supplemented with proper hygiene and, if indicated, medication.[146]

■ Contraindications

Infrared lamps are contraindicated in any conditions in which other forms of superficial heat are contraindicated (see Table 5–9 and At a Glance: Infrared Lamps, p 337). Because of the increased risk of burns associated with this modality, it should not be used over areas of sensory loss, including scars. Peripheral vascular disease and other circulatory impairments are contraindications to the use of infrared lamps because of the body's inability to dissipate heat. Infrared radiation should not be used over areas of sunburn.

■ Controversies in Treatment

The recent literature regarding traditional infrared heat treatments is scant, and the contemporary use of infrared radiation is rare. Infrared lamps are included in textbooks primarily for historical purposes.

Many of the effects associated with superficial heat treatments can also be associated with infrared radiation. A primary difference between this form of heat and other superficial heating agents, such as a moist heat pack, is that infrared lamps deliver a constant level of heat. This means that the temperature of the source is unchanging, and the only way to decrease the temperature gradient is for the skin to warm, potentially leading to burns.

Infrared radiation was once thought to assist in the healing of open wounds, such as turf burns or selected skin conditions. This practice actually deters the healing process because it dehydrates the exposed tissues even though blood flow is increased.[147]

▌ CLINICAL APPLICATION OF INFRARED LAMPS

■ Set-up and Application

Refer to manufacturer's operating instructions for the procedures specific to the unit being used.

Instrumentation

Power: Turns the unit ON and OFF (Note: the TIMER dial may also serve this purpose).

Timer: Sets the duration of the treatment, normally from 1 to 30 minutes.

Intensity: Adjusts the wattage of the heating element. The treatment intensity can also be adjusted by moving the lamp nearer or farther away from the target tissues.

Preparation of the Patient

1. Question the patient regarding the presence of any contraindications.
2. To prevent the concentration of heat, clean the area of any sweat, dirt, skin creams, or oils, and remove any jewelry.
3. Position the patient so that the energy of the lamp will strike the target tissues at a right angle.
4. If necessary, drape the patient for modesty.
5. If the treatment will be administered to the face, the patient should be fitted with infrared goggles.

Initiation of the Treatment

1. Warm up the lamp, if necessary.
2. Position the patient in a comfortable manner. Drape the body part so that only the area to be treated is exposed.
3. If a moist heat treatment is desired, place a damp terry cloth towel over the area. Replace the toweling as it dries out during the treatment.
4. Position a luminous lamp so that the source of the heat is approximately 24 inches away from the target tissues. Nonluminous lamps should be positioned approximately 32 inches from the target tissues. The intensity of the treatment can be increased by moving the lamp closer to the tissues and decreased by moving it farther away (see the Inverse Square Law in Appendix B).
5. Adjust the lamp so the energy will strike the tissues at a right angle (see the Cosine Law in Appendix B).
6. To prevent burns, instruct the patient not to move. Coming into contact with the reflector or wire guard can cause significant burns.
7. Check the patient's comfort periodically. The intensity of the treatment may be adjusted by moving the lamp toward the skin (increasing the temperature) or away from the skin (decreasing the temperature). Raised areas of the body area, such as the patella or lateral malleolus, will

At a Glance: **Infrared Lamps**

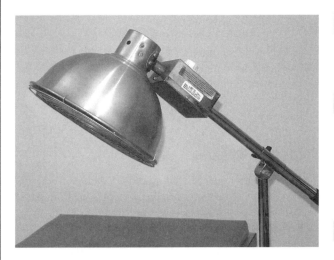

Used for

Superficial, dry heat used for drying superficial tissue and sedating sensory nerves. Although not common, infrared lamps have been used to:
■ Heat the skin
■ Dry certain **macerated** ■ dermatological conditions (use with caution and under a physician's direction).
Refer to Chapter 5 for a further description of superficial heating.

Treatment

The treatment time is 20 to 30 minutes and may be given as needed.

Indications

■ Subacute or chronic inflammatory conditions.
■ Skin infections.
■ Peripheral nerve injuries before electrical stimulation: Another modality should be considered if the patient lacks temperature perception.

Contraindications

■ Acute inflammatory conditions
■ Peripheral vascular disease
■ Areas with sensory loss
■ Over areas of scars
■ Sunburns

Precautions

■ The infrared heating element does not cool during the treatment, thus providing a constant level of energy. The unchanging temperature source increases the risk of burns. Check with the patient regularly.
■ Do not use on a sleeping or unconscious patient.

become hotter than other tissues because they are closer to the energy source.

8. Instruct the patient to summon assistance if the intensity of the treatment becomes too great.

Termination of the Treatment

1. To avoid patient contact with the lamp, remove the lamp prior to allowing the patient to move.
2. Check the patient's skin for signs of burns.
3. Dry, clean, and dress the area as needed.
4. Interview the patient to ascertain the effectiveness of the treatment.

▶ ULTRAVIOLET THERAPY

UV radiation has a shorter wavelength than visible light (see Fig. 19–1). Like infrared energy, UV light is unde-

tectable by the human eye. Energy in the near UV range—referred to as such because it is nearest to the visible light spectrum—has wavelengths ranging between 290 and 400 nm. The far UV range encompasses wavelengths between 180 and 290 nm.

There are three bands of therapeutic UV radiation, UV-A, UV-B, and UV-C (Table 19–1). UV light produces superficial chemical changes in the skin, with longer wavelengths (UV-A) penetrating more deeply into the skin than shorter wavelengths (UV-C). UV light in the B band is primarily responsible for the burning and blistering associated with doses above the minimal erythemal dose (MED; see Ultraviolet Treatment Dosage). The C band is more easily tolerated by the body, rarely causing burns or blistering, and for this reason, C-band lamps are used for killing bacteria.[148] Sunburn is an example of the effect of an overdose of UV-A and UV-B radiation.

Macerated: Skin that has been softened by soaking in water.

■ Ultraviolet Lamps

Clinically, UV light is produced by either a hot lamp or a cold lamp. The therapeutic effects, the band of UV light, and the procedures for use are different for each and are described below in more detail (see Set-up and Application). Selecting an UV lamp that produces the appropriate band allows for maximum benefit at the lowest treatment intensities.[148]

"Hot" UV lamps are commonly produced by argon gas and mercury vapor housed in a quartz tube. When a low-voltage (30 to 110 V), high-amperage (5 A) electrical current is introduced to the tube, the argon gas is heated, vaporizing and polarizing the mercury, producing UV light in all three bands and visible light in the violet spectrum (Fig. 19–3). A **Kromayer lamp** produces UV energy that is primarily in the UV-A and UV-B bands.[148]

"Cold" UV lamps use a high-voltage (3000 V), low-amperage (15 mA) current that produces only UV-C. Cold lamps are primarily used to kill bacteria, as seen with decubitus ulcers, for example. The energy produced by cold lamps is less than by hot lamps. Therefore, cold lamps are applied with the source of the UV energy closer to the body (approximately 1 in. from the tissues).

■ Ultraviolet Treatment Dosage

UV treatment dosages are determined relative to the MED, the least amount of UV exposure time required to produce redness (erythema) within 1 to 6 hours and disappear within 24 hours (Table 19–2). The MED for hot lamps must be determined for each patient and is specific for each lamp. The MED calculated for a patient using lamp "A" must not be assumed to be the same for the same patient using lamp "B." All cold lamps, however, use a standard MED value.

TABLE 19–1	Ultraviolet Bands and Their Associated Effects

Band	Wavelength	Effects
UV-A	320 to 400 nm	Erythema (reddening) without pigmentation (240 to 360 nm)
UV-B	290 to 320 nm	Erythema without pigmentation (240 to 360 nm)
		Erythema with pigmentation (290 to 300 nm)
		Skin tanning (299 nm)
		Formation of vitamin D (270 to 300 nm)
UV-C	180 to 290 nm	Formation of vitamin D (270 to 300 nm)
		Kills bacteria (260 to 270 nm)
		Skin tanning (254 nm)
		Note: Most naturally occurring UV-C from the sun is filtered from the earth by the ozone layer.

MED: Hot Lamp

The treatment dosage of large body areas is based on the MED applied at a standard distance of 30 in. (Box 19–1). For patients who are photosensitive, the distance can be increased. Moving the lamp closer to the tissues increases the intensity of the treatment.

The intensity of local treatments using hot lamps is based on the duration of the exposure and the distance of the lamp from the tissues (Box 19–2). Hot UV lamps should not be closer than 15 in from the tissues, moving the lamp inward significantly increases the treatment intensity.

MED: Cold Lamp

By convention, the MED for cold UV lamps is determined to be 12 to 15 seconds at a distance of 1 in. from the skin. Using the time factors presented in Table 19–2, the relative dosage for cold quartz lamps at 1 in. are computed to be: $E_1 = 30$ to 38 sec; $E_2 = 60$ to 75 sec; $E_3 = 120$ to 150 sec.

Adjusting the Treatment Dosage

Because of the biophysical changes associated with UV light exposure, the MED will increase with treatment. Increasing the treatment dosage is based on the intensity at which erythema is produced. The treatment duration should be increased by between 30 to 50 percent for each subsequent treatment. If the treatment duration reaches 3 to 5 minutes, the distance between the hot UV lamp and the tissue can be reduced. The decision about the percentage the treatment duration is increased is based on the patient's reaction to the UV light. Patients who display sensitivity to UV light (e.g., those who are fair skinned) should initially receive a 30-percent increase in the treatment dosage (e.g., first treatment = 120 sec; second treatment = 156 sec). Likewise, when the treatment duration reaches 3 minutes for UV-sensitive patients, the distance of the lamp from the skin should be decreased. Five to 10 seconds should be deducted from the treatment duration if the patient misses a treatment.

Referring to the inverse square law in Appendix B, decreasing the distance by one half, for example from 30 to 15 in. increases the intensity by a factor of four. Under these conditions, if the treatment duration was 5 min (300 sec) at 30 in., decreasing the distance to 15 in. would require a treatment duration of 72 sec to produce the same results. For patients who tolerate UV radiation well, the higher values of a 50-percent increase in treatment duration and a maximum duration of 5 min can be used.

■ Biophysical Effects of Ultraviolet Light Exposure

Depending on the amount of pigmentation, UV energy is absorbed between approximately 0.20 and 0.22 mm below

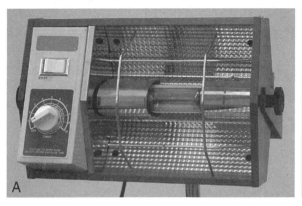
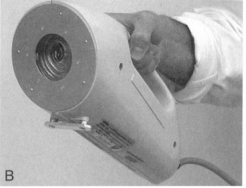

Figure 19–3. **Ultraviolet Bulbs.** (A) "Hot" ultraviolet lamp producing visible violet light and light in the ultraviolet A and B bands. (B) "Cold" ultraviolet lamp that produces invisible energy in the ultraviolet "C" band.

the skin's surface with longer UV bands affecting the tissues more than the shorter bands (see Table 19–1). Once within the tissues, UV energy causes a series of photochemical reactions (see Table 19–2). UV treatments have a latency period of at least 1 hour before effects are noted.

Given sufficient intensity and duration (dosage), UV radiation may damage cell proteins, **DNA** ■, and **RNA** ■. The skin reacts to this damage by initiating a series of local defensive responses. The most immediately visible of these is erythema. With time, the skin will pigment and darken ("tan") and the thickness of the epidermis will increase. The only systemic effect of UV exposure is the production of vitamin D.

UV light is also used to sterilize medical equipment, water, and food. These effects will not be addressed in this text.

■ Erythema

Erythema, best produced by UV with a wavelength of 297 nm (UV-B), represents the influx of arterial blood in the capillaries. **Photons** ■ from the UV light strike the skin, where they are absorbed by **melanin** ■ and cause photochemical reactions. Erythema may also be produced by the inflammation-induced release of prostaglandin precursors and histamine that increases vascular permeability. Vasodilation is also thought to be responsible for erythema,

TABLE 19–2	**Ultraviolet Treatment Dosage**	
Dose	*Description*	*Target Area*
Suberythemal (SED)	No erythema	Full body Vitamin D production
Minimal erythemal dose (MED)	Smallest dose that produces erythema within 1 to 6 hr and disappears within 24 hrs	Full body or local exposure
First degree erythemal dose (E_1)	Erythema lasts for 1 to 3 days. Some scaling of the skin is present. E_1 is approximately 2.5 times the MED.	Less than 20 percent of body area
Second degree erythemal dose (E_2)	Erythema with associated edema, peeling, and pigmentation. E_2 is approximately 5 times the MED.	Less than 250 cm^2
Third degree erythemal dose (E_3)	Severe erythema and burning with associated blistering, peeling, and edema. E_3 is approximately 10 times the MED.	Less than 25 cm^2

DNA: Deoxyribonucleic acid. Carries genetic information for all organisms except RNA.
Melanin: Pigmentation of the hair, skin, and eye produced by melanocytes.
Photon: A unit of light energy that has zero mass, no electrical charge, and an indefinite life span.
RNA: Ribonucleic acid. Controls protein synthesis.

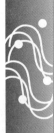

Box 19–1. Determining the Ultraviolet Minimal Erythemal Dose (MED)

MED Test Pattern

Patient: _____   Time Completed: _____

Time Redness
Appeared   Disappeared

30 Sec   _____   _____

30 Sec   _____   _____

15 Sec   _____   _____

15 Sec   _____   _____

15 Sec   _____   _____

15 Sec   _____   _____

Check the area that was exposed to the UV light once every hour and indicate the time that each of the shapes above first appears as a red area on your skin. Once a shape has appeared, note the time that it disappears. **Bring this card with you to your next appointment.**

(A)

The minimal erythemal dose (MED) is the least amount of ultraviolet exposure time required to produce redness within 1 to 6 hours and disappear within 24 hours (Note: there is no standard definition of the MED). This process is only required for hot quartz UV generators (typically those in the UV-A and UV-B range). The MED is device dependent, that is, each lamp will produce its own MED. Patients should only be treated with the unit that was used to calculate the MED and the MED for each patient must be calculated prior to administering the first bout in the treatment series. The MED test is used to determine the patient's sensitivity to UV light and determine treatment exposure.

The MED test is performed using a cardboard test strip, an erythrometer, in which six distinct shapes have been cut (A). A second cardboard strip covers all but the first opening (the square in the above example) and the surrounding skin is covered with a sheet. After exposure to the ultraviolet light, the next shape in the sequence is uncovered and the prior shapes are left exposed. At the end of the treatment, the first shape will have been exposed for 120 sec and the last shape (the inverted triangle) for 15 sec.

Following the test session, the patient regularly checks the treated area and notes the time that red shapes corresponding to those on the test strip appear on the skin. The initial ultraviolet exposure to determine the MED should be performed early in the morning to prevent sleep from interrupting the patient's monitoring of the results.

Box 19–1. Determining the Ultraviolet Minimal Erythemal Dose (MED) *(Continued)*

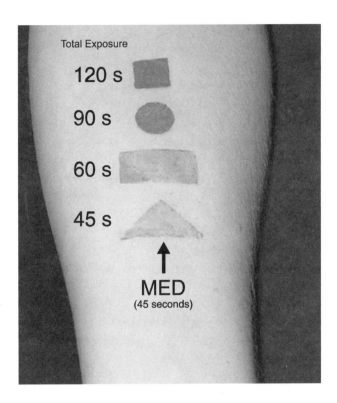

Technique

1. If needed, turn on the UV generator to allow it to warm up.
2. Identify an area of skin that has not previously been exposed to UV light, including recent sun exposure (e.g., low back, forearm, lower abdomen).
3. Remove any jewelry, clean and dry the area.
4. Position the patient so the UV light will strike the target tissues at a right angle.
5. Fit the patient with goggles. The clinician should wear goggles as well.
6. Affix the MED test strip (A) to the target tissue with tape.
7. Cover the surrounding area with a towel, assuring that no other skin area is exposed.
8. Cover all of the test patterns with a piece of thin cardboard.
9. Position the UV lamp 30 in. from the test strip so that the energy will strike the tissues at a right angle. Note the test distance in the patient's file.
10. Cover all but the first opening in the test strip. Open the shutters and expose the first test pattern to 30 sec. of UV light. Close the shutters.
11. Following the procedure described in Step 10, expose the second test pattern for 30 sec, leaving the first pattern uncovered.
12. Expose each of the remaining four test patterns for 15 sec each, leaving the prior patterns uncovered.
13. At the end of the test, the first pattern will have received 120 sec of UV exposure, the sixth pattern will receive 15 sec. The test increments can be decreased for light-skinned individuals who are prone to sunburn and increased for those who are more tolerant to sun exposure.
14. Instruct the patient to check the target area every hour and record when the redness for each symbol appears and disappears. The test strip can be used for this.
15. If no redness appears within 24 hours, repeat on a different body area using slightly increased exposure durations (e.g., 40, 40, 20, 20, 20, 20 sec).
16. Record the lamp used, the distance of the lamp from the skin, and the MED results in the patient's medical file.

Box 19–2. Local Treatment Dosages Using a Hot Quartz Generator

Local exposure treatment times are based on the distance of the lamp from the skin and are calculated using the formula:

$$T_2 = T_1 \left(\frac{(D_2)^2}{(D_1)^2} \right)$$

T_2 = New treatment exposure time
T_1 = Previous exposure
D_1 = Initial distance
D_2 = New distance

but its role appears to be secondary to other cellular level responses.[148, 149]

Therapeutically, erythema is most often triggered using UV-B exposure. Given a consistent intensity of UV-B, the constitutional skin color most influences the resulting magnitude of erythema.[150, 151] UV-B–induced erythema and vasodilation are the result of a series of chemical events rather than thermal changes. In response to UV-B, human keratinocytes and endothelial cells release nitrogen oxides that activates soluble guanylate cyclase, which, in turn, produces vasodilation and erythema.[152, 153]

Erythema formation is **latent** ■ . When applied at therapeutic dosages, the first sign of erythema does not appear for 1 to 2 hours following the treatment and continues to increase to its maximum intensity for 24 hours following the treatment, presumably because of the increased presence of prostaglandins. Erythema will persist for up to 48 hours following the treatment.[149]

Pigmentation

UV radiation with the wavelength of 254 nm or 299 nm causes melanin production in the deep layers of the skin. Melanin then diffuses to the superficial layers, causing the skin to darken ("tan") and the stratum corneum to thicken (see Epidermal Hyperplasia). Mild UV exposure and the subsequent darkening of the skin can reduce the risk of sunburn.

Epidermal Hyperplasia

Epidermal hyperplasia, the excessive proliferation of normal skin cells that results in a thickening of the skin's outer layer, is greatest following exposure to UV-B. Many of the mechanisms proposed to account for erythema and increased pigmentation may also be responsible for hyperplasia. Prostaglandin precursors cause increased epidural DNA synthesis and hyperplasia and is most pronounced following UV-B exposure.[154, 155]

Because the skin darkens and thickens following UV-A and UV-B exposure, less energy is absorbed by the deeper skin layers. As the skin darkens, the treatment dosages must be increased to affect deeper tissues.[148, 155]

Vitamin D Production

UV light is needed for the body to produce vitamin D. The body normally receives sufficient amounts of UV exposure from sunlight. **Rickets** ■ occurs when individuals are not exposed to sunlight for an extended time, resulting in decreased production of vitamin D. The lack of vitamin D decreases the intestine's ability to absorb and subsequently process calcium. In rare instances, patients may require full-body exposure to UV light to counter the effects of the lack of sunlight (e.g., bedridden patients).

● EFFECTS ON
The Injury Response Process

Wound Healing

Given sufficient intensity, UV energy activates the inflammatory response and triggers the release of histamine. Some evidence suggests that UV light may also stimulate the superficial growth of granulation tissue.[148] UV rays in the C-band, especially 260 nm to 270 nm, kill bacteria, and increase epithelialization with minimum erythema formation.[156–158] Cold lamps are applied at an intensity of E_3 (see Table 19–2).

Treatment of Psoriasis

Psoriasis, an intermittently appearing chronic condition, is the overproduction of epithelial cells that forms scales on the skin and is characterized by raised, red skin patches (Fig. 19–4). In addition to the cosmetic concerns, psoriasis can cause itching and pain as the scales crack, and the condition may be associated with psoriatic arthritis.

Latent: Delayed period between the stimulus and the response.

Rickets: Common in children, a vitamin D deficiency that results in inadequate deposition of lime salts, altering the shape, structure, and function of bone.

Chronic psoriasis is often treated with topical medications including corticosteroids and **retinoids** ■, **psoralen** ■, calcipotriene, and tazarotene that contain tar.[159–161] UV light in the A or B bands may be used in conjunction with these medications. The B band is most commonly used for treating psoriasis.[160, 162] Narrow-band UV-B administered twice per week produces optimum results with the minimum amount of patient risk.[162]

UV-A is administered in conjunction with a retinoid and psoralen, a treatment approach termed **PUVA**. This technique is often performed by dermatologists. UV-A is not an effective treatment for psoriasis unless the treatment is augmented by medications.[161] UV light in the C band is not used for treating psoriasis.[160] These regimens result in exfoliation of the tissues and are thought to damage the DNA that produces the excess skin cell growth associated with psoriasis.

■ Contraindications and Precautions in Ultraviolet Light Treatment

Similar to overexposure to the sun, too much UV exposure can produce severe burning, blistering, edema, and shock. There are relatively few absolute contraindications to UV exposure (see At a Glance: Ultraviolet Therapy, p 344). Patients who are prohibited from sunlight exposure should not be treated with UV light unless the protocol is specifically approved by the patient's physician.

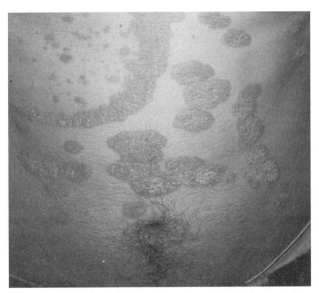

Figure 19–4. **Psoriasis.** During eruptions, psoriasis is characterized by red, raised areas of the skin that contains white, silver, or yellow scales. (From Goldsmith, LA, et al: Adult and Pediatric Dermatology. FA Davis, Philadelphia, 1997, p 258.)

UV radiation in the A band, and to a lesser extent the B band, is associated with skin cancer and other forms of cancer and liver disease. Although it is unlikely that normal treatment exposures are sufficient to cause melanoma in and of itself, therapeutic treatment could add to the cumulative effects of UV exposure from the sun and accelerate existing conditions. Therefore, UV treatments are absolutely contraindicated in the presence of skin cancer. Exposure to UV radiation can also worsen the skin discoloration associated with lupus and is contraindicated in the presence of kidney, liver, or cardiac disease and with patients with pulmonary tuberculosis.

UV light is injurious to the eyes and unprotected exposure can cause permanent damage to the lens, cornea, and lids. Both the patient and the clinician must wear approved UV-resistant goggles during the treatment. If the patient was prescribed psoralens or other medications that increase the sensitivity to UV light, the eyes should be protected for up to 12 hours following the treatment.[162]

Patients who are highly sensitive to sunlight, have little skin pigmentation, or are taking medications or eating foods that increase sunlight sensitivity must be managed with caution.

■ Controversies in Treatment

UV therapy is primarily limited to dermatology clinics and is rarely used in the orthopedic setting. Advances in medications and personal hygiene have decreased the role of UV in the treatment of open wounds and skin conditions.[146]

A comparison of wounds treated with UV light demonstrated no significant differences in wound strength, inflammation, or macroscopic or microscopic indicators of healing relative to a control group.[163] Repeated exposure to UV-A and UV-B alters the skin structure and can decrease the tensile strength of the wound.[164]

Consistent dosage is problematic in the application of UV therapy and is further complicated by the lack of a standard definition of the MED.

▶ CLINICAL APPLICATION OF ULTRAVIOLET LIGHT

■ Set-up and Application

Many UV generators produce **ozone** ■. Ozone-producing lamps should be used only in well-ventilated areas. This section describes the process of local UV treatment.

Ozone: Formed by the grouping of three oxygen atoms (O_3). Ozone is present in the atmosphere where it filters out ultraviolet light (especially in the C band), helping to prevent certain forms of cancer.

Psoralen: A group of substances that produce inflammation of the skin when exposed to sunlight or ultra violet light.

Retinoid: Topical medication consisting of retinoic acid. Used to treat psoriasis and severe acne.

At a Glance: **Ultraviolet Therapy**

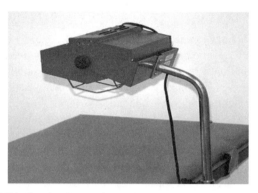

(A) "Hot" or luminous ultraviolet lamp produces energy in the ultraviolet "A" and "B" bands as well as visible violet light.

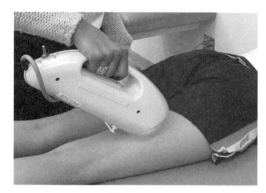

(B) "Cold" or nonluminous ultraviolet lamp that produces light in the "C" range.

Description

The use of electromagnetic energy that is below that of visible light to produce photo-chemical reactions in the skin. Each of the three ultraviolet bands (A, B, and C) produces unique effects. Ultraviolet therapy is used for:
- Wound healing
- Resolution of dermatitis
- Treatment of infection
- Treatment of psoriasis

Primary Effects

- Vasodilation of superficial arterioles, resulting in erythema.
- Destruction of bacteria.
- Production of cells in the **stratum basale,** resulting in increased thickness (hyperplasia) of the epidermis.
- Melanin production
- Vitamin D production

Treatment

The treatment duration is based on the MED. Treatments are given every other day.

Indications

- Psoriasis
- Folliculitis
- Acne vulgaris
- Pityriasis rosea
- Tineal infections
- Slow-healing open wounds
- Pressure sores
- **Uremic pruritus**
- Exfoliation
- Preventing sunburn (prior to sun exposure)

Contraindications

- Liver or kidney disease
- Certain cardiovascular conditions
- Diabetes mellitus
- Tuberculosis
- **Hyperthyroidism**
- Lupus
- Herpes simplex I and II
- **Albinism**
- **Porphyria**
- Fever
- Patients receiving x-ray therapy
- Patients prone to sunburn or sensitive to sunlight exposure
- Certain birth control pills

Precautions

- Certain medications (e.g., tetracycline, quinolones, psoralens), disease states (e.g., syphilis, kidney/liver disease, lupus, alcoholism), foods (e.g., shellfish, strawberries, eggs) can predispose the patient to sunburns. Identify if the patient has a history of sunburns and check with a physician regarding the history of burns or medications that the patient is taking.
- Exposure of the eyes to ultraviolet light can cause keratitis and conjunctivitis. Eye protection should always be worn by the patient and the clinician.
- Overexposure to ultraviolet radiation can result in protein shock.
- Ultraviolet radiation in the C band increases the risk of skin cancer.

Instrumentation

Shutters: During the warm-up period or when repositioning the unit, the shutters prevent the UV energy from leaving the lamp. During the treatment, the shutters help to direct the energy to the target tissues.

Power: Turns the power to the lamp ON or OFF.

Preparation of the Patient

1. Question the patient regarding the presence of any contraindications.
2. If required, turn on the UV generator to allow it to warm up. Close the shutters on hot lamps.
3. Calculate the treatment duration (see Box 19–2, Ultraviolet Treatment Dosage).
4. Clean the area of any sweat, dirt, skin creams, or oils, and remove any jewelry.
5. Cover the skin surface that is not being treated with sheets or towels. If the patient is extra sensitive to UV radiation, first apply a sun screen to the surrounding skin and then apply the protective drape. Areas that do not normally receive UV exposure (e.g., the nipples and genitals) are particularly sensitive to this treatment.
6. If multiple areas are being treated, avoid the possibility of double exposure.
7. Fit the patient with UV-resistant goggles. The clinician should also wear UV goggles while working with the patient and the generator is on.
8. Position the patient so that the UV light will fully strike the body area being treated.
9. If open wounds are being treated, cover the area using a sterile drape or dressing.
10. Although precooling the skin is sometimes used to increase the level of erythema, this technique has not been proved to be effective.[165]
11. The operator must avoid accidental self-exposure to the UV light.

Initiation of the Treatment—Hot Lamp

1. Position the UV lamp so that the light rays will strike the target tissues at a right angle at the distance from the skin used in determining the MED, normally 30 in. (see Box 19–1).
2. Determine the treatment dosage to be used during the treatment (see Box 19–2).
3. If practical, position the patient's head so that it is facing away from the lamp.
4. Open the shutters, and administer the treatment for the appropriate duration.
5. Although treatment durations are typically short, provide the patient with a means of immediately summoning assistance if help is required.

Initiation of the Treatment—Cold Lamp

1. Follow the steps described in "Preparation of the Patient."

2. Hold the lamp 1 in. from the target tissues so that the UV energy will strike the tissues evenly and at a right angle. Some hand-held lamps include spacers that will position the lamp a predetermined distance from the tissues.
3. Treat the wound for the appropriate duration based on the MED value.

Terminating the Treatment

1. Record the lamp used and the distance, duration, and other treatment parameters used in the patient's medical file.
2. Interview the patient regarding the treatment outcomes, keeping in mind that the effects of UV light are latent.
3. Instruct the patient to monitor the treated area in the hours following UV exposure and report back any adverse effects. The patient should be provided with an emergency contact number in case severe burning occurs.

■ Maintenance

Refer to the manufacturer's recommended maintenance schedule and procedures.

After Each Use

Clean the lamp's bulb and reflectors with 95-percent ethyl alcohol or other cleaner recommended by the manufacturer, with a lint-free cloth.

Annually or as Required

UV lamps lose their potency with use and time (due to the collection of dust and oils on the bulb). Most bulbs have an expected lifespan of 500 to 1000 hours.

1. Cold lamps: Check and if needed, change the lamp every 1000 hours of use (or annually).
2. Calibrate the UV output according to the manufacturer's recommendations or by a qualified service technician.

▶ THERAPEUTIC LASERS

Laser, an acronym for *L*ight *A*mplification by *S*timulated *E*mission of *R*adiation, uses highly organized light to emit photons that elicit physiological changes in the tissues. Therapeutic lasers are strictly controlled in the United States but are more frequently used in Canada and Europe. In the United States, an investigational device exemption from the Food and Drug Administration (FDA) is required for its use. For this reason, therapeutic laser devices are not available for general use, but have been approved for the treatment of certain pathologies including **carpal tunnel syndrome ▪** .

High-power (hot) lasers have an output of greater than 60 mW and create thermal changes in the tissues, causing the tissues to be destroyed, evaporated, or dehydrated or causing protein coagulation.[166] High-power lasers are used for surgery, capsular shrinkage, ocular surgery, and wrinkle and tattoo removal. Because of their destructive potential, high-power lasers are not found in the rehabilitation setting.

Therapeutic low-power (cold) lasers should not normally cause tissue destruction.[167] The energy produced by therapeutic lasers has a wavelength ranging from 1 nanometer (nm) to 1 mm. This range includes UV, visible, and infrared light. The frequency (wavelength) determines the color of the laser light. These terms can be used interchangeably.

Lasers produce a refined, homogeneous beam of light that is characterized by being monochromatic, coherent, and collimated. **Monochromatic** indicates that all of the light energy has the same wavelength and therefore has the same color. Sunlight passing through a prism creates a literal rainbow of colors because it has light of different wavelengths.

Laser light that is passed through a prism simply bends the ray and the color leaving the prism the same as that entering it. Light photons travel in individual waves having different wavelengths based on the color of the light. When all of the light waves are in phase, they are said to be **coherent** (Fig 19–5). Light from a light bulb spreads—diverges—as it travels. Laser light is **collimated** because it diverges very little as it travels through space.

Lasers are classified by the FDA's Center for Devices and Radiological Health (CDRH) based on the Accessible Emission Limit (AEL). The AEL is the maximum permissible power level for each class, ranging from 1 (minimum risk of causing harm) to 4 (extreme risk) (Table 19–3).

▪ Laser Output Parameters

Therapeutic (cold) lasers produce a maximum output of 90 mW or less, although this value may be higher in other countries.[168] The low power output is not sufficient to cause thermal changes in the tissues, so therapeutic benefits are thought to be related to photochemical events.

The magnitude of the tissue's reaction to laser light is based on the physical characteristics of the output wavelength/frequency (absorption, reflection, and transmission), the density of the power, the duration of the treatment, and the vascularity of the target tissues.[169] Effects that occur from the absorption of photons are termed the **direct effect**. An **indirect effect** is produced by chemical events caused by the interaction of the photons emitted from the laser and the tissues. The indirect effect

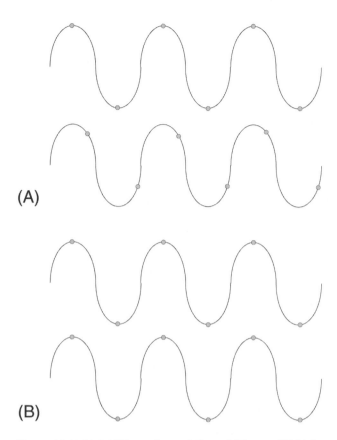

(A)

(B)

Figure 19–5. **Light Waves In and Out of Phase.** (A) Light having the same wavelength, but the photons are out of phase. (B) With coherent light the photons are in phase.

may produce changes that occur deeper in the tissues than those caused by the direct effect.

Therapeutic lasers require a base unit that houses the laser generator (Box 19–3). The output is delivered to the body through a fiber optic cable and a hand-held applicator. The laser medium (e.g., argon, helium-neon) determines the wavelength—and therefore the effects of—the laser output.

Frequency

As with all electromagnetic energy, wavelength and frequency are inversely related. Long wavelengths have a lower frequency than shorter wavelengths (see Appendix B). The depth of laser penetration is based on the wavelength and power of the output; the wavelength of the laser depends on the medium used. Wavelengths of 300 to 1000 nm penetrate up to 3.6 mm, shorter wavelengths penetrate less deeply. New evaluation methods have indicated that some low-power lasers can penetrate up to 2 cm deep, especially when applied over bony prominences such as the cervical spine and skull.[170]

Lasers of different frequencies are thought to produce different physiological effects. Table 19–4 presents a list of therapeutic lasers.

Carpal tunnel syndrome: Compression of the median nerve that produces pain, numbness, and weakness in the palm and ring and index fingers.

TABLE 19–3   Food and Drug Administration's Center for Devices and Radiological Health Laser Classification System

Classification	Description
1	These lasers are exempt from most control measures.
	The laser output is either safe to the human eye or contained within the device in a manner that keeps the laser from escaping.
	No special labeling is required.
2	Low-power lasers–visible light may be emitted.
	Output does not exceed 1 mW.
	The normal eye reflex (approximately 0.25 s) will protect the eye from direct contact with the laser output.
	Must be labeled with "CAUTION—Laser Radiation: Do not stare into beam."
2a	Visible laser is produced (e.g., a bar code scanner).
	Eye damage can occur if the laser enters the eye for more than 1000 seconds.
	The labeling is the same as for type 2 lasers.
3a	Produces an output up to 5 mW.
	Direct contact with the eye for short periods is not hazardous. Viewing the laser through magnifying optics such as eyeglasses can present a hazard.
	Must be labeled with "CAUTION—Laser Radiation: Do not stare into beam or view directly with optical instruments."
3b	Medium power lasers producing an output of 5 mW to 500 mW.
	Direct contact of the laser output with the eyes can result in damage
	Must be labeled with "DANGER—Visible and/or invisible laser radiation—avoid direct exposure to beam."
4	High power lasers having an output of greater than 500 mW.
	Direct or indirect contact with the skin and eyes can be hazardous.
	Toxic airborne contaminants may be produced.
	The output creates a fire hazard.
	Must be labeled with "DANGER—Visible and/or invisible laser radiation—avoid eye or skin expo sure to direct or scattered beam."

Helium neon (HeNe) lasers are created by exciting a mixture of helium and neon gases, producing a wavelength of 632.8 nm, within the visible red light range. The maximum output of HeNe lasers is usually 1 mW or less, and their energy can penetrate up to 0.8 to 15 mm deep.[171] The indirect effect may produce tissue changes deeper than 15 mm. HeNe lasers typically have an output in the range of 14 to 29 mJ (see Table 11–2).

Gallium arsenide (GaAs) laser is produced by a semiconductor diode chip with an output between 904 to 910 nm. This wavelength places the GaAs laser within the infrared spectrum and is invisible to the human eye and can penetrate the tissues up to 2 cm. GaAs lasers may produce up to 2 mW output that is often pulsed, delivering a significantly lower average power than HeNe lasers (see Power and Treatment Dosage). GaAs lasers may have a visible light pointing system and must have a light that illuminates when the laser output is being emitted.

Gallium aluminum arsenide (GaAlAs) laser uses three diodes, each producing 30 mW of power at a wavelength of 830 nm. The outputs of the three diodes combine to produce a total treatment output of 90 mW, theoretically producing a deeper depth of penetration.[172] Although multidiode systems produce an increased output, their dosage specifications are unclear.[168]

Power and Treatment Dosage

The measurement of laser output is similar to that used for therapeutic ultrasound. The power density of the treatment is expressed in milliwatts per square centimeter (mW/cm^2) and is based on the laser output (expressed in mW) and the surface area (circumference) of the emitted energy. This calculation is based on the formula:

$$\text{Power density (mW/cm}^2) = \frac{\text{Watts (mW)}}{\text{Target Area (cm}^2)}$$

Laser output can also be expressed in Joules, especially when pulsed laser output is used. This calculation takes into consideration the actual amount of time that the energy is being emitted and is expressed in terms of Joules per square centimeter (J/cm^2):

$$\text{Energy density (J/cm}^2) = \frac{\text{Watts (W)} \times \text{Time (Sec)}}{\text{Target Area (cm}^2)}$$

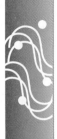

Box 19–3. Production of Laser

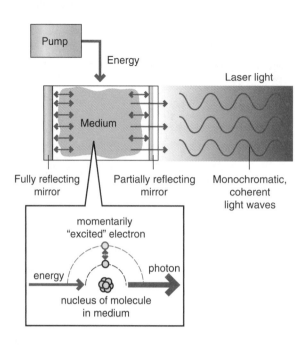

Laser production requires four essential components: (1) An active (amplifying) medium, (2) a mechanism for exciting the medium (a pump), (3) a reflective mirror, and (4) a partially reflective mirror that allows for some transmission of light and reflects the rest.

Lasers are referred to by the type of active medium (the atoms that are stimulated to produce the light) they use, HeNe or GaAs for example. The active medium is a solid, liquid, or gas that contains atoms, molecules, or ions that are capable of storing energy which, when stimulated, release their energy as light. Any subsequent increase in light energy through the lasing mechanism is known as **gain**.

Through a process known as **pumping**, energy is introduced into the active medium. For a solid medium, the pumping is obtained by irradiating the medium with a bright light; gaseous mediums are energized by passing an electrical current through the medium.

When a photon of light is absorbed by an atom (collectively including molecules and ions), an outer electron moves from its normal orbit, its **ground state,** to a higher orbit termed the **excited state**. By being moved to a higher orbit, the electron and therefore the atom, reaches a higher energy state. After a brief stay (less than a millionth of a second) in the higher orbit, the electron spontaneously returns to its ground state and in the process releases another photon. The released photon will have the same wavelength (and therefore frequency) as the photon that was absorbed.

Stimulated response occurs when a photon strikes an atom that is already in the excited state and causes the electron that is in the higher orbit to move to a lower one. In this case, instead of a single photon being released, two photons are released. Each of these photons has the same wavelength and is in phase with each other. When more atoms are in an excited state than in the ground state, a **population inversion,** more photons are emitted than absorbed, forming the basis for the emission of laser.

A laser generator consists of an **oscillator,** the active medium located between two mirrors. One mirror reflects 100 percent of the photons that strike it and the other mirror is partially reflective. Photons that reflect off the mirrors are reflected back into the medium for further amplification. Those photons that transmit through the partially reflective mirror form the laser output.

TABLE 19–4	Types of Therapeutic Lasers	
Name	*Abbreviation*	*Wavelength (nm)*
Argon	Ar	488
Gallium-arsenide	GaAs	904
Gallium aluminum arsenide	GaAlAs	830
Helium-neon	HeNe	632.8
Indium gallium aluminum phosphate	InGaAlPO$_4$	670

Acute conditions are treated with an output of less than 0.5 J/cm^2. The dosage for chronic conditions is normally less than 3.0 J/cm^2. Individual laser manufacturers publish recommended treatment intensity and durations, although the evidence base for making this decision is currently lacking.

● E FFECTS ON

The Injury Response Process

Laser energy can effectively stimulate tissues at depths up to 15 mm below the surface of the skin.[173, 174] When the photons are absorbed by the tissues, it is thought to alter molecular-level activity, including short-term stimulation of the electron transport chain, increased synthesis of adenosine triphosphate (ATP), and a reduction in intracellular pH.[168] These actions are theorized to affect pain-producing tissue, such as areas of muscle spasm, by restoring the normal properties of muscle tissue via the increased formation of ATP and increased enzyme activity.[174]

Wound Healing

Lasers have been used to assist in the healing of superficial wounds including ulcers, surgical incisions, and burns. The healing process is enhanced by the accelerated phagocytic activity and the selective destruction of bacteria.[175] The absorption of photons is believed to cause increased ATP synthesis that increases the cellular metabolism and encourages the release of free radicals.[175, 176] Cell membrane permeability is altered and there is an increase in fibroblast, lymphocyte, and macrophage activity.[177] Blood and lymph circulation is improved in the area surrounding the treatment area, promoting the growth of granulation tissue.[178] Laser therapy is also thought to increase collagen content and increase tensile strength of healing wounds.

The bactericidal effects of low-power lasers are enhanced by the preapplication of photosensitizers. These substances absorb light having a specific frequency and increase the intensity of the laser output to the point where membrane permeability is altered, free radicals and **singlet oxygen** ■ are produced, and selective cell death occurs.[175]

Because of their relatively low power output, HeNe lasers were less effective in destroying bacteria than indium gallium aluminum phosphate (InGaAlPO$_4$) lasers.[175]

Pain Reduction

Low-level laser therapy has been used to decrease acute and chronic pain. Pain reduction is believed to occur as a result of altering nerve conduction velocity or decreased muscle spasm. These pain control approaches have been augmented with the use of sympathetic blocks and antidepressant medication.[179] Although the underlying mechanism is not fully understood, low-intensity laser can reduce the rate and velocity of sensory nerve impulses.

Theories on how laser disrupts sensory nerve condition include effects similar to that seen during cold application but without the thermal changes.[171] Low-intensity laser having a wavelength of 830 nm and applied at 9.6 J/cm^2 [180] and HeNe applied at 19 mJ/cm^2 [171] reduced the rate of nerve conduction at the site of the treatment and distally. These effects had a significant latency period following the treatment.

Decreased skin resistance indicates the presence of local hypersensitive areas such as trigger points and acupuncture points. Helium neon laser applied to cervical trigger points [181] and acupuncture points corresponding to pain caused by fibromyalgia[182] resulted in increased skin resistance and decreased pain.

Laser therapy has demonstrated the ability to reduce the pain associated with postherpetic neuralgia[179] and to resolve neurapraxia.[178] Another possible explanation for pain reduction following laser treatment is a strong placebo effect.[183]

Fracture Healing

Many of the same biophysical effects that assist soft tissue healing may also enhance fracture healing and bone remodeling. These effects including increased capillary formation, calcium deposition, increased callus formation, and reduction of hematoma may be associated with the direct or indirect effect. Photons striking the tissues may create acoustic sound waves that affect the healing bone in a manner similar to ultrasonic bone growth stimulators.[177, 184]

Using an animal model, both GaAs and GaAlAs lasers applied daily at 4.0 J/cm^2 increased the density of the healing callus relative to a control group. However, the longer wavelength GaAs laser group had significantly denser callus than the GaAlAs group.[184] A higher power carbon dioxide (CO_2) laser increased the rate of hematoma absorption and the removal of necrotic tissue, leading to enhanced fracture healing in laboratory animals.[177]

Singlet oxygen: An uncharged form of oxygen that can selectively destroy cells.

At a Glance: Therapeutic "Cold" Lasers

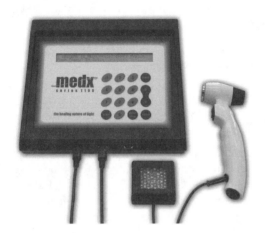

Description

Laser is a highly organized form of ultraviolet, visible, or infrared light. Photons that are absorbed by the cells produce direct changes in their function. Indirect effects occur secondary to photochemical events. Therapeutic laser has been used for the following conditions with varying results:

- Wound healing
- Decreasing inflammation
- Pain control (e.g., for arthritis)
- Stimulation of acupuncture points
- Treatment of carpal tunnel syndrome

Primary Effects

- Altered nerve conduction velocity
- Vasodilation
- Increased ATP production
- Increased collagen production
- Increased macrophage activity

Treatment

The treatment duration depends on the type of laser being used (e.g., helium neon), the pathology being treated, and the power of the output.

Indications

- Wound healing
- Fracture healing
- Musculoskeletal pain
- Osteoarthritis
- Rheumatoid arthritis

Contraindications

- Application to the eyes
- Over areas of hemorrhage in high intensities
- Over cancerous areas

Precautions

- Laser therapy should not be applied within 6 months of radiation therapy.
- Because of unknown effects, lasers should not be applied to the low back or abdomen during pregnancy, over unfused epiphyseal plates, or be administered to small children.
- The patient may experience dizziness during the treatment. If this occurs, discontinue the treatment. If the episode reoccurs, laser therapy should not be applied to the patient.

■ Contraindications and Precautions

Laser produces nonionizing radiation, greatly reducing the possibility of causing permanent damage to cellular structures or damaging DNA. The retina is sensitive to low-power laser exposure; even brief contact can result in permanent damage to the retina (see At a Glance: Therapeutic "Cold" Lasers, p 351). Depending on the type of laser being used, appropriate safety goggles should be worn by both the patient and the clinician (refer to the manufacturer's instructions for goggle requirements). Because of the risk of increased proliferation of cancerous cells, low-power laser therapy must not be applied to tumors or cancerous lesions.

■ Controversies in Treatment

Therapeutic laser therapy is a controversial treatment approach that is hindered by unclear treatment protocol, conflicting results, and unknown biophysical effects. This is further compounded by limited published research studies, which is partially attributable to its restricted use in the United States.

Although therapeutic laser has been used to control pain and otherwise alter nerve conduction velocity, research studies using various types of lasers and a range of output parameters have not significantly substantiated this effect.[168, 172, 173, 185] Several studies have concluded that laser treatment was not effective in treating musculoskeletal pain including myofascial pain,[186] lateral epicondylitis,[185] traumatic orthopedic pain,[187] rheumatoid arthritis,[183] and tooth extraction.[188] Two meta-analyses of the effect of laser therapy in treating orthopedic and skin conditions strongly suggest that this is not an effective modality in the treatment of these conditions.[189, 190]

A study investigating the effects of HeNe laser, GaAs laser, and standard treatment protocol on pain and range of motion associated with **tendinopathies** ■ demonstrated that all three treatment groups improved over a 2-week period, but the laser treatment groups had no significant benefits relative to the control group.[191]

Several studies investigating the effect of laser on wound healing have questioned the efficacy of this technique. Using human subjects, no significant difference in the healing rates of chronic venous leg ulcers was found between a group receiving standard treatment protocol augmented by HeNe laser (applied at 6 mW) and a group receiving standard treatment and sham laser.[192] A laboratory study investigating the healing characteristics of straight-line incisions in rat skin concluded that HeNe laser application demonstrated slight increases in tensile strength and other healing measures early, but these differences were only statistically significant, not clinically significant. There was no long-term difference in healing characteristics between irradiated and nonirradiated groups.[193]

Although cellular level effects and increased callus formation in fractures treated with GaAs and GaA1As,[184] and CO_2 [177] lasers, these effects were not replicated using the more common HeNe lasers applied at 2 or 4 J.[194]

▶ CLINICAL APPLICATION OF THERAPEUTIC LASERS

▇ Set-up and Application

Because of the investigational status of therapeutic lasers, the step-by-step set-up and application of therapeutic lasers are not described. The following sections discuss the application considerations.

Instrumentation

Although there is a limited number of laser units marketed in the United States, the available functions and types of laser output produced (e.g., HeNe, GaAs) creates diversity in the instrumentation. When units produced outside of the United States are considered, the difference in instrumentation becomes even greater.

Timer: Selects the duration of the treatment. On some units, the timer function may be overridden by selecting the MANUAL switch.

Frequency: For pulsed output, adjusts the frequency or duration, or both, of the laser pulses. Do not confuse this parameter with the output frequency of the laser.

Source: Selects the type of laser, typically HeNe or GaAs.

Power: Adjusts the output in watts. The total amount of energy is equal to the output wattage and the treatment duration (Joules = power × duration). The total output per unit of area is measured as Joules per square centimeter (J/cm^2).

Point locator: This function uses a low-voltage current to identify areas of low electrical resistance that correspond to acupuncture points, motor points, trigger points, and areas of pathology. An electrode from the unit is attached to the patient. The tip of the laser applicator serves as the electrode that completes the electrical circuit. The applicator is slowly moved over the target tissues until a decrease in resistance is found. That area is then treated.

● Chapter Highlights

- Light modalities are found on the electromagnetic spectrum. Infrared radiation has a wavelength greater than 780 nm; UV light has a wavelength of less than 380 nm. The range in between these values represents visible light.
- Although they are seldom used, infrared lamps provide superficial dry heat to the tissues.
- Infrared lamps are either in the near-infrared range (luminous lamps) or the far-infrared range (nonluminous lamps).
- UV light is formed by three primary bands: A, B, and C. The A and B bands produce various levels of reddening and skin pigmentation. The C band is primarily used for killing bacteria in wounds.
- Treatment dosages for UV light are based on the MED, the least amount of exposure required to produce reddening.
- Laser light is characterized by being monochromatic, coherent, and collimated. Cold lasers may be in the visible, UV, or infrared light spectrum.
- Therapeutic (cold) lasers are nonthermal devices that are designed to produce chemical changes in the skin.
- The primary effects of cold laser occur when the photons are absorbed by the tissues, altering molecular level function.
- The efficacy of therapeutic lasers has not been established.

Tendinopathy: Any disease or trauma involving a muscle's tendon, tissues surrounding the tendon, or the tendon's insertion into the bone.

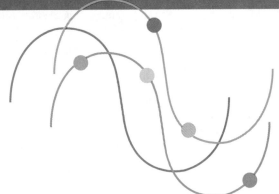

Chapter 20

Hyperbaric Oxygen Therapy

Hyperbaric oxygen therapy places the patient in a high-atmosphedic-pressure, high-oxygen environment. The high-oxygen intake increases the oxygen content in plasma and prevents ischemia and the high pressure causes gas bubbles to be displaced. Long used for treatment of the bends experienced by divers, the use of hyperbaric oxygen therapy has expanded to treat a wide range of musculoskeletal, neurological, and disease states. Hyperbaric oxygen chambers are "high-end" devices that are housed in select hospitals, private specialized clinics, and professional sports teams.

Hyperbaric oxygen (HBO) therapy (HBOT) was originally used for decompression sickness experienced by divers and gas **embolisms** ■ (Table 20–1).[195] The role of HBOT has evolved to include the treatment of crush injuries, compartment syndromes, severe burns, infection, traumatic brain injury, and strokes and has recently been used as an adjunctive treatment for orthopedic injuries such as sprains, strains, and large hematomas.[195–198] HBO is also used to enhance athletic performance by pre-loading the body with oxygen.[195] This technique will not be discussed in this chapter.

Although the efficacy for musculoskeletal injuries has not been established, many "high-end" users such as professional sports teams have begun to integrate HBOT into the standard treatment protocol for ligament sprains and contusions.

Hyperbaric oxygen can also be applied superficially to the extremities or torso (Fig. 20–1). Superficial HBOT is used to promote the healing of chronic wounds. These systems deliver HBO using less pressure than hyperbaric oxygen chambers and, in most cases, the patient does not breathe high oxygen concentrations.

■ Biophysical Principles

The body's inflammatory immune responses are impaired in a low-oxygen environment such as that which occurs during secondary hypoxic injury.[196] The underlying

---

Embolism: Blockage of a blood vessel by a blood clot or other foreign substance.

TABLE 20–1	Approved Uses of Hyperbaric Oxygen Therapy

Actinomycosis ■
Acute traumatic ischemia
Carbon monoxide poisoning
Compartment syndromes
Crush injury
Cyanide poisoning
Decompression sickness (the bends)
Intracranial abscess
Gas embolism
Myonecrosis ■
Necrotic infections
Necrotic open wounds
Osteomyelitis
Profound blood loss (anemia)
Radiation injury
Skin grafts and flaps
Thermal burns

principle of HBOT is to overload the body with oxygen to prevent ischemia and assist in the healing process. Under normal resting conditions, the body consumes approximately 5 mL of oxygen per 100 mL of blood. Ninety-seven percent of the oxygen attaches itself to hemoglobin and 3 percent dissolves in the plasma.[196]

During HBOT, the patient is placed in an environment where the barometric pressure is between 2.0 to 3 **atmospheres absolute** ■ (ATA) and breathes an atmosphere that is between 95 to 100 percent oxygen (relative to the 21 percent oxygen concentration in the air).[196, 199] The oxygen content of plasma is increased to as much as 6.6 mL of oxygen per 100 mL of blood (Henry's law), increasing tissue oxygen delivery to 26.7 mL per 100 mL of blood.[196] At 3 ATA, the plasma contains enough oxygen (6.8%) to sustain life without hemoglobin and is therefore able to supply ischemic areas with oxygen, preventing hypoxia.[199] Although its effect is unclear in the treatment of musculoskeletal pathology, the increased atmospheric pressure, usually in the range of 2.0 to 3.0 ATA, reduces the diameter and volume of gaseous bubbles in the body.[199]

The high oxygen concentration results in vasoconstriction, decreasing blood flow by 20 percent. However, the difference in oxygen concentration between the blood and the tissues is increased, forming a diffusion gradient that increases the rate of oxygen being delivered to the tissues.[196] Inflammation is decreased and hypoxia is avoided.[200] During hypoxia, fibroblasts are unable to synthesize collagen and osteoclastic activity is impaired. The increased oxygen content accelerates the formation of new blood vessels and increases the rate of epithelial cell function.[196]

Polymorphonuclear leukocyte (PMN) migration and phagocytic function is hindered during hypoxia. HBOT maintains PMN function and inhibits adhesion to the post-capillary venules, inhibiting reperfusion that aids the healing of crush injuries and compartment syndromes.[196]

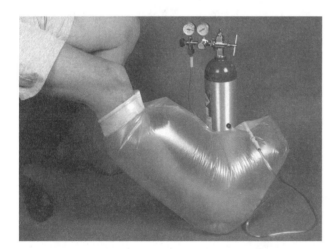

Figure 20–1. Superficial Hyperbaric Oxygen Therapy. This method of hyperbaric oxygen therapy is used to treat chronic, open wounds. (O2Boot, Courtesy of GWR Medical, Inc, Chadds Ford, PA).

● E F F E C T S O N

The Injury Response Process

This section addresses only the effect of HBOT on musculoskeletal conditions and wound healing. Information regarding the effects of HBOT on decompression sickness and other disease states can be located in other sources.[196, 199, 201, 202] For the treatment of musculoskeletal injuries, HBOT should be administered as soon as possible following the onset of injury (see: At a Glance: Hyperbaric Oxygen Therapy, p 355).[200, 203, 204]

Blood Flow

The increased concentration of oxygen in the blood stream produces a systemic vasoconstriction. However, the increased oxygen content within the blood increases the amount of oxygen delivered to the tissues. This effect may be most beneficial in poorly vascularized areas such as the Achilles tendon and rotator cuff tendons.[200]

Actinomycosis: A disease state of actin caused by a fungus.
Atmospheres absolute (ATA): Water (or air) pressure exerted on the body. One ATA is the standard pressure placed on the body at sea level. Each 33-ft immersion from sea level equals an increase of 1 ATA. For example, immersion to a depth of 33 feet exerts 2 ATA, 66 feet exerts 3 ATA, 99 feet exerts 4 ATA, and so on.
Myonecrosis: Death of muscle tissue.

Wound Healing

Wound healing is facilitated by increasing the partial pressure with which oxygen is supplied to the tissues.[205] Oxygen serves as a **catalyst** ■ to phagocytosis. Decreased oxygen levels, hypoxia, inhibits the activity of neutrophils. When the level of oxygen drops below 30 mm Hg, phagocytosis ceases. The hyperperfusion of oxygen in the blood stream maintains antimicrobial function in what would otherwise be a hypoxic or ischemic environment.[199] Wound healing is enhanced by increased levels of adenosine triphosphate (ATP).[196]

Tissue Regeneration

The effects associated with wound healing also assist in the regeneration and healing of other tissues. Increased oxygen delivery increases the rate of fibroblast proliferation and accelerates the growth of motoneurons' terminal axons.[199, 206] HBOT may also assist in the healing of fractures [207] and recovery from delayed-onset muscle soreness.[204]

■ Contraindications and Precautions

Atmospheric pressures greater than 1 ATA alter the volume of gas-filled structures in the body (see At a Glance: Hyperbaric Oxygen Therapy, p 355). As the pressure in the HBO chamber increases, the greater the pressure-related effects within the body. Changes in the body's flexible cavities, such as the abdomen, are generally mild. However, pressure changes within rigid spaces can cause more severe consequences. The inner ear and middle ear, **tympanic membrane** ■, and sinuses are at increased risk. Ruptures of the tympanic membrane during treatment in an HBO chamber have been reported, especially if the patient is suffering from a middle ear infection.[201] Decongestants can help reduce the risk of barotrauma to the ear and sinuses.

Certain cardiovascular and respiratory conditions also contraindicate the use of HBOT. Red blood cell (RBC) disorders such as congenital **spherocytosis** ■ can predispose the RBCs to collapse under the high atmospheric pressures. Patients suffering from asthma can be predisposed to the formation of cerebral arterial gas embolism as the pressure is reduced back to normal. A preexisting **pneumothorax** ■

will be decreased as the pressure is increased, but may expand to well beyond the pretreatment level as the pressure is reduced.[199]

Certain medications such as **Antabuse** ■ (disulfiram) and **Adriamycin** ■ (doxorubicin) can counter the effects of HBOT or produce unwanted consequences. Check with a physician regarding the effect of any prescribed medications that the patient may be using at the time of treatment.

A 100-percent oxygen environment and high pressure is toxic to the neurological system when the treatment is extended for several hours or days, as seen with the treatment of burns or decompression sickness (a significantly longer period than that used for musculoskeletal conditions) can trigger seizures. Should this occur, decrease the pressure within the chamber and reduce the percentage of oxygen that the patient is breathing.

■ Controversies in Treatment

Many of the benefits of HBOT are based on anecdotal claims. Few controlled research studies have examined the effect of this treatment on musculoskeletal injury. Although the science behind HBOT is sound, further research is needed to establish its efficacy.

To date, the only published controlled study regarding the effect of HBOT on musculoskeletal injury found no significant difference in the recovery time following ankle ligament sprains between a group receiving HBOT and those who did not. However, treatments were not initiated until 34 hours after the onset of injury.[203] The underlying theory of HBOT suggests that it is most beneficial when applied immediately following the injury.[200, 203, 204]

The topical application of HBO has proved advantageous in the treatment of chronic, open wounds.[205] The efficacy of this treatment approach is improved when HBOT is used as an adjunct to other therapeutic techniques.

■ Clinical Application of Hyperbaric Oxygen Therapy

The Undersea and Hyperbaric Medical Society recommends that all HBO treatments be administered in a hospital environment.[202] Because of the diversity in the types of HBO chambers and their relative rarity in clinical settings,

---

Adriamycin: An antibiotic medication.

Antabuse: A medication (generic name: disulfiram) used in treating alcoholism. Consumption of alcoholic drinks results in severe nausea and vomiting.

Catalyst: A substance that accelerates a chemical reaction.

Pneumothorax: The collection of air in the pleural cavity (a void between the lungs and rib cage) that inhibits the lung's ability to expand.

Spherocytosis: An anemic condition in which red blood cells assume a spheroid shape.

Tympanic membrane: The ear drum.

At a Glance: **Hyperbaric Oxygen Therapy**

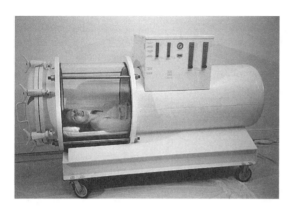

(By Michael Capria/Tampa Hyperbaric Enterprise, Inc.)

Description

Hyperbaric oxygen therapy involves placing the patient in a sealed chamber and increasing the atmospheric pressure to 2 to 3 times that of sea level and breathing pure (95% to 100%) oxygen. Hyperbaric oxygen therapy has traditionally been used to treat decompression sickness suffered by divers, carbon monoxide poisoning, and other conditions where the body's oxygen-carrying ability has been incapacitated. Its use has since expanded to treat ischemic conditions including acute musculoskeletal conditions.

Primary Effects

Increased pressure decreases the size and volume of blood-borne gas bubbles. Breathing pure oxygen oversaturates the blood plasma with oxygen (6.6 mL of oxygen per 100 mL of blood). The increased oxygen concentration results in a vasoconstriction but allows for a net increase in oxygen delivery to the tissues. This allows for phagocytic and fibroblastic activity in what would otherwise be a hypoxic environment.

Treatment

Using 100 percent oxygen at 2.5 atmospheres absolute:
90 to 100 min.
- or -
Three 30-minute sessions. Five-minute breaks between treatments breathing normal atmospheric oxygen.

Indications

- Muscle soreness
- Inflammatory conditions
- Sprains
- Strains
- Wound hypoxia
- Delayed onset muscle soreness
- Chronic open wounds, especially those that are necrotic
- Tendon lacerations, including surgical procedures
- Uncontrolled infection
- Osteomyelitis

See Table 20–1 for a list of approved uses of hyperbaric oxygen.

Contraindications

- Pregnancy
- Middle or inner ear infection
- Tympanic membrane rupture
- Upper respiratory infection
- Sinusitis or other sinus condition
- Severe lung disease
- Asthma
- High fever
- Seizure disorders
- Congenital spherocytosis
- Optic neuritis
- Pneumothorax
- Claustrophobia

Precautions

- The increased environmental pressure can produce abdominal cramping and flatulence.
- Pressure that is too great or a sudden increase or decrease in pressure within the chamber can cause the tympanic membrane to rupture, especially if the eustachian tube is blocked.
- Long-duration treatment can affect the central nervous system and lower the patient's seizure threshold during the treatment.[199]

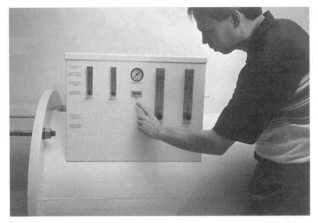

Figure 20–2. **Controls for a Hyperbaric Oxygen Chamber**. (By Michael Capria/Tampa Hyperbaric Enterprise, Inc.)

this section presents the clinical use of HBOT in an overview format. Specialized training should be obtained before operating any HBO unit.

Instrumentation

HBO chambers: Many HBO chambers are large enough to hold multiple people. Single-person chambers are most often used for orthopedic patients. Oxygen may be delivered through a face mask or, less commonly, filled within the chamber (the high concentration of oxygen creates an explosion hazard) (Fig. 20–2). Because of the explosion hazard, open flames and electrical equipment capable of producing a spark are prohibited from most HBO chambers. Some "clinical" units, such as those found with professional sporting teams, have accommodations that allow for music or videos to keep the patient occupied during the treatment.

Topical HBO administration: Relatively small, chronic open wounds can be treated using a topically applied patch that delivers 100-percent oxygen to the lesion. This method of HBO application does not use the high atmospheric pressure associated with HBO chambers.

Oxygen concentration: Regulates the amount of oxygen inhaled by the patient. This gauge normally ranges from 30- to 100-percent oxygen concentration. Most HBO treatments are administered at 95- to 100-percent oxygen concentration.

Pressure: Adjusts the atmospheric pressure in the chamber and measured in atmosphere absolute. One ATA equals air pressure at sea level. Most treatments are administered between 2.0 and 3.0 ATA. The pressure within the chamber must be gradually increased and decreased.

Set-up and Application

Preparation for the Treatment
If an oxygen mask is being used, fit it snugly over the patient's mouth and nose. Instruct the patient to breath normally.

Initiation of the Treatment
To avoid injury to the tympanic membrane, slowly increase the atmospheric pressure to the prescribed treatment range, usually between 2.0 and 3.0 ATA.

Termination of the Treatment
Slowly decrease the pressure within the chamber to that outside of the chamber. A rapid decrease in pressure can damage the tympanic membrane or, in rare circumstances, can cause decompression sickness.

Maintenance
After Each Use

1. Clean the interior of the HBO chamber.
2. Clean or replace the oxygen mask.

As Indicated

1. Calibrate the pressure gauge as recommended by the manufacturer.
2. A qualified technician should inspect, service, and calibrate the unit according to the timetable established by the manufacturer.

● Chapter Highlights

* HBO involves exposing the body to a high-pressure, high-oxygen environment.
* This treatment technique has long been used for treating decompression sickness ("the bends") and burns. It is now being used to aid in the healing of superficial wounds and for the treatment of musculoskeletal conditions.
* The high-oxygen environment oversaturates the blood with oxygen, increasing the oxygen supply to otherwise ischemic areas.
* The high-pressure environment creates the primary contraindication to the use of HBO chambers.
* Still in its early stage of research, the efficacy of HBOT in the treatment of musculoskeletal conditions has not been substantiated.

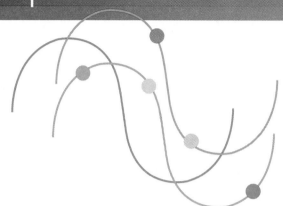

Chapter 21

Therapeutic Magnets

The body produces its own electromagnetic charges, the earth has magnetic fields, and proponents of magnet therapy theorize that static magnetic charges can restore the "harmony" between the two. The use of therapeutic magnets has been proposed for a wide range of musculoskeletal conditions, disease states, mental and cognitive disorders, and energy restoration. This chapter presents both the proposed effects of magnet therapy and the results of published research that supports or contradicts these claims.

Throughout recorded history, various forms of magnetic energy have been used to treat a broad range of ailments. Several of the modalities and treatment techniques described in this text use the property of magnetic fields as their basis: electrical stimulation, shortwave diathermy, iontophoresis, and bone growth generators for example. Each of these relies on the interaction of positive and negative charges to alter the body's physiology. The effects of static, relatively low-power magnets should not be confused with the effects of these other forms of electromagnetic energy.

Therapeutic magnets are often self-prescribed by the patient. The purpose of this chapter is to provide an overview of the reported effects of therapeutic magnets to help the clinician understand the patient's rationale for using therapeutic magnets and to better articulate other treatment options to the patient. It should not be construed as an endorsement of the efficacy of these devices.

Using wearable magnets to prevent or cure ailments is not new, having cycled in and out of popularity for centuries.[208] Many magnet therapy and electrical stimula-

tion techniques were the "invention" of charlatans whose primary objective was to bilk unsuspecting (and gullible) consumers of their money (Fig. 21–1). Governmental agencies and consumer protection advocates have taken great strides in reducing the quackery associated with many forms of medical fraud.[208] Although many forms of alternative medicine and alternative therapy are legitimate practices, misrepresentation and fraud are still commonplace.

Magnet therapy is sometimes referred to as "magnetotherapy." However, the use of this term can be confusing because it can be used to describe both static and pulsed magnetic fields, and the biophysical effects of each must be considered separately. Shortwave diathermy and electrical bone growth generators use pulsed electromagnetic fields.[209] This chapter focuses on low-power static magnetic fields (DC magnetic fields) that are produced by a magnet and worn on the body.

The current boom in alternative medicine practices has increased the popularity of therapeutic magnet therapy. However, anecdotal claims in the media have not yet been

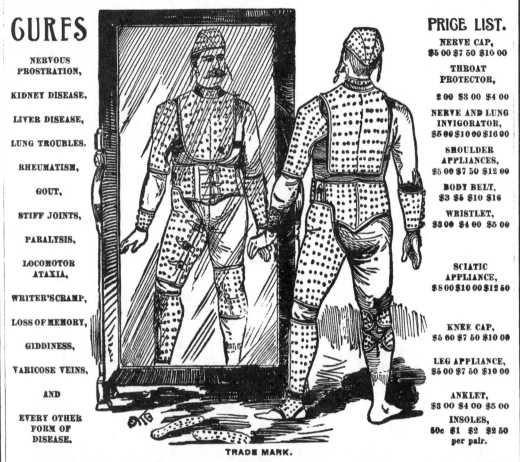

Figure 21–1. **An Advertisement for a Garment Fitted with Therapeutic Magnets.** This underwear (and sporty matching hat) was sold in 1902 to prevent and cure ailments. (Reproduced with permission from the Bakken Library and Museum, Minneapolis, MN.)

substantiated by controlled research studies. Even today, there is little, if any, first-hand knowledge, let alone agreement about how low-level magnetic fields affect human tissue. Evidence does suggest that electromagnetic energy caused by electrical power sources such as high-tension electrical wires does increase the risk of certain disease, including cancer. But these forms of electromagnetic fields are different than those produced by therapeutic magnets.[210]

As the evidence base regarding the therapeutic benefits of magnetic fields on the human body increases, their level of efficacy—and therefore their level of acceptance—in the medical field should follow. At the very least, the commercial magnets promoted for their medicinal properties are of insufficient power to cause further harm. In the worst case, patients may turn to these devices instead of seeking proper medical treatment.

■ Types of Magnets

Therapeutic magnets are available in a wide array of strengths, with many of the most popular having an advertised magnetic strength of 500 to 1000 Gauss (G) (Box 21–1). However, these magnets may not actually deliver their advertised power (see Controversies in Treatment). Magnets exceeding 1000 G are regulated by the United States Food and Drug Administration,[211] but the World Health Organization has determined that human exposure to static magnetic fields of up to 20,000 G is safe.[212]

There are two primary categories of permanent therapeutic magnets: unipolar and bipolar. These terms are based on the magnetic poles that are in contact with the body. A third classification, quadripolar, involves the placement of unipolar magnets so that opposite charges are in contact with the skin (e.g., positive-negative-positive-negative).

Unipolar Magnets

Unipolar magnets have only one pole touching the patient's skin, with the opposite pole facing away. Most therapeutic treatments have the negative pole (referred to as the north pole) touching the skin and the positive pole

(the south pole) facing away from the skin. Unipolar magnet therapy generally uses multiple magnets arranged on or around the target tissues (Fig. 21–2).

Bipolar Magnets

Bipolar magnet therapy has both the positive and negative poles in contact with the patient's skin. This type of magnet is formed from a flexible plastic and metal alloy similar to that used for refrigerator magnets but possesses a stronger magnetic field. Magnetic patterns of differing shapes such as concentric circles, triangles, and jagged lines are etched within the alloy so that the negative pole of one element corresponds with the positive pole of the next element (Fig. 21–3).

■ Polar Effects

Therapeutic magnets produce a direct current static magnetic field where the poles are always aligned in the same direction. Using cadavers as a model, magnets having a strength of 190 G at each pole can penetrate 5 cm into the tissues, although the strength of the field at this depth was not reported.[213]

The negative magnetic pole (north pole) is the "receptive pole" and may be indicated by a green marking. The positive pole (south pole) is the "active pole" and has a red marking. A school of thought suggests that the negative pole should be applied over areas that are overstimulated and the positive pole over understimulated tissues. The effects for the negative and positive pole advertised by magnet therapy proponents and manufacturers are presented in Table 21–1.

● EFFECTS ON
The Injury Response Process

The following sections describe the theoretical or advertised effects of therapeutic magnets. Refer to the Controversies in Treatment section of this chapter for further discussion on these topics.

The premise of exposing the body to low-intensity magnetic fields is to restore the natural magnetic fields and

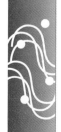

Box 21–1. **Magnetic Strength**

The strength of a magnetic field, inductance, is measured by units of Gauss or Tesla:

    1.0 Gauss is equal to 100 microTeslas (mT)
    10.0 Gauss is equal to 1 milliTeslas (mT)

It is difficult to conceptualize the strength of magnets. Comparatively, the earth's magnetic field exerts a force of 0.5 G, refrigerator magnets have a strength of approximately 4 G, and magnetic resonance imaging (MRI) devices exert a magnetic strength that exceeds 15,000 G. Most therapeutic magnets have a strength of 500 to 1000 G.

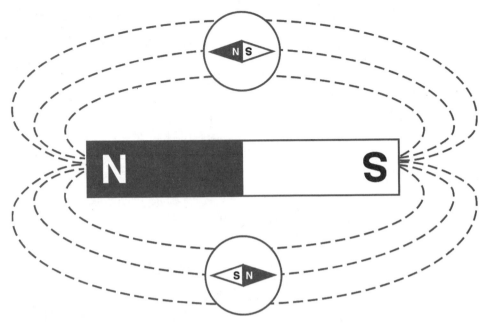

Figure 21-2. **Unipolar Therapeutic Magnets.** A magnetic field is created between the north (N) and south (S) poles. Given sufficient field strength, ions will align themselves along the magnetic field lines based on their charge.

realigning the body's biological energy. The biological injury potential that occurs after trauma is said to produce a positive electrical charge (see Wound Healing, Chapter 12, p 235). Placing the negative pole over the target tissues is said to inhibit the release of inflammatory mediators, increase blood flow, and decrease pain and muscle soreness. Manufacturers also claim that magnetic therapy can decrease edema; improve muscular strength, athletic performance, sleep, and emotional state (including depression); decrease the effect of jet lag; and have antibiotic properties.

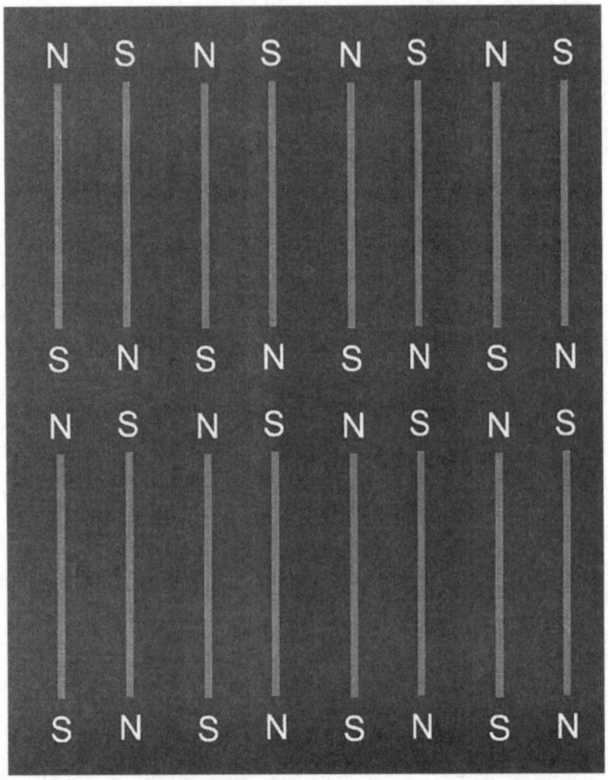

Tissue Heating

Some manufacturers claim that the application of therapeutic magnets can increase subcutaneous tissue temperature. The basis for tissue heating is the **Hall effect** in which

Figure 21-3. **Bipolar Therapeutic Magnets.** These magnets are etched with designs where the positive and negative poles are opposite to each other, theoretically balancing the polarity.

TABLE 21–1	Manufacturers' Claims of Healing Properties of Magnetic Poles*
Negative Polarity	*Positive Polarity*
Pain reduction	Increases energy
Anti-inflammatory effects	Stimulates the immune system
Promotes healing	Increases intercellular fluids
Assists coagulation	Increases intracellular fluids
Edema reduction	Causes vasodilation
Causes vasoconstriction	Assists fracture healing
Attracts oxygen to the area	
Restores acid/base balance	
Dissolves fat deposits	
Assists in restful sleep	
Central nervous system sedation	

These effects have not been substantiated.

a magnetic field causes ions having like charges to cluster together. As the ions move, they create friction and produce heat (Box 21–2).[211]

Slight intramuscular tissue temperature increases of 0.36°F (0.2°C) and skin temperature increases of 1.44°F (0.8°C) have been observed during therapeutic magnet application. These temperature increases are not within the therapeutic range, not statistically significant, and were most likely the result of the thermal insulating effect caused by the rubberized magnet being held against the skin.[211]

Blood Flow

The Hall effect that is theorized to cause tissue heating is also believed to result in increased blood flow (see Box 21–2). The temperature increase associated with the ionic motion would result in vasodilation and thereby increase blood flow to the treated area. This effect is therefore contingent on the magnet's ability to elevate tissue temperature. If the magnets do not increase tissue temperature, it is unlikely that there is a significant increase in blood flow.

The use of therapeutic magnets to increase blood flow is also based on research that demonstrated that magnetic fields can increase the flow of ionically charged fluids in glass capillary tubes. Theoretically, magnets of sufficient strength applied to the skin would likewise result in an increase in blood flow.[215] The increased tissue temperatures that would be expected to be associated with increased blood flow have not been documented.

Pain Reduction

Bipolar magnets, or the negative field of a unipolar magnet, have been used for pain reduction.[216] Several

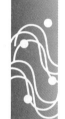

Box 21–2. The Hall Effect

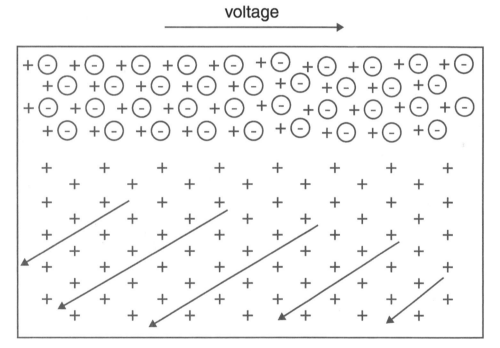

The Hall effect describes an electromotive force that causes charged particles to group together in the presence of a magnetic field.[211] If an electric current flows perpendicularly through a magnetic field, a transverse force is placed on charged particles. Similarly charged particles move through a concentration gradient and cluster together on one side of the conductor, creating a **Hall voltage.** The strength of the Hall voltage is proportional to the strength of the magnetic field.

Blood vessels are capable of conducting an electrical current. When a magnetic field of sufficient strength is applied perpendicularly to a blood vessel, the Hall effect will cause positively charged ions to move against their intended direction of flow toward the vessel walls. Hypothetically, a significantly strong Hall voltage will cause blood ions to oscillate and collide, causing friction that produces heat and causes vasodilation.[211, 214]

The Hall effect and Hall voltage are staples of electromagnetic science. However, these events have not been identified in living tissue using therapeutic magnets. The claim that the Hall effect occurs during therapeutic magnet use is, at best, dubious.

theories have been proposed to describe the mechanism of pain relief. A Hall voltage (see Box 21–2) could increase the nerve membrane's resting potential, theoretically making it more difficult to obtain nerve depolarization and slowing nerve conduction velocity.[214] This, in turn, would result in decreased pain. However, no rationale has been proposed to explain how this affects only nociceptors and not sensory or motor nerves.

Other possible mechanisms include indirect effects in the cerebral cortex or the subcortical areas, a change in the reticular system and its subsequent release in enkephalins, activation of the gate control theory caused by superficial heating, and increased blood flow.[214–216] Many studies have demonstrated that pain reduction obtained from therapeutic magnets is no better than that of a placebo. Pain reduction is probably obtained from psychological mechanisms rather than from physiological means.[217]

■ Contraindications and Precautions

Magnet therapy has few absolute contraindications, but the identification of these conditions is hindered by the relatively unknown effect of low-power magnetic fields. Many of the contraindicated conditions are inferred from exposure to high-power magnetic fields (see At a Glance: Therapeutic Magnets, p 363). Patients with implanted pacemakers should use therapeutic magnets with caution. The magnet should not be placed over the implanted pacemaker or along the leads to the heart because the strong magnetic fields can disrupt the pacemaker.[218]

Although the risk is probably minimal when using magnets of 1000 G or less, treatment over the lumbar or pelvic area during pregnancy should be avoided. The long-term effects of exposure to low-level static magnetic fields on a developing fetus have not been established.

Manufacturers warn about a "detoxification period" following the initial exposure to magnetic therapy, especially with the use of magnetic mattress pads. The rationale is that improved blood flow and restoration of the body's magnetic balance causes toxins to be removed from the body, at which time they cause pain, malaise, and discomfort until the toxins are completely flushed from the body.

Perhaps the gravest concern is when therapeutic magnets are used in lieu of proper treatment or medical care. For this reason, therapeutic magnets should not be used for pain or dysfunction stemming from an unknown origin. Although the use of therapeutic magnets as an adjunct to the treatment of aggressive diseases such as cancer may not be harmful, this method of treatment should not be used in place of other forms of medical treatment.

■ Controversies in Treatment

Few published studies provide a detailed rationale as to the underlying mechanisms affecting the body. Proponents of therapeutic magnets have interpolated the body's response to high-power electromagnetic stimulation, the effects of direct current stimulation on ionic properties on the body, and laboratory experiments of high-power magnetic fields on blood or ionic solutions and applied them to effects relatively low-power magnetic fields on living tissue. Although the base rationale for these effects may be sound, their actual effects on the human body have not been substantiated. Indeed, all but one peer-reviewed study demonstrated positive effects from the application of therapeutic magnets. A placebo-controlled study revealed that a single 45-minute application of a therapeutic magnet resulted in a statistically significant reduction in pain related to **postpolio syndrome** ■ relative to a control group.[216] Patients may also perceive an overall sense of well-being while on a therapeutic magnet regime.[213]

Some studies that used a placebo control group showed improvements in measures such as pain and range of motion, but no significant difference in the group receiving magnet therapy. There was no significant reduction in pain relative to a control group for rheumatoid arthritis-related pain,[213] chronic low back pain,[219] and exercise-induced muscle soreness.[214]

An investigation into the efficacy of therapeutic magnets in elevating intramuscular tissue temperatures concluded that the slight temperature increase (which was equal to that seen in a placebo group) was caused by the insulating effect of the object on the skin. By extension, the researchers also concluded that blood flow was not affected.[211] Even the strength of the fields used for magnetic resonance imaging (15,000 G) fails to trigger the Hall effect (see Box 21–2).[220]

Using magnets in a shoe insole, the strength of isometric quadriceps contractions were increased relative to a control group but were not significantly different from a placebo group, suggesting that any strength benefits were related to a placebo effect.[221]

The magnetic fields produced by these devices are often not uniform and less than advertised.[211, 221] These differences can be over 20 percent less than the advertised strength at the core of the magnet and up to 99 percent less around the magnet's periphery.[211]

A case can be made for the potentially beneficial (and also harmful) effects of the biological exposure to magnetic fields. However, the strength of this field and the duration of exposure required to produce meaningful changes has yet to be identified. For the principles of magnetic therapy to affect the body, they must have sufficient strength to affect the target tissues.

Postpolio syndrome: Musculoskeletal symptoms, including pain and atrophy, that affect patients 25 to 30 years after the original polio symptoms occurred.

At a Glance: **Therapeutic Magnets**

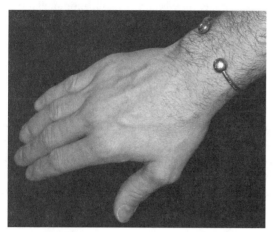

(A) Magnetic bracelet

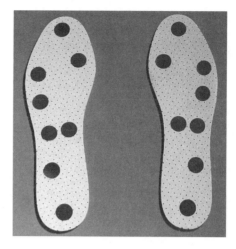

(B) Magnetic shoe insoles

Description

Therapeutic magnets are sold under the assumption that if the body is exposed to static, relatively low-intensity magnetic fields, the body's natural magnetic fields and natural biological energy will be restored. These effects have not been substantiated.

Therapeutic magnets may be affixed to the body using Neoprene or Velcro straps, worn as necklaces or bracelets, worn as shoe insoles, or used as mattress or chair pads.

Primary Effects

- Increased blood flow*
- Increased intramuscular temperature*
- Restoration of the body's normal magnetic balance*

Treatment Duration

- Pain reduction has been documented following a 45-minute treatment.[216]
- Most manufacturers recommend that the magnets be worn for as long as possible.
- Some patients wear the magnets continuously, removing them only to bathe.

Indications

Manufacturer's claims for use (partial list)*
- Fibromyalgia
- Pain reduction (acute and chronic)
- Healing of sprains and strains
- Inflammatory conditions
- Edema reduction
- Improving sleep
- Diminishing jet lag
- Improving athletic performance
- Improving emotional/mental state

Contraindications

- Over or near implanted pacemakers
- Over the pelvic and lumbar area during pregnancy
- Over cancerous areas

Note: The effects of magnet therapy, and therefore the contraindications, have not been definitively established.

Precautions

- Some patients may experience discomfort and **malaise** following exposure to therapeutic magnets, especially after sleeping on a magnetic mattress pad.
- An allergic reaction or skin irritation from bare metal magnets may occur.
- Therapeutic magnets should not be used in lieu of other mainstream therapies and medical techniques, especially for disease states requiring aggressive medical treatment (e.g., cancer, HIV).

*Unsubstantiated effects.

■ Clinical Application of Magnet Therapy

Therapeutic magnets are sold in many different shapes, sizes, and strengths. This section discusses the application of the most common types of therapeutic magnets, keeping in mind that the theories regarding how to use therapeutic magnets are even more diverse than the magnets themselves.

Instrumentation

Flexible magnets: Round, square, or oval. Conform to relatively large, regularly shaped areas such as the quadriceps, shoulder, wrist, and so on. Flexible magnets are usually bipolar. This type of magnet must be secured in place.

Solid magnets: These magnets are made from metal or ceramic and must be taped or wrapped in place. Solid magnets are usually monopolar.

Jewelry/ornamental magnets: These devices are worn, usually as bracelets or necklaces. Each side of the band corresponds to a magnetic pole.

Magnetic appliances: These forms of magnets work in conjunction with other items which are used during the patient's day-to-day activities. Magnetic shoe insoles, magnetic mattress pads, and chair backrests are some common examples of magnetic appliances.

Set-up and Application

There is relatively little formal preparation and set-up for the application of therapeutic magnets, especially in light of the fact that many of these devices are self-prescribed and purchased by the patient.

Preparation for the Treatment

1. To prevent the collection of dirt, grime, and body oils, clean the areas to be covered by the magnet and any device used to hold it in place.

2. Many flexible and solid magnets require a cloth be placed between the skin and the magnet. This cloth absorbs skin oils, thus protecting the magnet.

3. Flexible and solid magnets must be affixed to the patient's skin when they are to be worn throughout the course of the day. Double-sided tape, water-resistant medical tape, Velcro straps, and Neoprene sleeves are often used for this purpose. Some garments may contain pouches to hold the magnet.

4. Magnets may be placed on the skin and used to stimulate acupuncture points and are often used in conjunction with other therapeutic modalities such as massage.

5. Some proponents of magnet therapy recommend covering the magnet with gold foil or other form of barrier.

Treatment Protocol

The fundamental principle of magnet therapy is "the more, the longer, the better." Most proponents recommend wearing the magnets continuously. Strong magnets may be worn at night, and lesser powered magnets may be worn during the day. Many controlled research studies used protocols having a much shorter duration, such as 6 hours per day, 3 days a week for low back pain.[219]

Maintenance

Little maintenance is required for therapeutic magnets other than cleaning the magnet's surface. Wraps and sleeves used to hold the magnet in place should be laundered on a regular basis using the suggested protocol.

● Chapter Highlights

- There are two classifications of therapeutic magnets: (1) unipolar magnets, in which only one pole is in contact with the patient's body, and (2) bipolar magnets, in which both poles are in contact.
- The negative pole is thought to benefit overstimulated tissues (e.g., inflamed) and the positive pole understimulated tissues.
- Increased tissue temperature and changes in blood flow are proposed to occur secondary to the Hall effect, in which ions shift in response to the magnetic field. Subsequent movement creates friction that produces heat, which, in turn, causes vasodilation. The Hall effect has not been proved to occur when therapeutic magnets are applied to the human body.
- Most pain reduction is obtained by the placebo effect.
- Little, if any, conclusive research evidence supports the use of low-level static magnetic fields as a therapeutic treatment for musculoskeletal conditions.

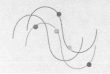

Section Five Review

Case Study: Bertha

Bertha is a 62-year-old female who sustained a right wrist fracture 6 weeks ago, which was medically managed with immobilization of a fiberglass cast. The cast was removed 3 days ago by the physician, and today you are the treating therapist for this patient. Her primary limitations are pain 4/10 rest, 10/10 activity; greater than 50% limited active and passive wrist range of motion, and poor strength due to pain and edema. Her edema measures 3 cm greater midpalm right versus left. She is medically healthy, except for history of ovarian cancer 20 years ago that was treated successfully.

What are some edema management options to consider in this situation?

What are the physiological effects on the injury response cycle from the application of this thermal agent?

What are the clinical symptoms that you hope to address with this intervention?

What other modalities may be appropriate over the following 2 weeks for this diagnosis? Why?

Case Study: Sam

Sam is a 40-year-old gentleman who is diagnosed with a herniated lumbar disk with left leg radiculopathy. He has mild osteoarthritis. His evaluation shows limited trunk active range of motion, moderate spasm in his lumbosacral paraspinals and pain that radiates into the left buttock. The physician would like him to receive a course of treatment of lumbar traction.

What are the indications for traction?

What are the physiological effects on the injury response cycle from the application of this agent?

What are the clinical symptoms that you hope to address with this intervention?

What other thermal modalities may be appropriate over the following 2 weeks for this diagnosis? Why?

Case Study: Mr. Smith

Mr. Smith is a 77-year-old gentleman with 10 years of progressive degenerative joint disease at the knee. He is currently 2 days out of surgery for a total knee arthroplasty. A continuous passive machine is requested by the physician.

What are three contraindications to the use of a continuous passive machine?

What are the physiological effects on the injury response cycle from the application of this thermal agent?

What are the clinical symptoms that you hope to address with this intervention?

Case Study: Continuation of Case Study from Section One

(The following discussion relates to Case Study 2, found on pages 93 through 96 of Section One.)

Two of the modalities presented in this section, cervical traction and massage, would be appropriate for our patient's cervical trauma.

Massage

Soft tissue massage using effleurage and pétrissage strokes can promote relaxation of the involved muscles. Depending on the clinician's preference, the patient could be placed in the supine, prone, or seated position, with the head resting on a table to promote relaxation. The massage strokes should run parallel to the muscle fibers to help lengthen them. The patient would further benefit from massage by increased local blood flow and decreased neuromuscular excitability. Deep, localized friction massage can be used to help break up trigger points.

Cervical Traction

Cervical traction would be used only in the later stages of this patient's treatment protocol. Recall that the patient has been diagnosed as having a cervical strain and sprain. If traction were used too soon after the injury, the force may cause further damage to the cervical ligaments. Likewise, the patient does not show signs of

365

radiating pain, decreasing the likelihood of cervical nerve root impingement.

Intermittent cervical traction, applied in two 5-minute intervals with a maximum of 25 pounds of tension, will assist in decreasing muscle spasm and pain, espe-cially if the treatment is preceded by the application of moist heat packs. Placing the patient in the supine position lowers the amount of tension needed to elongate the muscles by decreasing motor activity in the cervical musculature.

● ● ● Section Five Quiz

1. All of the following effects have been attributed to continuous passive motion (CPM) except:
   A. Increased nutrition to the meniscus
   B. Increased nutrition to the articular cartilage
   C. Increased tensile strength of tendons and allografts
   D. Increased nutrition to the anterior cruciate ligament

2. Intermittent cervical traction can be useful in reliev-ing the pain associated with intervertebral disk herni-ations. This reduction of pain occurs by reducing the bulge of the _____ through the _____.
   A. Fibrous pulposus and nucleus pulposus
   B. Annulus fibrosus and nucleus pulposus
   C. Nucleus pulposus and annulus fibrosus
   D. Nucleus pulposus and fibrous pulposus

3. When applying intermittent compression to an extremity, the pressure in the appliance should not exceed:
   A. The diastolic blood pressure
   B. The systolic blood pressure
   C. The difference between the diastolic and systolic blood pressure
   D. The resting heart rate

4. Electromyographic biofeedback measures:
   A. The amount of tension produced by a muscle group
   B. The amount of electrical activity within a muscle
   C. The amount of myelin activity within a muscle
   D. All of the above

5. Which of the following techniques produces the greatest amount of femoral blood flow?
   A. Pneumatic sleeve
   B. Manual calf compression
   C. Straight-leg raises
   D. Anatomic CPM

6. All of the following are indications for the use of intermittent compression except:
   A. Postsurgical edema
   B. Gangrene
   C. Lymphedema
   D. Venous stasis ulcers

7. Which of the following types of continuous passive motion designs provides for the most joint stability?
   A. Free linkage
   B. Anatomic
   C. Nonanatomic

8. Light having a wavelength of 780 to 12,500 nm would be classified as:
   A. Ultraviolet-A
   B. Ultraviolet-B
   C. Ultraviolet-C
   D. Infrared

9. A first-degree erythemal dose (E_1) should be applied to no more than:
   A. 50 percent of the patient's body area
   B. 20 percent of the patient's body area
   C. 250 cm^2
   D. 25 cm^2

10. Ultraviolet light is being used to treat an infected open wound. Which form of ultraviolet light would be most appropriate in this case?
    A. Ultraviolet-A
    B. Ultraviolet-B
    C. Ultraviolet-C
    D. All would be appropriate

11. Ultraviolet A was being applied for 60 seconds at a distance of 30 inches. Calculate the new treatment duration if the distance between the lamp and the skin were decreased to 20 inches.
    A. 70 seconds
    B. 50 seconds
    C. 27 seconds
    D. 15 seconds

12. Therapeutic laser is being applied at a total of 5 watts for 10 seconds over an area of 10 square centimeters. What is the energy density (J/cm^2)?
    A. 5 J/cm^2
    B. 25 J/cm^2
    C. 0.5 J/cm^2
    D. 50 J/cm^2

13. The depth that laser energy penetrates into the body is related to:
    A. Total watts
    B. Duty cycle
    C. Output frequency
    D. Total joules

14. The primary benefit of hyperbaric oxygen therapy is:
    A. Vasoconstriction
    B. Saturating the plasma with oxygen
    C. Vasodilation
    D. Decreased oxygen diffusion gradient

15. The patient's medical history reveals the use of Antabuse to treat alcoholism. Which of the following modalities would be contraindicated for this patient?
    A. Ultraviolet light
    B. Hyperbaric oxygen therapy
    C. Electromyographic biofeedback
    D. A and B
    E. B and C
    F. A and C

16. Pain reduction is thought to occur from exposure to this magnetic pole:
    A. Positive
    B. Negative

17. The body's fascia can be elongated using a _____ force.
    A. Quick, high-intensity
    B. Slow, high-intensity
    C. Quick, moderate-intensity
    D. Slow, moderate-intensity

18. The effectiveness of cervical traction is dependent on many factors, including the amount of force applied. Other factors include:
    A.
    B.
    C.
    D.

19. List two reasons why separation of the vertebral column occurs at a lower percentage of the patient's body weight in the reclining position than in the sitting position.
    A.
    B.

20. Match the following massage strokes to method of delivery:
    A. Pétrissage _____ Pounding of the skin
    B. Tapotement _____ Kneading of the skin
    C. Effleurage _____ Stroking of the skin

References

1. Muhe, E: Intermittent sequential high-pressure compression of the leg: A new method of preventing deep vein thrombosis. Am J Surg 147:781, 1984.
2. Olavi, A, et al: Edema and lower leg perfusion in patients with posttraumatic dysfunction. Acupunct Electrother Res 16:7, 1991.
3. Miranda, F, et al: Effect of sequential intermittent pneumatic compression on both leg lymphedema volume and on lymph transport as semi-quantitatively evaluated by lymphoscintigraphy. Lymphology, 34:135, 2001.
4. Rucinski, TJ, et al: The effects of intermittent compression on edema in postacute ankle sprains. J Orthop Sports Phys Ther 14:65, 1991.
5. Stöckle, U, et al: Fastest reduction of posttraumatic edema: Continuous cryotherapy or intermittent impulse compression? Foot Ankle Int 18:432, 1997.
6. Hopkins, JT, et al: Cryotherapy and transcutaneous electric neuromuscular stimulation decrease arthrogenic muscle inhibition of the vastus medialis after knee joint effusion. J Athletic Training 37:25, 2001.
7. Hopkins, JT and Ingersoll, CD: Arthrogenic muscle inhibition: A limiting factor in joint rehabilitation. J Sports Rehabil 9:135, 2000.
8. Hopkins, JT, et al: The effects of cryotherapy and TENS on arthrogenic muscle inhibition of the quadriceps. J Athletic Training 36:S49, 2001.
9. Boris, M, et al: The risk of genital edema after external pump compression for lower limb lymphedema. Lymphology 31:15, 1998.
10. Gilbart, MK, et al: Anterior tibial compartment pressures during intermittent sequential pneumatic compression therapy. Am J Sports Med 23:769, 1995.
11. Salter, RB: The biologic concept of continuous passive motion of synovial joints: The first 18 years of basic research. Clin Orthop 12, May, 1989.
12. McCarthy, MR, et al: The clinical use of continuous passive motion in physical therapy. J Orthop Sports Phys Ther 15:132, 1992.
13. Saringer, J: Engineering aspects of the design and construction of continuous passive motion devices for humans. In Salter, RB (ed): Continuous Passive Motion (CPM): A Biological Concept for the Healing and Regeneration of Articular Cartilage, Ligaments, and Tendons—From Origination to Research to Clinical Applications. Williams & Wilkins, Baltimore, 1993, pp 403–410.
14. Jordan, LR, et al: Early flexion routine: An alternative method of continuous passive motion. Clin Orthop 231, June, 1995.
15. Rosen, MA, et al: The efficacy of continuous passive motion in the rehabilitation of anterior cruciate ligament reconstructions. Am J Sports Med 20:122, 1992.
16. Ververeli, PA, et al: Continuous passive motion after total knee arthroplasty: Analysis of costs and benefits. Clin Orthop 208, December, 1995.
17. Diehm, SL: The power of CPM: Healing through motion. Patient Care 8:34, 1989.
18. O'Donoghue, PC, et al: Clinical use of continuous passive motion in athletic training. Athletic Training 26:200, 1991.

19. Williams, JM, et al: Continuous passive motion stimulates repair of rabbit knee cartilage after matrix proteoglycan loss. Clin Orthop 252, July, 1994.
20. McInnes, J, et al: A controlled evaluation of continuous passive motion in patients undergoing total knee arthroplasty. JAMA 268:1423, 1992.
21. O'Driscoll, SW and Nicholas, JG: Continuous passive motion (CPM): Theory and principles of clinical application. J Rehabil Res Dev 37:178, 2000.
22. Ring, D, et al: Continuous passive motion following metacarpophalangeal joint arthroplasty. J Hand Surg [Am] 23:505, 1998.
23. LaStayo, PC, et al: Continuous passive motion after repair of the rotator cuff. A prospective outcome study. J Bone Joint Surg Am 80:1002, 1998.
24. Gates, HS, et al: Anterior capsulotomy and continuous passive motion in the treatment of posttraumatic flexion contracture of the elbow: A prospective study. J Bone Joint Surg Am 74:1229, 1992.
25. Nadler, SF, et al: Continuous passive motion in the rehabilitation setting: A retrospective study. J Phys Med Rehabil 72:162, 1993.
26. Montgomery, F and Eliasson, M: Continuous passive motion compared to active physical therapy after knee arthroplasty: Similar hospitalization times in a randomized study of 68 patients. Acta Orthop Scand 67:7, 1996.
27. Chiarello, CM, et al: The effect of continuous passive motion duration and increment on range of motion in total knee arthroplasty patients. J Orthop Sports Phys Ther 25:119, 1997.
28. McNair, PJ, et al: Stretching at the ankle joint: Viscoelastic responses to holds and continuous passive motion. Med Sci Sports Exerc, 33:354, 2001.
30. London, N, et al: Continuous passive motion: Evaluation of a new portable low cost machine. Physiotherapy 85:610, 1999.
31. Chin, B, et al: Continuous passive motion after total knee arthroplasty. Am J Phys Med Rehabil 79:421, 2000.
32. Lachiewicz, PF: The role of continuous passive motion after total knee arthroplasty. Clin Orthop 380:144, 2000.
33. Flowers, KR and LaStayo, P: Effect of total end range time on improving passive range of motion. J Hand Ther 7:150, 1994.
34. Wright, A, et al: An investigation of the effect of continuous passive motion and lower limb passive movement on heart rate in normal volunteers. Physiother Theory Pract 9:13, 1993.
35. Gershuni, DH, et al: Regional nutrition and cellularity of the meniscus. Implications for tear and repair. Sports Med 5:322, 1988.
36. Kim, HKL, et al: The potential for regeneration of articular cartilage in defects created by chondral shaving and subchondral abrasion: An experimental investigation in rabbits. J Bone Joint Surg Am 73:1301, 1991.
37. Kim, HKW, et al: Effects of continuous passive motion and immobilization on synovitis and cartilage degeneration in antigen induced arthritis. J Rheumatol 22:1714, 1995.
38. Alfredson, H and Lorentzon, R: Superior results with continuous passive motion compared to active motion after periosteal transplantation. A retrospective study of human patella cartilage defect treatment. Knee Surge Sports Traumatol 7:232, 1999.
39. Mussa, R, et al: Condylar cartilage response to continuous passive motion in adult guinea pigs: A pilot study. Am J Orthod Dentofacial Orthop 115:360, 1999.
40. Moran, ME and Salter, RB: Biological resurfacing of full-thickness defects in patellar articular cartilage of the rabbit. Investigation of autogenous periosteal grafts subjected to continuous passive motion. J Bone Joint Surg Br 74:659, 1992.
41. Namba, RS, et al: Continuous passive motion versus immobilization: The effect on posttraumatic joint stiffness. Clin Orthop 218, June, 1991.
42. Von Schroeder, HP, et al: The changes in intramuscular pressure and femoral vein flow with continuous passive motion, pneumatic compression stockings, and leg manipulations. Clin Orthop 218, May, 1991.
43. Grumbine, NA, et al: Continuous passive motion following partial ankle joint arthroplasty. J Foot Surg 29:557, 1990.
44. Mullaji, AB and Shahane, MN: Continuous passive motion for prevention and rehabilitation of knee stiffness: A clinical evaluation. J Postgrad Med 35:204, 1989.
45. Giudice, ML: Effects of continuous passive motion and elevation on hand edema. Am J Occup Ther 44:914, 1990.
46. Dirette, D and Hinojosa, J: Effects of continuous passive motion to the edematous hands of two persons with flaccid hemiplegia. Am J Occup Ther 48:403, 1994.
47. Macdonald, SJ, et al: Prospective randomized clinical trial of continuous passive motion after total knee arthroplasty. Clin Orthop 380:30, 2000.
48. Barthelet, Y, et al: Effects of perioperative analgesic technique on the surgical outcome and duration of rehabilitation after major knee surgery. Anesthesiology 91:8, 1999.
49. Kannus, P: Immobilization or early mobilization after an acute soft-tissue injury? Phys Sports Med 28:55, 2000.
50. Skyhar, MJ, et al: Nutrition of the anterior cruciate ligament: Effects of continuous passive motion. Am J Sports Med 13:415, 1985.
51. Engstrom, B, et al: Continuous passive motion in rehabilitation after anterior cruciate ligament reconstruction. Knee Surg Sports Traumatol Arthrosc 3:18, 1995.
52. McCarthy, MR, et al: The effect of immediate continuous passive motion on pain during the inflammatory phase of soft tissue healing following anterior cruciate ligament reconstruction. J Orthop Sports Phys Ther 17:96, 1993.
53. Witherow, GE, et al: The use of continuous passive motion after arthroscopically assisted anterior cruciate ligament reconstruction: Help or hindrance? Knee Surg Sports Traumatol Arthrosc 1:68, 1993.
54. Zarnett, R, et al: The effect of continuous passive motion on knee ligament reconstruction with carbon fiber. J Bone Joint Surg Br 73:47, 1991.
55. Drez, D, et al: In vivo measurement of anterior tibial translation using continuous passive motion devices. Am J Sports Med 19:381, 1991.
56. McCarthy, MR, et al: Effects of continuous passive motion on anterior laxity following ACL reconstruction with autogenous patellar tendon grafts. J Sports Rehabil 2:171, 1993.
57. Wasilewski, SA, et al: Value of continuous passive motion in total knee arthroplasty. Orthopedics 13:291, 1990.
58. Yashar, AA, et al: Continuous passive motion with accelerated flexion after total knee arthroplasty. Clin Orthop 345:38, 1998.
59. Chen, B, et al: Continuous passive motion after total knee arthroplasty: A prospective study. Am J Phys Med Rehabil 79:421, 2000.
60. Sperber, A and Wredmark, T: Continuous passive motion in rehabilitation after anterior cruciate ligament reconstruction. Knee Surg Sports Traumatol 3:18, 1995.
61. Richmond, JC, et al: Continuous passive motion after arthroscopically assisted anterior cruciate ligament reconstruction: Comparison of short- versus long-term use. Arthroscopy 7:39, 1991.

62. Takai, S, et al: The effects of frequency and duration of controlled passive mobilization on tendon healing. J Orthop Res 9:705, 1991.

63. Graham, G and Loomer, RL: Anterior compartment syndrome in a patient with fracture of the tibial plateau treated by continuous passive motion and anticoagulants: Report of a case. Clin Orthop 197, May, 1985.

64. Cyriax, JH: Clinical applications of massage. In Rogoff, JB (ed): Manipulation, Traction, and Massage, ed 2. Williams & Wilkins, Baltimore, 1980.

65. Brasseau, L, et al: Deep transverse friction massage for treating tendinitis. Cochrane Database Syst Rev 1:CD003528, 2002.

66. Goldenberg, DL: Fibromyalgia, chronic fatigue syndrome, and myofascial pain syndrome. Curr Opin Rheumatol 3:247, 1991.

67. Wolfe, F, et al: The fibromyalgia and myofascial pain syndromes: A preliminary study of tender points and trigger points in persons with fibromyalgia, myofascial pain syndrome and no disease. J Rheumatol 19:944, 1992.

68. King, JC and Goddard, MJ: Pain rehabilitation: II. Chronic pain syndrome and myofascial pain. Arch Phys Med Rehabil 75:S9, 1994.

69. Ferrell-Torry, AT and Glick, OJ: The use of therapeutic massage as a nursing intervention to modify anxiety and the perception of cancer pain. Cancer Nurs 16:93, 1993.

70. Felhendler, D and Lisander, B: Effects of non-invasive stimulation of acupoints on the cardiovascular system. Complement Ther Med 7:231, 1999.

71. Delaney, JP, et al: The short-term effects of myofascial trigger point massage therapy on cardiac autonomic tone in healthy subjects. J Adv Nurs 37:364, 2002.

72. Morelli, M, et al: Changes in H-reflex amplitude during massage of triceps surae in healthy subjects. J Orthop Sports Phys Ther 12:55, 1990.

73. Sullivan, SJ, et al: Effects of massage on alpha motoneuron excitability. Phys Ther 71:555, 1991.

74. Morelli, M, et al: H-reflex modulation during manual muscle massage of human triceps surae. Arch Phys Med Rehabil 72:915, 1991.

75. Crosman, LJ, et al: The effects of massage to the hamstring muscle group on range of motion. J Orthop Sports Phys Ther 6:168, 1984.

76. Smith, LL, et al: The effects of athletic massage on delayed onset muscle soreness, creatine kinase, and neutrophil count: A preliminary report. J Orthop Sports Phys Ther 19:93, 1994.

77. Tiidus, PM and Shoemaker, JK: Effleurage massage, muscle blood flow and long-term post exercise strength recovery. Int J Sports Med 16:478, 1995.

78. Nalilbolff, BD and Tachiki, KH: Autonomic and skeletal muscle response to nonelectrical cutaneous stimulation. Percept Motor Skills 72:575, 1991.

79. Kriederman, B, et al: Limb volume reduction after physical treatment by compression and/or massage in a rodent model of peripheral lymphedema. Lymphology 35:23, 2002.

80. Howard, SB and Krishnagiri, S: The use of manual edema mobilization for the reduction of persistent edema in the upper limb. J Hand Ther 14:291, 2000.

81. Nixon, M, et al: Expanding the nursing repertoire: The effect of massage on post-operative pain. Australian J Adv Nursing 14:21, 1997.

82. Malkin, K: Use of massage in clinical practice. Br J Nurs 3:292, 1994.

83. Furlan, AD, et al: Massage for low back pain. Cochrane Database Syst Rev 2:CD001929, 2002.

84. Goldberg, J, et al: The effect of two intensities of massage on H-reflex amplitude. Phys Ther 72:449, 1992.

85. Goldberg, J, et al: The effect of therapeutic massage on H-reflex amplitude in persons with a spinal cord injury. Phys Ther 74:728, 1994.

86. Day, JA, et al: Effect of massage on serum level of a-endorphin and a-lipotropin in healthy adults. Phys Ther 67:926, 1987.

87. Goats, GC and Keir, KA: Connective tissue massage. Br J Sports Med 25:131, 1991.

88. Ching, M: The use of touch in nursing practice. Australian J Advanced Nursing 10:4, 1993.

89. Field, T, et al: Massage therapy reduces anxiety and enhances EEG pattern of alertness and math computations. Int J Neurosci 86:197, 1996.

90. Weinrich, SP and Weinrich, MC: The effect of massage on pain in cancer patients. Appl Nurs Res 3:140, 1990.

91. Ferrell, BA, et al: A randomized trial of walking versus physical methods for chronic pain management. Aging (Milano) 9:99, 1997.

92. Shoemaker, JK, et al: Failure of manual massage to alter limb blood flow: Measures by Doppler ultrasound. Med Sci Sports Exer 29:610, 1997.

93. Boone, T, et al: A physiologic evaluation of the sports massage. Athletic Training 26:51, 1991.

94. Harmer, PA: The effect of pre-performance massage on stride frequency in sprinters. Athletic Training 26:55, 1991.

95. Cafarelli, E, et al: Vibratory massage and short-term recovery from muscular fatigue. Int J Sports Med 11:474, 1990.

96. Tiidus, PM: Manual massage and recovery of muscle function following exercise. A literature review. J Orthop Sports Phys Ther, 25:107, 1997.

97. Martin, NA; Zoeller, RF; Robertson, RJ and Lephart, SM: The comparative effects of sports massage, active recovery, and rest in promoting blood lactate clearance after supramaximal leg exercise. J Athletic Training 33:30, 1998.

98. Striggle, JM, et al: Effects of vibrational massage on delayed onset muscle soreness and H-reflex amplitude. J Athletic Training 37(S):S-105, 2002.

99. Lehmann, JF, et al: Effect of therapeutic temperatures on tendon extensibility. Arch Phys Med Rehabil, 51:481, 1970.

100. LaBan, MM, et al: Intermittent cervical traction: A progenitor of lumbar radicular pain. Arch Phys Med Rehabil 73:295, 1992.

101. Saunders H: The use of spinal traction in the treatment of neck and back conditions. Clin Orthop Rel Res 179:31, 1983.

102. Oegema, TR: Biochemistry of the intervertebral disc. Clin Sports Med 12:419, 1993.

103. Carrigg, SY and Hillemeyer, LE: The effect of running-induced intervertebral disc compression on thoracolumbar vertebral column mobility in young, healthy males. J Orthop Sports Phys Ther 16:19, 1992.

104. Naylor, A and Shentall, R: Biochemical aspects of intervertebral discs in aging and disease. In Jayson, M (ed): The Lumbar Spine and Back Pain. Grune and Stratton, Inc, New York, 1976. pp 317–326.

105. Tekeoglu, I, et al: Distraction of lumbar vertebrae in gravitational traction. Spine 23:1061, 1998.

106. Moeti, P and Marchetti, G: Clinical outcome from mechanical intermittent cervical traction for the treatment of cervical radiculopathy: A case series. Phys Ther 31:2001.

107. Meszaros, TF, et al: Effect of 10%, 30%, and 60% body weight traction on the straight leg raise test of symptomatic patients with low back pain. J Orthop Sports Phys Ther 30:595, 2000.

108. Yang, KH and King, AI: Mechanism of facet load transmission as a hypothesis for low-back pain. Spine 9:557, 1984.

109. Judovich, B and Nobel, GR: Traction therapy: A study of resistance forces. Am J Surg 93:108, 1957.

110. Werners, R, et al: Randomized trial comparing interferential therapy with motorized lumbar traction and massage in the management of low back pain in a primary care setting. Spine 24:1579, 1999.

111. Wong, AM, et al: Clinical trial of a cervical traction modality with electromyographic biofeedback. Am J Phys Med Rehabil 76:19, 1997.

112. Walker, GL: Goodley polyaxial cervical traction: A new approach to a traditional treatment. Phys Ther 66:1255, 1986.

113. Wong, AM, et al: The traction angle and cervical intervertebral separation. Spine 17:136, 1992.

114. Harris, PR: Cervical traction: Review of literature and treatment guidelines. Phys Ther 57:910, 1977.

115. Jette, DU, et al: Effect of intermittent, supine cervical traction on the myoelectric activity of the upper trapezius muscle in subjects with neck pain. Phys Ther 65:1173, 1985.

116. Murphy, MJ: Effects of cervical traction on muscle activity. J Orthop Sports Phys Ther 13:220, 1991.

117. Bradnam, L, et al: Manual cervical traction reduces alpha-motoneuron excitability in normal subjects. Electromyogr Clin Neurophysiol 40:259, 2000.

118. DeLacerda, FG: Effect of angle of traction pull on upper trapezius muscle activity. J Orthop Sports Phys Ther 1:205, 1980.

119. Latimer, EA, et al: Tear of the cervical esophagus following hyperextension from manual traction: Case report. J Trauma 31:1448, 1991.

120. Simmers, TA, et al: Internal jugular vein thrombosis after cervical traction. J Int Med Res 241:333, 1997.

121. Bridger, RS, et al: Effect of lumbar traction on stature. Spine 15:522, 1990.

122. Letchuman, R and Deusinger, RH: Comparison of sacrospinalis myoelectric activity and pain levels in patients undergoing static and intermittent lumbar traction. Spine 18:1361, 1993.

123. Reilly, JP, et al: Effect of pelvic-femoral position on vertebral separation produced by lumbar traction. Phys Ther 59:282, 1979.

124. Saunders, HD: Unilateral lumbar traction. Phys Ther 61:221, 1981.

125. Ramos, G and Martin, W: Effects of vertebral axial decompression on intradiscal pressure. J Neurosurg 81:350, 1994.

126. Beurskens, AJ, et al: Efficacy of traction for nonspecific low back pain. 12-week and 6-month results of a randomized clinical trial. Spine 22:2756, 1997.

127. Beurskens, AJ, et al: Efficacy of traction for non-specific low back pain. A randomized clinical trial. Lancet 346:1596, 1995.

128. Onel, D, et al: Computer tomographic investigation of the effect of traction on lumbar disc herniations. Spine 14:82, 1989.

129. Ljunggren, AE, et al: Manual traction versus isometric exercises in patients with herniated intervertebral lumbar discs. Physiotherapy Theory and Practice 8:207, 1992.

130. Deets, D, et al: Cervical traction: A comparison of sitting and supine positions. Phys Ther 57:225, 1977.

131. Croce, RV: The effects of EMG biofeedback on strength acquisition. Biofeedback Self Regul 11:299, 1986.

132. Peek, CJ: A primer of biofeedback instrumentation. In Schwartz, MS (ed): Biofeedback: A Practitioner's Guide. Guilford Press, New York, 1987.

133. Araujo, RC, et al: On the inter- and intra-subject variability of the electromyographic signal in isometric contractions. Electromyogr Clin Neurophysiol 40:225, 2000.

134. Intiso, D, et al: Rehabilitation of walking with electromyographic biofeedback in drop-foot after stroke. Stroke 25:1189, 1994.

135. Coleborne, GR, et al: Feedback of ankle joint angle and soleus electromyography in the rehabilitation of hemiplegic gait. Arch Phys Med Rehabil 74:1100, 1993.

136. Utz, SW: The effect of instructions on cognitive strategies and performance in biofeedback. J Behav Med 17:291, 1994.

137. Segreto, J: The role of EMG awareness in EMG biofeedback learning. Biofeedback Self Regul 20:155, 1995.

138. Vander Linden, DW, et al: The effect of frequency of kinetic feedback on learning an isometric force production task in nondisabled subjects. Phys Ther 73:79, 1993.

139. Draper, V: Electromyographic biofeedback and recovery of quadriceps femoris muscle function following anterior cruciate ligament reconstruction. Phys Ther 70:25, 1990.

140. Wolf, SL: Neurophysiological factors in electromyographic feedback for neuromotor disturbances. In Basmajian, JV (ed): Biofeedback: Principles and Practice for Clinicians. Williams & Wilkins, Baltimore, 1983.

141. Ingersoll, CD and Knight, KL: Patellar location changes following EMG biofeedback or progressive resistive exercises. Med Sci Sports Exerc 23:1122, 1991.

142. Cummings, MS, et al: Flexibility development in sprinters using EMG biofeedback and relaxation training. Biofeedback Self Regul 9:395, 1984.

143. Flor, H and Birbaumer, N: Comparison of the efficacy of electromyographic biofeedback, cognitive-behavioral therapy, and conservative medical interventions in the treatment of chronic musculoskeletal pain. J Consult Clin Psychol 61:653, 1993.

144. Newton-John, TR, et al: Cognitive-behavioural therapy versus EMG biofeedback in the treatment of chronic low back pain. Behav Res Ther 33:691, 1995.

145. Valeyen, J, et al: Behavioural rehabilitation of chronic low back pain: Comparison of an operant treatment, an operant-cognitive treatment and an operant-respondent treatment. Br J Clin Psychol 34:95, 1995.

146. Rezabek, GH and Friedman, AD: Superficial fungal infections of the skin. Diagnosis and current treatment recommendations. Drugs 43:674, 1992.

147. Cummings, J: Role of light in wound healing. In Kloth, LC, et al (eds): Wound Healing: Alternatives in Management. FA Davis, Philadelphia, 1990, pp 287–301.

148. Nussbaum, EL, et al: Comparison of ultrasound/ ultraviolet-c laser for treatment of pressure ulcers in patients with spinal cord injury. Phys Ther 74:812, 1994.

149. Plummer, NA, et al: Inflammation in human skin induced by ultraviolet radiation. Postgrad Med J 53:656, 1977.

150. Leenutaphong, V: Relationship between skin color and cutaneous response to ultraviolet radiation in Thai. Photodermatol Photoimmunol Photomed 11:198, 1995.

151. Westerhof, W, et al: The relation between constitutional skin color and photosensitivity estimated from UV-induced erythema and pigmentation dose-response curves. J Investigative Dermatology Symposium Proceeding 94:812, 1990.

152. Deliconstantinos, G et al: Inhibition of ultraviolet B-induced skin erythema by *N*-nitro-L-arginine and *N*-monomethyl-L-arginine. J Dermatol Sci 15:23, 1997.

153. Kelfkens, G, et al: Skin temperature changes induced by ultraviolet A exposure: Implications for the mechanism of erythemogenesis. Photodermatol Photoimmunol Photomed 7:178, 1990.

154. Grim, PS, et al: Hyperbaric oxygen therapy. JAMA 263:2216, 1990.

155. Koivukangas, V and Oikarinen, A: Effects of PUVA and UVB treatments on restoration of epidermal barrier function and vascular response after suction blister injury in human skin in vivo. Photodermatol Photoimmunol Photomed 14:119, 1998.

156. Mertz, PM; Maiser, MR and Davis, SC: Effect of ultraviolet radiation-induced inflammation on epidermal wound healing. Wound Repair and Reproduction 3:311, 1995.

157. Taylor, GJ, et al: Wound disinfection with ultraviolet radiation. J Hosp Infect, 30:85, 1995.

158. Sullivan, PK and Conner-Kerr, TA: A comparative study of the effects of UVC irradiation on select procaryotic and eucaryotic wound pathogens. Ostomy Wound Management 46:28, 2000.

159. Arechalde, A and Saurat, JH: Management of psoriasis: The position of retinoid drugs. Biodrugs 13:327, 2000.

160. Lebwohl, M and Ali, S: Treatment of psoriasis. Part 1. Topical therapy and phototherapy. J Am Acad Dermatol 45:487, 2001.

161. Wan Po, AL, et al: A systematic review of treatments for severe psoriasis. Health Technol Assess 4:1, 2000.

162. Leenutaphong, V, et al: Comparison of phototherapy two times and four times a week with low doses of narrow-band ultraviolet B in Asian patients with psoriasis. Photodermatol Photoimmunol Photomed 16:202, 2000.

163. Nordback, I, et al: Effect of UV therapy on rat skin wound healing. J Surg Res 48:68, 1990.

164. Davidson, SF, et al: The effects of UV radiation on wound healing. Br J Plast Surg 44:210, 1991.

165. Shea, CR and Parrish, JA: Effects of temperature on ultraviolet-induced erythema of human skin. I. Convective cooling. Arch Dermatol Res 273:233, 1982.

166. Perkins, SA and Massie, JE: Patient satisfaction after thermal shrinkage of the glenohumeral-joint capsule. J Sports Rehabil 10:157, 2001.

167. Bischko, JJ: Use of the laser beam in acupuncture. Acupunct Electrother Res 5:29, 1980.

168. Bartlett, WP, et al: Effect of Gallium-aluminum-arsenide triple-diode laser irradiation on evoked motor and sensory action potentials of the median nerve. J Sports Rehabil 11:12, 2002.

169. Lehmann, JF and De Lateur, BJ: Laser as a physical treatment modality. In Lehmann, JF (ed): Therapeutic Heat and Cold, ed 4. Williams & Wilkins, Baltimore, 1990, p. 582.

170. Ohshiro, T, et al: Penetration depths of 830 nm diode laser irradiation of the head and neck assessed using a radiographic phantom model and wavelength-specific imaging film. Laser Therapy 8:197, 1996.

171. Snyder-Mackler, L and Bork, CE: Effect of helium-neon laser irradiation on peripheral sensory nerve latency. Phys Ther 68:223, 1988.

172. Bartlett, WP, et al: Effect of gallium aluminum arsenide triple-diode laser on median nerve latency in human subjects. J Sports Rehabil 8:99, 1999.

173. Greathouse, DG, et al: Effects of clinical infrared laser on superficial radial nerve conduction. Phys Ther 65:1184, 1985.

174. King, CE, et al: Effect of helium-neon laser auriculotherapy on experimental pain threshold. Phys Ther 70:24, 1990.

175. DeSimone, NA, et al: Bactericidal effect of 0.95-mW helium-neon and 5-mW indium-gallium-aluminum-phosphate laser irradiation at exposure times of 30, 60, and 120 seconds on photosensitized staphylococcus aureus and pseudomonas aeruginosa in vitro. Phys Ther 79:839, 1999.

176. Ricevuti, G, et al: In vivo and in vitro HeNe laser effects on phagocyte functions. Inflammation 13:507, 1989.

177. Tang, XM and Chai, BP: Effect of CO_2 laser irradiation on experimental fracture healing: A transmission electron microscope study. Lasers Surg Med 6:346, 1986.

178. Hamilton, GF, et al: The effects of helium-neon laser upon regeneration of the crushed peroneal nerve. J Orthop Sports Phys Ther 15:209, 1992.

179. Numazawa, R, et al: The role of laser therapy in intensive pain management of postherpetic neuralgia. Laser Therapy 8:143, 1996.

180. Baxter, GD, et al: Effects of low intensity infrared laser irradiation upon conduction in the human median nerve in vivo. Exp Physiol 79:227, 1994.

181. Snyder-Mackler, L, et al: Effects of helium-neon laser irradiation on skin resistance and pain in patients with trigger points in the neck or back. Phys Ther 69:336, 1989.

182. Sprott, H and Mueller, W: Efficiency of acupuncture in patients with fibromyalgia. Reumatologia—Warsaw, 32:414, 1994.

183. Heussler, JK, et al: A double blind randomized trial of low power laser treatment in rheumatoid arthritis. Ann Rheum Dis 52:703, 1993.

184. Glinkowski, W and Rowinski, J: Effect of low incident levels of infrared laser energy on the healing of experimental bone fractures. Laser Therapy 7:67, 1995.

185. Lundeberg, T, et al: Effect of laser versus placebo in tennis elbow. Scand J Rehabil Med 19:135, 1987.

186. Thorsen, H, et al: Low level laser therapy for myofascial pain in the neck and shoulder girdle. A double-blind cross-over study. Scand J Rheumatol 21:139, 1992.

187. Mulcahy, D, et al: Low level laser therapy: a prospective double blind trial of its use in an orthopaedic population. Injury 26:315, 1995.

188. Fernando, S, et al: A randomized double blind comparative study of low level laser therapy following surgical extraction of lower third molar teeth. Br J Oral Maxillofac Surg 31:170, 1993.

189. Gam, AN, et al: The effect of low-level laser therapy on musculoskeletal pain: A meta-analysis. Pain 52:63, 1993.

190. Beckerman, H, et al: The efficacy of laser therapy for musculoskeletal and skin disorders: A criteria-based meta-analysis of randomized clinical trials. Phys Ther 72:483, 1992.

191. Siebert, W, et al: What is the efficacy of soft and mid lasers in therapy of tendinopathies: A double-blind study. Arch Orthop Trauma Surg 106:358, 1987.

192. Lundeberg, T and Malm, M: Low-power HeNe laser treatment of venous leg ulcers. Ann Plastic Surg 27:537, 1991.

193. Surinchak, JS, et al: Effects of low level energy lasers on the healing of full thickness skin defects. Lasers Surg Med 2:267, 1983.

194. David, R, et al: Effect of low-power He-Ne laser on fracture healing in rats. Lasers Surg Med 19:458, 1996.

195. White, J: Alternative sports medicine. Phys Sports Med 26:92, 1998.

196. Delaney, JS and Montgomery, DL: How can hyperbaric oxygen contribute to treatment? Phys Sports Med 29:77, 2001.

197. Berg, E, et al: The use of adjunctive hyperbaric oxygen in treatment of orthopedic infections and problem wounds: An overview and case reports. J Invest Surg 2:409, 1989.

198. Strauss, MB and Bryant, B: Hyperbaric oxygen. Orthopedics 25:303, 2002.

199. Grim, PS, et al: Hyperbaric oxygen therapy. JAMA 263:2216, 1990.

200. Harrison, BC, et al: Treatment of exercise-induced muscle injury via hyperbaric oxygen therapy. Med Sci Sports Exerc 33:26, 2001.

201. Plafki, C, et al: Complications and side effects of hyperbaric oxygen therapy. Aviat Space Environ Med 71:194, 2000.

202. Undersea & Hyperbaric Medical Society. www.uhms.org. Last accessed 26 August 2002.

203. Borromeo, CN, et al: Hyperbaric oxygen therapy for acute ankle sprains. Am J Sports Med 25:619, 1997.

204. Staples, JR, et al: Effects of hyperbaric oxygen on a human model of injury. Am J Sports Med 27:600, 1999.

205. Uchino, F: Enhanced regeneration of terminal axons after hyperbaric oxygen therapy in a patient resembling progressive postpoliomyelitis muscular atrophy. Clin Neurol 34:48, 1994.

206. Ueng, SWN, et al: Bone healing of tibial lengthening is enhanced by hyperbaric oxygen therapy: A study of bone mineral density and torsional strength on rabbits. J Trauma 44:676, 1998.

207. Kalliainen, LK, et al: Topical oxygen as an adjunct to wound healing: a clinical case series. Pathophysiology 9:81, 2003.

208. Basford, JR: A historical perspective of the popular use of electric and magnetic therapy. Arch Phys Med Rehabil 82:1261, 2001.

209. Markov, MS and Colbert, AP: Magnetic and electromagnetic field therapy. J Back and Musculoskeletal Rehabil 15:17, 2001.

210. Macklis, RM: Magnetic healing, quackery, and the debate about the health effects of electromagnetic fields. Ann Intern Med 118:376, 1993.

211. Sweeney, KB, et al: Therapeutic magnets do not affect tissue temperatures. J Athletic Training 36:27, 2001.

212. World Health Organization. Magnetic fields. United Nations Environment Programme, The International Labour Organization. WHO, Geneva, 1987.

213. Segal, NA, et al: Two configurations of static magnetic fields for treating rheumatoid arthritis of the knee: A double-blind clinical trial. Arch Phys Med Rehabil 82:1453, 2001.

214. Borsa, PA and Liggett, CL: Flexible magnets are not effective in decreasing pain perception and recovery time after muscle microinjury. J Athletic Training 33:150, 1998.

215. Metz, G: Magnet mania. Training and Conditioning 7:46, 1997.

216. Vallbona, C, et al: Response of pain to static magnetic fields in postpolio patients: A double-blind pilot study. Arch Phys Med Rehabil 78:1200, 1997.

217. Hong, CZ, et al: Magnetic necklace: Its therapeutic effectiveness on neck and shoulder pain. Arch Phys Med Rehabil 63:462, 1982.

218. Villa, M, et al: Minireview: Biological effects of magnetic fields. Life Sci 49:85, 1991.

219. Collacott, EA, et al: Bipolar permanent magnets for the treatment of chronic low back pain. A pilot study. JAMA, 283:1322, 2000.

220. Shellock, FG: Biological effects and safety aspects of magnetic resonance imaging. Mag Reson Q, 5:243, 1986.

221. Lanza, NE; Stoklosa, DA; Cordova, ML; Edwards, JE and Swez, JA: The effects of static magnetic therapy on quadriceps muscle strength. J Athletic Training, 37(S):S-104, 2002.

Appendix A

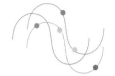

Trigger Points and Pain Patterns

"Trigger points" are small areas of localized sensitivity and pain found in muscles and connective tissue. They may be produced by trauma, can be a result of chronic strain, or may be developed as a result of stress from daily activities or postural habits. Although the pain and sensitivity are localized, reports in the literature suggest that the discomfort may be referred to other parts of the body ("referred pain") through the autonomic nervous system.

These areas may be located by palpation, with the aid of the eraser end of a pencil, or by means of electrical currents. It has been suggested that the combination of electrical stimulation and ultrasound is beneficial in both locating and treating the involved areas. A tetanizing current within the comfortable intensity range of the patient is normally used for both location and treatment, offering "massage-like" contraction to the muscles to which it is applied.[1, 2]

Illustrations are from Mettler Electronics Corporation, Anaheim, California, with permission.

References
1. Travel, J and Rinzier, SH: The myofascial genesis of pain. Postgrad Med II(5): May, 1952.
2. Sola, AE: Myofascial trigger point pain in the neck and shoulder girdle. Northwest Medicine 54:980, 1955.

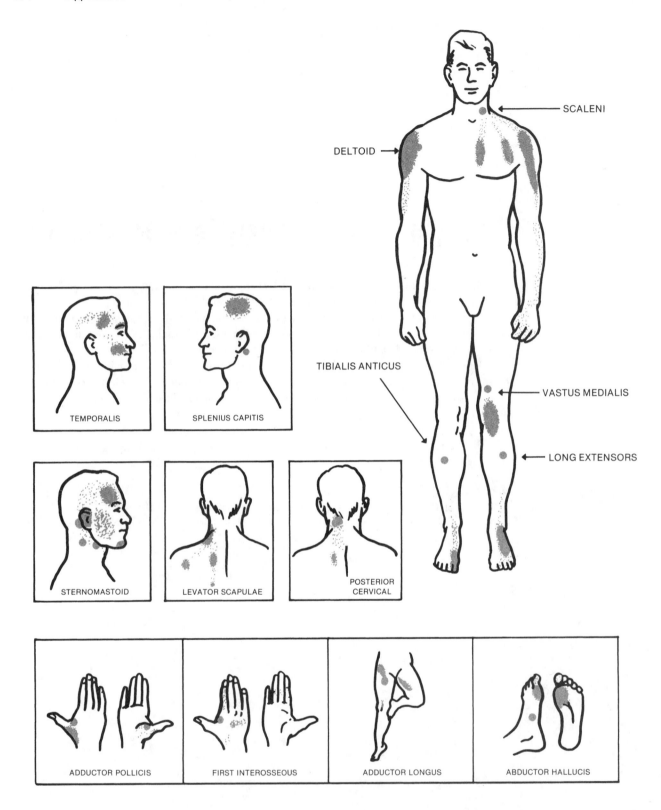

SCALENI

DELTOID

TEMPORALIS

SPLENIUS CAPITIS

STERNOMASTOID

LEVATOR SCAPULAE

POSTERIOR
CERVICAL

TIBIALIS ANTICUS

VASTUS MEDIALIS

LONG EXTENSORS

ADDUCTOR POLLICIS

FIRST INTEROSSEOUS

ADDUCTOR LONGUS

ABDUCTOR HALLUCIS

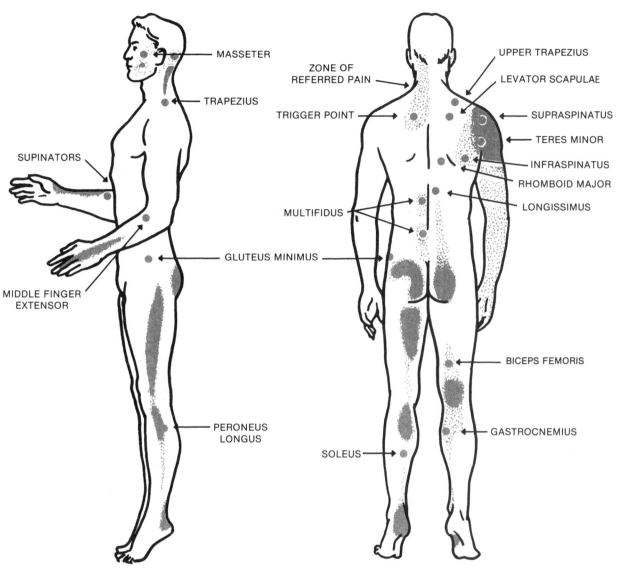

REFERENCES:
Travel, J. and Rinzier, S.H., "The Myofascial Genesis of Pain," POSTGRADUATE MEDICINE, Vol. II, No. 5, May, 1952.

Sola, A. E. "Myofascial Trigger Point Pain in the Neck and Shoulder Girdle," NORTHWEST MEDICINE, Vol. 54, pp. 980-984 September, 1955.

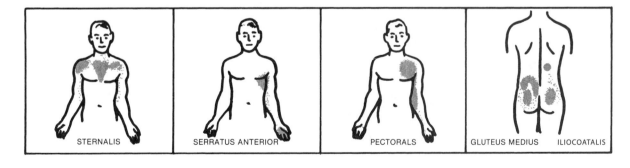

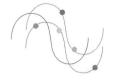

Appendix B

Physical Properties Governing Therapeutic Modalities

The laws of physics govern the energies used by therapeutic modalities. This appendix presents an overview of these physical properties. Modality-specific physical properties are discussed in the relevant chapters of this text.

■ The Electromagnetic Spectrum

Various forms of energy are constantly bombarding us: the light from the sun, the heat from a fire, and the waves emitted from radio transmitters. This energy, known as **electromagnetic radiation,** is produced by virtually every element in the universe and is characterized by the following traits:

- Transports energy through space
- Requires no transmission medium
- Travels through a vacuum at a constant rate of 300 million meters per second
- Does not have mass and is composed of pure energy

Each form of energy is ordered on the electromagnetic spectrum on the basis of its wavelength or frequency (Fig. B–1).

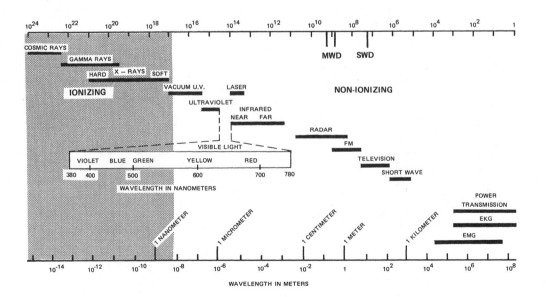

Figure B–1. **A Graphical Representation of the Electromagnetic Spectrum.** (Adapted from Illuminating Engineering Society of North America Lighting Handbook, New York, ed 8, 1993.)

TABLE B-1	Units of Measure for Wavelengths Relative to the Meter (39.37 in.)	
Name	*Symbol*	*Wavelength*
Angstrom	Å	10210 m
Nanometer	nm	1029 m
Micrometer	mm	1026 m
Millimeter	mm	1023 m
Centimeter	cm	1022 m
Meter	m	—
Kilometer	km	103 m

Regions of the Electromagnetic Spectrum

The energy's wavelength uniquely defines each portion of the electromagnetic spectrum. The reference measure for wavelength is the meter (Table B–1).

Ionizing Range

Energy within the ionizing range of the electromagnetic spectrum is characterized by the relative ease with which atoms can release free electrons, protons, or neutrons. Ionizing radiation can easily penetrate the tissues and deposit its energy within the cells. If this energy is sufficiently high, the cell loses its ability to divide, eventually killing the cell.

Energy within the ionizing range is used diagnostically in obtaining radiographs (below the threshold required for cell death) and therapeutically in radiation treatment for some forms of cancer (above the threshold). Because ionizing radiation is hazardous, the total dose of exposure must be tightly monitored and controlled. Energy found in this portion of the electromagnetic spectrum is used by physicians only under closely controlled circumstances.

The Light Spectrum

This portion of the spectrum encompasses ultraviolet, visible, and infrared light energy. Electromagnetic radiation possessing a wavelength between 380 and 780 nm forms the spectrum of **visible "white" light.** White light is the combination of seven colors, each representing a different wavelength on the spectrum. These seven colors, ranked from the shortest to the longest wavelength, are violet, indigo, blue, green, yellow, orange, and red.

Light energy having a wavelength greater than 780 nm is termed **infrared light** or infrared energy. Because this wavelength is greater than the upper limits of what the human eye is capable of detecting, infrared energy is invisible. Any object possessing a temperature greater than absolute zero emits infrared energy proportional to its temperature. Hotter sources transmit more infrared energy because they possess a shorter wavelength than cooler objects.

The infrared spectrum is divided into two distinct sections. The near infrared is the portion of the spectrum that is closest to visible light, with wavelengths ranging between 780 and 1500 nm. The far-infrared portion is located between 1500 and 12,500 nm. Energy in the near infrared range is capable of producing thermal effects 5 to 10 mm deep in tissue, whereas far infrared energy results in more superficial heating of the skin (less than 2 mm deep).

Light with a wavelength shorter than visible light is **ultraviolet light**. Like infrared energy, ultraviolet light is undetectable by the human eye. Energy in the near ultraviolet range has wavelengths ranging between 290 and 400 nm, whereas the far ultraviolet range encompasses wavelengths between 180 and 290 nm. Both of these forms of ultraviolet light produce superficial chemical changes in the skin. Sunburn is an example of the effect of an overdose of ultraviolet radiation.

Many therapeutic modalities use energy within the light range of the electromagnetic spectrum. Ultraviolet light is used for the treatment of certain skin conditions. Depending on the relative temperatures involved, transfer of infrared energy is used to heat or cool the body's tissues. Medical lasers produce beams of energy in the ultraviolet, visible, and infrared light regions that can result in either tissue destruction or therapeutic effects within the tissues.

Diathermy and Electrical Currents

Electromagnetic radiation of longer wavelengths has an intensity sufficient to cause an increase in tissue temperature. Collectively known as diathermy, these types of electromagnetic energies create a magnetic field that is changed into heat through the process of conversion. The two most common types of therapeutic diathermy are microwave and shortwave diathermy.

In the range above shortwave diathermy and extending on to infinity are electrical stimulating currents. These devices use the direct flow of electrons and ions to elicit physiological changes within the tissues. It should be noted that the physical manipulations done to the electrical current do not allow for its precise location on the electromagnetic spectrum. The exception to this is uninterrupted direct current, possessing the theoretical wavelength of infinity.

■ Physical Laws Governing the Application of Therapeutic Modalities

The efficacy of a particular treatment depends on the proper choice and application of a modality. The modality must be capable of producing the desired physiological changes at the intended tissue depth. A superficial heating agent has little positive effect on a deep-seated injury. The proper modality will not produce optimal results if it is applied incorrectly.

For physiological changes to occur, the energy applied to the body must be absorbed by the tissues. Across the electromagnetic spectrum, there is little correlation between wavelength and the ability to penetrate the body's tissues.[1] Both x-rays and radio waves penetrate the tissues despite their polar positions on the spectrum.

Heat Transfer

Conductive heat transfer to or from the body is governed by the laws of thermodynamics. The amount of energy exchanged during a cold or superficial heat treatment can be calculated using the following equation:

$$H = k \, A \, t \, (\Delta T / \Delta L)$$

where:

    H   = Total heat transfer

    k = Thermal conductivity of the tissues
    A   = Area through which the energy is being transmitted
    t   = Total time that the modality is applied
    ΔT = Temperature gradient between the modality and the tissues
    ΔL = Distance separating the thermal gradient

When applying modalities such as moist heat or ice packs, the area (A) represents the surface area where the modality contacts the skin. Increasing the surface area increases the amount of energy exchanged. The thermal conductivity (k) differs from tissue layer to tissue layer, with adipose tissue representing the lowest exchange rate. The distance separating the thermal gradient (ΔL) is the distance from the modality to the target tissues.

Adding an insulating layer between the modality and the skin reduces the energy exchange two ways. Insulators have a low thermal capacity that decreases the amount of energy exchanged. The insulating material also increases the distance between the modality and the skin, increasing the value of ΔL, thus reducing the total energy exchange.

Cosine Law

Electromagnetic energy is most efficiently transmitted to the tissues when it strikes the body at a right angle (90 degrees). Because this angle (the angle of incidence) deviates away from 90 degrees, the efficiency of the energy affecting the tissues is decreased by the cosine of the angle. The cosine law defines this relationship as:

$$\text{Effective energy} = \text{Energy} \times \text{Cosine of the angle of incidence}$$

With radiant energy, a difference of ± 10 degrees from the right angle is considered within acceptable limits during treatment.[2]

Inverse Square Law

The intensity of radiant energy depends on the distance between the source and the tissues and is described by the inverse square law. The intensity of the energy striking the tissues is proportional to the square of the distance between the source of the energy and the tissues:

$$E = Es/D^2$$

where:

E = the amount of energy received by the tissue

Es = the amount of energy produced by the source

D^2 = the square of the distance between the target and the source

Doubling the distance between the tissue and the energy decreases the intensity at the tissue by a factor of four (Fig. B–2).

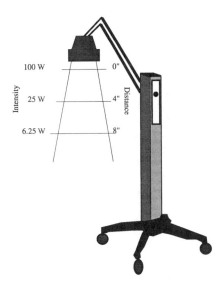

Figure B-2. **An Example of the Inverse-square Law.** Each time the distance between the source of infrared energy and the tissue is doubled, the intensity of the energy delivered to the tissue is reduced by a factor of four.

Arndt-Schultz Principle

To enable energy to affect the body, it must be absorbed by the tissues at a level sufficient to stimulate a physiological response. As described by the general adaptation syndrome (see Chap. 1), if the amount of energy absorbed is too little, no reaction takes place, and if the amount of energy is too great, damage results. This concept applied to the application of therapeutic modalities is known as the Arndt-Schultz principle and is translated into clinical practice through the application of the proper modality at the proper intensity for the appropriate duration.

Law of Grotthus-Draper

The law of Grotthus-Draper describes an inverse relationship between the penetration and absorption of energy by which any energy that penetrates the body and is not absorbed by one tissue layer is passed along to the next layer. The more energy is absorbed by the superficial tissues, the less remains to be transmitted to underlying tissues.

Consider, for example, the application of moist heat to the quadriceps muscle group. Some of the energy is absorbed by the skin, decreasing the amount of energy delivered to the adipose tissue. Some of the remaining energy is absorbed by the adipose tissue, leaving only a fraction of the initial energy left to heat the muscle. This example also illustrates the fact that adipose tissue can act as an insulator, inhibiting the thermal heating of muscle. This concept applies to most therapeutic modalities, with the difference being the layer or layers in which the majority of energy loss occurs.

■ Measures

Distance Conversion

The basis of measurement in the metric system is the meter (m), a distance of 39.37 inches. The exact distance of 1 m is the wavelength associated with a specific frequency in the electromagnetic spectrum. The inch, according to history, was derived from the length of the middle phalanx of a king's index finger.

Comparison between English and SI Measures of Length

Millimeters	Centimeters	Meters	Inches	Feet	Yards
1 mm = 1.0	0.1	0.001	0.03937	0.00328	0.0011
1 cm = 10.0	1.0	0.01	0.3937	0.03281	0.0109
1 in. = 25.4	2.54	0.0254	1.0	0.0833	0.0278
1 ft = 304.8	30.48	0.3048	12.0	1.0	0.333
1 yd = 914.4	91.44	0.9144	36.0	3.0	1.0
1 m = 1000.0	100.0	1.0	39.37	3.2808	1.0936

Source: Adapted from Venes, D and Thomas, CL (eds): Taber's Cyclopedic Medical Dictionary, ed 19. FA Davis, Philadelphia, 1997, p 2378.

To convert English measures to meters, multiply the unit by the following conversion constants. To convert meters to the English system, divide by the constant.

English Measure	Constant
Inches	0.0254
Feet	0.3048

Weight and Mass Conversion

English Measure	Constant
Ounces	0.0283495
Pounds	0.4535924

Temperature Conversion

To convert Fahrenheit to centigrade:

$$C° = (F° - 32) \times 5/9$$

To convert centigrade to Fahrenheit:

$$F° = (C° \times 9/5) + 32$$

References
1. Kloth, LC and Ziskin, MC: Diathermy and pulsed electromagnetic fields. In Michlovitz, SL (ed): Thermal Agents in Rehabilitation, ed 2. FA Davis, Philadelphia, 1990, pp 170–199.
2. Griffin, JE and Karselis, TC: Physical Agents for Physical Therapists, ed 3. Charles C Thomas, Springfield, IL, 1988, pp 229–263.

Appendix C

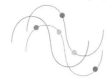

Motor Points

A motor point is the place in a muscle where the muscle is most easily excited with a minimum amount of electrical stimulation; the motor point is usually located near the center of the muscle mass, where the motor nerve enters the muscle. For each muscle, the motor point may vary from patient to patient, or even at different times for the same patient, depending on the pathology. The accompanying charts are guides to the motor points.

Illustrations are from Mettler Corporation, Anaheim, California, with permission.

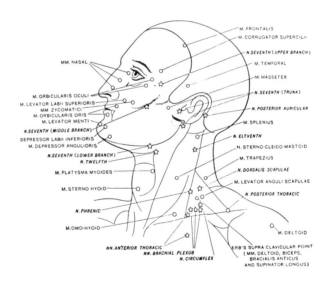

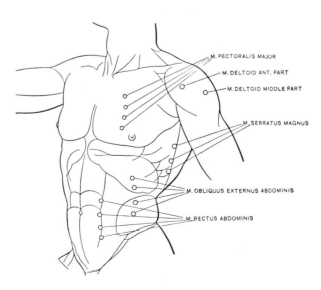

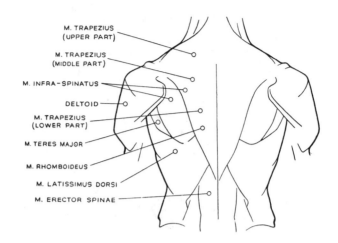

M. TRAPEZIUS
(UPPER PART)

M. TRAPEZIUS
(MIDDLE PART)

M. INFRA-SPINATUS

DELTOID

M. TRAPEZIUS
(LOWER PART)

M. TERES MAJOR

M. RHOMBOIDEUS

M. LATISSIMUS DORSI

M. ERECTOR SPINAE

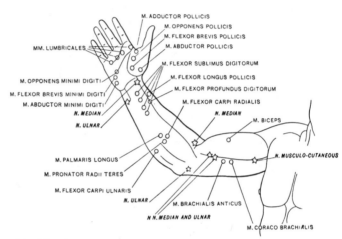

M. ADDUCTOR POLLICIS
M. OPPONENS POLLICIS
M. FLEXOR BREVIS POLLICIS
M. ABDUCTOR POLLICIS

MM. LUMBRICALES

M. FLEXOR SUBLIMUS DIGITORUM

M. OPPONENS MINIMI DIGITI
M. FLEXOR LONGUS POLLICIS

M. FLEXOR BREVIS MINIMI DIGITI
M. FLEXOR PROFUNDUS DIGITORUM

M. ABDUCTOR MINIMI DIGITI
M. FLEXOR CARPI RADIALIS

N. MEDIAN
N. MEDIAN   M. BICEPS

N. ULNAR

M. PALMARIS LONGUS
N. MUSCULO-CUTANEOUS

M. PRONATOR RADII TERES

M. FLEXOR CARPI ULNARIS

N. ULNAR
M. BRACHIALIS ANTICUS

N N. MEDIAN AND ULNAR

M. CORACO BRACHIALIS

M = Muscle
N = Nerves

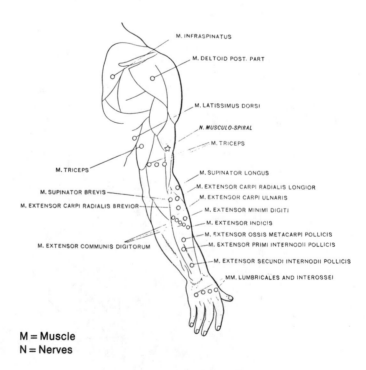

M. INFRASPINATUS

M. DELTOID POST. PART

M. LATISSIMUS DORSI

N. MUSCULO-SPIRAL

M. TRICEPS

M. TRICEPS

M. SUPINATOR LONGUS

M. EXTENSOR CARPI RADIALIS LONGIOR

M. SUPINATOR BREVIS
M. EXTENSOR CARPI ULNARIS

M. EXTENSOR CARPI RADIALIS BREVIOR
M. EXTENSOR MINIMI DIGITI

M. EXTENSOR INDICIS

M. EXTENSOR OSSIS METACARPI POLLICIS

M. EXTENSOR PRIMI INTERNODII POLLICIS

M. EXTENSOR COMMUNIS DIGITORUM

M. EXTENSOR SECUNDI INTERNODII POLLICIS

MM. LUMBRICALES AND INTEROSSEI

M = Muscle
N = Nerves

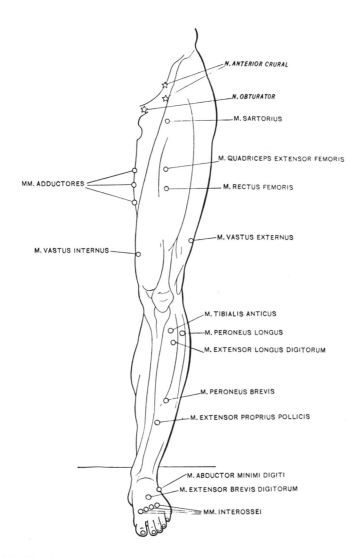

N. ANTERIOR CRURAL

N. OBTURATOR

M. SARTORIUS

M. QUADRICEPS EXTENSOR FEMORIS

M. RECTUS FEMORIS

MM. ADDUCTORES

M. VASTUS EXTERNUS

M. VASTUS INTERNUS

M. TIBIALIS ANTICUS

M. PERONEUS LONGUS

M. EXTENSOR LONGUS DIGITORUM

M. PERONEUS BREVIS

M. EXTENSOR PROPRIUS POLLICIS

M. ABDUCTOR MINIMI DIGITI

M. EXTENSOR BREVIS DIGITORUM

MM. INTEROSSEI

M = Muscle
N = Nerve

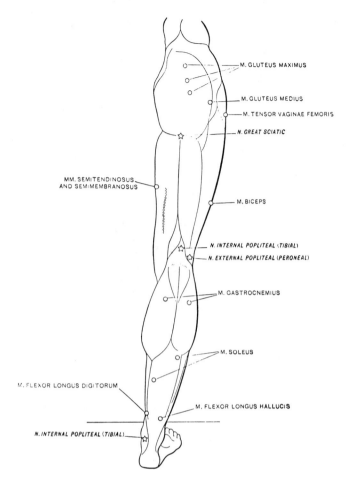

M. GLUTEUS MAXIMUS

M. GLUTEUS MEDIUS

M. TENSOR VAGINAE FEMORIS

N. GREAT SCIATIC

MM. SEMITENDINOSUS AND SEMIMEMBRANOSUS

M. BICEPS

N. INTERNAL POPLITEAL (TIBIAL)

N. EXTERNAL POPLITEAL (PERONEAL)

M. GASTROCNEMIUS

M. SOLEUS

M. FLEXOR LONGUS DIGITORUM

M. FLEXOR LONGUS HALLUCIS

N. INTERNAL POPLITEAL (TIBIAL)

M = Muscle
N = Nerve

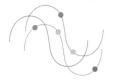

Appendix D

Medical Shorthand

The following represent examples of medical shorthand for note taking and medical records. Because of both the similarities and differences between different abbreviations, facilities should develop an approved institutional list of abbreviations and have them readily available for staff and administrators.

■ Therapeutic Modalities or Treatments

CWP	Cold whirlpool	MT	Manual therapy
EMS	Electrical muscle stimulation	MWD	Microwave diathermy
ES	Electrical stimulation	RICE	Rest, ice, compression, elevation
HP	Hot pack		
HT	Hubbard tank	SWD	Shortwave diathermy
HVPS	High-voltage pulsed stimulation	TENS	Transcutaneous electrical nerve stimulation
HWP	Hot whirlpool		
ICE	Ice, compression, elevation	TFM	Transverse friction massage
IFS	Interferential stimulation	TX	Traction
IM	Ice massage	US	Ultrasound
MENS	Microcurrent electrical neuromuscular stimulation	UV	Ultraviolet
		WP	Whirlpool

■ Dosage/Administration

AC	Before meals	PER OS, PO	By mouth
AD LIB	At discretion/as desired	PRN	Whenever necessary
ASA	Aspirin	Q	Every
ASAP	As soon as possible	QD	Every day
BID	Twice daily	QH	Every hour
BIW	Biweekly	QID	Four times a day
MAX	Maximum	QOD	Every other day
MED	Minimal erythemal dose (ultraviolet light) Medium	QN	Every night
		Q#HR	Every X hours (e.g., Q3HR = every 3 hours)
MIN	Minimal	SED	Suberythemal dose (ultraviolet light)
MOD	Moderate		
NOC	Night, nocturnal	SIG	Directions for use
NPO	Nothing by mouth	SOS	When necessary, if necessary
OD	Once daily	ST	Start
PC	After meals	TID	Three times a day
PCA	Patient-controlled anesthesia	TIW	Three times a week
PER	By or through	W/cm^2	Watts per square centimeter

Range of Motion, Exercise, and Activity

//	Parallel bars	NWB	Non–weight-bearing
AAROM	Active assistive (assisted) range of motion	OOB	Out of bed
		OOW	Out of work
ABD	Abduction	PWB	Partial weight-bearing
ADD	Adduction	PNF	Proprioceptive neuromuscular facilitation
ADL	Activities of daily living		
amb	ambulation	PREs	Progressive resistance exercises
AP	Ankle pumps	PROM	Passive range of motion
AROM	Active range of motion	PRON	Pronation
BR	Bed rest	QS	Quadriceps muscle sets
CWI	Crutch walking instruction/exercise	REHAB	Rehabilitation
EV	Eversion	REPs	Repetitions
EXT	Extension	ROM	Range of motion
FARM	Full active range of motion	ROT	Rotate, rotational
FLX	Flexion	RROM	Resistive range of motion
FWB	Full weight-bearing	RTW	Return to work
GT	Gait training	SB	Side bending
HEP	Home exercise program	SLR	Straight-leg raise
INV	Inversion	SUP	Supination
MMT	Manual muscle test	TTW	Toe touch weight-bearing
MVT	Movement	WBAT	Weight-bearing as tolerated

Surgical and Medical Procedures

ACLR	Anterior cruciate ligament reconstruction	OREF	Open reduction, external fixation
BX	Biopsy	ORIF	Open reduction, internal fixation
CBC	Complete blood count	THA	Total hip arthroplasty
CT/CAT	Computer assisted tomography	THR	Total hip replacement
CTR	Carpal tunnel release	TKA	Total knee arthroplasty
MRI	Magnetic resonance imaging	TKR	Total knee replacement

Assistive Devices and Braces

AFO	Ankle-foot orthosis	LAC	Long arm cast
CR	Crutches	LLC	Long leg cast
CW	Crutch walking	SAC	Short arm cast
HAC	Half arm cast	WC	Walking cast
HLC	Half leg cast	w/c	Wheelchair
KAFO	Knee-ankle-foot orthosis		

Measurements and Time

+, pos	Positive	C	Centigrade, Celsius
–, neg	Negative	cm	Centimeter
<	Less than	cont.	Continue
=	Equals	DA	Developmental age
>	Greater than	doa	Date of admission
a.m.	Morning (just after midnight to just before noon)	doi	Date of injury
		dos	Date of surgery
BLA	Baseline assessment	DTD	Dated

ft	Foot/feet		mo	Month
GA	Gestational age		oz	Ounce
g	Gram		PTA	Prior to admission
h, hr	Hour		p.m.	Afternoon (just past noon to just prior to midnight)
hs	At bedtime			
ht.	Height		sec	Seconds
H&P	History and physical		stat	Immediately
in.	Inch		TBSP	Tablespoon
kg	Kilogram		TSP	Teaspoon
L, l	Liter		UNK	Unknown
lb	Pounds		wk	Week
m	Meter		wt	Weight
min	Minutes		WNL	Within normal limits
mg	Milligram		X	Number of times performed (e.g., 2×)
mL	Milliliter		yr	Year
mm	Millimeter		y/o	Years old

■ Grades

1	First degree		N	Normal
2	Second degree		P	Poor
3	Third degree		T	Trace
ABN	Abnormal		N/A	Not applicable
F	Fair		WNL	Within normal limits
G	Good			

■ Body Area

Ⓛ	Left		FT	Foot/feet
Ⓡ	Right		GH	Glenohumeral joint
ACJ	Acromioclavicular joint		INF	Inferior
ACL	Anterior cruciate ligament		JT	Joint
AE	Above elbow		L	Lumbar spine
AIIS	Anterior inferior iliac spine		L#	Lumbar spine level (e.g., L1, L2)
AK	Above knee		LB	Low back (lumbar)
ANT	Anterior		LCL	Lateral collateral ligament
AP	Anteroposterior		LE	Lower extremity
ASIS	Anterosuperior iliac spine		MCL	Medial collateral ligament
ATF	Anterior talofibular ligament		P	Proximal
B	Bilateral/both		P/#	Proximal range (e.g., p/3 = proximal third)
BE	Below elbow			
Bilat.	Bilaterally		PA	Posteroanterior
BK	Below knee		PCL	Posterior cruciate ligament
BLE	Bilateral lower extremities		PIP	Proximal interphalangeal joint
C	Cervical spine		PSIS	Posterior superior iliac spine
C#	Cervical spine level (e.g., C1, C2)		PTF	Posterior talofibular ligament
CF	Calcaneofibular ligament		SCJ	Sternoclavicular joint
CV	Cardiovascular		T	Thoracic spine
D	Distal		T#	Thoracic spine level (e.g., T1, T2)
D/#	Distal range (e.g., d/1 = distal third)		UE	Upper extremity
DIP	Distal interphalangeal joint			

General Note Taking

p̄	After
~	Approximately
ā, a	Before
Δ	Change
↓	Down, decreasing
„	Female
,	Male
1°	Primary
2°	Secondary
3°	Tertiary
↑	Up, increasing
c̄	With
s̄	Without
A:	Assessment
ADM	Admission
AMA	Against medical advice
c/o	Complains of
CC	Chief complaint
cc	Cubic centimeter
D/C	Discontinue
DNK	Did not keep appointment
Dx	Diagnosis
EVAL	Evaluation
FH	Family history
Hx, hx	History
IC	Informed consent
imp.	Impression
IN SITU	In its natural place
indep	Independent
LTG	Long-term goals
M&R	Measure and record
MA	Medical assistance
Meds	Medication
MRN	Medical record number
N/A	Not applicable

NKA	No known allergies
NKI	No known injuries/illnesses
O.P., OP	Outpatient
O.R., OR	Operating room
O:	Objective
P:	Plan
PATH	Pathology
PALP	Palpation
PE	Physical examination/evaluation
PH	Past history
PMH	Prior medical history
POMR	Problem-oriented medical record
POSS	Possible
POST	Following, after
POSTOP	After surgery
PREOP	Before surgery
PROG	Progress/progressing
re:	Regarding, relating, pertaining
RE-ADM	Re-admission
RO, r/o	Rule out
Rx	Treatment, prescription
S/P	Status post (condition following)
S:	Subjective
SCP	Standard care plan
SOP	Standard operating procedure
SOAP	Subjective, objective, assessment plan format of note taking
SSN	Social security number
STG	Short term goals
Sx	Symptoms
t.o.	Telephone order
TPR	Temperature, pulse, and respiration
v.s.	Vital signs
vo	Verbal orders

Injuries and Diseases

AIDS	Acquired immunodeficiency syndrome
AODM	Adult onset diabetes mellitus
ARF	Acute renal failure
CA	Cancer
CAD	Coronary artery disease
COLD	Chronic obstructive lung disease
COPD	Chronic obstructive pulmonary disease
CP	Cerebral palsy
CVA	Cerebrovascular accident
DDD	Degenerative disc disease
DJD	Degenerative joint disease
DM	Diabetes mellitus
DVT	Deep vein thrombosis
FUO	Fever, unknown origin
FX	Fracture
HA, H/A	Headache

HBP	High blood pressure
HCVD	Hypertensive cardiovascular disease
HI	Head injury
HIV	Human immunodeficiency virus
HNP	Herniated nucleus pulposus
HTN	Hypertension
LAC	Laceration
LBP	Low back pain
LOC	Loss of consciousness
MCA	Motorcycle accident
MI	Myocardial infarction
MS	Multiple sclerosis
MTBI	Mild traumatic brain injury
NIDD	Non–insulin-dependent diabetes
OA	Osteoarthritis
PARA	Paraplegic

PID	Pelvic inflammatory disease	SCI	Spinal cord injury
PFJS	Patellofemoral joint syndrome	SIW	Self-inflicted wound
PNI	Peripheral nerve injury	SOB	Shortness of breath
PVD	Peripheral vascular disease	SPR	Sprain
QUAD	Quadriplegic	STR	Strain
RA	Rheumatoid arthritis	TBI	Traumatic brain injury

Personnel

AT, ATC	Athletic trainer	OTC	Orthopedic technologist, certified
COTA	Certified occupational therapy assistant	PA, P.A.	Physician assistant
CVT	Cardiovascular technologist	PT	Physical therapist/physical therapy
DC	Doctor of chiropractic	PTA	Physical therapy assistant
DO	Doctor of osteopathy	Pt, pt	Patient
EENT	Eye, ears, nose, and throat	RD	Registered dietitian
ENT	Ears, nose, and throat	RN	Registered nurse
GYN	Gynecology	RNC	Registered nurse, certified
MD	Medical doctor	RT	Respiratory therapist
MT	Massage therapist	RTR	Registered technologist, Radiology
OB	Obstetrics		
OT	Occupational therapist/occupational therapy		

Appendix E

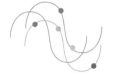

Case Study Discussion

■ Section Two

Cold therapy application is the modality of choice. The ideal combination of ice, compression, and elevation to limit postinjury fluid collection may best be attained with ice bags or conventional gel ice packs.

The physiological changes are to reduce the release of inflammatory mediators, decrease prostaglandin synthesis, and decrease capillary permeability.

The clinical symptoms in this case are from a prevention standpoint, because the injury just occurred. The ice application is aimed at limiting swelling accumulation, minimizing pain, limiting muscle spasm, and limiting range of motion loss.

The application of ice may be implemented after acute reinjury episodes ("rolling" ankle incident, or exercise or activity in excess), to reduce pain on a "bad" day, to reduce muscle spasm, or to assist in restoration of range of motion.

Other thermal modalities can include ice immersion, whirlpool (cold-warm temperature), and ice massage. The ice immersion allows range of motion to be performed simultaneously to increase patient's active role in recovery; the whirlpool will allow range of motion exercise, and the temperature can be increased as the injury moves into the subacute phase of recovery to enhance metabolism to promote healing; and ice massage works best for small, uneven local regions of injury (such as the lateral ligaments or foot intrinsics) where the trauma primarily occurred. Thermal ultrasound may be an option if inflammation has resolved, but low intensity is recommended owing to high bone-to-soft tissue ratio in the injured region.

■ Section Three

Shortwave diathermy induction coil drum is the best option owing to large surface area of involved tissues, marked muscle spasm, and the open wound in the lumbar region. The clinician should be certain that there is no metal within the field of the shortwave diathermy. If the patient has scoliosis with a rod implanted in his spine, for example, the treatment may need application of a sterile dressing to minimize the risk of infection and sterile towels used as a hot pack cover.

During heating, the following physiological responses are stimulated: local cellular metabolism, blood flow, fibroblastic activity, collagen deposition, and new capillary growth.

Heating agents may place the patient at higher risk for infection with contact from nonsterile towels or hot pack covers. Ultrasound can only be applied to a portion of the problem area, due to the wound.

Clinically, treatment is addressing marked muscle spasm, range of motion loss, pain, and wound healing.

■ Section Four

In a clinical setting, the best option for this patient varies tremendously according to the clinician's previous success rate, patient preference, and concurrent treatment approaches implemented. Much success comes from removing the source, the computer workstation ergonomics. Until the work station is adjusted for proper body mechanics, the problems are unlikely to resolve. Modality options could include thermal ultrasound, massage, cryostretch (e.g., spray and stretch), and neuromuscular or interferential electrical stimulation.

Physiologically, the main effect would be to reduce the muscle spasm by inhibiting muscle contraction.

The clinical symptoms that should be addressed are range of motion, pain, spasm, tenderness, and muscle strength and endurance.

■ Section Five

Commentary—Bertha

Edema management can be addressed with massage, electrical stimulation, and warm and cold thermal agents. The physiological effects are to assist venous and lymphatic return, reduce viscosity of fluid, removal of cellular debris, and increase delivery of nutrients for the healing of the soft tissues. Clinical goals would be based on her deficits, and treatment is rendered to reduce edema, improve range of motion, decrease pain, and improve function. Owing to her history of cancer, ultrasound should be avoided. Interferential electrical stimulation and heat packs would be appropriate.

Commentary—Sam

Indications include muscle spasm, degenerative disc disease, nerve root compression, capsulitis of the vertebral joint, and herniated intervertebral disks. Traction can be used to try to interrupt the pain-spasm-pain cycle. The pressure on the nerve roots should be reduced by the distraction force of the traction unit. Clinically, the centralization of symptoms is a sign of progress, by one man's opinion. The clinical symptoms that should be reduced are pain, range of motion, and radicular pain. Other modalities to ease the muscle spasm, without compromising the disc pressure, could include heat therapy, electrical stimulation, ice packs, and ultrasound, if symptoms are localized to a small area.

Commentary—Mr. Smith

Contraindications include peripheral vascular disease, deep vein thrombosis, dermatitis, gangrene, and compartment syndromes. Constant, gentle range of motion will increase remodeling of collagen in orderly fashion and promote nutrient exchange. Clinical gains are expected in range of motion, edema reduction, pain management, and diminished soft tissue spasm.

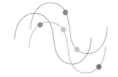

Quiz Answers

■ Section One

1 – B	11 – B
2 – C	12 – C
3 – C	13 – A
4 – B	14 – D
5 – A	15 – C
6 – A	16 – D
7 – C	17 – B
8 – C	18 – C
9 – D	19 – A
10 – D	20 – D

■ Section Two

1 – B	11 – D
2 – D	12 – B
3 – B	13 – C
4 – D	14 – C
5 – D	15 – B
6 – B	16 – B
7 – C	17 – B
8 – B	18 – A
9 – A	19:
10 – D	

Step	Effect
Rest	Prevents further physical trauma
Ice	Decreases the cell's metabolism, thereby reducing the amount of secondary hypoxic injury and secondary enzymatic injury.
Compression	Reduces the pressure gradient, reduces hemorrhage, and limits the collection of edema.
Elevation	Decreases local blood pressure and encourages venous and lymphatic return.
20:	Several mechanisms account for the longer-lasting effects of cold application relative to heat application. (1) The temperature gradient between the skin is greater with cold modalities than heat modalities, thus increasing the rate and magnitude of energy exchange. (2) Cold application decreases blood flow, thereby limiting re-warming the tissues; heat application increases blood flow which continually brings in relatively cool blood. (3) Cold penetrates deeper than heat, which

decreases the overall temperature gradient and slows tissue re-warming. (4) Perspiration occurs during heat application, regulating the local temperature.

Section Three

1 – C	10 – D
2 – B	11 – B
3 – D	12 – B
4 – D	13 – C
5 – A	14 – C
6 – A	15 – A
7 – C	16 – A
8 – B	17 – B
9 – A	18 – A

19: Any of the following:
Hydration
Age
Composition
Vascularity
Thickness

20:

	Ultrasound	*Shortwave Diathermy*
Type of energy	Acoustical	Electromagnetic
Tissue heated	Collagen-rich	C: Adipose tissue, skin
		I: Muscle, blood vessels
Volume of tissue heated	Small (20 cm^2)	Large (200 cm^2)
Temperature increase	1 MHz: More than 6.3°F (3.5°C)	C: More than 7°F (3.9°C) (Adipose tissue)
	3 MHz: More than 14.9°F (8.3°C)	I: More than 18°F (10°C) (intramuscular tissue)
Heat retention	Short (approximately 3 minutes)	Long (approximately 9 minutes)

Section Four

1 – C	11 – B
2 – D	12 – B
3 – C	13 – D
4 – B	14 – A
5 – D	15 – A
6 – A	16 – C
7 – D	17 – B
8 – A	18 – D
9 – A	19 – A
10 – C	20 – B

■ Section Five

1 – D
2 – C
3 – A
4 – B
5 – C
6 – B
7 – B
8 – D
9 – B

10 – C
11 – C
12 – A
13 – C
14 – B
15 – D
16 – B
17 – D

18:

Position of the cervical spine
Position of the patient
Angle of pull
Duration of treatment
Constant or intermittent traction

19:

The force of gravity is eliminated
The cervical muscles are placed in a more relaxed position

20:

B
A
C

Book Glossary

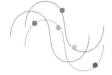

Absolute refractory period: The period after a nerve's depolarization during which a subsequent depolarization cannot occur, used for recharging the electrical potential.

Absolute zero: Theoretically, the lowest possible temperature, equal to –273°C or –460°F. At this point, all atomic and molecular motion ceases.

Absorption: The process of a medium collecting thermal energy and changing it to kinetic energy.

Accommodation: The decrease in a nerve's action potential frequency over time when exposed to an unchanging depolarization stimulus.

Acetylcholine: Neurotransmitter responsible for transmitting motor nerve impulses.

Acoustical interface: A surface where two materials of different densities meet.

Acoustical spectrum: Energy transmitted through mechanical waves.

Acoustical streaming: The unidirectional flow of fluids within the tissues caused by the application of therapeutic ultrasound.

Actin: A contractile muscle protein.

Actinomycosis: A disease state of actin caused by a fungus.

Action potential: The change in the electrical potential of a nerve or muscle fiber when stimulated.

Activities of daily living: Fundamental skills required for a certain lifestyle, including mobility, self-care, and grooming.

Acupuncture points: Points on the skin theorized to control systemic functions. These points lie along 12 main channels, eight secondary channels, and a network of subchannels.

Acute: Of recent onset. The period after an injury when the local inflammatory response is still active.

ADA: See Americans with Disabilities Act.

A-delta fibers: A type of nerve that transmits painful information that is often interpreted by the brain as burning or stinging pain.

Adenosine triphosphate (ATP): An important source of energy for intracellular metabolism.

Adriamycin: An antibiotic medication.

Aerobic: Requiring the presence of oxygen.

Afferent: Carrying impulses toward a central structure, for example, the brain.

Alarm stage: The first stage in the general adaptation syndrome in which the body readies its defensive systems.

Albinism: A condition in which the individual lacks pigmentation of the skin, hair, and eyes. The skin is prone to sunburns and the eyes are particularly sensitive to light (photophobia).

Allograft: A replacement or augmentation of a biological structure with a synthetic one.

Alpha-motoneurons: Efferent motor neurons that innervate muscle fibers.

ALS: See anterior lateral system.

Alternating current: The uninterrupted flow of electrons marked by a change in the direction and magnitude of the movement.

Americans with Disabilities Act: Legislation passed in 1990 (Public Law 101-336) that protects the right of disabled individuals by creating standards to ensure access and prohibit discrimination in transportation, accommodation, public services, and so on.

Amino acids: Building blocks of protein.

Amperage: The rate of flow of an electrical current. One ampere is equal to the rate of flow of 1 coulomb per second.

Amplitude: The maximum departure of a wave from the baseline.

Amplitude ramp: The gradual rise or fall in a pulse train's amplitude.

Anaerobic: Able to survive in the absence of oxygen. Anaerobic systems derive their energy through the breakdown of adenosine triphosphate (ATP) into adenosine diphosphate (ADP).

Analgesia: Absence of the sense of pain.

Analgesic: A pain-reducing substance.

Analog: A readout on a continuously variable scale. A clock with hands is a type of analog display.

Anesthesia: A loss of, or decrease in, sensation.

Angstrom (Å): A distance equal to 10^{-10} m or one-billionth of a meter.

Annulus fibrosus: The dense, inflexible outer layers of an intervertebral disk.

Anode: The positive pole of an electrical circuit. It has a low concentration of electrons and is the opposite of the cathode.

Antabuse: A medication (generic name: disulfiram) used in treating alcoholism. Consumption of alcoholic drinks results in severe nausea and vomiting.

Antalgic gait: A gait resulting from pain on weight bearing. The stance phase of gait is shortened on the affected side.

Anterior lateral fasciculus: The large bundle of fibers in the anterolateral spinal cord and brain stem that carry second-order pain fibers to the brain stem and thalamus.

Anterior lateral system: The ascending fiber system that conveys pain and temperature sensation from spinal cord to the thalamus.

Antibiotic: A substance that inhibits the growth of, or kills, microorganisms.

Arndt-Schultz principle: A principle stating that for energy to affect the body, it must be absorbed by the tissues at a level sufficient to stimulate a physiological response.

Arteriole: A small artery leading to a capillary at its distal end.

Arthrofibrosis: The repair and replacement of inflamed joint tissue by connective tissues.

Arthrogenic muscle inhibition: Denervation of a muscle or muscle group caused by joint swelling.

Arthroplasty: Surgical reconstruction or replacement of an articular joint.

Asymmetrical: Lacking symmetry (e.g., two halves of unequal size or shape).

Atmospheres absolute (ATA): Water (or air) pressure exerted on the body. One ATA is the standard pressure placed on the body at sea level. Each 33-ft immersion from sea level equals an increase of 1 ATA. For example, immersion to a depth of 33 feet exerts 2 ATA, 66 feet exerts 3 ATA, 99 feet exerts 4 ATA and so on.

ATP: See adenosine triphosphate.

Attenuation: The decrease in a wave's intensity resulting from the absorption, reflection, and refraction of energy.

Autoclave: A device used to sterilize medical instruments using steam heat at 250°F (121°C).

Average current: The average amplitude of a current. When the current can be represented by a sine wave, the average current is calculated by multiplying the amplitude by 0.637.

Axon: The stem of a nerve.

Axonotmesis: Damage to nerve tissue without physical severing of the nerve.

Bacterium (_plural_ bacteria): A microscopic organism.

Basement membrane: Extracellular material that separates the base of epithelial cells from connective tissue.

Basic fibroblast growth factor (bFGF): Increases the size of the callus and mechanical strength of the repair during fracture healing.

Battery (criminal): The unwanted touching of one person by another.

Beam nonuniformity ratio (BNR): The ratio between the highest intensity in an ultrasonic beam and the output reported on the meter.

Beat pattern: The frequency formed when two electrical circuits of two different frequencies are mixed.

β-Endorphin: A neurohormone similar to morphine.

Bilateral: On both sides of the body.

Biphasic current: A pulsed current possessing two phases, each of which occurs on opposite sides of the electrical baseline. The bidirectional flow of electrons that is marked by discrete periods of noncurrent flow.

Bipolar stimulation: Electrical stimulation using electrodes of approximately equal surface area from each lead. The

resulting current density under the electrodes from each lead is approximately equal.

Breach of duty: A departure from the implied duty based on the reasonable and prudent doctrine.

Calorie: The amount of energy needed to raise the temperature of 1 g of water by 1°C. One calorie equals 4.1860 joules of energy.

Capacitance: The frequency-dependent ability to store a charge. The symbol for capacitance is (C) and is expressed in farads (F).

Capillary filtration pressure: The pressure that moves the contents of a capillary outward to the tissues.

Cardinal signs of inflammation: Heat, redness, swelling, pain, and loss of function in the area; used as a gauge in determining the extent and stage of the injury response process.

Carotid sinus: An enlargement of the carotid artery near the branch of the internal carotid artery, located distal to the inferior arch of the mandible. Baroreceptors at this site monitor and assist in the regulation of blood pressure.

Carpal tunnel syndrome: Compression of the median nerve that produces pain, numbness, and weakness in the palm and ring and index fingers.

Catalyst: A substance that accelerates a chemical reaction.

Cathode: The negative pole of an electrical circuit. It has a high concentration of electrons and carries the opposite charge to the anode.

Cavitation: The formation of microscopic bubbles during the application of therapeutic ultrasound.

C fiber: A type of nerve that transmits painful information that is often interpreted by the brain as throbbing or aching.

Change of state: Transformation from one physical state to another (e.g., ice to water).

Channel (electrical): An electrical circuit consisting of two poles that operate independently of other circuits.

Chassis: The framework to which electrical components are attached.

Chemosensitive receptors: Nerves that are excited by the presence of certain chemical substances.

Chemotaxis: Movement of living protoplasm toward or away from a chemical stimulus.

Chronic: Continuing for a long period; with injury, extending past the primary hemorrhage and inflammation cycle.

Cingulate gyrus: A large region of the cerebral cortex that lies superior to the corpus callosum. It is important in affective responses to pain.

Circuit, closed: A complete pathway that allows electrons to flow to and from the electrical source.

Circuit, open: An incomplete pathway that does not allow electrons to flow to or from the electrical source.

Circumferential compression: Compression applied in a manner that provides even pressure around the circumference of the body part.

Coagulation: The process of blood clotting.

Cold-induced vasodilation: An unsubstantiated theory suggesting that cold application results in a net increase in the cross-sectional diameter of blood vessels.

Collagen: A protein-based connective tissue.

Collagenase: A substance that causes collagen to break down.

Collateral compression: A form of compression that provides pressure on only two sides of the body part.

Collimated: Possessing a beam of parallel rays or waves that form a column of energy.

Commission: Response to a situation in a manner that is not reasonable and prudent.

Compartment syndrome: Increased pressure within a muscular compartment, causing decreased blood flow to and from the distal extremity, decreased distal nerve function, and decreased local muscular blood perfusion and pain.

Compression (mechanical): An external force applied to the body (e.g., an elastic wrap) that serves to decrease the pressure gradient between the blood vessels and tissue.

Compression (ultrasonic): A decrease in the size of a cell during high-pressure peaks.

Conduction: The transfer of heat from a high temperature to a low temperature between two objects that are touching each other.

Conductive properties: The ability of a tissue to transfer heat (from a high temperature to a low temperature) or electrical energy.

Conductor (electrical): A material having the ability to transmit electricity. Conductors have many free electrons and provide relatively little resistance to electrical flow. Within the body, tissues having a high water content are considered conductors.

Connective tissue: Tissue that supports and connects other tissue types.

Consensual touching: A situation in which the person being touched has agreed to be touched. Consensual agreements negate the charge of battery.

Constructive interference: Two waves that, perfectly synchronized, combine to produce a single wave of greater amplitude.

Continuous interference: Two waves that are slightly out of phase interacting to produce a single wave whose amplitude and/or frequency varies.

Contracture: A condition resulting from the loss of a tissue's ability to lengthen.

Contraindicate: To make inadvisable.

Contralateral: Pertaining to the opposite side of the body. The left side is contralateral to the right.

Convection: The cooling of one object and the subsequent heating of another by the circulation of a fluid, usually water, or air.

Convergent: Two or more input routes reduced to a single route.

Conversion: Transformation of high-frequency electrical energy into heat.

Cortisol: A cortisone-like substance produced in the body.

Cosine law: A law stating that, as an angle deviates away from 90 degrees, the effective energy is reduced by the multiple of the cosine of the angle: Effective energy = Energy × Cosine of the angle. A deviation of ±10 degrees is considered within acceptable limits for therapeutic treatments.

Coulomb: The amount of charge produced by 6.25×10^{18} electrons (negative charge) or protons (positive charge).

Coulomb's law: A law stating that opposite charges attract and like charges repel each other.

Counterirritant: A substance causing irritation of superficial sensory nerves to reduce the transmission of pain from underlying nerves.

CPT Codes: See Current procedural terminology codes.

Crepitus: A grinding or crunching sound or sensation.

Cryoglobulinemia: A condition in which abnormal blood proteins, cryoglobulins, group together when exposed to cold. This condition can lead to skin color changes, hives, subcutaneous hemorrhage, and other disorders.

Cryokinetics: A treatment technique that involves moving the injured body part while it is being treated with cold, thus decreasing pain while increasing range of motion.

Cryotherapy: The application of therapeutic cold to living tissues.

Current procedural terminology codes: Codes used to describe the care provided for the patient and used for billing purposes.

Cyanosis (cyanotic): A blue-gray discoloration of the skin caused by a lack of oxygen.

Cyclooxygenase-2 (COX-2): Inflammatory agent that encourages bone healing.

Cytokine: A protein produced by white blood cells.

DC/ML: See Dorsal columns/Medial lemniscus.

Defamation of character: Mistruths said about a person that cause harm.

Degassed water: Water that has boiled for 30 to 45 minutes and then allowed to sit undisturbed for 4 to 24 hours, allowing gaseous bubbles to escape.

Degeneration (muscular): The decrease in size and strength of a muscle that occurs secondary to atrophy.

Delayed-onset muscle soreness: Residual muscle soreness, caused secondary to damage of the muscle cells, that appears within 24 hours after heavy muscular activity, particularly with eccentric muscle actions.

Dementia: The progressive loss of cognitive and intellectual functions without impairment of perception or consciousness. Symptoms include disorientation, memory impairment, impaired judgment, and impaired intellectual ability.

Dendrite: Synaptic connections of a nerve arising from a body.

Denervation: Lack of the proper nerve supply or nerve function to, for example, an area or muscle group.

Deoxyribonucleic acid: Carries genetic information for all organisms except RNA.

Dependent position: An arrangement in which the body part is placed lower than the heart, increasing the intravascular pressure.

Dermal ulcer: A slowly healing or nonhealing break in the skin.

Dermatome: A segmental skin area supplied by a single nerve root.

Destructive interference: Two waves that are exactly out of phase, interacting to cancel each other out.

Diagnosis: The determination of the nature and scope of an injury or illness.

Dialysis: An external device that is used to assist or replace the kidney's function of filtering blood.

Diapedesis: Part of the inflammatory response characterized by movement of white blood cells and other substances through gaps formed in vascular walls to enter the tissues.

Diastolic blood pressure: The lowest level of pressure in the arteries. For example, when a blood pressure reading is given as 120/80, 80 represents the diastolic value.

Diathermy: A classification of therapeutic modality that uses high-frequency electrical energy to heat subcutaneous tissues.

Dipole: A pair of equal and opposite charges separated by a distance.

Direct access: Health-care services can be provided without physician referral. Note that a physician referral is often required for third-party reimbursement.

Direct current: The uninterrupted, one-directional flow of electrons.

Disposition: The patient's current physical status and projected course of recovery.

Divergence: The spreading of a beam or wave.

DNA: See Deoxyribonucleic acid.

Doctrine: A statement of fundamental government policy.

Dorsal columns/medial lemniscal system: The ascending fiber system that conveys fine touch and proprioception from spinal cord to the thalamus.

Dorsal columns: The large bundle of fibers in the dorsal spinal cord formed by ascending primary afferent fibers that carry touch and proprioceptive sensation.

Dorsolateral fasciculus: The small bundle of fibers in the dorsolateral spinal cord formed by ascending primary afferent fibers that carry pain and temperature sensation.

Due care: An established responsibility for an individual to respond to a given situation in a certain manner.

Duty cycle: The ration between the pulse duration and the pulse interval: Duty cycle = Pulse duration/(Pulse duration + Pulse interval) $\times$ 100.

Dynamometer: A device used for measuring muscular strength.

Dyskinesia: A defect in the ability to perform voluntary joint movement.

Ecchymosis: A blue-black discoloration of the skin caused by movement of blood into the tissues. In the later stages, the color may appear as a greenish-brown or yellow.

Ectopic: Outside or away from its normal position; in an abnormal position or sequence.

Eddy: A circular current of fluid, often moving against the main flow.

Edema: An excessive accumulation of serous fluids.

Effective radiating area (ERA): The portion of an ultrasonic transducer's (sound head) surface that emits ultrasonic energy.

Efferent: Carrying impulses away from a central structure. Nerves leaving the central nervous system are efferent nerves.

Efficacy: The ability of a modality or treatment regimen to produce the intended effects.

Effleurage: Massage using long, deep strokes.

Electromagnetic field: The lines of force created by positive and negative poles.

Electromagnetic radiation: Energy found on the electromagnetic spectrum capable of traveling near the speed of light and exhibiting both electrical and magnetic properties.

Electromagnetic spectrum: A continuum ordered by the wavelength or frequency of the energy produced.

Electromyogram: A recording of the electrical charges associated with the contraction of a muscle.

Electron: A negatively charged atomic particle.

Electro-osmotic: Pertaining to the movement of ions as a result of electrical charges. Positive ions move away from the positive pole toward the negative pole; negative ions move away from the negative pole toward the positive pole.

Electrostatic field: A field created by static electricity.

Electropiezo: The vibration caused by an alternating current being passed through a crystal.

Embolism: Blockage of a blood vessel by a blood clot or other foreign substance.

Emigration: Passage of white blood corpuscles through the walls of capillaries and veins during inflammation.

Encapsulated receptor: A sensory receptor formed by a nerve fiber and surrounding connective tissue cells.

Endogenous opiates: Pain-inhibiting substances produced in the brain. These include endorphins and enkephalins.

Endorphin: A morphine-like neurohormone produced from b-lipotropin in the pituitary. Endorphins are thought to increase the pain threshold by binding to receptor sites.

Endothelial cells: Flat cells lining the blood and lymphatic vessels and the heart.

Enkephalin: A substance released by the body that reduces the perception of pain by bonding to pain receptor sites.

Enthesopathy: Pathology of the bony attachment of tendon, ligament, or joint capsule.

Epicritic pain: Pain that is well localized.

Epidemiology: The study of the distribution, rates, and causes of injuries and illness within a specified population. This information may then be used to prevent future occurrence.

Epiphyseal plates: Growth plates of bones.

Epithelial tissue: Tissue that forms the outer skin and lines the body's cavities. This type of tissue has a high potential to regenerate.

Ergometer: A device used to measure the amount of work performed by the legs or arms.

Evaporation: The change from a liquid to a gas state.

Exhaustion stage: The third and final stage in the general adaptation syndrome; the stage when cell death occurs.

External fixation: A fracture-setting technique incorporating the use of metal rods that extend through the skin and are attached to a device outside the body.

Extracellular: Outside the cell membrane.

Extravasation: To exude from or pass out of a vessel into the tissues, said of blood, lymph, or urine.

Exudate: Fluid that collects in a cavity and has a high concentration of cells, protein, and other solid matter.

Far infrared: The portion of the light spectrum located between 1500 and 12,500 nm.

Far ultraviolet: The portion of the light spectrum located between 180 and 290 nm.

Farad: A measure of the storage capability of capacitors. One farad stores a charge of 1 coulomb when 1 V is applied.

Fascia: Fibrous connective tissue found in muscle, beneath the skin, and in the viscera.

Fascia, deep: Found within muscle, this type of fascia is high in collagen content. The fascial fibers are arranged parallel to the line of stress.

Fascia, superficial: Found between the skin and underlying muscle. Superficial fascia has a random, loose fibrous arrangement.

Fibrin: A filamentous protein formed by the action of thrombin on fibrinogen.

Fibrinogen: A protein present in the blood plasma, essential for the clotting of blood.

Fibrinolysis: Pathological breaking up of fibrin.

Fibromyalgia: Chronic inflammation of a muscle or connective tissue.

Fibrosis: An abnormally large formation of inelastic fibrous tissue.

First-order neurons: Sensory nerves that course outside the central nervous system and have their bodies in a dorsal root ganglion.

Flux: A residual electromagnetic field created by two unlike charges.

Focal compression: Applying direct pressure to soft tissue surrounded by prominent structures.

Footcandle: A measure of light equal to 1 lumen per square foot. One lumen is the amount of light emitted by one international candle.

Foramen: An opening (e.g., in a bone) to allow the passage of blood vessels or nerves.

Free nerve endings: The unencapsulated receptor of pain and thermal primary afferent fibers. Unlike the encapsulated receptor organs, free nerve endings have no connective tissue capsule and appear to be bare nerve fibers. Within their membranes, however, are thermal, mechanical, and chemical receptor molecules.

Free radical: A highly reactive molecule having an odd number of electrons. Free radical production plays an important role in the progression of an ischemic injury.

Frequency: The number of times an event occurs in 1 second; measured in hertz (cycles per second) or pulses per second.

Fresnel zone: See Near field.

Functional scoliosis: Lateral curvature of the spinal column in the frontal plane caused as the spinal column attempts to compensate for postural deficits such as leg length discrepancy. Functional scoliosis is also known as protective scoliosis.

GaAs laser: Laser produced by the excitation of gallium arsenide.

Gallium arsenide lasers: See GaAs laser.

Galvanic current: A low-voltage direct current.

Galvanic effect: The migration of ions as the result of the application of a galvanic current.

Gamma globulin: An infection-fighting blood protein.

Gamma-motoneurons: Efferent motor nerves that innervate the intrafusal fibers of a muscle spindle.

Gauss: A unit of magnetic strength.

General adaptation syndrome: A theory stating that the body has a common mechanism for adapting to stress. The three stages of this response are alarm, resistance, and exhaustion.

Glycolytic pathway: A complex chemical reaction that yields adenosine triphosphate (ATP) from glucose.

Golgi tendon organ: A sensory nerve ending found in tendons and aponeuroses that detects tension within the muscle. When the tension reaches a threshold, muscle activity of the contracting muscle is inhibited and the antagonistic muscle is facilitated.

Granulation tissue: Delicate tissue composed of fibroblasts, collagen, and capillaries formed during the revascularization phase of wound healing.

Granuloma: A hard mass of fibrous tissue.

Gross negligence: Total failure to provide what would normally be deemed proper in a given situation.

Grotthus-Draper, Law of: A law stating that there is an inverse relationship between the amount of penetration and absorption. The more energy that is absorbed by the superficial tissues, the less that remains to be transmitted to underlying tissues.

Ground: An electrical connection that provides a path for leaked current to return safely to the earth.

Ground fault: A disruption in the electrical circuitry where the current exits from the normal path.

Ground-fault interrupter: An interrupter that discontinues the current flow when a ground fault is detected.

Ground substance: Material occupying the intercellular spaces in bone, fibrous connective tissue, cartilage, or bone (also known as matrix).

Growth factors: Substances that stimulate the production of specific types of cells.

Habituation: A function of the central nervous system that filters out nonmeaningful information.

Half-layer value: The depth, measured in cm, at which 50 percent of the ultrasonic energy has been absorbed by the tissues.

Heat capacity: See Thermal capacity.

Health Insurance Portability and Accountability Act: Federal legislation that ensures patient confidentiality during the electronic transfer of medical records.

Helium neon laser: See HeNe laser.

Hemarthrosis: Blood in a joint.

Hematoma: A mass of blood confined to a limited area, resulting from the subcutaneous leakage of blood.

Hemorrhage: Bleeding from veins, arteries, or capillaries.

HeNe laser: Laser produced by the excitation of helium and neon atoms.

Henry: A measure of inductance (H). One henry induces an electromagnetic force of 1 V when the current changes at a rate of 1 A per second.

Heparin: An inflammatory mediator produced by the mast cells of the liver. It inhibits the clotting process by preventing the transformation of prothrombin into thrombin.

Hertz (Hz): The number of cycles per second.

High frequency (electrical stimulation): An electrical current having a frequency greater than 100,000 cps.

High TENS: The application of transcutaneous electrical nerve stimulation possessing high-frequency, short-duration pulses and applied at the sensory level.

HIPAA: See Health Insurance Portability and Accountability Act.

Histamine: A blood-thinning chemical released from damaged tissue during the inflammatory process. Its primary function is vasodilation of arterioles and increased vascular permeability in venules.

Hives: See urticaria.

Homeostasis: State of equilibrium in the body and its systems that provides a stable internal environment.

Homunculus: A map of the body's surface across a brain region, usually a gyrus of the cerebral cortex.

Hunting response: A vascular response to cold application marked by a series of vasoconstrictions and vasodilations. This response has been shown to occur only in limited body areas.

Hydrocortisone: An anti-inflammatory drug that closely resembles cortisol.

Hydropic: Relating to edema; an excessive amount of fluid.

Hydrostatic: Relating to the pressure of liquids in equilibrium or to the pressure they exert.

Hydrostatic pressure: The pressure of blood within the capillary.

Hyperalgesia, primary: Pain resulting from a lowering of the nerve's threshold.

Hyperalgesia, secondary: The spreading of pain caused by chemical mediators being released into the painful tissues.

Hyperemia: A red discoloration of the skin caused by increased blood flow. The skin turns white when pressure is applied.

Hypermobile: An abnormally large amount of motion.

Hypersensitive: Abnormally increased sensitivity; a condition in which there is an exaggerated response by the body to a stimulus.

Hypertension: High blood pressure.

Hyperthermia: Increased core temperature.

Hyperthyroidism: Metabolic disorder characterized by the overproduction of endocrine hormones and includes conditions such as Graves' disease and gonad tumors.

Hypertrophic: Increased size.

Hypertrophy: To develop an increase in bulk, for example, in the cross-sectional area of muscle.

Hypomobile: An abnormal limitation of normal motion.

Hyporeflexia: Diminished function of the reflexes.

Hypotension: Low blood pressure.

Hypothalamus: The body's thermoregulatory center.

Hypothermia: Decreased core temperature.

Hypoxia: Lack of an adequate supply of oxygen.

ICD codes: See International Classification of Disease codes.

Immediate treatment: Used in the initial management of orthopedic injuries. Immediate treatment is composed of four components: rest, ice, compression, and elevation.

Impedance: The resistance to flow of an alternating current resulting from inductance and capacitance.

Impedance plethysmography: A determination of blood flow based on the amount of electrical resistance in the area.

Inductance: The degree to which a varying current can induce voltage, expressed in henries (H).

Induration: The hardening of tissue often caused by the deposition of fibroconnective cells.

Infection: A disease state produced by the invasion of a contaminating organism.

Inflammation: Tissue reaction to injury.

Inflammatory response, acute: The stage of the body's response to injury that attempts to isolate and localize the trauma.

Inflammatory response, maturation phase: The stage of injury response during which the body attempts to restore the orientation and function of the injured tissues.

Inflammatory response, proliferation phase: The stage of injury response during which the body prepares to rebuild the damaged tissues.

Infrapatellar: The distal portion of the patella including the patellar tendon.

Infrared light: Electromagnetic energy possessing a wavelength between 780 and 12,500 nm. Infrared light is invisible to the human eye.

Injury potential: Disruption of a tissue's normal electrical balance as a result of injury.

Innervate: Normal and sufficient nerve supply to a muscle, body area, and so on.

Institutional Review Board (IRB): An institutional agency that oversees medical investigations involving humans or animals by assuring compliance with federal regulations. In research involving humans, the IRB functions to protect the rights and health of the subjects.

Interferon gamma: A group of proteins released by white blood cells and fibroblasts when devouring the unwanted tissues. The gamma classification is also referred to as "angry macrophages" because of their heightened phagocytic activity.

Interleukin-8 (IL-8): Primarily produced by endothelial cells and macrophages, IL-8 enables immune cells into the tissues and acts as a chemotaxic for neutrophils.

Internal capsule: A massive band of ascending and descending fibers in the forebrain that connect the cerebral cortex to thalamus, brain stem, and spinal cord.

Internal fixation devices: Wires, screws, plates, or pins used to repair fractures.

International Classification of Disease codes (ICD): Standard nomenclature used to code injury and disease. ICD codes are used for research and reimbursement purposes.

Interneuron: A neuron connecting two nerves.

Interpulse interval: The elapsed time between the conclusion of one pulse and the start of the next.

Interstitial: Between the tissues.

Intra-articular: Within a joint.

Intracellular: Within the membrane of a cell.

Intramedullary rod: An internal fixation device placed with the marrow of fractured bone.

Intrapulse interval: The period within a discrete pulse when the current is not flowing. The duration of the intrapulse interval cannot exceed the duration of the interpulse interval.

Intrauterine device (IUD): A plastic or metal coil inserted within the uterus to prevent pregnancy.

Inverse square law: A law stating that the intensity of the energy striking the tissues is proportional to the square of the distance between the source of the energy and the tissues: Energy received = Energy at the source ÷ Distance from the source squared.

Ion: An atom, or group of atoms, with a net charge other than zero.

Iontophoresis: Introduction of ions into the body through the use of an electrical current.

Ipsilateral: On the same side of the body.

Ischemia: Local and temporary deficiency of blood supply caused by obstruction of circulation to a part.

Isoelectric point: The point at which positive and negative electrical points are equal. The electrical baseline of zero.

Isokinetic contraction: A muscle contraction against a variable resistance where limb moves through the range of motion at a constant speed.

Isometric contractions: Muscle contraction without appreciable joint motion.

Isotonic contractions: Muscle contraction through a range of motion against a constant resistance.

Joule: Basic unit of work in the International System of Units. One joule equals 0.74 foot-pounds of work. Joules = Coulombs × Volts.

Keloid: A nodular, firm, movable, and tender mass of dense, irregularly distributed collagen scar tissue in the dermis and subcutaneous tissue. Common in the African-American population, keloid scarring tends to occur after trauma or surgery.

Keratin: A dry, fibrous protein that replaces cytoplasm in the cells of the stratum corneum.

Kilohertz (kHz): One thousand cycles per second.

Kinetic energy: The energy possessed by an object by virtue of its motion.

Kinins: A group of polypeptides that dilate arterioles, serve as strong chemotactics, and produce pain. They are primarily involved in the inflammatory process in the early stages of vascular response.

Labile cells: Cells located in the skin, intestinal tract, and blood possessing good regenerative abilities.

Lactic acid: A cellular waste product produced by muscular contraction or cell metabolism. A fatiguing carbohydrate.

Laminectomy: Surgical removal of the lamina from a vertebra.

Laser: Acronym for *L*ight *A*mplification by *S*timulated *E*mission of *R*adiation. A highly organized beam of light.

Latent: Delayed period between the stimulus and the response.

Legal guardian: An individual who is legally responsible for the care of an infant or minor.

Leukocytes: White blood cells that serve as scavengers.

Leukotrienes: Fatty acids that cause smooth muscle contraction, increase vascular permeability, and attract neutrophils.

Libel: Defamation of character by the written word.

Limbic system: System in the brain that controls emotion.

Lipid: A broad category of fatlike substances.

Lissauer's tract: See dorsolateral fasciculus.

Lordosis: The forward curvature of the cervical and lumbar spine.

Low frequency (electrical stimulation): An electrical current having a frequency of less than 1000 cps.

Low TENS: The application of transcutaneous electrical nerve stimulation using low-frequency, long-duration pulses, applied at a motor-level intensity.

Lucid: Of clear and rational mind.

Luminous infrared: See Near infrared.

Lupus: A chronic disorder of the body's immune system that affects the skin, joints, internal organs, and neurological system.

Lymphangitis: Inflammation of the lymphatic vessels draining an extremity. This condition is most often associated with inflammation or infection.

Lymphatic return: A return process similar to that of the venous network but specializing in the removal of interstitial fluids.

Lymphedema: Swelling of the lymph nodes caused by blockage of the vessels by protein-rich substances.

Macerated: Skin that has been softened by soaking in water.

Macrophage: A cell having the ability to devour particles; a phagocyte.

Magnetic resonance image (MRI): A view of the body's internal structures obtained through the use of magnetic and radio fields.

Malaise: Discomfort, mental fogginess, or disorientation. Often associated with infection or fever.

Malfeasance: The performance of an unlawful or improper act.

Malpractice: Negligence on the part of a professional person serving in the line of duty.

Malunion fracture: The faulty or incorrect healing of bone.

Margination: A state in which platelets and leukocytes, normally flowing in the blood stream, begin to tumble along the walls of the vessel.

Master points: Points that, according to the theory of acupuncture, connect skin areas to deeper energy channels. Stimulating master points results in systemic changes.

McGill Pain Questionnaire: One of many pain rating scales, a method using pictures, scales, and words to describe the location, type, and magnitude of pain.

Mechanoreceptors: See Mechanosensitive receptors.

Mechanosensitive receptors: Nerve endings that are sensitive to mechanical pressure.

Medial lemniscus: The large bundle of fibers in the dorsal spinal cord formed by ascending second-order axons that carry touch and proprioceptive sensation.

Mediators: Chemicals that act through indirect means.

Medium: A material used to promote the transfer of energy. An object or substance that permits the transmission of energy through it.

Medium frequency (electrical stimulation): An electrical current having a frequency of 1000 to 100,000 cps.

Megahertz (MHz): One million cycles per second.

Melanin: Pigmentation of the hair, skin, and eye produced by melanocytes.

Meningitis: Inflammation of the membranes of the brain or spinal cord.

Meridians: In acupuncture, primary pathways through which the body's energy flows.

Messenger RNA (mRNA): Serves as the blueprint for protein synthesis.

Metabolism: The sum of physical and chemical reactions taking place within the body.

Metabolite: A by-product of metabolism.

Mho: The measure of a material's electrical conductance; the mathematical reciprocal of electrical resistance.

Microcoulomb: The charge produced by 10^{-6} electrons.

Micrometer(μm): 1/1,000,000 of a meter.

Microstreaming: During ultrasound application, the localized flow of fluids resulting from cavitation.

Microvolt (μV): One microvolt equals 1/1,000,000 of a volt.

Midline and intralaminar nuclei: Several medially placed thalamic nuclei that receive ascending pain information from the anterior lateral fasciculus and reticular nuclei.

Millivolt (mV): One millivolt equals 1/1000 of a volt.

Misfeasance: The improper performance of an otherwise lawful act.

Modality: The application of a form of energy to the body that elicits an involuntary response.

Modulate: To regulate or adjust.

Modulation: Regulation or adjustment.

Monochromatic: Light that consists of only one color.

Monocyte: A white blood cell that matures to become a macrophage.

Monophasic current: The unidirectional flow of electrons that is interrupted by discrete periods of noncurrent flow.

Monopolar stimulation: The application of electrical stimulation in which the current density under one set of electrodes (the active electrodes) is much greater than that under the other electrode (the dispersive electrode). All of the effects of the treatment should be experienced only under the active electrodes.

Motor-level stimulation: Electrical stimulation applied at an output intensity that produces a visible muscle contraction without activating pain fibers.

Motor nerve: A nerve that provides impulses to muscles.

Motor point: An area on the skin used to stimulate motor nerves.

Motor unit: A group of skeletal muscle fibers that are innervated by a single motor nerve.

Mottling: A blotchy discoloration of the skin.

Muscle, cardiac: Muscle associated with the heart and responsible for the pumping of blood.

Muscle guarding: A voluntary or subconscious contraction of a muscle to protect an injured area.

Muscle, skeletal: Responsible for the movement of the body's joints.

Muscle, smooth: Contractile tissue that is associated with the body's hollow organs. Smooth muscle is not under voluntary control.

Muscle spindle: An organ located within the muscular tissue that detects the rate and magnitude of a muscle contraction.

Muscular tissue: Tissue composed of smooth (found in the internal organs) cardiac and skeletal muscle; has the ability to actively shorten and passively lengthen.

Myelin: A fatty layer around nerves.

Myelinated: Having a fatlike outer coating (myelin) that serves as insulation for nerves.

Myocardial: Pertaining to the middle layer of the heart walls.

Myofibroblasts: Fibroblasts that have contractile properties.

Myonecrosis: Death of muscle tissue.

Myosin: Noncontractile muscle protein.

Myositis: Inflammation of muscular tissue.

Myositis ossificans: Ossification or deposition of bone in muscle fascia, resulting in pain and swelling.

Nanometer: One-billionth (10^{-9}) of a meter.

Nanosecond: One-billionth (10^{-9}) of a second.

Near field: The portion of an ultrasonic beam that is close to the sound head.

Near infrared: The range of infrared light that is closest to visible light, with wavelengths ranging between 770 and 1500 nm on the electromagnetic spectrum. Also known as luminous infrared.

Near ultraviolet: The range of light having wavelengths between 290 and 390 nm on the electromagnetic spectrum. This is the portion of the ultraviolet spectrum that is located the closest to visible light.

Necrosin: Increases the permeability of a cell membrane.

Necrosis: Cell death.

Negligence, gross: Intentional and conscious act or omission committed by an individual, with reckless disregard for the consequences.

Negligence, ordinary: Departure from the standard of care or duty. See also omission and commission.

Neoplasm: Abnormal tissue such as a tumor that grows at the expense of healthy organisms.

Neoprene: A synthetic rubber material.

Nervous tissue: Tissue possessing the ability to conduct electrochemical impulses.

Neuralgia: Pain following the path of a nerve; a hypersensitive nerve.

Neurapraxia: A temporary loss of function in a peripheral nerve.

Neurological: Pertaining to the nervous system.

Neuroma: Swelling or other mass formation around a nerve (Neuro = nerve; oma = tumor).

Neuropathy: Destruction, trauma, or inhibition of a nerve.

Neutron: An electrically neutral particle found in the center of an atom.

Nociceptive stimulus: Impulse giving rise to the sensation of pain.

Nociceptors: Specialized receptors on nerves that transmit pain impulses.

Nonfeasance: Failure to act when there is a duty to act.

Nonunion fracture: Fracture that fails to heal spontaneously within a normal time frame.

Norepinephrine: A hormone that causes vasoconstriction.

Normative data: Information that can be used to describe a specific population.

Noxious: Harmful, injurious, or painful. Capable of producing pain.

Noxious-level stimulation: Application of electrical stimulation that produces pain; caused by activation of C fibers.

Noxious-level TENS: Brief, intense electrical stimulation (above the threshold of pain) that is thought to activate the release of endogenous opiates.

Nucleus cuneatus: A nucleus in the caudal medulla that relays fine touch and proprioceptive information from the upper body to the thalamus.

Nucleus gracilis: A nucleus in the caudal medulla that relays fine touch and proprioceptive information from the lower body to the thalamus.

Nucleus pulposus: The gelatinous middle of an intervertebral disk.

Numbness: Lack of sensation in a body part.

Occiput: The posterior base of the skull.

Occupational Safety and Health Administration (OSHA): A federal agency responsible for ensuring safe working conditions. This agency has enforcement powers and is capable of levying fines against employers.

Ohm: Unit of electrical resistance required to develop 0.24 calories of heat when 1 A of current is applied for 1 second.

Ohm's law: A law stating that current is directly proportional to resistance: Amperage = Voltage/Resistance (I = V/R).

Omission: Failure to respond to a situation in which actions are necessary to limit or reduce harm.

Ordinary negligence: Failure to act as a reasonable and prudent person would act under similar circumstances.

Organelle: A specialized portion of a cell that performs a specific function, such as the mitochondria and the Golgi apparatus.

Orthotics: The use of orthopedic devices for correcting deformity or malalignment.

Osteoarthritis: Degeneration of a joint's articular surface.

Osteoblast: A cell involved in the formation of new bone.

Osteoclast: A cell that absorbs and removes unwanted bone.

Osteogenesis: Healing of fracture sites through the formation of callus, followed by the deposition of collagen and bone salts.

Osteomyelitis: Inflammation of the bone marrow and adjacent bone.

Osteophyte: A branching bony outgrowth.

Osteoporosis: A porous condition resulting in thinning of bone. Most commonly seen (but not exclusively) in postmenopausal women.

Outcome measures: Data that are used to evaluate the efficacy of a treatment program or protocol.

Overload principle: A principle stating that for strength gains to occur, the body must be subjected to more stress than it is accustomed to. This is accomplished by increasing the load, frequency, or duration of exercise.

Oxyhemoglobin: Hemoglobin that is carrying oxygen found in the arterial system.

Ozone: Formed by the grouping of three oxygen atoms (O_3). Ozone is present in the atmosphere, where it filters out ultraviolet light (especially in the C band), helping to prevent certain forms of cancer.

Pacinian corpuscles (pacinian receptors): Large encapsulated receptor organs found in the skin and deeper tissues. These rapid adapting receptors are best activated by an alternating stimulus, for example, a tuning fork. Within the joints, they assist in relaying proprioceptive information.

Pain threshold: The level of noxious stimulus required to alert the individual to possible tissue damage.

Pain tolerance: The amount of time an individual can endure pain.

Pallor: Lack of color in the skin.

Paradoxical (Paradox): Two seemingly contradictory statements that are nonetheless true.

Parallel circuit: An electrical circuit in which electrons have more than one route to follow.

Pathology: Changes in structure or function caused by disease or trauma.

Pavementing: Adherence of platelets to the vessel walls in multiple layers to form a patch over the injury site.

Peak-to-peak value: The sum of a pulse's maximum deviation above and below the baseline.

Penetration: Depth at which energy absorption takes place.

Perfusion: Local blood flow that supplies tissues and organs with oxygen and nutrients.

Periaqueductal gray nucleus: A midbrain nucleus that lies around the cerebral aqueduct. This nucleus regulates pain sensation through descending multisynaptic projections to the dorsal horn.

Periosteal pain: A deep-seated ache resulting from overly intense application of ultrasonic energy that irritates the bone's periosteum.

Prepatellar: Around the patella.

Peripheral vascular disease: A syndrome describing an insufficiency of arteries and/or veins for maintaining proper circulation (also known as PVD).

pH (potential of hydrogen): A measure of acidity or alkalinity (bases). A neutral solution has a pH of 7. Acids have a pH of less than 7; bases have a pH greater than 7.

Phagocyte: A classification of scavenger cells that ingest and destroy unwanted substances in the body.

Phagocytosis: The ingestion and digestion of bacteria and particles by phagocytes.

Phase: Individual sections of a single pulse that remain on one side of the baseline for a period.

Phase duration: The amount of time for a single phase to complete its route. During monopolar application, the terms "phase duration" and "pulse duration" are equivalent. The phase duration must be sufficient to cause depolarization.

Phonophoresis: The introduction of medication into the body through the use of ultrasonic energy.

Phosphocreatine system: A compound that is important in muscle metabolism.

Photon: A unit of light energy that has zero mass, no electrical charge, and an indefinite life span.

Physical medicine codes: Billing codes used to describe rehabilitation and treatment services rendered.

Physis: The growth plate of bone.

Piezoelectric crystal: A crystal that produces positive and negative electrical charges when it is compressed or expanded.

Pitting edema: An exudate-rich form of edema characterized by being easily indented by pressure (hence, "pitting").

Placebo: A substance of no objective curative value given to a patient to satisfy a need for treatment or used as a control treatment in an experimental study. Interestingly, this word means *I shall please* in Latin.

Platelet: A free-flowing cell fragment in the blood stream.

Pneumothorax: The collection of air in the pleural cavity (a void between the lungs and rib cage) that inhibits the lung's ability to expand.

Policies and procedures manual: An administrative manual that describes the operation of a department or agency.

Polymodal: Capable of being depolarized by different types of stimuli.

Polymorph: A type of white blood cell; a granulocyte.

Porphyria: Inherited disorder of hemoglobin, myoglobin, or cytochromes that results in light sensitivity and other complaints.

Postpolio syndrome: Musculoskeletal symptoms, including pain and atrophy, that affect patients 25 to 30 years after the original polio symptoms occurred.

Potential of hydrogen: See pH.

Power (electrical): See Watt.

Precedent: A previous ruling that serves as a guide in future legal action.

Precursor: A substance that is formed before changing into its final state or substance.

Primary afferent fiber: The complete nerve fiber—both peripheral and central process—of a first-order neuron.

Primary hyperalgesia: Increased pain sensation near the site of injury.

Pronation: An inward flattening and tilting of the foot, resulting in the lowering of the medial longitudinal arch.

Propagation: Transmission through a medium.

Prothrombin: A chemical found in the blood that reacts with an enzyme to produce thrombin.

Proton: A positively charged atomic particle.

Protopathic pain: Poorly localized pain sensation.

Psoralen: A group of substances that produce inflammation of the skin when exposed to sunlight or ultraviolet light.

Psychogenic: Pain of mental rather than physical origin.

Pulsatile current: See pulsed current.

Pulse charge: The number of coulombs contained in one electrical pulse.

Pulse duration: The amount of time from the initial nonzero charge to the return to a zero charge, including the intrapulse interval.

Pulse frequency: The number of electrical pulses that occur in a 1-second period.

Pulse interval (ultrasound): The amount of time between ultrasonic pulses.

Pulse length (ultrasound): The amount of time from the initial nonzero charge to the return to a zero charge, forming one complete cycle.

Pulse period: The period of time between the initiation of a pulse and the initiation of the subsequent pulse, including the phase duration(s), intrapulse interval, and interpulse interval.

Pulse width: See Pulse duration.

Pulsed current: A flow of electrons marked by discrete periods of nonelectron flow.

Q10 effect: Describes the relationship between tissue temperature and cell metabolism. For each 10°C increase in temperature, the cell's metabolism increases by a factor of 2 to 3.

Quadripolar stimulation: Electrical stimulation applied with two channels.

Radiant energy: Heat that is gained or lost through radiation.

Radiation: The transfer of electromagnetic energy that does not require the presence of a medium.

Radicular: Distally radiating pain caused by spinal nerve root involvement.

Range of motion: The distance, measured in degrees, that a limb moves in one plane (e.g., flexion-extension, adduction-abduction).

Raynaud's phenomenon: A vascular reaction to cold application or stress that results in a white, red, or blue discoloration of the extremities. The fingers and toes are the first to be affected.

Rebound vasoconstriction: A reflex constriction of blood vessels caused by prolonged exposure to extreme temperatures.

Reflection: The return of waves from an object.

Refraction: The bending of a wave as it passes through an object.

Regeneration (tissue): Restoration of damaged tissues with cells of the same type and function as the damaged cells.

Reimbursement: Payment for services rendered.

Replacement (tissue): Replacement of damaged tissues by cells of a different type from the original.

Resistance stage: The second stage in the general adaptation syndrome. During this stage, the body adapts to the stresses placed on it.

Resistor (electrical): A material that has few free electrons and opposes the flow of electricity. Within the body, tissues having a low water content are considered resistors.

Resonating: Vibrating.

Respondeat superior: See Vicarious liability.

Reticular nuclei (reticular formation): A diffuse network of cells and fibers located in the brain stem. The reticular formation influences alertness, waking, sleeping, and certain reflexes.

Retinaculum: A fibrous membrane that holds an organ or body part in place.

Retinoid: Topical medication consisting of retinoic acid. Used to treat psoriasis and severe acne.

Rheobase: The minimum amount of voltage under the negative pole that is required for depolarization when a direct current is applied to living tissues.

Ribonucleic acid: Controls protein synthesis.

Rickets: Common in children, a vitamin D deficiency that results in inadequate deposition of lime salts, altering the shape, structure, and function of bone.

RNA: See Ribonucleic acid.

Root-mean-square (RMS) value: A conversion of the electrical power delivered by an alternating current into the equivalent direct current power, calculated by multiplying the peak value by 0.707.

Salicylates: A family of analgesic compounds that includes aspirin.

Satellite cell: Spindle-shaped cell that assists in the repair of skeletal muscle.

Sclerotome: A portion of bone that is supplied by a spinal nerve root.

Scoliosis: Lateral curvature of the spinal column in the frontal plane. See also Functional scoliosis and Structural scoliosis.

Secondary hypoxic injury: Cell death resulting from a lack of oxygen.

Second-order neuron: A nerve having its body located in the spinal cord. It connects second- and third-order neurons (nerves having their bodies in the thalamus and extending into the cerebral cortex).

Sedation: The result of calming nerve endings.

Sedative: An agent that causes sedation.

Self-treatment: Treatment or rehabilitation performed by the patient without direct supervision, including home treatment programs.

Sensitization: The process of being made sensitive to a specific substance.

Sensory-level stimulation: Electrical stimulation applied at an intensity at which sensory nerves are stimulated without also producing a muscle contraction.

Sequential compression: Compression of an extremity characterized by a distal to proximal flow.

Series circuit: A circuit in which the current has only one path to follow.

Serotonin: A substance that causes local vasodilation and increases permeability of the capillaries.

Sham: A device that has no physiological effect on the body (e.g., an ultrasound unit with the output intensity set to zero). Sham devices are often used during research to determine the actual biophysical effects of a treatment by comparing the results of an actual treatment to a patient who is receiving no treatment.

Silica: A finely ground form of sand capable of holding water.

Singlet oxygen: An uncharged form of oxygen that can selectively destroy cells.

Slander: Defamation of character by the spoken word.

Somatic: Pertaining to the body.

Somatic receptive field: Area to which a stimulus is applied to obtain the optimum response.

Somatosensory cortex: An area in the cerebral cortex, located in the postcentral gyrus of the parietal lobe, that is important in the perception of touch and proprioception and in the localization of pain sensation.

Specific gravity: The ratio of the density of a substance to the density of pure water taken as a standard when both densities are obtained by weighing in air.

Specific heat: The ratio of a substance's thermal capacity to that of water, which has a thermal capacity of 1. The specific heats of the three states of water are: ice 0.50, water 1, and steam 0.48.

Spherocytosis: An anemic condition in which red blood cells assume a spheroid shape.

Spondylolisthesis: Forward slippage of the lower lumbar vertebrae on the vertebrae above.

Spondylolysis: The breaking down of a vertebral structure.

Sprain: A stretching or tearing of ligaments.

Stable cavitation: The gentle expansion and contraction of bubbles formed during ultrasound application.

Stabile cells: Cells possessing some ability to regenerate.

Standard of practice: The criteria against which an individual's performance is measured.

Standard precautions: See Universal precautions.

Standing orders: A "blanket prescription" from a physician describing how injuries are to be managed when the physician is not present.

Standing wave: A single-frequency wave formed by the collision of two waves of equal frequency and speed traveling in opposite directions. The energy with a standing wave cannot be transmitted from one area to another and is focused in a confined area.

States of matter: The three forms of physical matter: solid, liquid, and gas. Using water as example, we see the three states of matter as ice, water, and steam.

Statute of limitations: A legal time limit allowed for the filing of a lawsuit.

Strain: A stretching or tearing of tendons or muscles.

Stratum basale: The deepest layer of the lining of the uterus.

Stratum corneum: The outermost, nonliving portion of the epidermis.

Stress: A force that disrupts the normal homeostasis of a system.

Structural scoliosis: Lateral curvature of the spinal column caused by malformed vertebrae and/or intervertebral discs.

Subacute: Between the acute and chronic stages of the inflammatory stages.

Subcutaneous: Beneath the skin.

Subjective: Symptoms stated by the patient that are not externally apparent, such as pain. Personal beliefs and attitudes may alter subjective symptoms.

Substance P: A neurotransmitter thought to be responsible for the transmission of pain-producing impulses.

Summation: An overlap of muscle contractions that is caused by electrical stimulation.

Synapse: The junction at which two nerves communicate.

Synapse, chemical: The junction between two nerves that is characterized by a synaptic cleft. Chemical neurotransmitters carry the impulse from one nerve to the next.

Synapse, electrical: The junction between two nerves that is characterized by a gap junction. The nervous impulse is transferred directly to the subsequent nerve.

Synapse, excitatory: The release of the neurotransmitter tends to activate the postsynaptic nerve.

Synapse, inhibitory: The release of the neurotransmitter increases the nerve's resting potential, decreasing the probability that the nervous impulse will be propagated.

Synovitis: Inflammation of the synovial membrane.

Synovium: Membrane lining the capsule of a joint.

Systemic: Affecting the body as a whole.

T cell: A transmission cell that connects sensory nerves to the central nervous system. Not to be confused with T cells found in the immune system. See Tract cell.

Temporal average intensity: The average amount of power delivered to the body during pulsed ultrasound.

Tendinitis: Inflammation of the tendon.

Tendinopathy: Any disease or trauma involving a muscle's tendon, tissues surrounding the tendon, or the tendon's insertion into the bone.

Tendinosis: Degeneration of a tendon from repetitive microtrauma or collagen degeneration within a tendon.

Tensile strength: The ability of a structure to withstand a pulling force along its length. Resistance to tear.

Tesla: A unit of magnetic strength. 1 Tesla = 1000 Gauss.

Tetany: Total contraction of a muscle achieved through the recruitment and contraction of all motor units.

Thalamus: Gray matter located at the base of the brain.

Therapeutic: Having healing properties.

Thermal capacity: The number of heat units required to raise a unit of mass by 1°C.

Thermal conductivity: The quantity of heat (in calories per second) passing through a 1 cm thick by 1 cm wide substance having a temperature gradient of 1°C.

Thermolysis: Chemical decomposition caused by heating.

Thermoreceptors: Sensory receptors that detect temperature.

Thermotherapy: The application of therapeutic heat to living tissues.

Third-order neuron: A nerve having its body located in the thalamus and extending into the cerebral cortex.

Thoracic duct: A central collection point for the lymphatic system. The contents of the thoracic duct are routed into the left subclavian vein, where it returns to the blood system.

Thrombin: An enzyme formed in the blood of a damaged area.

Thrombophlebitis: Inflammation of the veins.

Thrombosis: The formation or presence of a blood clot within the vascular system.

Tissue hydrostatic pressure: The pressure that moves fluids from the tissues into the capillaries.

Tonic contraction: Prolonged contraction of a muscle.

Tract cell: Second-order neuron of the pain and temperature pathways. The axons of these cells cross the midline of the spinal cord and ascend in the anterior lateral fasciculus. Tract cells are sometimes called T cells, but this should not be confused with the T cells of the immune system. See T cell.

Transcutaneous: Through the skin.

Transdermally (transdermal): Introduction of medication to the subcutaneous tissues through unbroken skin.

Transducer: A device that converts one form of energy to another.

Transduction: The process of converting a stimulus into action potentials.

Transfer: Assisted patient mobility, such as when moving from a wheelchair to a bed.

Transient cavitation: See Unstable cavitation.

Translation: Sliding or gliding of opposing articular surfaces.

Trigger point: A localized area of spasm within a muscle.

Turf burn: A deep abrasion caused by friction between the skin and artificial playing surfaces.

Twitch contraction: Repeated muscle contraction characterized by the fibers returning to their original length subsequent to the next contraction. Twitch contractions are distinguishable from each other.

Tympanic membrane: The ear drum.

Type I muscle fibers: Muscle fibers that generate a relatively low level of force but can sustain contractions for a long period. Geared to aerobic activity, these muscle fibers are also referred to as tonic or slow-twitch fibers.

Type II muscle fibers: Muscle fibers that generate a large amount of force in a short time. Geared to anaerobic activity, they are also referred to as phasic or fast-twitch fibers.

Ultraviolet light: Energy on the electromagnetic spectrum having a wavelength between 180 and 390 nm. Ultraviolet light is invisible to the human eye.

Universal precautions: A series of steps, established by OSHA, that individuals should take to avoid accidental exposure to blood-borne pathogens.

Unstable cavitation: The violent oscillation and subsequent rupture of bubbles during ultrasound application at too high an intensity.

Upper motor neuron lesion: A spinal cord lesion resulting in paralysis, loss of voluntary movement, spasticity, sensory loss, and pathological reflexes.

Uremic pruritus: Itching caused by increased blood content in urine.

Urticaria: Skin vascular reaction to an irritant characterized by red, itchy areas, wheals, or papules. Commonly referred to as hives.

Valence shell: An imaginary shell in which the electrons responsible for chemical reactivity orbit around the nucleus of an atom.

Vascular endothelial growth factor (VEGF): Encourages capillary formation that precedes bone healing.

Vasoconstriction: Reduction in a blood vessel's diameter, resulting in a decrease in blood flow.

Vasodilation: Increase in a blood vessel's diameter, resulting in an increase in blood flow.

Vasomotor: Muscles and their associated nerves acting on arteries and veins that cause constriction and/or dilation.

Venous stasis ulcer: Ischemic necrosis and ulceration of tissue, especially that overlying bony prominences, caused by prolonged pressure. Also referred to as decubitus ulcers or bed sores.

Ventral posterior lateral nucleus: A nucleus in the posterior thalamus that receives fibers from the anterior lateral fasciculus and medial lemniscus.

Ventral white commissure: The bundle of fibers in the spinal cord through which second-order pain fibers cross the midline before entering the anterior lateral fasciculus.

Venule: A small vein exiting from a capillary.

Vicarious liability: Liability of employers for the acts of their employees.

Visceral: Pertaining to organs of the body.

Viscosity: The resistance of a fluid to flow.

Visible light: Electromagnetic energy possessing a wavelength between 390 and 760 nm. Visible light is a combination of violet, indigo, blue, green, yellow, orange, and red.

Vitamin D: Needed for bone formation and normal endocrine, intestine, and brain function.

Voltage: A measure of the potential for electrons to flow.

Volumetric measurement: Determination of the size of a body part by measuring the amount of water it displaces.

Wallerian degeneration: Gradual physiological breakdown of a nerve axon that has been severed from its body.

Watt: A unit of electrical power. For an electrical current: Watts = Voltage × Amperage.

Weaning: Decreasing dependence on a substance or device by gradually reducing its use.

White light: See visible light.

Wide dynamic range cells (neurons): Neurons in the spinal cord and thalamus that respond to a broad range of mechanical pressures. They respond to both touch and pain.

Withdrawal reflex: A multisynaptic spinal reflex that is normally elicited by a noxious stimulus. Muscle groups are activated so that the body is moved away from the damaging stimulus.

Work hardening: Job-specific exercises used to prevent work-related injuries or to rehabilitate injured workers.

X-ray: An electromagnetic wave 0.05 to 100 Å in length that is able to penetrate most solid matter.

Index

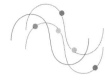

Note: Page numbers followed by f indicate figures; page numbers followed by t indicate tables; page numbers followed by b refer to boxed material.
Italicized page numbers refer to special text presented "at a glance."